Edda Klipp, Wolfram Liebermeister,
Christoph Wierling, Axel Kowald,
Hans Lehrach, and Ralf Herwig

Systems Biology

Related Titles

Helms, V.

Principles of Computational Cell Biology

From Protein Complexes to Cellular Networks

2008
Softcover
ISBN: 978-3-527-31555-0

Baxevanis, A. D., Ouellette, B. F. F. (eds.)

Bioinformatics

A Practical Guide to the Analysis of Genes and Proteins

560 pages
2004
Hardcover
ISBN: 978-0-471-47878-2

*Edda Klipp, Wolfram Liebermeister, Christoph Wierling,
Axel Kowald, Hans Lehrach, and Ralf Herwig*

Systems Biology

A Textbook

WILEY-VCH

WILEY-VCH Verlag GmbH & Co. KGaA

The Authors

Prof. Edda Klipp
Humboldt-Universität Berlin
Institut für Biologie
Theoretische Biophysik
Invalidenstr. 42
10115 Berlin

Dr. Wolfram Liebermeister
Humboldt-Universität Berlin
Institut für Biologie
Theoretische Biophysik
Invalidenstr. 42
10115 Berlin

Dr. Christoph Wierling
MPI für Molekulare Genetik
Ihnestr. 73
14195 Berlin
Germany

Dr. Axel Kowald
Protagen AG
Otto-Hahn-Str. 15
44227 Dortmund

Prof. Hans Lehrach
MPI für Molekulare Genetik
Ihnestr. 73
14195 Berlin
Germany

Prof. Ralf Herwig
MPI für Molekulare Genetik
Ihnestr. 73
14195 Berlin
Germany

Cover
The cover pictures were provided with kind permission by Santiago Ortiz and Dr. Michael Erlowitz

Library of Congress Card No.: applied for

British Library Cataloguing-in-Publication Data
A catalogue record for this book is available from the British Library.

Bibliographic information published by the Deutsche Nationalbibliothek
The Deutsche Nationalbibliothek lists this publication in the Deutsche Nationalbibliografie; detailed bibliographic data are available on the Internet at http://dnb.d-nb.de.

Typesetting Thomson Digital, Noida, India
Printing Strauss GmbH, Mörlenbach
Binding Litges & Dopf GmbH, Heppenheim
Cover Design Adam-Design, Weinheim

Printed in the Federal Republic of Germany
Printed on acid-free paper

ISBN: 978-3-527-31874-2

Contents

Systems Biology: A Textbook. Edda Klipp, Wolfram Liebermeister, Christoph Wierling, Axel Kowald, Hans Lehrach, and Ralf Herwig

ISBN: 978-3-527-31874-2

Preface

Life is probably the most complex phenomenon in the universe. We see kids growing, people aging, plants blooming, and microbes degrading their remains. We use yeast for brewery and bakery, and doctors prescribe drugs to cure diseases. But can we understand how life works? Since the 19th century, the processes of life have no longer been explained by special "living forces," but by the laws of physics and chemistry. By studying the structure and physiology of living systems more and more in detail, researchers from different disciplines have revealed how the mystery of life arises from the structural and functional organization of cells and from the continuous refinement by mutation and selection.

In recent years, new imaging techniques have opened a completely new perception of the cellular microcosm. If we zoom into the cell, we can observe how structures are built, maintained, and reproduced while various sensing and regulation systems help the cell to respond appropriately to environmental changes. But along with all these fascinating observations, many open questions remain. Why do we age? How does a cell know when to divide? How can severe diseases such as cancer or genetic disorders be cured? How can we convince – i.e., manipulate – microbes to produce a desirable substance? How can the life sciences contribute to environmental safety and sustainable technologies?

This book provides you with a number of tools and approaches that can help you to think in more detail about such questions from a theoretical point of view. A key to tackle such questions is to combine biological experiments with computational modeling in an approach called systems biology: it is the combined study of biological systems through (i) investigating the components of cellular networks and their interactions, (ii) applying experimental high-throughput and whole-genome techniques, and (iii) integrating computational methods with experimental efforts.

The systemic approach in biology is not new, but it recently gained new thrust due to the emergence of powerful experimental and computational methods. It is based on the accumulation of an increasingly detailed biological knowledge, on the emergence of new experimental techniques in genomics and proteomics, on a tradition of mathematical modeling of biological processes, on the exponentially growing computer power (as prerequisite for databases and the calculation of large

Systems Biology: A Textbook. Edda Klipp, Wolfram Liebermeister, Christoph Wierling, Axel Kowald, Hans Lehrach, and Ralf Herwig

ISBN: 978-3-527-31874-2

systems), and on the Internet as the central medium for a quick and comprehensive exchange of information.

Systems Biology has influenced modern biology in two major ways: on the one hand, it offers computational tools for analyzing, integrating and interpreting biological data and hypotheses. On the other hand, it has induced the formulation of new theoretical concepts and the application of existing ones to new questions. Such concepts are, for example, the theory of dynamical systems, control theory, the analysis of molecular noise, robustness and fragility of dynamic systems, and statistical network analysis. As systems biology is still evolving as a scientific field, a central issue is the standardization of experiments, of data exchange, and of mathematical models.

In this book, we attempt to give a survey of this rapidly developing field. We will show you how to formulate your own model of biological processes, how to analyze such models, how to use data and other available information for making your model more precise – and how to interpret the results. This book is designed as an introductory course for students of biology, biophysics and bioinformatics, and for senior scientists approaching Systems Biology from a different discipline. Its nine chapters contain material for about 30 lectures and are organized as follows.

Chapter 1 – Introduction (E. Klipp, W. Liebermeister, A. Kowald, 1 lecture)

Introduction to the subject. Elementary concepts and definitions are presented. Read this if you want to start right from the beginning.

Chapter 2 – Modeling of Biochemical Systems (E. Klipp, C. Wierling, 4 lectures)

This chapter describes kinetic models for biochemical reaction networks, the most common computational technique in Systems Biology. It includes kinetic laws, stoichiometric analysis, elementary flux modes, and metabolic control analysis. Introduces tools and data formats necessary for modeling.

Chapter 3 – Specific Biochemical Systems (E. Klipp, C. Wierling, W. Liebermeister, 5 lectures)

Using specific examples from metabolism, signaling, and cell cycle, a number of popular modeling techniques are discussed. The aim of this chapter is to make the reader familiar with both modeling techniques and biological phenomena.

Chapter 4 – Model Fitting (W. Liebermeister, A. Kowald, 4 lectures)

Models in systems biology usually contain a large number of parameters. Assigning appropriate numerical values to these parameters is an important step in the creation of a quantitative model. This chapter shows how numerical values can be obtained from the literature or by fitting a model to experimental data. It also discusses how model structures can be simplified and how they can be chosen if several different models can potentially describe the experimental observations.

Chapter 5 – Analysis of High-Throughput Data (R. Herwig, 2 lectures)

Several techniques that have been developed in recent years produce large quantities of data (e.g., DNA and protein chips, yeast two-hybrid, mass spectrometry). But such large quantities often go together with a reduced quality of the individual measurement. This chapter describes techniques that can be used to handle this type of data appropriately.

Chapter 6 – Gene Expression Models (R. Herwig, W. Liebermeister, E. Klipp, 3 lectures)

Thousands of gene products are necessary to create a living cell, and the regulation of gene expression is a very complex and important task to keep a cell alive. This chapter discusses how the regulation of gene expression can be modeled, how different input signals can be integrated, and how the structure of gene networks can be inferred from experimental data.

Chapter 7 – Stochastic Systems and Variability (W. Liebermeister, 4 lectures)

Random fluctuations in transcription, translation and metabolic reactions make mathematics complicated, computation costly and interpretation of results not straight forward. But since experimentalists find intriguing examples for macroscopic consequences of random fluctuation at the molecular level, the incorporation of these effects into the simulations becomes more and more important. This chapter gives an overview where and how stochasticity enters cellular life.

Chapter 8 – Network Structures, Dynamics and Function (W. Liebermeister, 3 lectures)

Many complex systems in biology can be represented as networks (reaction networks, interaction networks, regulatory networks). Studying the structure, dynamics, and function of such networks helps to understand design principles of living cells. In this chapter, important network structures such as motifs and modules as well as the dynamics resulting from them are discussed.

Chapter 9 – Optimality and Evolution (W. Liebermeister, E. Klipp, 3 lectures)

Theoretical research suggests that constraints of the evolutionary process should have left their marks in the construction and regulation of genes and metabolic pathways. In some cases, the function of biological systems can be well understood by models based on an optimality hypothesis. This chapter discusses the merits and limitations of such optimality approaches.

Various aspects of systems biology – the biological systems themselves, types of mathematical models to describe them, and practical techniques – reappear in different contexts in various parts of the book. The following diagram, which shows the contents of the book sorted by a number of different aspects, may serve as an orientation.

Biological systems

- Metabolism (3.1, 8.1, 9.1)
- Transcription (6.1, 6.2, 8.2)
- Genetic network (6.3, 6.4, 8.1, 8.2)
- Signaling systems (3.2, 7.4, 8.2)
- Cell cycle (3.3)
- Development (3.4)
- Apoptosis (3.5)

Perspectives on biological function

- Qualitative behavior (2.3, 3.3)
- Parameter sensitivity/robustness (7.3, 7.4)
- Robustness against failure (7.4)
- Modularity (8.3)
- Optimality (9.1, 9.2)
- Evolution (9.3)
- Game-theoretical requirements (9.3)

Model types with different levels of abstraction

- Thermodynymic/many particles (7.1)
- Kinetic models (2.1, 2.3)
- Dynamical systems (2.3)
- Optimization/control theory (2.3, 9.1, 9.2)

Mathematical frameworks to describe cell states

- Topological (8.1)
- Structural stoichiometric (2.2)
- Deterministic linear (15)
- Deterministic kinetic (2.1, 2.3)
- Spatial (3.4)
- Discrete (6.3, 6.4)
- Stochastic dynamics (7.1, 7.2, 14)
- Uncertain parameters (7.3)

Modeling skills

- Model building (2.1 – 2.4)
- Model reduction and combination (4.3)
- Data collection (4.1, 5.1)
- Statistical data analysis (5.2)
- Parameter estimation (4.2)
- Model testing and selection (4.4)
- Local sensitivity/control theory (2.3, 7.3)
- Global sensitivity/uncertainty analysis (7.3)
- Parameter optimization (9.1, 9.2)
- Optimal control (9.2)

Practical issues in modeling

- Data formats (2.4)
- Data sources (2.4, 16)
- Modeling software (2.4, 17)
- Experimental techniques (11)
- Statistical methods (4.2, 4.4, 13)

At the end of the regular course material, you will find a number of additional chapters that summarize important biological and mathematical methods. The first chapters deal with to cell biology (chapter 10, C. Wierling) and molecular biological methods (chapter 11, A. Kowald). For looking up mathematical and statistical definitions and methods, turn to chapters 12 and 13 (R. Herwig, A. Kowald). Chapters 14 and 15 (W. Liebermeister) concentrate on random processes and control theory. The final chapters provide an overview over useful databases (chapter 16, C. Wierling) as well as a huge list of available software tools including a short description of their purposes (chapter 17, A. Kowald).

Further material is available on an accompanying website

(www.wiley-vch.de/home/systemsbiology)

Beside additional and more specialized topics, the website also contains solutions to the exercises and problems presented in the book.

We give our thanks to a number of people who helped us in finishing this book. We are especially grateful to Dr. Ulrich Liebermeister, Prof. Dr. Hans Meinhardt, Dr. Timo Reis, Dr. Ulrike Baur, Clemens Kreutz, Dr. Jose Egea, Dr. Maria Rodriguez-Fernandez, Dr. Wilhelm Huisinga, Sabine Hummert, Guy Shinar, Nadav Kashtan, Dr. Ron Milo, Adrian Jinich, Elad Noor, Niv Antonovsky, Bente Kofahl, Dr. Simon Borger, Martina Fröhlich, Christian Waltermann, Susanne Gerber, Thomas Spießer, Szymon Stoma, Christian Diener, Axel Rasche, Hendrik Hache, Dr. Michal Ruth Schweiger, and Elisabeth Maschke-Dutz for reading and commenting on the manuscript.

We thank the Max Planck Society for support and encouragement. We are grateful to the European Commission for funding via different European projects (MEST-CT2004-514169, LSHG-CT-2005-518254, LSHG-CT-2005-018942, LSHG-CT-2006-037469, LSHG-CT-2006-035995-2 NEST-2005-Path2-043310, HEALTH-F4-2007-200767, and LSHB-CT-2006-037712). Further funding was obtained from the Sysmo project "Translucent" and from the German Research Foundation (IRTG 1360) E.K. thanks with love her sons Moritz and Richard for patience and incentive and the Systems Biology community for motivation. W.L. wishes to thank his daughters Hannah and Marlene for various insights and inspiration. A.K. likes to thank Prof. Dr. H.E. Meyer for support and hospitality. This book is dedicated to our teacher Prof. Dr. Reinhart Heinrich (1946–2006), whose works on metabolic control theory in the 1970s paved the way to systems biology and who greatly inspired our minds.

Part One
Introduction to Systems Biology

Systems Biology: A Textbook. Edda Klipp, Wolfram Liebermeister, Christoph Wierling, Axel Kowald, Hans Lehrach, and Ralf Herwig

ISBN: 978-3-527-31874-2

1
Introduction

1.1
Biology in Time and Space

Biological systems like organisms, cells, or biomolecules are highly organized in their structure and function. They have developed during evolution and can only be fully understood in this context. To study them and to apply mathematical, computational, or theoretical concepts, we have to be aware of the following circumstances.

The continuous reproduction of cell compounds necessary for living and the respective flow of information is captured by the central dogma of molecular biology, which can be summarized as follows: genes code for mRNA, mRNA serves as template for proteins, and proteins perform cellular work. Although information is stored in the genes in form of DNA sequence, it is made available only through the cellular machinery that can decode this sequence and can translate it into structure and function. In this book, this will be explained from various perspectives.

A description of biological entities and their properties encompasses different levels of organization and different time scales. We can study biological phenomena at the level of populations, individuals, tissues, organs, cells, and compartments down to molecules and atoms. Length scales range from the order of meter (e.g., the size of whale or human) to micrometer for many cell types, down to picometer for atom sizes. Time scales include millions of years for evolutionary processes, annual and daily cycles, seconds for many biochemical reactions, and femtoseconds for molecular vibrations. Figure 1.1 gives an overview about scales.

In a unified view of cellular networks, each action of a cell involves different levels of cellular organization, including genes, proteins, metabolism, or signaling pathways. Therefore, the current description of the individual networks must be integrated into a larger framework.

Many current approaches pay tribute to the fact that biological items are subject to evolution. The structure and organization of organisms and their cellular machinery has developed during evolution to fulfill major functions such as growth, proliferation, and survival under changing conditions. If parts of the organism or of the cell fail to perform their function, the individual might become unable to survive or replicate.

Systems Biology: A Textbook. Edda Klipp, Wolfram Liebermeister, Christoph Wierling, Axel Kowald, Hans Lehrach, and Ralf Herwig

ISBN: 978-3-527-31874-2

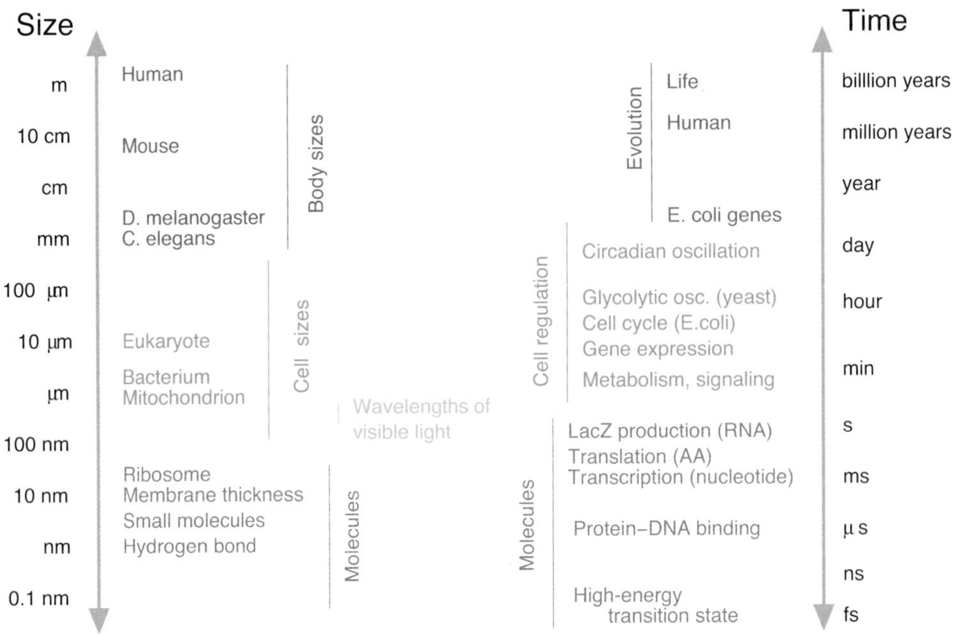

Figure 1.1 Length and time scales in biology. Data from the BioNumbers database http://bionumbers.hms.harvard.edu.

One consequence of evolution is the similarity of biological organisms from different species. This similarity allows for the use of model organisms and for the critical transfer of insights gained from one cell type to other cell types. Applications include, e.g., prediction of protein function from similarity, prediction of network properties from optimality principles, reconstruction of phylogenetic trees, or the identification of regulatory DNA sequences through cross-species comparisons. But the evolutionary process also leads to genetic variations within species. Therefore, personalized medicine and research is an important new challenge for biomedical research.

1.2
Models and Modeling

If we observe biological processes, we are confronted with various complex processes that cannot be explained from first principles and the outcome of which cannot reliably be foreseen from intuition. Even if general biochemical principles are well established (e.g., the central dogma of transcription and translation, the biochemistry of enzyme-catalyzed reactions), the biochemistry of individual molecules and systems is often unknown and can vary considerably between species. Experiments lead to biological hypotheses about individual processes, but it often remains unclear if these hypotheses can be combined into a larger coherent picture because it is often difficult to foresee the global behavior of a complex system from knowledge of its parts. Mathematical modeling and computer simulations can help us understand the internal nature and dynamics of these processes and to arrive at predictions about their future development and the effect of interactions with the environment.

1.2.1
What is a Model?

The answer to this question will differ among communities of researchers. In a broad sense, a model is an abstract representation of objects or processes that explains features of these objects or processes (Figure 1.2). A biochemical reaction network can be represented by a graphical sketch showing dots for metabolites and arrows for reactions; the same network could also be described by a system of differential equations, which allows simulating and predicting the dynamic behavior of that network. If a model is used for simulations, it needs to be ensured that it faithfully predicts the system's behavior – at least those aspects that are supposed to be covered by the model. Systems biology models are often based on well-established physical laws that justify their general form, for instance, the thermodynamics of chemical reactions; besides this, a computational model needs to make specific statements about a system of interest – which are partially justified by experiments and biochemical knowledge, and partially by mere extrapolation from other systems. Such a model can summarize established knowledge about a system in a coherent mathematical formulation. In experimental biology, the term "model" is also used to denote a species that is especially suitable for experiments, for example, a genetically modified mouse may serve as a model for human genetic disorders.

1.2.2
Purpose and Adequateness of Models

Modeling is a subjective and selective procedure. A model represents only specific aspects of reality but, if done properly, this is sufficient since the intention of modeling is to answer particular questions. If the only aim is to predict system outputs from given input signals, a model should display the correct input–output relation, while its interior can be regarded as a black box. But if instead a detailed biological mechanism has to be elucidated, then the system's structure and the relations between its parts must be described realistically. Some models are meant to be generally applicable to many similar objects (e.g., Michaelis–Menten kinetics holds for many enzymes, the promoter–operator concept is applicable to many genes, and gene regulatory motifs are common), while others are specifically tailored to one particular object (e.g., the 3D structure of a protein, the sequence of a gene, or a model of deteriorating mitochondria during aging). The mathematical part can be kept as simple as possible to allow for easy implementation and comprehensible results. Or it can be modeled very realistically and be much more complicated. None of the characteristics mentioned above makes a model wrong or right, but they determine whether a model is appropriate to the problem to be solved. The phrase "essentially,

(a) Biological system

(b) Mental model

(c) Model scheme

Activation

X
Protein X

Y
Protein Y

(d) Process model

$$0 \rightarrow X \; : \quad a_1 = v_0 \text{ (const.)}$$
$$X \rightarrow 0 \; : \quad a_2 = \kappa_x \cdot [X]$$
$$0 \rightarrow Y \; : \quad a_3 = f_y \cdot [X]$$
$$Y \rightarrow 0 \; : \quad a_4 = \kappa_y \cdot [Y]$$

(e) Dynamical model

$$\mathrm{d}x/\mathrm{d}t = v_0 - \kappa_x x$$
$$\mathrm{d}y/\mathrm{d}t = f_y x - \kappa_y y$$
$$x(0) = x_0$$
$$y(0) = y_0$$

(f) Quantitative results

Concentration

Time

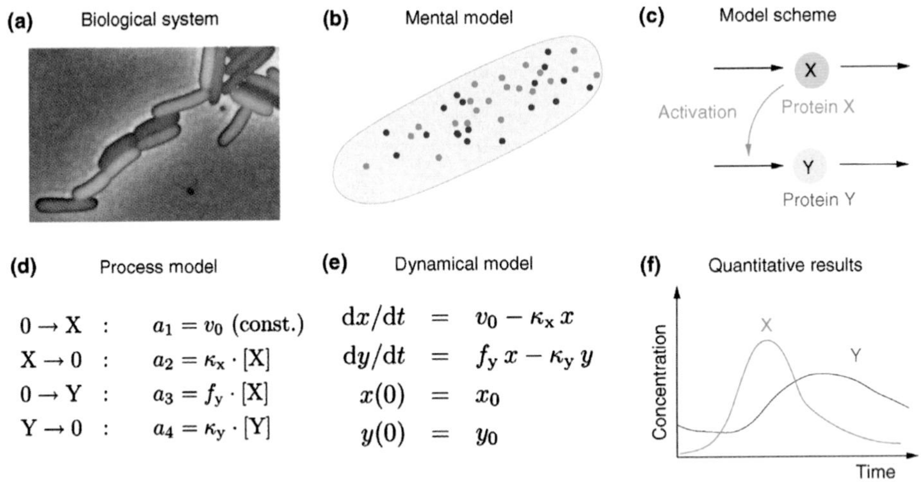

Figure 1.2 Typical abstraction steps in mathematical modeling. (a) *Escherichia coli* bacteria produce thousands of different proteins. If a specific protein type is fluorescently labeled, cells glow under the microscope according to the concentration of this enzyme (Courtesy of M. Elowitz). (b) In a simplified mental model, we assume that cells contain two enzymes of interest, X (red) and Y (blue) and that the molecules (dots) can freely diffuse within the cell. All other substances are disregarded for the sake of simplicity. (c) The interactions between the two protein types can be drawn in a wiring scheme: each protein can be produced or degraded (black arrows). In addition, we assume that proteins of type X can increase the production of protein Y. (d) All individual processes to be considered are listed together with their rates *a* (occurrence per time). The mathematical expressions for the rates are based on a simplified picture of the actual chemical processes. (e) The list of processes can be translated into different sorts of dynamic models; in this case, deterministic rate equations for the protein concentrations *x* and *y*. (f) By solving the model equations, predictions for the time-dependent concentrations can be obtained. If these predictions do not agree with experimental data, it indicates that the model is wrong or too much simplified. In both cases, it has to be refined.

all models are wrong, but some are useful" coined by the statistician George Box is indeed an appropriate guideline for model building.

1.2.3
Advantages of Computational Modeling

Models gain their reference to reality from comparison with experiments, and their benefits therefore depend on the quality of the experiments used. Nevertheless, modeling combined with experimentation has a lot of advantages compared to purely experimental studies:

- Modeling drives conceptual clarification. It requires verbal hypotheses to be made specific and conceptually rigorous.

- Modeling highlights gaps in knowledge or understanding. During the process of model formulation, unspecified components or interactions have to be determined.

- Modeling provides independence of the modeled object.
- Time and space may be stretched or compressed *ad libitum*.
- Solution algorithms and computer programs can be used independently of the concrete system.
- Modeling is cheap compared to experiments.
- Models exert by themselves no harm on animals or plants and help to reduce ethical problems in experiments. They do not pollute the environment.
- Modeling can assist experimentation. With an adequate model, one may test different scenarios that are not accessible by experiment. One may follow time courses of compounds that cannot be measured in an experiment. One may impose perturbations that are not feasible in the real system. One may cause precise perturbations without directly changing other system components, which is usually impossible in real systems. Model simulations can be repeated often and for many different conditions.
- Model results can often be presented in precise mathematical terms that allow for generalization. Graphical representation and visualization make it easier to understand the system.
- Finally, modeling allows for making well-founded and testable predictions.

The attempt to formulate current knowledge and open problems in mathematical terms often uncovers a lack of knowledge and requirements for clarification. Furthermore, computational models can be used to test whether proposed explanations of biological phenomena are feasible. Computational models serve as repositories of current knowledge, both established and hypothetical, about how systems might operate. At the same time, they provide researchers with quantitative descriptions of this knowledge and allow them to simulate the biological process, which serves as a rigorous consistency test.

1.3 Basic Notions for Computational Models

1.3.1 Model Scope

Systems biology models consist of mathematical elements that describe properties of a biological system, for instance, mathematical variables describing the concentrations of metabolites. As a model can only describe certain aspects of the system, all other properties of the system (e.g., concentrations of other substances or the environment of a cell) are neglected or simplified. It is important – and to some extent, an art – to construct models in such ways that the disregarded properties do not compromise the basic results of the model.

1.3.2
Model Statements

Besides the model elements, a model can contain various kinds of statements and equations describing facts about the model elements, most notably, their temporal behavior. In kinetic models, the basic modeling paradigm considered in this book, the dynamics is determined by a set of ordinary differential equations describing the substance balances. Statements in other model types may have the form of equality or inequality constraints (e.g., in flux balance analysis), maximality postulates, stochastic processes, or probabilistic statements about quantities that vary in time or between cells.

1.3.3
System State

In dynamical systems theory, a system is characterized by its *state*, a snapshot of the system at a given time. The state of the system is described by the set of variables that must be kept track of in a model: in deterministic models, it needs to contain enough information to predict the behavior of the system for all future times. Each modeling framework defines what is meant by the state of the system. In kinetic rate equation models, for example, the state is a list of substance concentrations. In the corresponding stochastic model, it is a probability distribution or a list of the current number of molecules of a species. In a Boolean model of gene regulation, the state is a string of bits indicating for each gene whether it is expressed ("1") or not expressed ("0"). Also the temporal behavior can be described in fundamentally different ways. In a *dynamical system*, the future states are determined by the current state, while in a *stochastic process*, the future states are not precisely predetermined. Instead, each possibly future history has a certain probability to occur.

1.3.4
Variables, Parameters, and Constants

The quantities in a model can be classified as variables, parameters, and constants. A *constant* is a quantity with a fixed value, such as the natural number e or Avogadro's number (number of molecules per mole). *Parameters* are quantities that have a given value, such as the K_m value of an enzyme in a reaction. This value depends on the method used and on the experimental conditions and may change. *Variables* are quantities with a changeable value for which the model establishes relations. A subset of variables, the *state variables*, describes the system behavior completely. They can assume independent values and each of them is necessary to define the system state. Their number is equivalent to the dimension of the system. For example, the diameter d and volume V of a sphere obey the relation $V = \pi d^3/6$, where π and 6 are constants, V and d are variables, but only one of them is a state variable since the relation between them uniquely determines the other one.

Whether a quantity is a variable or a parameter depends on the model. In reaction kinetics, the enzyme concentration appears as a parameter. However, the enzyme concentration itself may change due to gene expression or protein degradation and in an extended model, it may be described by a variable.

1.3.5 Model Behavior

Two fundamental factors that determine the behavior of a system are (i) influences from the environment (input) and (ii) processes within the system. The system structure, that is, the relation among variables, parameters, and constants, determines how endogenous and exogenous forces are processed. However, different system structures may still produce similar system behavior (output); therefore, measurements of the system output often do not suffice to choose between alternative models and to determine the system's internal organization.

1.3.6 Model Classification

For modeling, processes are classified with respect to a set of criteria.

- A structural or *qualitative* model (e.g., a network graph) specifies the interactions among model elements. A *quantitative* model assigns values to the elements and to their interactions, which may or may not change.
- In a *deterministic* model, the system evolution through all following states can be predicted from the knowledge of the current state. *Stochastic* descriptions give instead a probability distribution for the successive states.
- The nature of values that time, state, or space may assume distinguishes a *discrete* model (where values are taken from a discrete set) from a *continuous* model (where values belong to a continuum).
- *Reversible* processes can proceed in a forward and backward direction. Irreversibility means that only one direction is possible.
- *Periodicity* indicates that the system assumes a series of states in the time interval $\{t, t + \Delta t\}$ and again in the time interval $\{t + i\Delta t, t + (i + 1)\Delta t\}$ for $i = 1,2,\ldots$.

1.3.7 Steady States

The concept of stationary states is important for the modeling of dynamical systems. *Stationary states* (other terms are *steady states* or *fixed points*) are determined by the fact that the values of all state variables remain constant in time. The asymptotic behavior of dynamic systems, that is, the behavior after a sufficiently long time, is often stationary. Other types of asymptotic behavior are oscillatory or chaotic regimes.

The consideration of steady states is actually an abstraction that is based on a separation of time scales. In nature, everything flows. Fast and slow processes – ranging from formation and breakage of chemical bonds within nanoseconds to growth of individuals within years – are coupled in the biological world. While fast processes often reach a quasi-steady state after a short transition period, the change of the value of slow variables is often negligible in the time window of consideration. Thus, each steady state can be regarded as a quasi-steady state of a system that is embedded in a larger nonstationary environment. Despite this idealization, the concept of stationary states is important in kinetic modeling because it points to typical behavioral modes of the system under study and it often simplifies the mathematical problems.

Other theoretical concepts in systems biology are only rough representations of their biological counterparts. For example, the representation of gene regulatory networks by Boolean networks, the description of complex enzyme kinetics by simple mass action laws, or the representation of multifarious reaction schemes by black boxes proved to be helpful simplification. Although being a simplification, these models elucidate possible network properties and help to check the reliability of basic assumptions and to discover possible design principles in nature. Simplified models can be used to test mathematically formulated hypothesis about system dynamics, and such models are easier to understand and to apply to different questions.

1.3.8
Model Assignment is not Unique

Biological phenomena can be described in mathematical terms. Models developed during the last decades range from the description of glycolytic oscillations with ordinary differential equations to population dynamics models with difference equations, stochastic equations for signaling pathways, and Boolean networks for gene expression. But it is important to realize that a certain process can be described in more than one way: a biological object can be investigated with different experimental methods and each biological process can be described with different (mathematical) models. Sometimes, a modeling framework represents a simplified limiting case (e.g., kinetic models as limiting case of stochastic models). On the other hand, the same mathematical formalism may be applied to various biological instances: statistical network analysis, for example, can be applied to cellular-transcription networks, the circuitry of nerve cells, or food webs.

The choice of a mathematical model or an algorithm to describe a biological object depends on the problem, the purpose, and the intention of the investigator. Modeling has to reflect essential properties of the system and different models may highlight different aspects of the same system. This ambiguity has the advantage that different ways of studying a problem also provide different insights into the system. However, the diversity of modeling approaches makes it still very difficult to merge established models (e.g., for individual metabolic pathways) into larger supermodels (e.g., models of complete cell metabolism).

1.4
Data Integration

Systems biology has evolved rapidly in the last years driven by the new high-throughput technologies. The most important impulse was given by the large sequencing projects such as the human genome project, which resulted in the full sequence of the human and other genomes [1, 2]. Proteomics technologies have been used to identify the translation status of complete cells (2D-gels, mass spectrometry) and to elucidate protein–protein interaction networks involving thousands of components [3]. However, to validate such diverse high-throughput data, one needs to correlate and integrate such information. Thus, an important part of systems biology is data integration.

On the lowest level of complexity, data integration implies common schemes for data storage, data representation, and data transfer. For particular experimental techniques, this has already been established, for example, in the field of transcriptomics with minimum information about a microarray experiment [4], in proteomics with proteomics experiment data repositories [5], and the Human Proteome Organization consortium [6]. On a more complex level, schemes have been defined for biological models and pathways such as Systems Biology Markup Language (SBML) [7] and CellML [8], which use an XML-like language style.

Data integration on the next level of complexity consists of data correlation. This is a growing research field as researchers combine information from multiple diverse data sets to learn about and explain natural processes [9, 10]. For example, methods have been developed to integrate the results of transcriptome or proteome experiments with genome sequence annotations. In the case of complex disease conditions, it is clear that only integrated approaches can link clinical, genetic, behavioral, and environmental data with diverse types of molecular phenotype information and identify correlative associations. Such correlations, if found, are the key to identifying biomarkers and processes that are either causative or indicative of the disease. Importantly, the identification of biomarkers (e.g., proteins, metabolites) associated with the disease will open up the possibility to generate and test hypotheses on the biological processes and genes involved in this condition. The evaluation of disease-relevant data is a multistep procedure involving a complex pipeline of analysis and data handling tools such as data normalization, quality control, multivariate statistics, correlation analysis, visualization techniques, and intelligent database systems [11]. Several pioneering approaches have indicated the power of integrating data sets from different levels: for example, the correlation of gene membership of expression clusters and promoter sequence motifs [12]; the combination of transcriptome and quantitative proteomics data in order to construct models of cellular pathways [10]; and the identification of novel metabolite-transcript correlations [13]. Finally, data can be used to build and refine dynamical models, which represent an even higher level of data integration.

1.5 Standards

As experimental techniques generate rapidly growing amounts of data and large models need to be developed and exchanged, standards for both experimental procedures and modeling are a central practical issue in systems biology. Information exchange necessitates a common language about biological aspects. One seminal example is the gene ontology which provides a controlled vocabulary that can be applied to all organisms, even as the knowledge about genes and proteins continues to accumulate. The SBML [7] has been established as exchange language for mathematical models of biochemical reaction networks. A series of "minimum-information-about" statements based on community agreement defines standards for certain types of experiments. *M*inimum *i*nformation *r*equested *i*n the *a*nnotation of biochemical *m*odels (MIRIAM) [14] describes standards for this specific type of systems biology models.

References

1 Lander, E.S. *et al.* (2001b) Initial sequencing and analysis of the human genome. *Nature*, **409**, 860–921.

2 Venter, J.C. *et al.* (2001a) The sequence of the human genome. *Science*, **291**, 1304–1351.

3 von Mering, C. *et al.* (2002) Comparative assessment of large-scale data sets of protein–protein interactions. *Nature*, **417**, 399–403.

4 Brazma, A. *et al.* (2001) Minimum information about a microarray experiment (MIAME)-toward standards for microarray data. *Nature Genetics*, **29**, 365–371.

5 Taylor, C.F. *et al.* (2003) A systematic approach to modeling, capturing, and disseminating proteomics experimental data. *Nature Biotechnology*, **21**, 247–254.

6 Hermjakob, H. *et al.* (2004) The HUPO PSI's molecular interaction format – a community standard for the representation of protein interaction data. *Nature Biotechnology*, **22**, 177–183.

7 Hucka, M. *et al.* (2003) The systems biology markup language (SBML): a medium for representation and exchange of biochemical network models. *Bioinformatics*, **19**, 524–531.

8 Lloyd, C.M. *et al.* (2004) CellML: its future present and past. *Progress in Biophysics and Molecular Biology*, **85**, 433–450.

9 Gitton, Y. *et al.* (2002) A gene expression map of human chromosome 21 orthologues in the mouse. *Nature*, **420**, 586–590.

10 Ideker, T. *et al.* (2001) Integrated genomic and proteomic analyses of a systematically perturbed metabolic network. *Science*, **292**, 929–934.

11 Kanehisa, M. and Bork, P. (2003) Bioinformatics in the post-sequence era. *Nature Genetics*, **33** (Suppl), 305–310.

12 Tavazoie, S. *et al.* (1999) Systematic determination of genetic network architecture. *Nature Genetics*, **22**, 281–285.

13 Urbanczyk-Wochniak, E. *et al.* (2003) Parallel analysis of transcript and metabolic profiles: a new approach in systems biology. *EMBO Reports*, **4**, 989–993.

14 Le Novere, N. *et al.* (2005) Minimum information requested in the annotation of biochemical models (MIRIAM). *Nature Biotechnology*, **23**, 1509–1515.

2
Modeling of Biochemical Systems

2.1
Kinetic Modeling of Enzymatic Reactions

Summary

The rate of an enzymatic reaction, i.e., the velocity by which the execution of the reaction changes the concentrations of its substrates, is determined by concentrations of its substrates, concentration of the catalyzing enzyme, concentrations of possible modifiers, and by certain parameters. We introduce different kinetic laws for reversible and irreversible reactions, for reactions with varying numbers of substrates, and for reactions that are subject to inhibition or activation. The derivations of the rate laws are shown and the resulting restrictions for their validity and applicability. Saturation and sigmoidal kinetics are explained. The connection to thermodynamics is shown.

Deterministic kinetic modeling of individual biochemical reactions has a long history. The Michaelis–Menten model for the rate of an irreversible one-substrate reaction is an integral part of biochemistry, and the K_m value is a major characteristic of the interaction between enzyme and substrate. Biochemical reactions are catalyzed by enzymes, i.e., specific proteins which often function in complex with cofactors. They have a catalytic center, are usually highly specific, and remain unchanged by the reaction. One enzyme molecule can catalyze thousands of reactions per second (this so-called turnover number ranges from $10^2\,s^{-1}$ to $10^7\,s^{-1}$). Enzyme catalysis leads to a rate acceleration of about 10^6- up to 10^{12}-fold compared to the noncatalyzed, spontaneous reaction.

In this chapter, we make you familiar with the basic concepts of the mass action rate law. We will show how you can derive and apply more advanced kinetic expressions. The effect of enzyme inhibitors and activators will be discussed. The thermodynamic foundations and constraints are introduced.

The basic quantities are the concentration S of a substance S, i.e., the number n of molecules (or, alternatively, moles) of this substance per volume V, and the rate v of a reaction, i.e., the change of concentration S per time t. This type of modeling is

Systems Biology: A Textbook. Edda Klipp, Wolfram Liebermeister, Christoph Wierling, Axel Kowald, Hans Lehrach, and Ralf Herwig

ISBN: 978-3-527-31874-2

macroscopic and phenomenological, compared to the microscopic approach, where single molecules and their interactions are considered. Chemical and biochemical kinetics rely on the assumption that the reaction rate v at a certain point in time and space can be expressed as a unique function of the concentrations of all substances at this point in time and space. Classical enzyme kinetics assumes for sake of simplicity a spatial homogeneity (the "well-stirred" test tube) and no direct dependency of the rate on time

$$v(t) = v(S(t)). \tag{2.1}$$

In more advanced modeling approaches, longing toward whole-cell modeling, spatial inhomogeneities are taken into account, paying tribute to the fact that many components are membrane-bound or that cellular structures hinder the free movement of molecules. But, in the most cases, one can assume that diffusion is rapid enough to allow for an even distribution of all substances in space.

2.1.1 The Law of Mass Action

Biochemical kinetics is based on the mass action law, introduced by Guldberg and Waage in the nineteenth century [1–3]. It states that the reaction rate is proportional to the probability of a collision of the reactants. This probability is in turn proportional to the concentration of reactants to the power of the molecularity, that is the number in which they enter the specific reaction. For a simple reaction such as

$$S_1 + S_2 \rightleftharpoons 2P, \tag{2.2}$$

the reaction rate reads

$$v = v_+ - v_- = k_+ S_1 \cdot S_2 - k_- P^2. \tag{2.3}$$

where v is the net rate; v_+ and v_- are the rates of the forward and backward reactions; and k_+ and k_- are the *kinetic* or *rate constants*, i.e., the respective proportionality factors.

The molecularity is 1 for S_1 and for S_2 and 2 for P, respectively. If we measure the concentration in mol l^{-1} (or M) and the time in seconds (s), then the rate has the unit M s^{-1}. Accordingly, the rate constants for bimolecular reactions have the unit M^{-1} s^{-1}. Rate constants of monomolecular reactions have the dimension s^{-1}. The general mass action rate law for a reaction transforming m_i substrates with concentrations S_i into m_j products with concentrations P_j reads

$$v = v_+ - v_- = k_+ \prod_{i=1}^{m_i} S_i^{n_i} - k_- \prod_{j=1}^{m_j} P_j^{n_j}, \tag{2.4}$$

where n_i and n_j denote the respective molecularities of S_i and P_j in this reaction.

The equilibrium constant K_{eq} (we will also use the simpler symbol q) characterizes the ratio of substrate and product concentrations in equilibrium (S_{eq} and P_{eq}), i.e., the state with equal forward and backward rate. The rate constants are related to K_{eq} in the following way:

$$K_{eq} = \frac{k_+}{k_-} = \frac{\prod_{j=1}^{m_j} P_{j,eq}^{n_j}}{\prod_{i=1}^{m_i} S_{i,eq}^{n_i}} \tag{2.5}$$

The relation between the thermodynamic and the kinetic description of biochemical reactions will be outlined in Section 2.1.2.

The equilibrium constant for the reaction given in Eq. (2.2) is $K_{eq} = P_{eq}^2/(S_{1,eq} \cdot S_{2,eq})$. The dynamics of the concentrations away from equilibrium is described by the ODEs.

$$\frac{d}{dt}S_1 = \frac{d}{dt}S_2 = -v \quad \text{and} \quad \frac{d}{dt}P = 2v. \tag{2.6}$$

The time course of S_1, S_2, and P is obtained by integration of these ODEs (see Section 2.3).

Example 2.1

The kinetics of a simple decay like

$$S \rightarrow \tag{2.7}$$

is described by $v = kS$ and $dS/dt = -kS$. Integration of this ODE from time $t = 0$ with the initial concentration S_0 to an arbitrary time t with concentration $S(t)$, $\int_{S_0}^{S} dS/S = -\int_{t=0}^{t} k\,dt$, yields the temporal expression $S(t) = S_0 e^{-kt}$.

2.1.2 Reaction Kinetics and Thermodynamics

An important purpose of metabolism is to extract energy from nutrients, which is necessary for the synthesis of molecules, growth, and proliferation. We distinguish between energy-supplying reactions, energy-demanding reactions, and energetically neutral reactions. The principles of reversible thermodynamics and their application to chemical reactions allow understanding of energy circulation in the cell.

A biochemical process is characterized by the direction of the reaction, by whether it occurs spontaneously or not, and by the position of the equilibrium. The first law of thermodynamics, i.e., the law of energy conservation, tells us that the total energy of a closed system remains constant during any process. The second law of thermodynamics states that a process occurs spontaneous only if it increases the total entropy of the system. Unfortunately, entropy is usually not directly measurable. A more suitable measure is the Gibbs free energy G, which is the energy capable of carrying out work under isotherm–isobar conditions, i.e., at constant temperature and constant pressure. The change of the free energy is given as

$$\Delta G = \Delta H - T\Delta S, \tag{2.8}$$

where ΔH is the change in enthalpy, ΔS the change in entropy, and T the absolute temperature in Kelvin. ΔG is a measure for the driving force, the spontaneity of a chemical reaction. The reaction proceeds spontaneous under release of energy, if $\Delta G < 0$ (exergonic process). If $\Delta G > 0$, then the reaction is energetically not favorable and will not occur spontaneously (endergonic process). $\Delta G = 0$ means that the system has reached its equilibrium. Endergonic reactions may proceed if they obtain energy from a strictly exergonic reaction by energetic coupling. In tables, free energy is usually given for standard conditions (ΔG°), i.e., for a concentration of the reaction partners of 1 M, a temperature of $T = 298$ K, and, for gaseous reactions, a pressure of $p = 98$, 1 kPa = 1 atm. The unit is kJ mol^{-1}. Free energy differences satisfy a set of relations as follows. The free energy difference for a reaction can be calculated from the balance of free energies of formation of its products and substrates:

$$\Delta G = \sum G_P - \sum G_S. \tag{2.9}$$

The enzyme cannot change the free energies of the substrates and products of a reaction, neither their difference, but it changes the way the reaction proceeds microscopically, the so-called reaction path, thereby lowering the activation energy for the reaction. The *Transition State Theory* explains this as follows. During the course of a reaction, the metabolites must pass one or more transition states of maximal free energy, in which bonds are solved or newly formed. The transition state is unstable; the respective molecule configuration is called an activated complex. It has a lifetime of around one molecule vibration, 10^{-14}–10^{-13} s, and it can hardly be experimentally verified. The difference $\Delta G^\#$ of free energy between the reactants and the activated complex determines the dynamics of a reaction: the higher this difference, the lower the probability that the molecules may pass this barrier and the lower the rate of the reaction. The value of $\Delta G^\#$ depends on the type of altered bonds, on steric, electronic, or hydrophobic demands, and on temperature.

Figure 2.1 presents a simplified view of the reaction course. The substrate and the product are situated in local minima of the free energy; the active complex is assigned to the local maximum. The free energy difference ΔG is proportional to the logarithm of the equilibrium constant K_{eq} of the respective reaction:

$$\Delta G = -RT \ln K_{eq}, \tag{2.10}$$

where R is the gas constant, 8.314 J mol^{-1} K^{-1}. The value of $\Delta G^\#$ corresponds to the kinetic constant k_+ of the forward reaction (Eqs. (2.3)–(2.5)) by $\Delta G^\# = -RT \ln k_+$, while $\Delta G^\# + \Delta G$ is related to the rate constant k_- of the backward reaction.

The interaction of the reactants with an enzyme may alter the reaction path and, thereby, lead to lower values of $\Delta G^\#$ as well as higher values of the kinetic constants. Furthermore, the free energy may assume more local minima and maxima along the path of reaction. They are related to unstable intermediary complexes. Values for the difference of free energy for some biologically important reactions are given in Table 2.1.

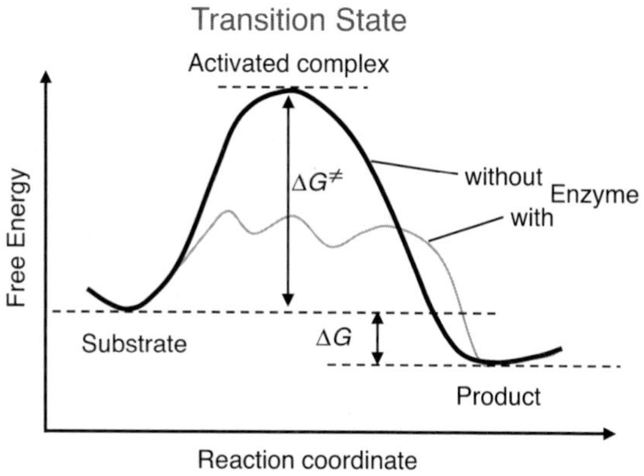

Figure 2.1 Change of free energy along the course of a reaction. The substrate and the product are situated in local minima of the free energy; the active complex is assigned to the local maximum. The enzyme may change the reaction path and thereby lower the barrier of free energy.

A biochemical reaction is reversible if it may proceed in both directions, leading to a positive or negative sign of the rate v. The actual direction depends on the current reactant concentrations. In theory, every reaction should be reversible. In practice, we can consider many reactions as irreversible since (i) reactants in cellular environment cannot assume any concentration, (ii) coupling of a chemical conversion to ATP consumption leads to a severe drop in free energy and therefore makes a reaction reversal energetically unfavorable, and (iii) for compound destruction, such as protein degradation, reversal by chance is extremely unlikely.

The detailed consideration of enzyme mechanisms by applying the mass action law for the single events has led to a number of standard kinetic descriptions, which will be explained in the following.

Table 2.1 Values of $\Delta G^{0'}$ and K_{eq} for some important reactions[a].

Reactions	$\Delta G^{0'}$ **(kJ mol^{-1})**
$2H_2 + O_2 \rightarrow 2H_2O$	−474
$2H_2O_2 \rightarrow 2H_2O + O_2$	−99
$PP_i + H_2O \rightarrow 2P_i$	−33.49
$ATP + H_2O \rightarrow ADP + P_i$	−30.56
Glucose-6-phosphate + H_2O → Glucose + P_i	−13.82
Glucose + P_i → Glucose-6-phosphate + H_2O	+13.82
Glucose-1-phosphate → Glucose-6-phosphate	−7.12
Glucose-6-phosphate → Fructose-6-phosphate	+1.67
Glucose + $6O_2$ → $6CO_2$ + $6H_2O$	−2890

[a] *Source:* ZITAT: Lehninger, A.L. Biochemistry, 2nd edition, New York, Worth, 1975, p. 397.

2.1.3
Michaelis–Menten Kinetics

Brown [4] proposed an enzymatic mechanism for invertase, catalyzing the cleavage of saccharose to glucose and fructose. This mechanism holds in general for all one-substrate reactions without backward reaction and effectors, such as

$$E + S \underset{k_{-1}}{\overset{k_1}{\rightleftharpoons}} ES \xrightarrow{k_2} E + P. \tag{2.11}$$

It comprises a reversible formation of an enzyme–substrate complex ES from the free enzyme E and the substrate S and an irreversible release of the product P. The ODE system for the dynamics of this reaction reads

$$\frac{dS}{dt} = -k_1 E \cdot S + k_{-1} ES, \tag{2.12}$$

$$\frac{dES}{dt} = k_1 E \cdot S - (k_{-1} + k_2) ES, \tag{2.13}$$

$$\frac{dE}{dt} = -k_1 E \cdot S + (k_{-1} + k_2) ES, \tag{2.14}$$

$$\frac{dP}{dt} = k_2 ES. \tag{2.15}$$

The reaction rate is equal to the negative decay rate of the substrate as well as to the rate of product formation:

$$v = -\frac{dS}{dt} = \frac{dP}{dt}. \tag{2.16}$$

This ODE system (Eqs. (2.12)–(2.16)) cannot be solved analytically. Different assumptions have been used to simplify this system in a satisfactory way. Michaelis and Menten [5] considered a *quasi-equilibrium* between the free enzyme and the enzyme–substrate complex, meaning that the reversible conversion of E and S to ES is much faster than the decomposition of ES into E and P, or in terms of the kinetic constants,

$$k_1, k_{-1} \gg k_2. \tag{2.17}$$

Briggs and Haldane [6] assumed that during the course of reaction a state is reached where the concentration of the ES complex remains constant, the so-called quasi-steady state. This assumption is justified only if the initial substrate concentration is much larger than the enzyme concentration, $S(t=0) \gg E$, otherwise such a state will never be reached. In mathematical terms, we obtain

$$\frac{dES}{dt} = 0. \tag{2.18}$$

In the following, we derive an expression for the reaction rate from the ODE system (2.12)–(2.15) and the quasi-steady-state assumption for ES. First, adding Eqs. (2.13) and (2.14) results in

$$\frac{dES}{dt}+\frac{dE}{dt}=0 \quad \text{or} \quad E_{total}=E+ES=\text{constant}. \tag{2.19}$$

This expression shows that enzyme is neither produced nor consumed in this reaction; it may be free or part of the complex, but its total concentration remains constant. Introducing (2.19) into (2.13) under the steady-state assumption (2.18) yields

$$ES=\frac{k_1 E_{total} S}{k_1 S+k_{-1}+k_2}=\frac{E_{total} S}{S+(k_{-1}+k_2)/k_1}. \tag{2.20}$$

For the reaction rate, this gives

$$v=\frac{k_2 E_{total} S}{S+((k_{-1}+k_2)/k_1)}. \tag{2.21}$$

In enzyme kinetics, it is convention to present Eq. (2.21) in a simpler form, which is important in theory and practice

$$v=\frac{V_{max} S}{S+K_m}. \tag{2.22}$$

Equation (2.22) is the expression for Michaelis–Menten kinetics. The parameters have the following meaning: the *maximal velocity*,

$$V_{max}=k_2 E_{total}, \tag{2.23}$$

is the maximal rate that can be attained, when the enzyme is completely saturated with substrate. The *Michaelis constant*,

$$K_m=\frac{k_{-1}+k_2}{k_1}, \tag{2.24}$$

is equal to the substrate concentration that yields the half-maximal reaction rate. For the quasi-equilibrium assumption (Eq. (2.17)), it holds that $K_m \cong k_{-1}/k_1$. The maximum velocity divided by the enzyme concentration (here $k_2=v_{max}/E_{total}$) is often called the turnover number, k_{cat}. The meaning of the parameters is illustrated in the plot of rate versus substrate concentration (Figure 2.2).

2.1.3.1 How to Derive a Rate Equation

Below, we will present some enzyme kinetic standard examples to derive a rate equation. Individual mechanisms for your specific enzyme of interest may be more complicated or merely differ from these standards. Therefore, we summarize here the general way of deriving a rate equation.

1. Draw a wiring diagram of all steps to consider (e.g., Eq. (2.11)). It contains all substrates and products (S and P) and *n* free or bound enzyme species (E and ES).

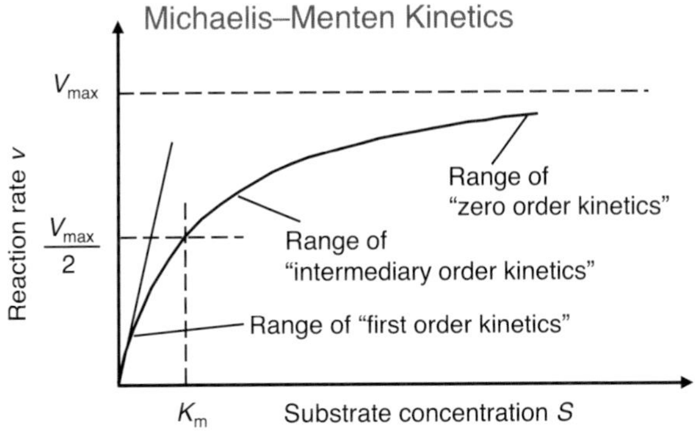

Figure 2.2 Dependence of reaction rate v on substrate concentration S in Michaelis–Menten kinetics. V_{max} denotes the maximal reaction rate that can be reached for large substrate concentration. K_m is the substrate concentration that leads to half-maximal reaction rate. For low substrate concentration, v increases almost linearly with S, while for high substrate concentrations v is almost independent of S.

2. The right sites of the ODEs for the concentrations changes sum up the rates of all steps leading to or away from a certain substance (e.g., Eqs. (2.12)–(2.15)). The rates follow mass action kinetics (Eq. (2.3)).
3. The sum of all enzyme-containing species is equal to the total enzyme concentration E_{total} (the right site of all differential equations for enzyme species sums up to zero). This constitutes one equation.
4. The assumption of quasi-steady state for $n-1$ enzyme species (i.e., setting the right sites of the respective ODEs equal to zero) together with (3.) result in n algebraic equations for the concentrations of the n enzyme species.
5. The reaction rate is equal to the rate of product formation (e.g., Eq. (2.16)). Insert the respective concentrations of enzyme species resulting from (4.).

2.1.3.2 **Parameter Estimation and Linearization of the Michaelis–Menten Equation**

To assess the values of the parameters V_{max} and K_m for an isolated enzyme, one measures the initial rate for different initial concentrations of the substrate. Since the rate is a nonlinear function of the substrate concentration, one has to determine the parameters by nonlinear regression. Another way is to transform Eq. (2.22) to a linear relation between variables and then apply linear regression.

The advantage of the transformed equations is that one may read the parameter value more or less directly from the graph obtained by linear regression of the measurement data. In the plot by Lineweaver and Burk [7] (Table 2.2), the values for V_{max} and K_m can be obtained from the intersections of the graph with the ordinate and the abscissa, respectively. The Lineweaver–Burk plot is also helpful to easily discriminate different types of inhibition (see below). The drawback of the transformed equations is that they may be sensitive to errors for small or high substrate

Table 2.2 Different approaches for the linearization of Michaelis–Menten enzyme kinetics.

	Lineweaver–Burk	Eadie–Hofstee	Hanes–Woolf
Transformed equation	$\frac{1}{v} = \frac{K_m}{V_{max}} \frac{1}{S} + \frac{1}{V_{max}}$	$v = V_{max} - K_m \frac{v}{S}$	$\frac{S}{v} = \frac{S}{V_{max}} + \frac{K_m}{V_{max}}$
New variables	$\frac{1}{v}, \frac{1}{S}$	$v, \frac{v}{S}$	$\frac{S}{v}, S$
Graphical representation	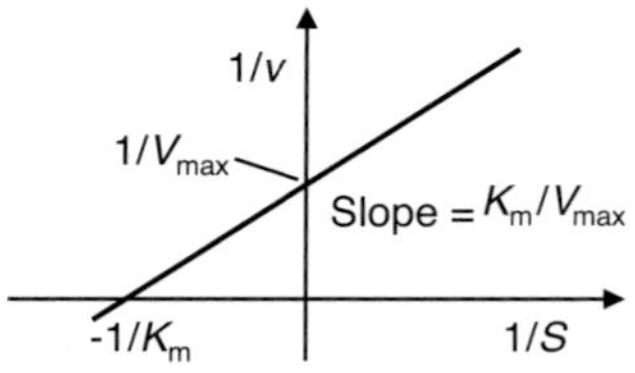	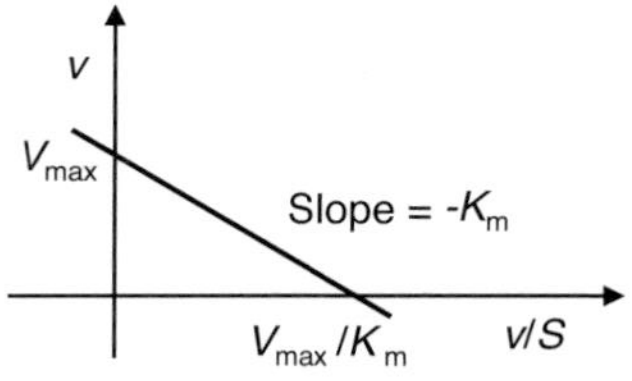	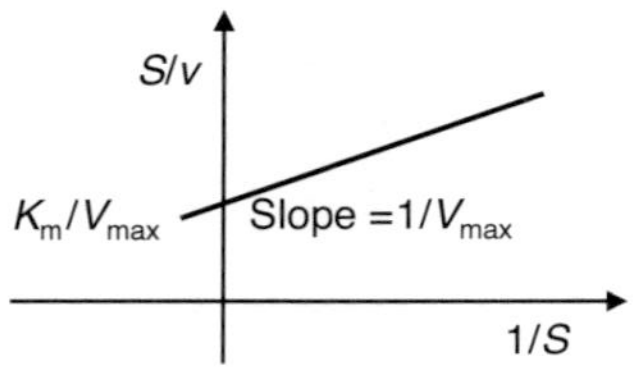

concentrations or rates. Eadie and Hofstee [8] and Hanes and Woolf [9] have introduced other types of linearization to overcome this limitation.

2.1.3.3 The Michaelis–Menten Equation for Reversible Reactions

In practice, many reactions are reversible. The enzyme may catalyze the reaction in both directions. Consider the following mechanism:

$$\mathrm{E}+\mathrm{S} \underset{k_{-1}}{\overset{k_1}{\rightleftarrows}} \mathrm{ES} \underset{k_{-2}}{\overset{k_2}{\rightleftarrows}} \mathrm{E}+\mathrm{P} \tag{2.25}$$

The product formation is given by

$$\frac{\mathrm{d}P}{\mathrm{d}t} = k_2 ES - k_{-2} E \cdot P = v. \tag{2.26}$$

The respective rate equation reads

$$\begin{aligned} v &= E_{\mathrm{total}} \frac{Sq-P}{Sk_1/(k_{-1}k_{-2}) + 1/k_{-2} + k_2/(k_{-1}k_{-2}) + P/k_{-1}} \\ &= \frac{(V_{\max}^{\mathrm{for}}/K_{\mathrm{m}S})S - (V_{\max}^{\mathrm{back}}/K_{\mathrm{m}P})P}{1 + S/K_{\mathrm{m}S} + P/K_{\mathrm{m}P}}. \end{aligned} \tag{2.27}$$

While the parameters $k_{\pm 1}$ and $k_{\pm 2}$ are the kinetic constants of the individual reaction steps, the phenomenological parameters $V_{\max}^{\mathrm{for}}$ and $V_{\max}^{\mathrm{back}}$ denote the maximal velocity in forward or backward direction, respectively, under zero product or substrate concentration, and the phenomenological parameters $K_{\mathrm{m}S}$ and $K_{\mathrm{m}P}$ denote the substrate or product concentration causing half maximal forward or backward rate. They are related in the following way [10]:

$$K_{\mathrm{eq}} = \frac{V_{\max}^{\mathrm{for}} K_{\mathrm{m}P}}{V_{\max}^{\mathrm{back}} K_{\mathrm{m}S}}. \tag{2.28}$$

2.1.4 Regulation of Enzyme Activity by Effectors

Enzymes may immensely increase the rate of a reaction, but this is not their only function. Enzymes are involved in metabolic regulation in various ways. Their production and degradation is often adapted to the current requirements of the cell. Furthermore, they may be targets of effectors, both inhibitors and activators.

The effectors are small molecules, or proteins, or other compounds that influence the performance of the enzymatic reaction. The interaction of effector and enzyme changes the reaction rate. Such regulatory interactions that are crucial for the fine-tuning of metabolism will be considered here [11].

Basic types of inhibition are distinguished by the state, in which the enzyme may bind the effector (i.e., the free enzyme E, the enzyme–substrate complex ES, or both), and by the ability of different complexes to release the product. The general pattern of inhibition is schematically represented in Figure 2.3. The different types result, if some of the interactions may not occur.

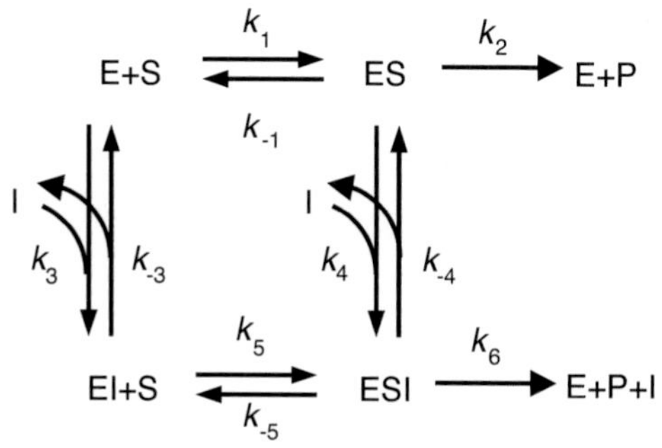

Figure 2.3 General scheme of inhibition in Michaelis–Menten kinetics. Reactions 1 and 2 belong to the standard scheme of Michaelis–Menten kinetics. Competitive inhibition is given, if in addition reaction 3 (and not reactions 4, 5, or 6) occurs. Uncompetitive inhibition involves reactions 1, 2, and 4, and noncompetitive inhibition comprises reactions 1, 2, 3, 4, and 5. Occurrence of reaction 6 indicates partial inhibition.

The rate equations are derived according to the following scheme:

1. Consider binding equilibriums between compounds and their complexes:

$$K_{\mathrm{m}} \cong \frac{k_{-1}}{k_1} = \frac{E \cdot S}{ES}, \; K_{\mathrm{I},3} = \frac{k_{-3}}{k_3} = \frac{E \cdot I}{EI}, \; K_{\mathrm{I},4} = \frac{k_{-4}}{k_4} = \frac{ES \cdot I}{ESI}, \; K_{\mathrm{I},5} = \frac{k_{-5}}{k_5} = \frac{EI \cdot S}{ESI}. \tag{2.29}$$

Note that, if all reactions may occur, the Wegscheider condition [12] holds in the form

$$\frac{k_1 k_4}{k_{-1} k_{-4}} = \frac{k_3 k_5}{k_{-3} k_{-5}}, \tag{2.30}$$

which means that the difference in the free energies between two compounds (e.g., E and ESI) is independent of the choice of the reaction path (here via ES or via EI).

2. Take into account the moiety conservation for the total enzyme (include only those complexes, which occur in the course of reaction):

$$E_{\mathrm{total}} = E + ES + EI + ESI. \tag{2.31}$$

3. The reaction rate is equal to the rate of product formation

$$v = \frac{\mathrm{d}P}{\mathrm{d}t} = k_2 ES + k_6 ESI. \tag{2.32}$$

Equations (2.29)–(2.31) constitute four independent equations for the four unknown concentrations of E, ES, EI, and ESI. Their solution can be inserted into Eq. (2.32). The effect of the inhibitor depends on the concentrations of substrate and inhibitor and on the relative affinities to the enzyme. Table 2.3 lists the different types of inhibition for irreversible and reversible Michaelis–Menten kinetics together with the respective rate equations.

Table 2.3 Types of inhibition for irreversible and reversible Michaelis–Menten kinetics[a].

Name	Implementation	Equation – irreversible case	Equation – reversible case	Characteristics
Competitive inhibition	I binds only to free E; P-release only from ES complex $k_{\pm 4} = k_{\pm 5} = k_6 = 0$	$v = \frac{V_{max} S}{K_m \cdot i_3 + S}$	$v = \frac{V^f_{max}(S/K_{mS}) - V^r_{max}(P/K_{mP})}{(S/K_{mS}) + (P/K_{mP}) + i_3}$	K_m changes, V_{max} remains same. S and I compete for the binding place; high S may out compete I.
Uncompetitive inhibition	I binds only to the ES complex; P-release only from ES complex $k_{\pm 3} = k_{\pm 5} = k_6 = 0$	$v = \frac{V_{max} S}{K_m + S \cdot i_4}$	$v = \frac{V^f_{max}(S/K_{mS}) - V^r_{max}(P/K_{mP})}{1 + ((S/K_{mS}) + (P/K_{mP}))i_4}$	K_m and V_{max} change, but their ratio remains same. S may not out compete I
Noncompetitive inhibition	I binds to E and ES; P-release only from ES $K_{I,3} = K_{I,4}$, $k_6 = 0$	$v = \frac{V_{max} S}{(K_m + S) i_3}$	$v = \frac{V^f_{max}(S/K_{mS}) - V^r_{max}(P/K_{mP})}{(1 + (S/K_{mS}) + (P/K_{mP}))i_4}$	K_m remains, V_{max} changes. S may not out compete I
Mixed inhibition	I binds to E and ES; P-release only from ES $K_{I,3} \neq K_{I,4}$, $k_6 = 0$	$v = \frac{V_{max} S}{K_m \cdot i_4 + S \cdot i_3}$		K_m and V_{max} change. $K_{I,3} > K_{I,4}$: competitive–noncompetitive inhibition $K_{I,3} < K_{I,4}$: noncompetitive–uncompetitive inhibition
Partial Inhibition	I may bind to E and ES; P-release from ES and ESI $K_{I,3} \neq K_{I,4}$, $K_6 \neq 0$	$v = \frac{V_{max} S[1 + \{(k_6 I)/(k_2 K_{I,3})\}]}{K_m i_4 + S i_3}$		K_m and V_{max} change. if $k_6 > k_2$: activation instead of inhibition.

[a] These abbreviations are used: $K_{I,3} = \frac{k_{-3}}{k_3}$, $K_{I,4} = \frac{k_{-4}}{k_4}$, $i_3 = 1 + \frac{I}{K_{I,3}}$, $i_4 = 1 + \frac{I}{K_{I,4}}$.

In the case of *competitive* inhibition, the inhibitor competes with the substrate for the binding site (or inhibits substrate binding by binding elsewhere to the enzyme) without being transformed itself. An example for this type is the inhibition of succinate dehydrogenase by malonate. The enzyme converts succinate to fumarate forming a double bond. Malonate has two carboxyl groups, like the proper substrates, and may bind to the enzyme, but the formation of a double bond cannot take place. Since substrates and inhibitor compete for the binding sites, a high concentration of one of them may displace the other one. For very high substrate concentrations, the same maximal velocity as without inhibitor is reached, but the effective K_m value is increased.

In the case of *uncompetitive* inhibition, the inhibitor binds only to the ES complex. The reason may be that the substrate binding caused a conformational change, which opened a new binding site. Since S and I do not compete for binding sites, an increase in the concentration of S cannot displace the inhibitor. In the presence of inhibitor, the original maximal rate cannot be reached (lower V_{max}). For example, an inhibitor concentration of $I = K_{I,4}$ halves the K_m-value as well as V_{max}. Uncompetitive inhibition occurs rarely for one-substrate reactions, but more frequently in the case of two substrates. One example is inhibition of arylsulphatase by hydracine.

Noncompetitive inhibition is present, if substrate binding to the enzyme does not alter the binding of the inhibitor. There must be different binding sites for substrate and inhibitor. In the classical case, the inhibitor has the same affinity to the enzyme with or without bound substrate. If the affinity changes, this is called mixed inhibition. A standard example is inhibition of chymotrypsion by H^+-ions.

If the product may also be formed from the enzyme–substrate–inhibitor complex, the inhibition is only partial. For high rates of product release (high values of k_6), this can even result in an activating instead of an inhibiting effect.

The general types of inhibition, competitive, uncompetitive, and noncompetitive inhibition also apply for the reversible Michaelis–Menten mechanism. The respective rate equations are also listed in Table 2.3.

2.1.4.1 Substrate Inhibition

A common characteristic of enzymatic reaction is the increase of the reaction rate with increasing substrate concentration S up to the maximal velocity V_{max}. But in some cases, a decrease of the rate above a certain value of S is recorded. A possible reason is the binding of a further substrate molecule to the enzyme–substrate complex yielding the complex ESS that cannot form a product. This kind of inhibition is reversible if the second substrate can be released. The rate equation can be derived using the scheme of uncompetitive inhibition by replacing the inhibitor by another substrate. It reads

$$v = k_2 ES = \frac{V_{max} S}{K_m + S(1 + (S/K_I))}. \tag{2.33}$$

This expression has an optimum, i.e., a maximal value of v, at

$$S_{opt} = \sqrt{K_m K_I} \quad \text{with} \quad v_{opt} = \frac{V_{max}}{1 + 2\sqrt{K_m/K_I}}. \tag{2.34}$$

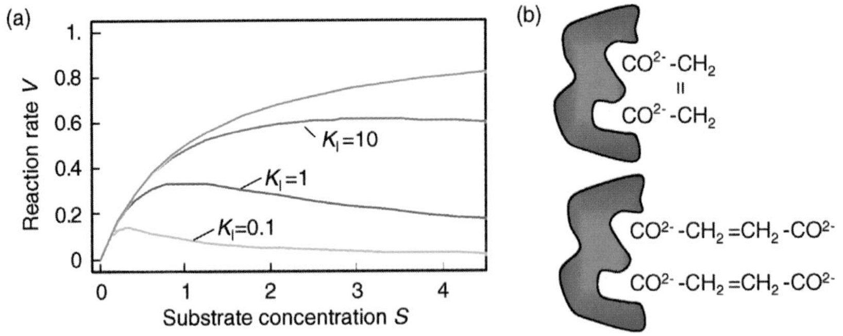

Figure 2.4 Plot of reaction rate v against substrate concentration S for an enzyme with substrate inhibition. The upper curve shows Michaelis–Menten kinetics without inhibition, the lower curves show kinetics for the indicated values of binding constant K_I. Parameter values: $V_{max} = 1$, $K_m = 1$. The left part visualizes a possible mechanism for substrate inhibition: The enzyme (gray item) has two binding pockets to bind different parts of a substrate molecule (upper scheme). In case of high substrate concentration, two different molecules may enter the binding pockets, thereby preventing the specific reaction (lower scheme).

The dependence of v on S is shown in Figure 2.4. A typical example for substrate inhibition is the binding of two succinate molecules to malonate dehydrogenase, which possesses two binding pockets for the carboxyl group. This is schematically represented in Figure 2.4.

2.1.4.2 Binding of Ligands to Proteins

Every molecule that binds to a protein is a ligand, irrespective of whether it is subject of a reaction or not. Below we consider binding to monomer and oligomer proteins. In oligomers, there may be interactions between the binding sites on the subunits.

Consider binding of one ligand (**S**) to a protein (**E**) with only one binding site:

$$E + S \rightleftharpoons ES \tag{2.35}$$

The binding constant K_B is given by

$$K_B = \left(\frac{ES}{E \cdot S}\right)_{eq}. \tag{2.36}$$

The reciprocal of K_B is the dissociation constant K_D. The fractional saturation Y of the protein is determined by the number of subunits that have bound ligands, divided by the total number of subunits. The fractional saturation for one subunit is

$$Y = \frac{ES}{E_{total}} = \frac{ES}{ES + E} = \frac{K_B \cdot S}{K_B \cdot S + 1}. \tag{2.37}$$

The plot of Y versus S at constant total enzyme concentration is a hyperbola, like the plot of v versus S in the Michaelis–Menten kinetics (Eq. (2.22)). At a process where the binding of S to E is the first step followed by product release and where the initial concentration of S is much higher than the initial concentration of E, the rate is proportional to the concentration of ES and it holds

$$\frac{v}{V_{max}} = \frac{ES}{E_{total}} = Y. \tag{2.38}$$

If the protein has several binding sites, then interactions may occur between these sites, i.e., the affinity to further ligands may change after binding of one or more ligands. This phenomenon is called *cooperativity*. Positive or negative cooperativity denote increase or decrease in the affinity of the protein to a further ligand, respectively. Homotropic or heterotropic cooperativity denotes that the binding to a certain ligand influences the affinity of the protein to a further ligand of the same or another type, respectively.

2.1.4.3 Positive Homotropic Cooperativity and the Hill Equation

Consider a dimeric protein with two identical binding sites. The binding to the first ligand facilitates the binding to the second ligand.

$$\begin{aligned} &E_2 + S \xrightarrow{\text{slow}} E_2S \\ &E_2S + S \xrightarrow{\text{fast}} E_2S_2 \end{aligned} \tag{2.39}$$

where E is the monomer and E_2 is the dimer. The fractional saturation is given by

$$Y = \frac{E_2S + 2 \cdot E_2S_2}{2 \cdot E_{2,total}} = \frac{E_2S + 2 \cdot E_2S_2}{2 \cdot E_2 + 2 \cdot E_2S + 2 \cdot E_2S_2}. \tag{2.40}$$

If the affinity to the second ligand is strongly increase by binding to the first ligand, then E_2S will react with S as soon as it is formed and the concentration of E_2S can be neglected. In the case of complete *cooperativity*, i.e., every protein is either empty or fully bound, Eq. (2.39) reduces to

$$E_2 + 2S \rightarrow E_2S_2 \tag{2.41}$$

The binding constant reads

$$K_B = \frac{E_2S_2}{E_2 \cdot S^2}, \tag{2.42}$$

and the fractional saturation is

$$Y = \frac{2 \cdot E_2S_2}{2 \cdot E_{2,total}} = \frac{E_2S_2}{E_2 + E_2S_2} = \frac{K_B \cdot S^2}{1 + K_B \cdot S^2}. \tag{2.43}$$

Generally, for a protein with n subunits, it holds:

$$v = V_{max} \cdot Y = \frac{V_{max} \cdot K_B \cdot S^n}{1 + K_B \cdot S^n}. \tag{2.44}$$

This is the general form of the *Hill equation*. To derive it, we assumed complete homotropic cooperativity. The plot of the fractional saturation Y versus substrate concentration S is a sigmoid curve with the inflection point at $1/K_B$. The quantity n (often "h" is used instead) is termed the *Hill coefficient*.

The derivation of this expression was based on experimental findings concerning the binding of oxygen to hemoglobin (Hb) [13, 14]. In 1904, Bohr *et al.* found that the plot of the fractional saturation of Hb with oxygen against the oxygen partial pressure had a sigmoid shape. Hill (1913) explained this with interactions between the binding sites located at the Hb subunits [14]. At this time, it was already known that every subunit Hb binds one molecule of oxygen. Hill assumed complete cooperativity and predicted an experimental Hill coefficient of 2.8. Today it is known that Hb has four binding sites, but that the cooperativity is not complete. The sigmoid binding characteristic has the advantage that Hb binds strongly to oxygen in the lung with a high oxygen partial pressure while it can release O_2 easily in the body with low oxygen partial pressure.

2.1.4.4 The Monod–Wyman–Changeux Model for Sigmoid Kinetics

The Monod model [15] explains sigmoid enzyme kinetics by taking into account the interaction of subunits of an enzyme. We will show here the main characteristics and assumptions of this kinetics. The full derivation is given in the web material. It uses the following assumptions: (i) the enzyme consists of n identical subunits, (ii) each subunit can assume an active (R) or an inactive (T) conformation, (iii) all subunits change their conformations at the same time (concerted change), and (iv) the equilibrium between the R and the T conformation is given by an allosteric constant

$$L = \frac{T_0}{R_0}. \tag{2.45}$$

The binding constants for the active and inactive conformations are given by K_R and K_T, respectively. If substrate molecules can only bind to the active form, i.e., if $K_T = 0$, the rate can be expressed as

$$V = \frac{V_{max} K_R S}{(1 + K_R S)} \frac{1}{[1 + \{L/((1 + K_R S)^n)\}]}, \tag{2.46}$$

where the first factor $(V_{max} K_R S)/(1 + K_R S)$ corresponds to the Michaelis–Menten rate expression, while the second factor $[1 + (L/(1 + K_R S)^n)]^{-1}$ is a regulatory factor (Figure 2.5).

For $L = 0$, the plot v versus S is hyperbola as in Michaelis–Menten kinetics. For $L > 0$, we obtain a sigmoid curve shifted to the right. A typical value for the allosteric constant is $L \cong 10^4$.

Up to now we considered in the model of Monod, Wyman, and Changeux only homotropic and positive effects. But this model is also well suited to explain the dependence of the reaction rate on activators and inhibitors. Activators A bind only to the active conformation and inhibitors I bind only to the inactive conformation. This shifts the equilibrium to the respective conformation. Effectively, the binding to effectors changes L:

$$L' = L \frac{(1 + K_I I)^n}{(1 + K_A A)^n}, \tag{2.47}$$

where K_I and K_A denote binding constants. The interaction with effectors is a heterotropic effect. An activator weakens the sigmoidity, while an inhibitor strengthens it.

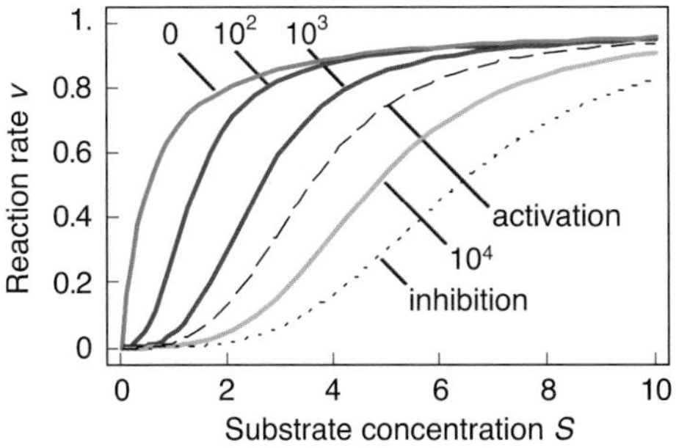

Figure 2.5 Model of Monod, Wyman, and Changeux: Dependence of the reaction rate on substrate concentration for different values of the allosteric constant L, according to equation. The binding constants for the active and inactive conformations are given by K_R and K_T, respectively. If substrate molecules can only bind to the active form, i.e., if $K_T = 0$, the rate can be expressed as $V = \frac{V_{max} K_R S}{(1 + K_R S)} \frac{1}{[1 + \{L/((1 + K_R S)^n)\}]}$, (2.46). Parameters: $V_{max} = 1$, $n = 4$, $K_R = 2$, $K_T = 0$. The value of L is indicated at the curves. Obviously, increasing value of L causes stronger sigmoidity. The influence of activators or inhibitors (compare Eq. (2.47)) is illustrated with the dotted line for $K_I I = 2$ and with the dashed line for $K_A A = 2$ ($L = 10^4$ in both cases).

A typical example for an enzyme with sigmoid kinetics that can be described with the Monod model is the enzyme phosphofructokinase, which catalyzes the transformation of fructose-6-phosphate and ATP to fructose-1,6-bisphosphate. AMP, NH_4, and K^+ are activators, ATP is an inhibitor.

2.1.5
Generalized Mass Action Kinetics

Mass action kinetics (see Section 2.1.1) has experienced refinements in different ways. The fact that experimental results frequently do not show the linear dependence of rate on concentrations as assumed in mass action laws is acknowledged in power law kinetics used in the S-systems approach [16]. Here, the rate reads

$$\frac{v_j}{v_j^0} = k_j \prod_{i=1}^{n} \left(\frac{S_i}{S_i^0}\right)^{g_{j,i}}, \tag{2.48}$$

where the concentrations S_i and rates v_j are normalized to some standard value denoted by superscript 0, and $g_{i,j}$ is a real number instead of an integer as in Eq. (2.4). The normalization yields dimensionless quantities. The power law kinetics can be considered as a generalization of the mass action rate law. The exponent $g_{i,j}$ is equal to the concentration elasticities, i.e., the scaled derivatives of rates with respect to substrate concentrations (see Section 2.3, Eq. (2.107)). Substrates and effectors (their concentrations both denoted by S_i) enter expression (2.48) in the same formal way, but the respective exponents $g_{i,j}$ will be different. The exponents $g_{i,j}$ will be positive for substrates and activators, but should assume a negative value for inhibitors.

2.1.6
Approximate Kinetic Formats

In metabolic modeling studies, approximate kinetic formats are used (for a recent review, see [17]). They preassume that each reaction rate v_j is proportional to the enzyme concentration E_j. The rates, enzyme concentrations, and substrate concentrations are normalized with respect to a reference state, which is usually a steady state. This leads to the general expression

$$\frac{v_j}{v_j^0} = \frac{E_j}{E_j^0} \cdot f\left(\frac{S}{S^0}, \varepsilon_c^0\right), \tag{2.49}$$

where ε_c is the matrix of concentration elasticities as explained in Section 2.3. One example is the so-called lin-log kinetics

$$\frac{\boldsymbol{v}}{\boldsymbol{v}^0} = \frac{\boldsymbol{E}}{\boldsymbol{E}^0}\left(\boldsymbol{I} + \varepsilon_c^0 \ln \frac{\boldsymbol{S}}{\boldsymbol{S}^0}\right), \tag{2.50}$$

where $\boldsymbol{I}$ is the $r \times r$ identity matrix. Another example is an approximation of the power-law kinetics

$$\ln \frac{\boldsymbol{v}}{\boldsymbol{v}^0} = \ln \frac{\boldsymbol{E}}{\boldsymbol{E}^0} + \varepsilon_c^0 \ln \frac{\boldsymbol{S}}{\boldsymbol{S}^0}. \tag{2.51}$$

Approximative kinetics simplify the determination of model parameters and, especially, of concentration elasticities, since Eq. (2.51) is a set of linear equations in the elasticity coefficients.

2.1.7
Convenience Kinetics

The convenience kinetics [18] has been introduced to ease parameter estimation and to have a kinetic mechanism, where all parameters are independent of each other and not related via the Haldane relation (Eq. (2.28)). It is a generalized form of Michaelis–Menten kinetics that covers all possible stoichiometries, and describes enzyme regulation by activators and inhibitors. For a reaction with stoichiometry

$$n_{-1}S_1 + n_{-2}S_2 + \cdots \leftrightarrow n_{+1}P_1 + n_{+2}P_2 + \cdots, \tag{2.52}$$

it reads

$$v = E_{\text{total}} \cdot f_{\text{reg}} \cdot \frac{k_{\text{cat}}^{\text{for}} \prod_i (S_i/K_{\text{m},S_i})^{n_{-i}} - k_{\text{cat}}^{\text{back}} \prod_j (P_j/K_{\text{m},P_j})^{n_{+j}}}{\prod_i (1 + (S_i/K_{\text{m},S_i}) + \cdots + (S_i/K_{\text{m},S_i})^{n_{-i}}) + \prod_j (1 + (P_j/K_{\text{m},P_j}) + \cdots + (P_j/K_{\text{m},P_j})^{n_{+j}}) - 1}, \tag{2.53}$$

with enzyme concentration E_{total} and turnover rates $k_{\text{cat}}^{\text{for}}$ and $k_{\text{cat}}^{\text{back}}$. The regulatory prefactor f_{reg} is either 1 (in case of no regulation) or a product of terms $M/(K_A + M)$ or $1 + M/K_A$ for activators and $K_I/(K_I + M)$ for inhibitors. Activation constants K_A and inhibition constants K_I are measured in concentration units. M is the concentration of the modifier.

In analogy to Michaelis–Menten kinetics, K_m values denote substrate concentrations, at which the reaction rate is half-maximal if the reaction products are absent; K_I and K_A values denote concentrations, at which the inhibitor or activator has its half-maximal effect. In this respect, many parameters in convenience kinetics are comparable to the kinetic constants measured in enzyme assays. This is important for parameter estimation (see Section 4.2).

To facilitate thermodynamic independence of the parameters, we introduce new system parameters that can be varied independently, without violating any thermodynamic constraints (see Section 2.1.1). For each reaction, we define the velocity constant $K_V = (k_{cat}^{for} \cdot k_{cat}^{back})^{1/2}$ (geometric mean of the turnover rates in both directions). Given the equilibrium and velocity constants, the turnover rates can be written as $k_{cat}^{for} = K_V(K_{eq})^{-1/2}$, $k_{cat}^{back} = K_V(K_{eq})^{1/2}$. The equilibrium constants K_{eq} can be expressed by independent parameters such as the Gibbs free energies of formation: for each substance i, we define the dimensionless energy constant $K_i^G = \exp(G_i(0)/(RT))$ with Boltzmann's gas constant $R = 8.314\,\mathrm{J}\,(\mathrm{mol}^{-1}\,\mathrm{K}^{-1})$ and absolute temperature T. The equilibrium constants then satisfy $\ln K_{eq} = -N^T \ln K^G$.

2.2 Structural Analysis of Biochemical Systems

Summary

We discuss basic structural and dynamic properties of biochemical reaction networks. We introduce a stoichiometric description of networks and learn how moieties and fluxes are balanced within networks.

The *basic elements* of a metabolic or regulatory network model are

1. the compounds with their concentrations or activities and
2. the reactions or transport processes changing the concentrations or activities of the compounds.

In biological environments, reactions are usually catalyzed by enzymes, and transport steps are carried out by transport proteins or pores, thus they can be assigned to identifiable biochemical compounds. In the following, we will mainly refer to metabolic networks. However, the analysis can also be applied to regulatory networks, if different activity states or complexes of regulatory molecules are considered as individual compounds that are converted into each other by modifying reactions.

2.2.1 System Equations

Stoichiometric coefficients denote the proportion of substrate and product molecules involved in a reaction. For example, for the reaction

$$S_1 + S_2 \rightleftharpoons 2P, \tag{2.54}$$

the stoichiometric coefficients of S_1, S_2, and P are −1, −1, and 2, respectively. The assignment of stoichiometric coefficients is not unique. We could also argue that for the production of one mole P, half a mole of each S_1 and S_2 have to be used and, therefore, choose −1/2, −1/2, and 1. Or, if we change the direction of the reaction, then we may choose 1, 1, and −2.

The change of concentrations in time can be described using ODEs. For the reaction depicted in Eq. (2.54) and the first choice of stoichiometric coefficients, we obtain

$$\frac{dS_1}{dt} = -v, \quad \frac{dS_2}{dt} = -v, \quad \text{and} \quad \frac{dP}{dt} = 2v. \tag{2.55}$$

This means that the degradation of S_1 with rate v is accompanied by the degradation of S_2 with the same rate and by the production of P with the double rate.

For a metabolic network consisting of m substances and r reactions, the system dynamics is described by the *system equations* (or *balance equations*, since the balance of substrate production and degradation is considered) [19, 20]:

$$\frac{dS_i}{dt} = \sum_{j=1}^{r} n_{ij} v_j \quad \text{for} \quad i = 1, \ldots, m. \tag{2.56}$$

The quantities n_{ij} are the stoichiometric coefficients of the ith metabolite in the jth reaction. Here, we assume that the reactions are the only reason for concentration changes and that no mass flow occurs due to convection or to diffusion. The balance equations (2.56) can also be applied, if the system consists of several compartments. In this case, every compound in different compartments has to be considered as an individual compound and transport steps are formally considered as reactions transferring the compound belonging to one compartment into the same compound belonging to the other compartment. In case, volume differences must be considered (see Section 3.4).

The stoichiometric coefficients n_{ij} assigned to the compounds S_i and the reactions v_j can be comprehended into the *stoichiometric matrix*

$$\mathbf{N} = \{n_{ij}\} \quad \text{for} \quad i = 1, \ldots, m \quad \text{and} \quad j = 1, \ldots, r, \tag{2.57}$$

where each column belongs to a reaction and each row to a compound. Table 2.4 shows some examples for reaction networks and their respective stoichiometric matrices.

Note that all reactions may be reversible. In order to determine the signs is $\mathbf{N}$, the direction of the arrows is artificially assigned as positive "from left to right" and "from top down." If the net flow of a reaction proceeds in the opposite direction as the arrow indicates, the value of rate v is negative.

Table 2.4 Different reaction networks and their stoichiometric matrices[a].

	Network	Stoichiometric matrix
N1	$S_1 + S_2 + S_3 \overset{v_1}{\longleftrightarrow} S_4 + 2S_5$	$N = \begin{pmatrix} -1 \\ -1 \\ -1 \\ 1 \\ 2 \end{pmatrix}$
N2	$\xrightarrow{v_1} S_1 \xrightarrow{v_2} S_2 \xrightarrow{v_3} S_3 \xrightarrow{v_4} S_4 \xrightarrow{v_5}$	$N = \begin{pmatrix} 1 & -1 & 0 & 0 & 0 \\ 0 & 1 & -1 & 0 & 0 \\ 0 & 0 & 1 & -1 & 0 \\ 0 & 0 & 0 & 1 & -1 \end{pmatrix}$
N3	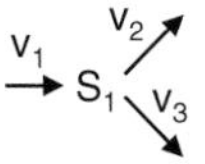	$N = \begin{pmatrix} 1 & -1 & -1 \end{pmatrix}$
N4	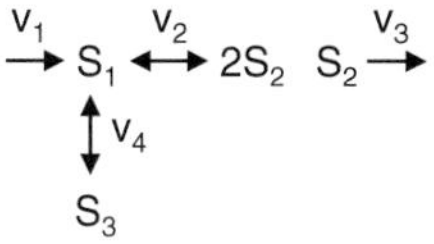	$N = \begin{pmatrix} 1 & -1 & 0 & -1 \\ 0 & 2 & -1 & 0 \\ 0 & 0 & 0 & 1 \end{pmatrix}$
N5	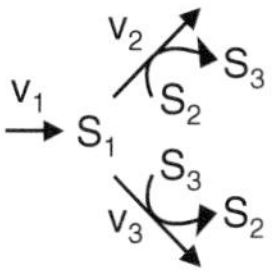	$N = \begin{pmatrix} 1 & -1 & -1 \\ 0 & -1 & 1 \\ 0 & 1 & -1 \end{pmatrix}$
N6	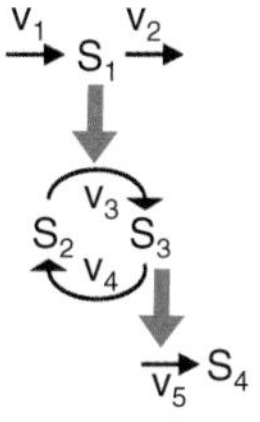	$N = \begin{pmatrix} 1 & -1 & 0 & 0 & 0 \\ 0 & 0 & -1 & 1 & 0 \\ 0 & 0 & 1 & -1 & 0 \\ 0 & 0 & 0 & 0 & 1 \end{pmatrix}$

[a] Note that external metabolites are neither drawn in the network nor included in the stoichiometric matrix. Thin arrows denote reactions, bold arrows denote activation.

Altogether, the mathematical description of the metabolic system consists of a vector $\boldsymbol{S} = (S_1, S_2, S_n)^{\mathrm{T}}$ of concentrations values, a vector $\boldsymbol{v} = (v_1, v_2, \ldots, v_r)^{\mathrm{T}}$ of reaction rates, a parameter vector $\boldsymbol{p} = (p_1, p_2, \ldots, p_m)^{\mathrm{T}}$, and the stoichiometric matrix $\boldsymbol{N}$. If the system is in steady state, we can also consider the vector $\boldsymbol{J} = (J_1, J_2, \ldots, J_r)^{\mathrm{T}}$ containing the steady-state fluxes. With these notions, the balance equation reads

$$\frac{\mathrm{d}\boldsymbol{S}}{\mathrm{d}t} = \boldsymbol{N}\boldsymbol{v}, \tag{2.58}$$

a compact form that is suited for various types of analysis.

2.2.2 Information Encoded in the Stoichiometric Matrix N

The stoichiometric matrix contains important information about the structure of the metabolic network. Using the stoichiometric matrix, we may calculate which combinations of individual fluxes are possible in steady state (i.e., calculate the admissible steady-state flux space). We may easily find out dead ends and unbranched reaction pathways. In addition, we may find out the conservation relations for the included reactants.

In steady state, it holds that

$$\frac{dS}{dt} = \boldsymbol{N}\boldsymbol{v} = \boldsymbol{0}. \tag{2.59}$$

The right equality sign denotes a linear equation system for determination of the rates $\boldsymbol{v}$. From linear algebra, it is known that this equation has nontrivial solutions only for Rank $\boldsymbol{N} < r$. A kernel matrix $\boldsymbol{K}$ fulfilling

$$\boldsymbol{NK} = \boldsymbol{0} \tag{2.60}$$

shows the respective linear dependencies [21]. The choice of the kernel is not unique. It can be determined using the Gauss Algorithm (see mathematical textbooks). It contains as columns r–Rank $\boldsymbol{N}$ basis vectors. Every possible set $\boldsymbol{J}$ of steady-state fluxes can be expressed as linear combination of the columns $\boldsymbol{k}_i$ of $\boldsymbol{K}$

$$\boldsymbol{J} = \sum_{i=1}^{r-\text{Rank}\,\boldsymbol{N}} \alpha_i \cdot \boldsymbol{k}_i. \tag{2.61}$$

The coefficients must have units corresponding to the units of reaction rates ($\mathrm{M\,s^{-1}}$ or $\mathrm{mol\,l^{-1}\,s^{-1}}$).

Example 2.2

For the network N2 in Table 2.4, we have $r = 5$ reactions and Rank $\boldsymbol{N} = 4$. The kernel matrix contains just $1 = 5 - 4$ basis vectors, which are multiples of $k = (1 \quad 1 \quad 1 \quad 1 \quad 1)^T$. This means that in steady state, the flux through all reactions must be equal. Network N3 comprises $r = 3$ reactions and has Rank $\boldsymbol{N} = 1$. Each representation of the kernel matrix contains $3 - 1 = 2$ basis vectors, e.g.,

$$\boldsymbol{K} = (\boldsymbol{k}_1 \quad \boldsymbol{k}_2) \quad \text{with} \quad \boldsymbol{k}_1 = \begin{pmatrix} 1 \\ -1 \\ 0 \end{pmatrix}, \quad \boldsymbol{k}_2 = \begin{pmatrix} 1 \\ 0 \\ 1 \end{pmatrix}, \tag{2.62}$$

and for the steady-state flux holds

$$\boldsymbol{J} = \alpha_1 \cdot \boldsymbol{k}_1 + \alpha_2 \cdot \boldsymbol{k}_2. \tag{2.63}$$

Network N6 can present a small signaling cascade. It has five reactions and Rank $\mathbf{N} = 3$. The resulting two basis vectors of the kernel are linear combinations of

$$\mathbf{k}_1 = \begin{pmatrix} 1 & 1 & 0 & 0 & 0 \end{pmatrix}^{\mathrm{T}}, \quad \mathbf{k}_2 = \begin{pmatrix} 0 & 0 & 1 & 1 & 0 \end{pmatrix}^{\mathrm{T}}. \tag{2.64}$$

If we calculate the possible steady-state fluxes according to Eq. (2.63), we can easily see that in every steady state, it holds that production and degradation of S_1 are balanced ($J_1 = J_2$) and that the fluxes through the cycle are equal ($J_3 = J_4$). In addition, J_5 must be equal to zero, otherwise S_4 would accumulate. One could prevent the last effect by also including the degradation of S_4 into the network.

If the entries in a certain row are zero in all basis vectors, we have found an equilibrium reaction. In any steady state, the net rate of this reaction must be zero. For the reaction system N4 in Table 2.4, it holds that $r = 4$ and Rank $\mathbf{N} = 3$. Its kernel consists of only one column $K = \begin{pmatrix} 1 & 1 & 1 & 0 \end{pmatrix}^{\mathrm{T}}$. Hence, $v_4 = \sum_{i=1}^{1} \alpha \cdot 0 = 0$. In any steady state, the rates of production and degradation of S_3 must equal.

If all basis vectors contain the same entries for a set of rows, this indicates an unbranched reaction path. In each steady state, the net rate of all respective reactions is equal.

Example 2.3

Consider the reaction scheme

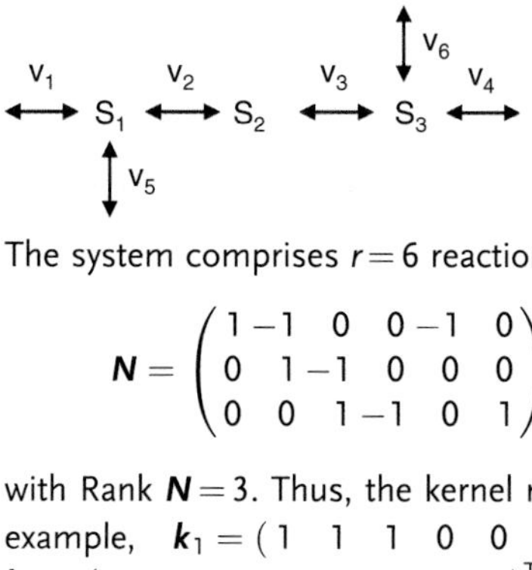

(2.65)

The system comprises $r = 6$ reactions. The stoichiometric matrix reads

$$\mathbf{N} = \begin{pmatrix} 1 & -1 & 0 & 0 & -1 & 0 \\ 0 & 1 & -1 & 0 & 0 & 0 \\ 0 & 0 & 1 & -1 & 0 & 1 \end{pmatrix}$$

with Rank $\mathbf{N} = 3$. Thus, the kernel matrix is spanned by three basis vectors, for example, $\mathbf{k}_1 = \begin{pmatrix} 1 & 1 & 1 & 0 & 0 & -1 \end{pmatrix}^{\mathrm{T}}$, $\mathbf{k}_2 = \begin{pmatrix} 1 & 0 & 0 & 0 & 1 & 0 \end{pmatrix}^{\mathrm{T}}$, and $\mathbf{k}_3 = \begin{pmatrix} -1 & -1 & -1 & -1 & 0 & 0 \end{pmatrix}^{\mathrm{T}}$. The entries for the second and third reactions are always equal, thus in any steady state, the fluxes through reactions 2 and 3 must be equal.

Up to now, we have not been concerned about (ir)reversibility of reactions in the network. If a certain reaction is considered irreversible, this has no consequences for the stoichiometric matrix $\mathbf{N}$ but rather for the kernel $\mathbf{K}$. The set of vectors belonging to $\mathbf{K}$ is restricted by the condition that some values may not become negative (or positive – depending on the definition of flux direction).

2.2.3
Elementary Flux Modes and Extreme Pathways

The definition of the term "pathway" in a metabolic network is not straightforward. A descriptive definition of a pathway is a set of subsequent reactions that are linked by common metabolites. Typical examples include glycolysis or different amino acid synthesis pathways. More detailed inspection of metabolic maps like the *Boehringer Chart* [22] shows that metabolism is highly interconnected. Pathways that are known for a long time from biochemical experience are already hard to recognize, and it is even harder to find out new pathways, for example in metabolic maps that have been reconstructed from sequenced genomes of bacteria.

This problem has been elaborated in the concept of *elementary flux modes* [21, 23–27]. Here, the stoichiometry of a metabolic network is investigated to find out which direct routes are possible that lead from one external metabolite to another external metabolite. The approach takes into account that some reactions are reversible, while others are irreversible.

A *flux mode* $\boldsymbol{M}$ is set of flux vectors that represent such direct routes through the metabolic networks. In mathematical terms, it is defined as the set

$$M = \{\boldsymbol{v} \in R^r | \boldsymbol{v} = \lambda \boldsymbol{v}^*, \lambda > 0\}, \tag{2.66}$$

where $\boldsymbol{v}^*$ is an r-dimensional vector (unequal to the null vector) fulfilling two conditions: (i) steady state, i.e., Eq. (2.59), and (ii) sign restriction, i.e., the flux directions in $\boldsymbol{v}^*$ fulfill the prescribed irreversibility relations.

A flux mode $\boldsymbol{M}$ comprising $\boldsymbol{v}$ is called reversible if the set $\boldsymbol{M}'$ comprising $-\boldsymbol{v}$ is also a flux mode. A flux mode is an elementary flux mode if it uses a minimal set of reactions and cannot be further decomposed, i.e., the vector $\boldsymbol{v}$ cannot be represented as nonnegative linear combination of two vectors that fulfill conditions (i) and (ii) but contain more zero entries than $\boldsymbol{v}$. An elementary flux mode is a minimal set of enzymes that could operate at steady state, with all the irreversible reactions used in the appropriate direction. The number of elementary flux modes is at least as high as the number of basis vectors of the null space.

Example 2.4

The systems (A) and (B) differ by the (ir)reversibility of reaction 2.

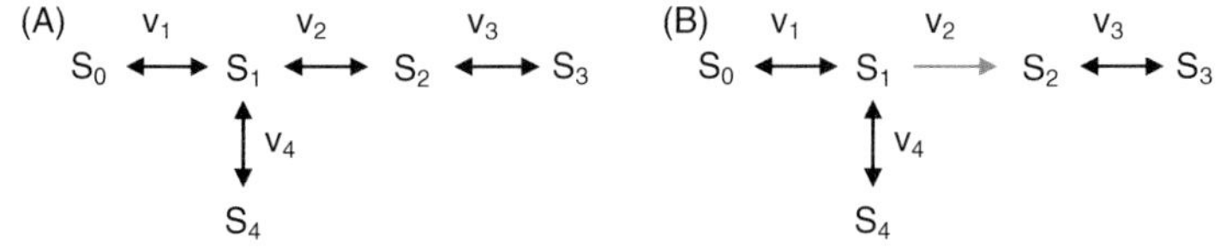

(2.67)

The elementary flux modes connect the external metabolites S_0 and S_3, S_0 and S_4, or S_3 and S_4. The stoichiometric matrix and the flux modes read for case (A) and case (B)

$$\boldsymbol{N} = \begin{pmatrix} 1 & -1 & 0 & -1 \\ 0 & 1 & -1 & 0 \end{pmatrix}, \quad \boldsymbol{\nu}^A = \begin{pmatrix} 1 \\ 1 \\ 1 \\ 0 \end{pmatrix}, \begin{pmatrix} 1 \\ 0 \\ 0 \\ 1 \end{pmatrix}, \begin{pmatrix} 0 \\ -1 \\ -1 \\ 1 \end{pmatrix}, \begin{pmatrix} -1 \\ -1 \\ -1 \\ 0 \end{pmatrix}, \begin{pmatrix} -1 \\ 0 \\ 0 \\ -1 \end{pmatrix}, \begin{pmatrix} 0 \\ 1 \\ 1 \\ -1 \end{pmatrix},$$
$$\text{and } \boldsymbol{\nu}^B = \begin{pmatrix} 1 \\ 1 \\ 1 \\ 0 \end{pmatrix}, \begin{pmatrix} 1 \\ 0 \\ 0 \\ 1 \end{pmatrix}, \begin{pmatrix} -1 \\ 0 \\ 0 \\ -1 \end{pmatrix}, \begin{pmatrix} 0 \\ 1 \\ 1 \\ -1 \end{pmatrix}. \tag{2.68}$$

The possible routes are illustrated in Figure 2.6.

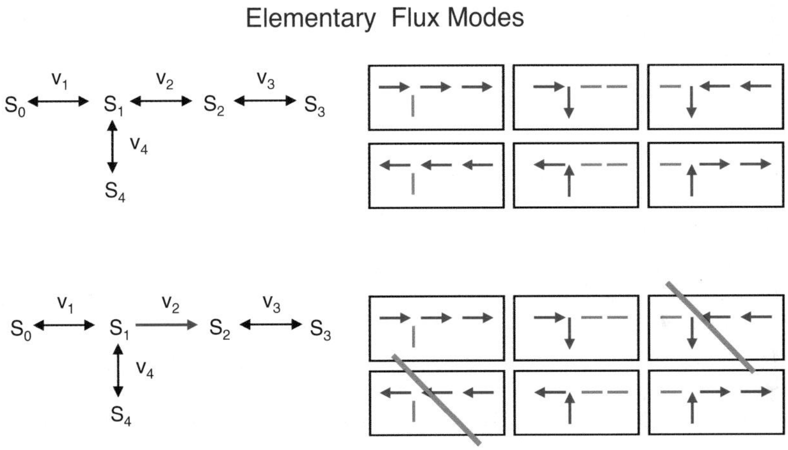

Figure 2.6 Schematic representation of elementary flux modes for the reaction network depicted in Eq. (2.67).

2.2.3.1 **Flux Cone**

The stoichiometric analysis of biochemical network analysis can be modified by considering only irreversible reactions (e.g., by splitting reversible reactions into two irreversible ones). Based on such a unidirectional representation, the basis vectors (Eq. (2.61)) form a convex cone in the flux space. This mapping relates stoichiometric analysis to the concepts of convex geometry as follows. The steady-state assumption requires that a flux vector is an element of the null space of the stoichiometry matrix $\boldsymbol{N}$ spanned by matrix $\boldsymbol{K}$. A row of $\boldsymbol{K}$ can be interpreted as a hyperplane in flux space. The intersection of all these hyperplanes forms the null space. From thermodynamic

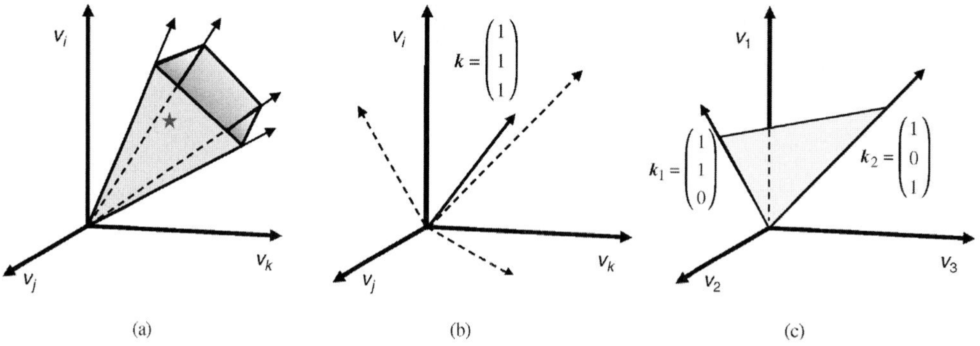

Figure 2.7 Flux cone: schematic representation of the subspace of feasible steady states within the space spanned by all positive-valued vectors for rates of irreversible reactions, v_i, $i = 1, \ldots, r$. Only three dimensions are shown. Feasible solutions are linear combinations of basis vectors of matrix $\boldsymbol{K}$ (see text). (a) Illustrative representation of the flux cone for a higher dimensional system (with r–Rank $(\boldsymbol{N}) = 4$)). The basis vectors of $\boldsymbol{K}$ are rays starting at the origin. The line connecting the four rays indicates possible limits for real flux distributions set by constraints. The little star indicates one special feasible solution for the fluxes. (b) The flux cone for an unbranched reaction chain of arbitrary length, such as the network N2 in Table 2.4, is just a ray since $\boldsymbol{K}$ is represented by a single basis vector containing only 1s. (c) The flux cone for network N3 in Table 2.4 is the plane spanned by the basis vectors $\boldsymbol{k}_1 = (1 \quad 1 \quad 0)^T$, $\boldsymbol{k}_2 = (1 \quad 0 \quad 1)^T$.

considerations, some of the reactions can be assumed to proceed only in one direction so that the backward reaction can be neglected. Provided that all reactions are unidirectional or irreversible, the intersection of the null space with the semipositive orthant of the flux space forms a polyhedral cone, the flux cone. The intersection procedure results in a set of rays or edges starting at 0, which fully describe the cone. The edges are represented by vectors and any admissible steady state of the system is a positive combination of these vectors. An illustration is presented in Figure 2.7.

The set of elementary flux modes is uniquely defined. Pfeiffer *et al.* [23] developed a software ("Metatool") to calculate the elementary flux modes for metabolic networks. The concept of *extreme pathways* [28–30] is analogous to the concept of elementary flux modes, but here all reactions are constrained by flux directionality, while the concept of elementary flux modes allows for reversible reactions. To achieve this, reversible reactions are broken down into their forward and backward components. This way, the set of extreme pathways is a subset of the set of elementary flux modes and the extreme pathways are systemically independent.

Elementary flux modes and extreme pathways can be used to understand the range of metabolic pathways in a network, to test a set of enzymes for production of a desired product and detect nonredundant pathways, to reconstruct metabolism from annotated genome sequences and analyze the effect of enzyme deficiency, to reduce drug effects, and to identify drug targets. A specific application, the flux balance analysis, will be explained in Section 8.1.

2.2.4
Conservation Relations: Null Space of N^T

If a substance is neither added to nor removed from the reaction system (neither produced nor degraded), its total concentration remains constant. This also holds if the substance interacts with other compounds by forming complexes. We have seen already as an example the constancy of the total enzyme concentration (Eq. (2.19)) when deriving the Michaelis–Menten rate equation. This was based on the assumption that enzyme production and degradation takes place on a much faster timescale than the catalyzed reaction.

For the mathematical derivation of the conservation relations [21], we consider a matrix $\boldsymbol{G}$ fulfilling

$$\boldsymbol{GN} = 0. \tag{2.69}$$

Due to Eq. (2.58), it follows

$$\boldsymbol{G\dot{S}} = \boldsymbol{GNv} = 0. \tag{2.70}$$

Integrating this equation leads directly to the conservation relations

$$\boldsymbol{GS} = \text{constant}. \tag{2.71}$$

The number of independent rows of $\boldsymbol{G}$ is equal to n–Rank $\boldsymbol{N}$, where n is the number of metabolites in the system. $\boldsymbol{G}^T$ is the kernel matrix of N^T, hence it has similar properties as $\boldsymbol{K}$. Matrix $\boldsymbol{G}$ can also be found using the Gauss algorithm. It is not unique, but every linear combination of its rows is again a valid solution. There is a simplest representation $\boldsymbol{G} = (\; \boldsymbol{G}_0 \quad \boldsymbol{I}_{n-\text{Rank}\,\boldsymbol{N}} \;)$. Finding this representation may be helpful for a simple statement of conservation relations, but this may necessitate renumbering and reordering of metabolite concentrations (see below).

Example 2.5

Consider a set of two reactions comprising a kinase and a phosphatase reaction

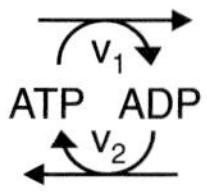

(2.72)

The metabolite concentration vector reads $\boldsymbol{S} = (\,ATP \quad ADP\,)^T$, the stoichiometric matrix is $\boldsymbol{N} = \begin{pmatrix} -1 & 1 \\ 1 & -1 \end{pmatrix}$ yielding $\boldsymbol{G} = (\,1 \quad 1\,)$. From the condition $\boldsymbol{GS}$ = constant, it follows $ATP + ADP$ = constant. Thus, we have a conservation of adenine nucleotides in this system. The actual values of $ATP + ADP$ must be determined from the initial conditions.

Example 2.6

For the following model of the upper part of glycolysis

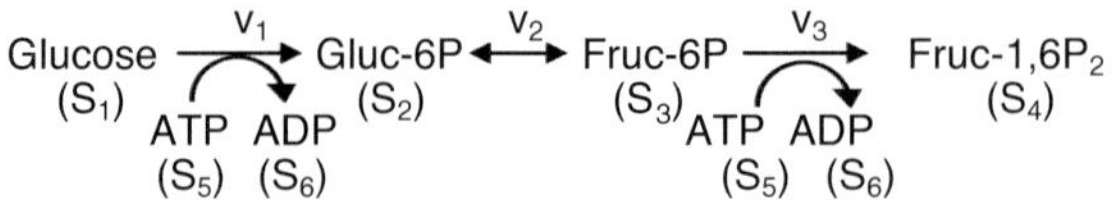

(2.73)

the stoichiometric matrix $\boldsymbol{N}$ (note the transpose!) and a possible representation of the conservation matrix $\boldsymbol{G}$ are given by

$$\boldsymbol{N}^{\mathrm{T}} = \begin{pmatrix} -1 & 1 & 0 & 0 & -1 & 1 \\ 0 & -1 & 1 & 0 & 0 & 0 \\ 0 & 0 & -1 & 1 & -1 & 1 \end{pmatrix} \quad \text{and} \quad \boldsymbol{G} = \begin{pmatrix} 2 & 1 & 1 & 0 & 0 & 1 \\ 0 & 0 & 0 & 0 & 1 & 1 \\ 1 & 1 & 1 & 1 & 0 & 0 \end{pmatrix} = \begin{pmatrix} \boldsymbol{g}_1 \\ \boldsymbol{g}_2 \\ \boldsymbol{g}_3 \end{pmatrix}. \tag{2.74}$$

The interpretation of the second and third row is straightforward, showing the conservation of adenine nucleotides ($\boldsymbol{g}_2$, $ADP + ATP =$ constant) and the conservation of sugars ($\boldsymbol{g}_3$), respectively. The interpretation of the first row is less intuitive. If we construct the linear combination $\boldsymbol{g}_4 = -\boldsymbol{g}_1 + 3\cdot\boldsymbol{g}_2 + 2\cdot\boldsymbol{g}_3 = (0\ \ 1\ \ 1\ \ 2\ \ 3\ \ 2)$, we find the conservation of phosphate groups.

Importantly, conservation relations can be used to simplify the system of differential equations $\dot{\boldsymbol{S}} = \boldsymbol{N}\boldsymbol{v}$ describing the dynamics of our reaction system. The idea is to eliminate linear dependent differential equations and to replace them by appropriate algebraic equations. Below the procedure is explained systematically [20].

First we have to rearrange the rows in the stoichiometric matrix $\boldsymbol{N}$ as well as in the concentration vector $\boldsymbol{S}$ such that a set of independent rows is on top and the dependent rows are at the bottom. Then the matrix $\boldsymbol{N}$ is split into the independent part $\boldsymbol{N}_{\mathrm{R}}$ and the dependent part $\boldsymbol{N}'$ and a *link matrix* $\boldsymbol{L}$ is introduced in the following way:

$$\boldsymbol{N} = \begin{pmatrix} \boldsymbol{N}_{\mathrm{R}} \\ \boldsymbol{N}' \end{pmatrix} = \boldsymbol{L}\boldsymbol{N}_{\mathrm{R}} = \begin{pmatrix} \boldsymbol{I}_{\mathrm{Rank}\ N} \\ \boldsymbol{L}' \end{pmatrix} \boldsymbol{N}_{\mathrm{R}}. \tag{2.75}$$

$\boldsymbol{I}_{\mathrm{Rank}\ N}$ is the identity matrix of size Rank $\boldsymbol{N}$. The differential equation system may be rewritten accordingly

$$\dot{\boldsymbol{S}} = \begin{pmatrix} \dot{\boldsymbol{S}}_{\mathrm{indep}} \\ \dot{\boldsymbol{S}}_{\mathrm{dep}} \end{pmatrix} = \begin{pmatrix} \boldsymbol{I}_{\mathrm{Rank}\ N} \\ \boldsymbol{L}' \end{pmatrix} \boldsymbol{N}_{\mathrm{R}}\boldsymbol{v}, \tag{2.76}$$

and the dependent concentrations fulfil

$$\dot{S}_{\text{dep}} = L' \cdot \dot{S}_{\text{indep}}. \tag{2.77}$$

Integration leads to

$$S_{\text{dep}} = L' \cdot S_{\text{indep}} + \text{constant}. \tag{2.78}$$

This relation is fulfilled during the entire time course. Thus, we may replace the original system by a reduced differential equation system

$$\dot{S}_{\text{indep}} = N_{\text{R}} \boldsymbol{v}, \tag{2.79}$$

supplemented with the set of algebraic equations (2.78).

Example 2.7

For the reaction system,

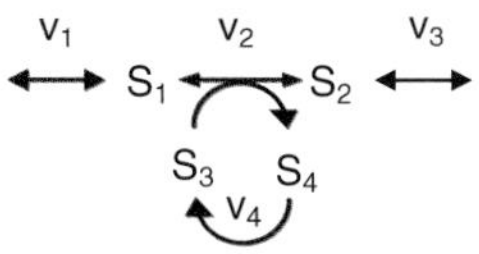

(2.80)

the stoichiometric matrix, the reduced stoichiometric matrix, and the link matrix read

$$\boldsymbol{N} = \begin{pmatrix} 1 & -1 & 0 & 0 \\ 0 & 1 & -1 & 0 \\ 0 & -1 & 0 & 1 \\ 0 & 1 & 0 & -1 \end{pmatrix}, \quad \boldsymbol{N}_{\text{R}} = \begin{pmatrix} 1 & -1 & 0 & 0 \\ 0 & 1 & -1 & 0 \\ 0 & -1 & 0 & 1 \end{pmatrix},$$

$$\boldsymbol{L} = \begin{pmatrix} 1 & 0 & 0 \\ 0 & 1 & 0 \\ 0 & 0 & 1 \\ 0 & 0 & -1 \end{pmatrix}, \quad \boldsymbol{L}' = \begin{pmatrix} 0 & 0 & -1 \end{pmatrix}$$

The conservation relation $S_3 + S_4 = \text{constant}$ is expressed by $\boldsymbol{G} = \begin{pmatrix} 0 & 0 & 1 & 1 \end{pmatrix}$. The ODE system

$$\begin{aligned} \dot{S}_1 &= \nu_1 - \nu_2 \\ \dot{S}_2 &= \nu_2 - \nu_3 \\ \dot{S}_3 &= \nu_4 - \nu_2 \\ \dot{S}_4 &= \nu_2 - \nu_4 \end{aligned}$$

can be replaced by the differential-algebraic system

$$\begin{aligned}\dot{S}_1 &= v_1 - v_2 \\ \dot{S}_2 &= v_2 - v_3 \\ \dot{S}_3 &= v_4 - v_2 \\ S_3 + S_4 &= \text{constant}\end{aligned},$$

which has one differential equation less.

Eukaryotic cells contain a variety of organelles like nucleus, mitochondria, or vacuoles, which are separated by membranes. Reaction pathways may cross the compartment boundaries. If a substance S occurs in two different compartments, e.g., in the cytosol and in mitochondria, the respective concentrations can be assigned to two different variables, S^{C1} and S^{C2}. Formally, the transport across the membrane can be considered as a reaction with rate v. It is important to note that both compartments have different volumes V^{C1} and V^{C2}. Thus, transport of a certain amount of S with rate v from compartment $C1$ into the compartment $C2$ changes the concentrations differently:

$$V^{C1} \cdot \frac{\mathrm{d}}{\mathrm{d}t} S^{C1} = -v \quad \text{and} \quad V^{C2} \cdot \frac{\mathrm{d}}{\mathrm{d}t} S^{C2} = v, \tag{2.81}$$

where $V \cdot S$ denotes substance amount in moles. Compartmental models are discussed in more detail in Section 3.4.

2.3 Kinetic Models of Biochemical Systems

Summary

An important problem in the modeling of biological systems is to characterize the dependence of certain properties on time and space. One frequently applied strategy is the description of the change of state variables by differential equations. If only temporal changes are considered, ODEs are used. For changes in time and space, partial differential equations (PDEs) are appropriate. In this chapter, we will deal with the solution, analysis, a numerical integration of ODEs, and with basic concepts of dynamical systems theory as state space, trajectory, steady states, and stability.

2.3.1 Describing Dynamics with ODEs

The time behavior of biological systems in a deterministic approach can be described by a set of differential equations

$$\frac{\mathrm{d}x_i}{\mathrm{d}t} = \dot{x}_i = f_i(x_1, \ldots, x_n, p_1, \ldots, p_l, t) \quad i = 1, \ldots, n, \tag{2.82}$$

where x_i are the variables, e.g., concentrations, and p_j are the parameters, e.g., enzyme concentrations or kinetic constants, and t is the time. We will use the notions dx/dt and $\dot{x}$ interchangeably. In vector notation, Eq. (2.82) reads

$$\frac{\mathrm{d}}{\mathrm{d}t}\boldsymbol{x} = \dot{\boldsymbol{x}} = f(\boldsymbol{x}, \boldsymbol{p}, t), \tag{2.83}$$

with $\boldsymbol{x} = (x_1, \ldots, x_n)^{\mathrm{T}}$, $\boldsymbol{f} = (f_1, \ldots, f_n)^{\mathrm{T}}$, and $\boldsymbol{p} = (p_1, \ldots, p_l)^{\mathrm{T}}$. For biochemical reaction systems, the functions f_i are frequently given by the contribution of producing and degrading reactions as described for the balance equations in Section 1.2.

2.3.1.1 Notations

ODEs depend on one variable (e.g., time t). Otherwise, they are called PDEs. PDEs are not considered here.

An implicit ODE

$$F(t, x, x', \ldots, x^{(n)}) = 0 \tag{2.84}$$

includes the variable t, the unknown function x, and its derivatives up to nth order. An explicit ODE of nth order has the form

$$x^{(n)} = f(t, x, x', \ldots, x^{(n-1)}). \tag{2.85}$$

The highest derivative (here n) determines the order of the ODE.

Studying the time behavior of our system, we may be interested in finding solutions of the ODE, i.e., finding an n times differentiable function x fulfilling Eq. (2.85). Such a solution may depend on parameters, so-called integration constants, and represents a set of curves. A solution of an ODE of nth order depending on n integration parameters is a *general* solution. Specifying the integration constants, for example, by specifying n initial conditions (for $n = 1$: $x(t = 0) = x^0$) leads to a special or *particular* solution.

We will not show here all possibilities of solving ODEs, instead we will focus on some cases relevant for the following chapters.

If the right-hand sides of the ODEs are not explicitly dependent on time t ($\dot{x} = \boldsymbol{f}(\boldsymbol{x}, \boldsymbol{p})$), the system is called autonomous. Otherwise it is nonautonomous. This case will not be considered here.

The system state is a snapshot of the system at a given time that contains enough information to predict the behavior of the system for all future times. The state of the system is described by the set of variables. The set of all possible states is the state space. The number n of independent variables is equal to the dimension of the state space. For $n = 2$, the two-dimensional state space can be called phase plane.

A particular solution of the ODE system $\dot{\boldsymbol{x}} = \boldsymbol{f}(\boldsymbol{x}, \boldsymbol{p}, t)$, determined from the general solution by specifying parameter values $\boldsymbol{p}$ and initial conditions $\boldsymbol{x}(t_0) = \boldsymbol{x}^0$, describes a path through the state space and is called trajectory.

Stationary states or steady states are points $\bar{\boldsymbol{x}}$ in the phase plane, where the condition $\dot{\boldsymbol{x}} = 0 (\dot{x}_1 = 0, \ldots, \dot{x}_n = 0)$ is met. At steady state, the system of n differential equations is represented by a system of n algebraic equations for n variables.

The equation system $\dot{x} = 0$ can have multiple solutions referring to multiple steady states. The change of number or stability of steady states upon changes of parameter values $\boldsymbol{p}$ is called a bifurcation.

Linear systems of ODEs have linear functions of the variables as right-hand sides, such as

$$\begin{aligned} \frac{dx_1}{dt} &= a_{11}x_1 + a_{12}x_2 + z_1 \\ \frac{dx_2}{dt} &= a_{21}x_1 + a_{22}x_2 + z_2 \end{aligned}, \tag{2.86}$$

or in general $\dot{\boldsymbol{x}} = \boldsymbol{A}\boldsymbol{x} + \boldsymbol{z}$. The matrix $\boldsymbol{A} = \{a_{ik}\}$ is the system matrix containing the system coefficients $a_{ik} = a_{ik}(\boldsymbol{p})$ and the vector $\boldsymbol{z} = (z_1, \ldots, Z_n)^{\mathrm{T}}$ contains inhomogeneities. The linear system is *homogeneous* if $\boldsymbol{z} = 0$ holds. Linear systems can be solved analytically. Although in real-world problems, the functions are usually nonlinear, linear systems are important as linear approximations in the investigation of steady states.

Example 2.8

The simple linear system

$$\frac{dx_1}{dt} = a_{12}x_2, \quad \frac{dx_2}{dt} = -x_1 \tag{2.87}$$

has the general solution

$$x_1 = \frac{1}{2}e^{-i\sqrt{a_{12}t}}\left(1 + e^{2i\sqrt{a_{12}t}}\right)C_1 - \frac{1}{2}ie^{-i\sqrt{a_{12}t}}\left(-1 + e^{2i\sqrt{a_{12}t}}\right)\sqrt{a_{12}}C_2$$

$$x_2 = \frac{i}{2\sqrt{a_{12}}}e^{-i\sqrt{a_{12}t}}\left(1 + e^{2i\sqrt{a_{12}t}}\right)C_1 + \frac{1}{2}e^{-i\sqrt{a_{12}t}}\left(1 + e^{2i\sqrt{a_{12}t}}\right)C_2$$

with the integration constants C_1 and C_2. Choosing $a_{12} = 1$ simplifies the system to $x_1 = C_1 \cos t + C_2 \sin t$ and $x_2 = C_2 \cos t - C_1 \sin t$. Specification of the initial conditions to $x_1(0) = 2$, $x_2(0) = 1$ gives the particular solution $x_1 = 2\cos t + \sin t$ and $x_2 = \cos t - 2\sin t$. The solution can be presented in the phase plane or directly as functions of time (Figure 2.8).

2.3.1.2 Linearization of Autonomous Systems

In order to investigate the behavior of a system close to steady state, it may be useful to linearize it. Considering the deviation $\hat{x}(t)$ from steady state with $\boldsymbol{x}(t) = \bar{\boldsymbol{x}} + \hat{\boldsymbol{x}}(t)$, it follows

$$\dot{\boldsymbol{x}} = \boldsymbol{f}(\bar{\boldsymbol{x}} + \hat{\boldsymbol{x}}(t)) = \frac{\mathrm{d}}{\mathrm{d}t}(\bar{\boldsymbol{x}} + \hat{\boldsymbol{x}}(t)) = \frac{\mathrm{d}}{\mathrm{d}t}\hat{\boldsymbol{x}}(t). \tag{2.88}$$

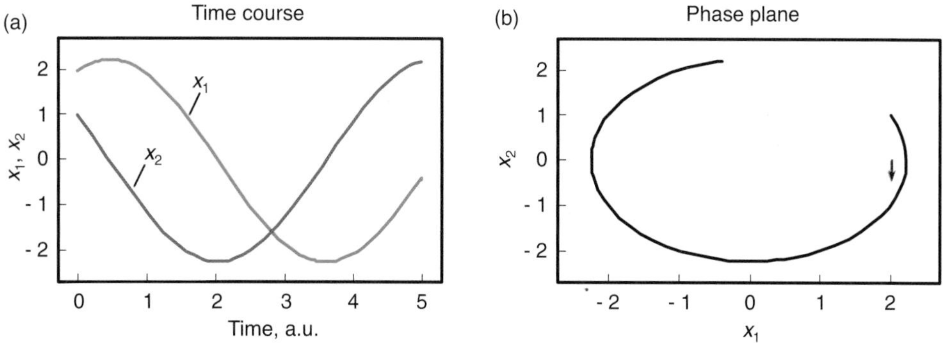

Figure 2.8 Phase plane and time course for the linear system of ODEs represented in Eq. (2.87). In time course panel: gray line $x_1(t)$, black line $x_2(t)$. Parameters: $a_{12} = 1$, $x_1(0) = 1$, $x_2(0) = 2$.

Taylor expansion of the temporal change of the deviation, $(\mathrm{d}/\mathrm{d}t)\hat{x}_i = f_i(\bar{x}_1 + \hat{x}_1, \ldots, \bar{x}_n + \hat{x}_n)$, gives

$$\frac{\mathrm{d}}{\mathrm{d}t}\hat{x}_i = f_i(\bar{x}_1, \ldots, \bar{x}_n) + \sum_{j=1}^{n} \frac{\partial f_i}{\partial x_j}\hat{x}_j + \frac{1}{2}\sum_{j=1}^{n}\sum_{k=1}^{n}\frac{\partial^2 f_i}{\partial x_j \partial x_k}\hat{x}_j\hat{x}_k + \cdots . \tag{2.89}$$

Since we consider steady state, it holds $f_i(\bar{x}_1, \ldots, \bar{x}_n) = 0$. Neglecting terms of higher order, we have

$$\frac{\mathrm{d}}{\mathrm{d}t}\hat{x}_i = \sum_{j=1}^{n}\frac{\partial f_i}{\partial x_j}\hat{x}_j = \sum_{j=1}^{n} a_{ij}\hat{x}_j. \tag{2.90}$$

The coefficients $a_{ij} = \partial f_i/\partial x_j$ are calculated at steady state and are constant. They form the so-called *Jacobian* matrix:

$$J = \{a_{ij}\} = \begin{pmatrix} \frac{\partial f_1}{\partial x_1} & \frac{\partial f_1}{\partial x_2} & \cdots & \frac{\partial f_1}{\partial x_n} \\ \frac{\partial f_2}{\partial x_1} & \frac{\partial f_2}{\partial x_2} & \cdots & \frac{\partial f_2}{\partial x_n} \\ \vdots & \vdots & \ddots & \vdots \\ \frac{\partial f_n}{\partial x_1} & \frac{\partial f_n}{\partial x_2} & \cdots & \frac{\partial f_n}{\partial x_n} \end{pmatrix}. \tag{2.91}$$

For linear systems, it holds $\boldsymbol{J} = \boldsymbol{A}$.

2.3.1.3 Solution of Linear ODE Systems

We are interested in two different types of problems: describing the temporal evolution of the system and finding its steady state. The problem of finding the steady state $\bar{\boldsymbol{x}}$ of a linear ODE system, $\dot{\boldsymbol{x}} = 0$, implies solution of $\boldsymbol{A}\bar{\boldsymbol{x}} + \boldsymbol{z} = \boldsymbol{0}$. The problem can be solved by inversion of the system matrix $\boldsymbol{A}$:

$$\bar{\boldsymbol{x}} = -\boldsymbol{A}^{-1}\boldsymbol{z}. \tag{2.92}$$

The time course solution of homogeneous linear ODEs is described in the following. The systems can be solved with an exponential function as ansatz. In the simplest case $n = 1$, we have

$$\frac{dx_1}{dt} = a_{11}x_1. \tag{2.93}$$

Introducing the ansatz $x_1(t) = b_1 e^{\lambda t}$ with constant b_1 into Eq. (2.93) yields $b_1 \lambda e^{\lambda t} = a_{11} b_1 e^{\lambda t}$, which is true, if $\lambda = a_{11}$. This leads to the general solution $x_1(t) = b_1 e^{a11t}$. To find a particular solution, we must specify the initial conditions $x_1(t=0) = x_1^{(0)} = b_1 e^{a_{11}t}|_{t=0} = b_1$. Thus, the solution is

$$x_1(t) = x_1^{(0)} e^{a_{11}t}. \tag{2.94}$$

For a linear homogeneous system of n differential equations, $\dot{\boldsymbol{x}} = \boldsymbol{A}\boldsymbol{x}$, the approach is $\boldsymbol{x} = \boldsymbol{b}e^{\lambda t}$. This gives $\dot{\boldsymbol{x}} = \boldsymbol{b}\lambda e^{\lambda t} = \boldsymbol{A}\boldsymbol{b}e^{\lambda t}$. The scalar factor $e^{\lambda t}$ can be cancelled out, leading to $\boldsymbol{b}\lambda = \boldsymbol{A}\boldsymbol{b}$ or the characteristic equation

$$(\boldsymbol{A} - \lambda \boldsymbol{I}_n)\boldsymbol{b} = 0. \tag{2.95}$$

For homogeneous linear ODE systems, the *superposition principle* holds: if $\boldsymbol{x}_1$ and $\boldsymbol{x}_2$ are solutions of this ODE system, then also their linear combination is a solution. This leads to the general solution of the homogeneous linear ODE system:

$$\boldsymbol{x}(t) = \sum_{i=1}^{n} c_i \boldsymbol{b}^{(i)} e^{\lambda_i t}, \tag{2.96}$$

where $\boldsymbol{b}^{(i)}$ is the eigenvectors of the system matrix $\boldsymbol{A}$ corresponding to the eigenvalues λ_i. A particular solution specifying the coefficients c_i can be found considering the initial conditions $\boldsymbol{x}(t=0) = \boldsymbol{x}^{(0)} = \sum_{j=1}^{n} c_i \boldsymbol{b}^{(i)}$. This constitutes an inhomogeneous linear equation system to be solved for c_i.

For the solution of inhomogeneous linear ODEs, the system $\dot{\boldsymbol{x}} = \boldsymbol{A}\boldsymbol{x} + \boldsymbol{z}$ can be transformed into a homogeneous system by the coordination transformation $\hat{\boldsymbol{x}} = \boldsymbol{x} - \bar{\boldsymbol{x}}$. Since $(d/dt)\bar{\boldsymbol{x}} = \boldsymbol{A}\bar{\boldsymbol{x}} + \boldsymbol{z} = 0$, it holds $(d/dt)\hat{\boldsymbol{x}} = \boldsymbol{A}\hat{\boldsymbol{x}}$. Therefore, we can use the solution algorithm for homogeneous systems for the transformed system.

2.3.1.4 Stability of Steady States

If a system is at steady state, it should stay there – until an external perturbation occurs. Depending on the system behavior after perturbation, steady states are either

- *stable* – the system returns to this state
- *unstable* – the system leaves this state
- *metastable* – the system behavior is indifferent

A steady state is *asymptotically* stable, if it is stable and solutions based on nearby initial conditions tend to this state for $t \to \infty$. *Local* stability describes the behavior after small perturbations, *global* stability after any perturbation.

To investigate, whether a steady state $\bar{\boldsymbol{x}}$ of the ODE system $\dot{\boldsymbol{x}} = \boldsymbol{f}(\boldsymbol{x})$ is asymptotically stable, we consider the linearized system $d\hat{\boldsymbol{x}}/dt = \boldsymbol{A}\hat{\boldsymbol{x}}$ with $\hat{\boldsymbol{x}}(t) = \boldsymbol{x}(t) - \bar{\boldsymbol{x}}$. The steady state $\bar{\boldsymbol{x}}$ is asymptotically stable, if the Jacobian $\boldsymbol{A}$ has n eigenvalues with strictly negative real parts each. The steady state is unstable, if at least one eigenvalue has a positive real part. This will now be explained in more detail for 1- and 2D systems.

We start with 1D systems, i.e., $n = 1$, and assume without loss of generality $\bar{x}_1 = 0$. The system $\dot{x}_1 = f_1(x_1)$ yields the linearized system $\dot{x}_1 = (\partial f_1/\partial x_1)|_{\bar{x}_1} x_1 = a_{11}x_1$. The Jacobian matrix $A = \{a_{11}\}$ has only one eigenvalue $\lambda_1 = a_{11}$. The solution is $x_1(t) = x_1^{(0)} e^{\lambda_1 t}$. It is obvious that $e^{\lambda 1t}$ increases for $\lambda_1 > 0$ and the system runs away from the steady state. For $\lambda_1 < 0$, the deviation from steady state decreases and $x_1(t) \to \bar{x}_1$ for $t \to \infty$. For $\lambda_1 = 0$, consideration of the linearized system allows no conclusion about stability of the original system because higher order terms in Eq. (2.89) play a role.

Consider the 2D case, $n = 2$. For the general (linear or nonlinear) system

$$\begin{aligned} \dot{x}_1 &= f_1(x_1, x_2) \\ \dot{x}_2 &= f_2(x_1, x_2) \end{aligned}, \tag{2.97}$$

we can compute the linearized system

$$\begin{aligned} \dot{x}_1 &= \left.\frac{\partial f_1}{\partial x_1}\right|_{\bar{x}} x_1 + \left.\frac{\partial f_1}{\partial x_2}\right|_{\bar{x}} x_2 \\ \dot{x}_2 &= \left.\frac{\partial f_2}{\partial x_1}\right|_{\bar{x}} x_1 + \left.\frac{\partial f_2}{\partial x_2}\right|_{\bar{x}} x_2 \end{aligned} \quad \text{or } \dot{\boldsymbol{x}} = \begin{pmatrix} \left.\frac{\partial f_1}{\partial x_1}\right|_{\bar{x}} & \left.\frac{\partial f_1}{\partial x_2}\right|_{\bar{x}} \\ \left.\frac{\partial f_2}{\partial x_1}\right|_{\bar{x}} & \left.\frac{\partial f_2}{\partial x_2}\right|_{\bar{x}} \end{pmatrix} \boldsymbol{x} = \begin{pmatrix} a_{11} & a_{12} \\ a_{21} & a_{22} \end{pmatrix} \boldsymbol{x} = \boldsymbol{A}\boldsymbol{x}. \tag{2.98}$$

To find the eigenvalues of $\boldsymbol{A}$, we have to solve the characteristic polynomial

$$\lambda^2 - \underbrace{(a_{11} + a_{22})}_{\text{Tr } \boldsymbol{A}} \lambda + \underbrace{a_{11}a_{22} - a_{12}a_{21}}_{\text{Det } \boldsymbol{A}} = 0, \tag{2.99}$$

with Tr $\boldsymbol{A}$ the trace and Det $\boldsymbol{A}$ the determinant of $\boldsymbol{A}$, and get

$$\lambda_{1/2} = \frac{\text{Tr } \boldsymbol{A}}{2} \pm \sqrt{\frac{(\text{Tr } \boldsymbol{A})^2}{4} - \text{Det } \boldsymbol{A}}. \tag{2.100}$$

The eigenvalues are either real for $(\text{Tr } \boldsymbol{A})^2/4 - \text{Det } \boldsymbol{A} \geq 0$ or complex (otherwise). For complex eigenvalues, the solution contains oscillatory parts.

For stability, it is necessary that Tr $\boldsymbol{A} < 0$ and Det $\boldsymbol{A} \geq 0$. Depending on the sign of the eigenvalues, steady states of a 2D system may have the following characteristics:

1. $\lambda_1 < 0$, $\lambda_2 < 0$, both real: stable node
2. $\lambda_1 > 0$, $\lambda_2 > 0$, both real: unstable node
3. $\lambda_1 > 0$, $\lambda_2 < 0$, both real: saddle point, unstable
4. $Re(\lambda_1) < 0$, $Re(\lambda_2) < 0$, both complex with negative real parts: stable focus
5. $Re(\lambda_1) > 0$, $Re(\lambda_2) > 0$, both complex with positive real parts: unstable focus
6. $Re(\lambda_1) = Re(\lambda_2) = 0$, both complex with zero real parts: center, unstable.

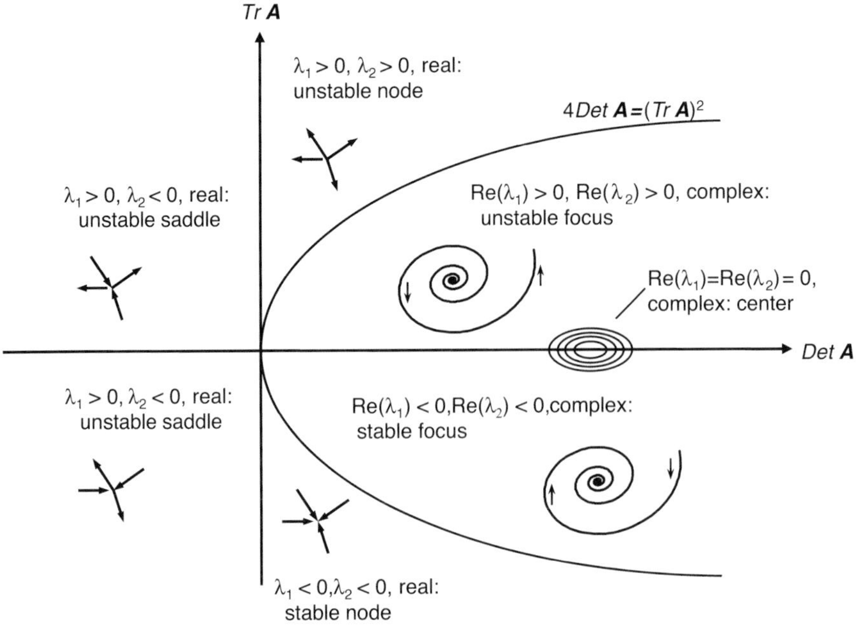

Figure 2.9 Stability of steady states in two-dimensional systems: the character of steady-state solutions is represented depending on the value of the determinant (x-axis) and the trace (y-axis) of the Jacobian matrix. Phase plane behavior of trajectories in the different cases is schematically represented.

Graphical representation of stability depending on trace and determinant is given in Figure 2.9.

Up to now, we considered only the linearized system. For the stability of the original system, the following holds. If the steady state of the linearized system is asymptotically stable, then the steady state of the complete system is also asymptotically stable. If the steady state of the linearized system is a saddle point, an unstable node or an unstable focus, then the steady state of the complete system is also unstable. This means that statements about the stability remain true, but the character of the steady state is not necessarily kept. For the center, no statement on the stability of the complete system is possible.

Routh–Hurwitz Theorem [31] For systems with $n > 2$ differential equations, we obtain the characteristic polynomial

$$c_n\lambda^n + c_{n-1}\lambda^{n-1} + \cdots + c_1\lambda + c_0 = 0. \tag{2.101}$$

This is a polynomial of degree n, which frequently cannot be solved analytically (at least for $n > 4$). We can use the Hurwitz criterion to test whether the real parts of all eigenvalues are negative. We have to form the Hurwitz matrix $\boldsymbol{H}$, containing the coefficients of the characteristic polynomial:

$$H=\begin{pmatrix} c_{n-1} & c_{n-3} & c_{n-5} & \cdots & 0 \\ c_n & c_{n-2} & c_{n-4} & \cdots & 0 \\ 0 & c_{n-1} & c_{n-3} & \cdots & 0 \\ 0 & c_n & c_{n-2} & \cdots & 0 \\ \vdots & \vdots & \vdots & \ddots & \vdots \\ 0 & 0 & 0 & \cdots & c_0 \end{pmatrix}=\{h_{ik}\} \text{ with } h_{ik}=\begin{cases} c_{n+i-2k}, & \text{if } 0\le 2k-i\le n \\ 0, \text{else} \end{cases}. \tag{2.102}$$

It has been shown that all solutions of the characteristic polynomial have negative real parts, if all coefficients c_i of the polynomial as well as all principal leading minors of $\boldsymbol{H}$ have positive values.

2.3.1.5 Global Stability of Steady States

A state is globally stable, if the trajectories for all initial conditions approach it for $t \to \infty$. The stability of a steady state of an ODE system can be tested with a method proposed by Lyapunov:

Shift the steady state into the point of origin by coordination transformation $\hat{\boldsymbol{x}} = \boldsymbol{x}-\bar{\boldsymbol{x}}$.

Find a function $V_L(x_1, \ldots, x_n)$, called Lyapunov function, with the following properties:

(1) $V_L(x_1, \ldots, x_n)$ has continuous derivatives with respect to all variables x_i.
(2) $V_L(x_1, \ldots, x_n)$ satisfies $V_L(x_1, \ldots, x_n) = 0$ for $x_i = 0$ and is positive definite elsewhere, i.e., $V_L(x_1, \ldots, x_n) > 0$ for $x_i \neq 0$.
(3) The time derivative of $V_L(\boldsymbol{x}(t))$ is given by

$$\frac{dV_L}{dt}=\sum_{i=1}^{n}\frac{\partial V_L}{\partial x_i}\frac{dx_i}{dt}=\sum_{i=1}^{n}\frac{\partial V_L}{\partial x_i}f_i(x_1,\ldots,x_n). \tag{2.103}$$

A steady state $\bar{\boldsymbol{x}} = 0$ is stable, if the time derivative of $V_L(\boldsymbol{x}(t))$ in a certain region around this state has no positive values. The steady state is asymptotically stable, if the time derivative of $V_L(\boldsymbol{x}(t))$ in this region is negative definite, i.e., $dV_L/dt = 0$ for $x_i = 0$ and $dV_L/dt < 0$ for $x_i \neq 0$.

Example 2.9

The system $\dot{x}_1 = -x_1$, $\dot{x}_2 = -x_2$ has the solution $x_1(t) = x_1^{(0)}e^{-t}$, $x_2(t) = x_2^{(0)}e^{-t}$ and the state $x_1 = x_2 = 0$ is asymptotically stable.

The global stability can also be shown using the positive definite function $V_L = x_1^2 + x_2^2$ as Lyapunov function. It holds $dV_L/dt = (\partial V_L/\partial x_1)\dot{x}_1 + (\partial V_L/\partial x_2)\dot{x}_2 = 2x_1(-x_1) + 2x_2(-x_2)$, which is negative definite.

2.3.1.6 Limit Cycles

Oscillatory behavior is a typical phenomenon in biology. The cause of the oscillation may be different either imposed by external influences or encoded by internal

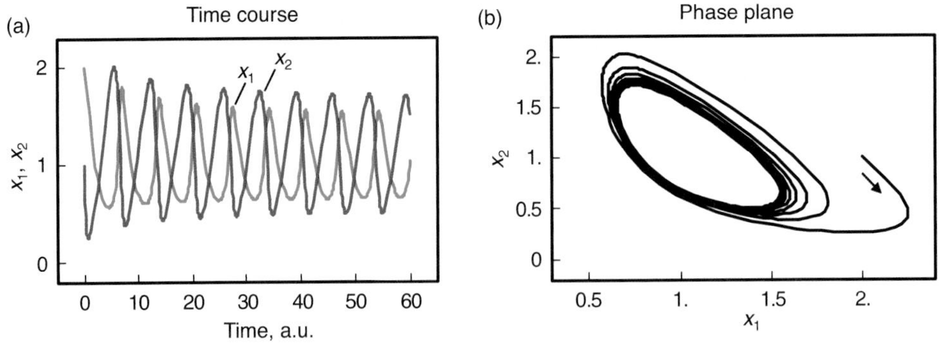

Figure 2.10 Solution of the Equation system in Example 2.10 represented as time course (left panel) and in phase plane (right panel). Initial conditions $x_1(0) = 2$, $x_2(0) = 1$.

structures and parameters. Internally caused stable oscillations can be found if we have a limit cycle in the phase space.

A *limit cycle* is an isolated closed trajectory. All trajectories in its vicinity are periodic solutions winding toward (stable limit cycle) or away from (unstable) the limit cycle for $t \to \infty$.

Example 2.10

The nonlinear system $\dot{x}_1 = x_1^2 x_2 - x_1$, $\dot{x}_2 = p - x_1^2 x_2$ has a steady state at $\bar{x}_1 = p$, $\bar{x}_2 = 1/p$. If we choose, e.g., $p = 0.98$, this steady state is unstable since $\text{Tr}\,\mathbf{A} = 1 - p^2 > 0$ (Figure 2.10).

For 2D systems, there are two criteria to check whether a limit cycle exists. Consider the system of differential equations

$$\begin{aligned} \dot{x}_1 &= f_1(x_1, x_2) \\ \dot{x}_2 &= f_2(x_1, x_2) \end{aligned} . \tag{2.104}$$

The *negative criterion of Bendixson* states: if the expression $\text{Tr}\,A = \partial f_1/\partial x_1 + \partial f_2/\partial x_2$ does not change its sign in a certain region of the phase plane, then there is no closed trajectory in this area. Hence, a necessary condition for the existence of a limit cycle is the change of the sign of Tr A.

Example 2.11

Example 2.10 holds $\text{Tr}\,A = (2x_1x_2 - 1) + (-x_1^2)$. Therefore, $\text{Tr}\,A = 0$ is fulfilled at $x_2 = (x_1^2 + 1)/(2x_1)$ and $\text{Tr}\,\mathbf{A}$ may assume positive or negative values for varying x_1, x_2, and the necessary condition for the existence of a limit cycle is met.

The criterion of Poincaré–Bendixson states: if a trajectory in the 2D phase plane remains within a finite region without approaching a singular point (a steady state), then this trajectory is either a limit cycle or it approaches a limit cycle. This criterion provides a sufficient condition for the existence of a limit cycle. Nevertheless, the limit cycle trajectory can be computed analytically only in very rare cases.

2.3.2 Metabolic Control Analysis

Metabolic control analysis (MCA) is a powerful quantitative and qualitative framework for studying the relationship between steady-state properties of a network of biochemical reaction and the properties of the individual reactions. It investigates the sensitivity of steady-state properties of the network to small parameter changes. MCA is a useful tool for theoretical and experimental analysis of control and regulation in cellular systems.

MCA was independently founded by two different groups in the 1970s [32, 33] and was further developed by many different groups upon the application to different metabolic systems. A milestone in its formalization was provided by Reder [20]. Originally intended for metabolic networks, MCA has nowadays found applications also for signaling pathways, gene expression models, and hierarchical networks [34–38].

Metabolic networks are very complex systems that are highly regulated and exhibit a lot of interactions such as feedback inhibition or common substrates such as ATP for different reactions. Many mechanisms and regulatory properties of isolated enzymatic reactions are known. The development of MCA was motivated by a series of questions like the following: Can one predict properties or behavior of metabolic networks from the knowledge about their parts, the isolated reactions? Which individual steps control a flux or a steady-state concentration? Is there a rate-limiting step? Which effectors or modifications have the most prominent effect on the reaction rate? In biotechnological production processes, it is of interest which enzyme(s) should be activated in order to increase the rate of synthesis of a desired metabolite. There are also related problems in health care. Concerning metabolic disorders involving overproduction of a metabolite, which reactions should be modified in order to down-regulate this metabolite while perturbing the rest of the metabolism as weakly as possible?

In metabolic networks, the steady-state variables, i.e., the fluxes and the metabolite concentrations, depend on the value of parameters such as enzyme concentrations, kinetic constants (like Michaelis constants and maximal activities), and other model-specific parameters. The relations between steady-state variables and kinetic parameters are usually nonlinear. Up to now, there is no general theory that predicts the effect of large parameter changes in a network. The approach presented here is, basically, restricted to small parameter changes. Mathematically, the system is linearized at steady state, which yields exact results, if the parameter changes are infinitesimally small.

In this section, we will first define a set of mathematical expressions that are useful to quantify control in biochemical reaction networks. Later we will show the relations between these functions and their application for prediction of reaction network behavior.

2.3.2.1 The Coefficients of Control Analysis

Biochemical reaction systems are networks of metabolites connected by chemical reactions. Their behavior is determined by the properties of their components – the individual reactions and their kinetics – as well as by the network structure – the involvement of compounds in different reaction or in brief: the stoichiometry. Hence, the effect of a perturbation exerted on a reaction in this network will depend on both – the local properties of this reaction and the embedding of this reaction in the global network.

Let $y(x)$ denotes a quantity that depends on another quantity x. The effect of the change Δx on y is expressed in terms of sensitivity coefficients:

$$c_x^y = \left(\frac{x}{y}\frac{\Delta y}{\Delta x}\right)_{\Delta x \to 0}. \tag{2.105}$$

In practical applications, Δx might be, e.g., identified with 1% change of x and Δy with the percentage change of y. The factor x/y is a normalization factor that makes the coefficient independent of units and of the magnitude of x and y. In the limiting case $\Delta x \to 0$, the coefficient defined in Eq. (2.105) can be written as

$$c_x^y = \frac{x}{y}\frac{\partial y}{\partial x} = \frac{\partial \ln y}{\partial \ln x}. \tag{2.106}$$

Both right-hand expressions are mathematically equivalent.

Two distinct types of coefficients, local and global coefficients, reflect the relations among local and global effects of changes. *Elasticity coefficients* are local coefficients pertaining to individual reactions. They can be calculated in any given state. *Control coefficients* and *response coefficients* are global quantities. They refer to a given steady state of the entire system. After a perturbation of x, the relaxation of y to new steady state is considered.

The general form of the coefficients in control analysis as defined in Eq. (2.106) contains the normalization x/y. The normalization has the advantage that we get rid of units and can compare, e.g., fluxes belonging to different branches of a network. The drawback of the normalization is that x/y is not defined as soon as $y = 0$, which may happen for certain parameter combinations. In those cases, it is favorable to work with nonnormalized coefficients. Throughout this chapter, we will consider usually normalized quantities. If we use nonnormalized coefficients, they are flagged as $\tilde{c}$. In general, the use of one or the other type of coefficient is also a matter of personal choice of the modeler.

Changes reflected by the different coefficients are illustrated in Figure 2.11.

2.3.2.2 The Elasticity Coefficients

An elasticity coefficient quantifies the sensitivity of a reaction rate to the change of a concentration or a parameter while all other arguments of the kinetic law are kept

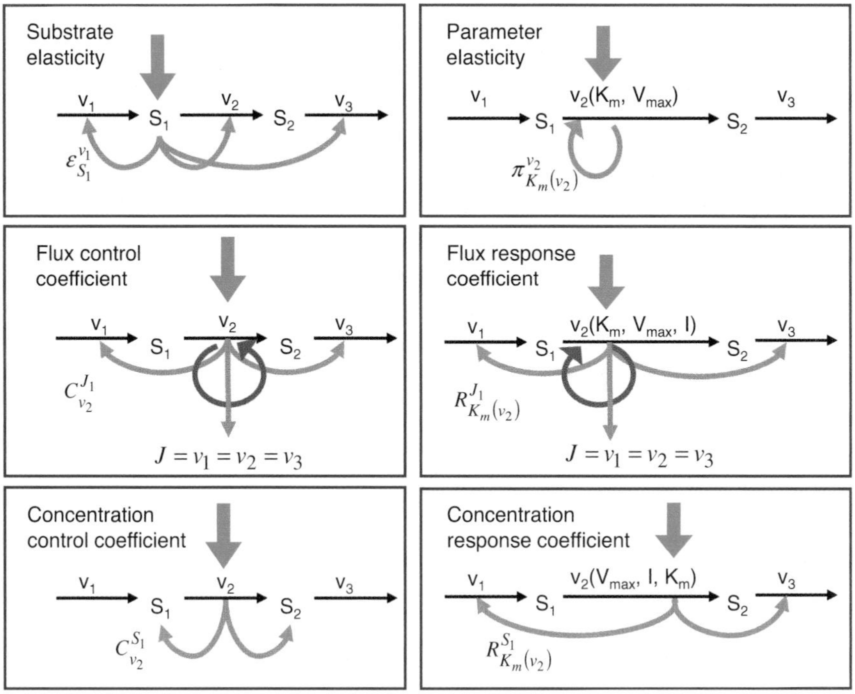

Figure 2.11 Schematic representation of perturbation and effects quantified by different coefficients of metabolic control analysis.

fixed. It measures the direct effect on the reaction velocity, while the rest of the network is not taken into consideration. The sensitivity of the rate v_k of a reaction to the change of the concentration S_i of a metabolite is calculated by the *ε-elasticity*:

$$\varepsilon_i^k = \frac{S_i}{v_k}\frac{\partial v_k}{\partial S_i}. \tag{2.107}$$

The *π-elasticity* is defined with respect to parameters p_m such as kinetic constants, concentrations of enzymes, or concentrations of external metabolites as follows:

$$\pi_m^k = \frac{p_m}{v_k}\frac{\partial v_k}{\partial p_m}. \tag{2.108}$$

Example 2.12

In Michaelis–Menten kinetics, the rate v of a reaction depends on the substrate concentration S in the form $v = V_{max}S/(K_m + S)$ (Eq. (2.22)). The sensitivity is given by the elasticity $\varepsilon_S^v = \partial \ln v / \partial \ln S$. Since the Michaelis–Menten equation defines a mathematical dependency of v on S, it is easy to calculate that

$$\varepsilon_S^v = \frac{S}{v}\frac{\partial}{\partial S}\left(\frac{V_{max}S}{K_m + S}\right) = \frac{S}{v}\frac{V_{max}(K_m + S) - V_{max}S}{(K_m + S)^2} = \frac{S}{K_m + S}. \quad (2.109)$$

The normalized ε-elasticity in the case of mass action kinetics can be calculated similarly and is always 1. Whenever the rate does not depend directly on a concentration (e.g., for a metabolite of a reaction system that is not involved in the considered reaction), the elasticity is zero.

Example 2.13

Typical values of elasticity coefficients will be explained for an isolated reaction transforming substrate S into product P. The reaction is catalyzed by enzyme E with the inhibitor I, and the activator A as depicted below

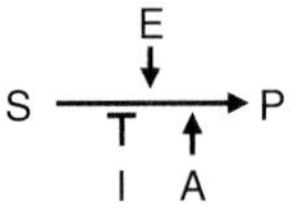

(2.110)

Usually, the elasticity coefficients for metabolite concentrations are in the following range:

$$\varepsilon_S^v = \frac{S}{v}\frac{\partial v}{\partial S} > 0 \quad \text{and} \quad \varepsilon_P^v = \frac{P}{v}\frac{\partial v}{\partial P} \leq 0. \quad (2.111)$$

In most cases, the rate increases with the concentration of the substrate (compare, e.g., Eq. (2.109)) and decreases with the concentration of the product. An exception from $\varepsilon_S^v > 0$ occurs in the case of substrate inhibition (Eq. (2.33)), where the elasticity will become negative for $S > S_{opt}$. The relation $\varepsilon_P^v = 0$ holds, if the reaction is irreversible or if the product concentration is kept zero by external mechanisms. The elasticity coefficients with respect to effectors I or A should obey

$$\varepsilon_A^v = \frac{A}{v}\frac{\partial v}{\partial A} > 0 \quad \text{and} \quad \varepsilon_I^v = \frac{I}{v}\frac{\partial v}{\partial I} < 0, \quad (2.112)$$

since this is essentially what the notions activator and inhibitor mean.

For the most kinetic laws, the reaction rate v is proportional to the enzyme concentration E. For example, E is a multiplicative factor in the mass action rate law as well as in the maximal rate of the Michaelis–Menten rate law. Therefore, it holds that

$$\varepsilon_E^v = \frac{\partial \ln v}{\partial \ln E} = 1. \quad (2.113)$$

More complicated interactions between enzymes and substrates such as metabolic channeling (direct transfer of the metabolite from one enzyme to the next without release to the medium) may lead to exceptions from this rule.

2.3.2.3 Control Coefficients

When defining control coefficients, we refer to a stable steady state of the metabolic system characterized by steady-state concentrations $\boldsymbol{S}^{st} = \boldsymbol{S}^{st}(\boldsymbol{p})$ and steady-state fluxes $\boldsymbol{J} = \boldsymbol{v}(\boldsymbol{S}^{st}(\boldsymbol{p}), \boldsymbol{p})$. Any sufficiently small perturbation of an individual reaction rate, $v_k \to v_k + \Delta v_k$, by a parameter change $p_k \to p_k + \Delta p_k$ drives the system to a new steady state in close proximity with $\boldsymbol{J} \to \boldsymbol{J} + \Delta \boldsymbol{J}$ and $\boldsymbol{S}^{st} \to \boldsymbol{S}^{st} + \Delta \boldsymbol{S}$. A measure for the change of fluxes and concentrations are the control coefficients.

The *flux control coefficient* for the control of rate v_k over flux J_j is defined as

$$C_k^j = \frac{v_k}{J_j} \frac{\partial J_j / \partial p_k}{\partial v_k / \partial p_k}. \tag{2.114}$$

The control coefficients quantify the control that a certain reaction v_k exerts on the steady-state flux J_j. It should be noted that the rate change, Δv_k, is caused by the change of a parameter p_k that has a direct effect solely on v_k. Thus, it holds

$$\frac{\partial v_k}{\partial p_k} \neq 0 \quad \text{and} \quad \frac{\partial v_l}{\partial p_k} = 0 \quad (l \neq k). \tag{2.115}$$

Such a parameter might be the enzyme concentration, a kinetic constant, or the concentration of a specific inhibitor or effector.

In a more compact form the flux control coefficients read

$$C_k^j = \frac{v_k}{J_j} \frac{\partial J_j}{\partial v_k}. \tag{2.116}$$

Equivalently, the *concentration control coefficient* of concentrations S_i^{st} with respect to v_k reads

$$C_k^i = \frac{v_k}{S_i^{st}} \frac{\partial S_i^{st}}{\partial v_k}. \tag{2.117}$$

2.3.2.4 Response Coefficients

The steady state is determined by the values of the parameters. A third type of coefficients expresses the direct dependence of steady-state variables on parameters. The response coefficients are defined as

$$R_m^j = \frac{p_m}{J_j} \frac{\partial J_j}{\partial p_m} \quad \text{and} \quad R_m^i = \frac{p_m}{S_i^{st}} \frac{\partial S_i^{st}}{\partial p_m}, \tag{2.118}$$

where the first coefficient expresses the response of the flux to a parameter perturbation, while the latter describes the response of a steady-state concentration.

2.3.2.5 Matrix Representation of the Coefficients

Control, response, and elasticity coefficients are defined with respect to all rates, steady-state concentrations, fluxes, or parameters in the metabolic system and in the respective model. They can be arranged in matrices:

$$\boldsymbol{C}^J = \{C_k^j\},\ \boldsymbol{C}^S = \{C_k^i\},\ \boldsymbol{R}^J = \{R_m^j\},\ \boldsymbol{R}^S = \{R_m^i\},\ \boldsymbol{\varepsilon} = \{\varepsilon_i^k\},\ \boldsymbol{\pi} = \{\pi_m^k\}. \tag{2.119}$$

Matrix representation can also be chosen for all types of nonnormalized coefficients. The arrangement in matrices allows us to apply matrix algebra in control analysis. In particular, the matrices of normalized control coefficients can be calculated from the matrices of nonnormalized control coefficient as follows:

$$\begin{array}{ll} \boldsymbol{C}^J = (\mathrm{dg}\boldsymbol{J})^{-1} \cdot \tilde{\boldsymbol{C}}^J \cdot \mathrm{dg}\boldsymbol{J} & \boldsymbol{C}^S = (\mathrm{dg}\boldsymbol{S}^{\mathrm{st}})^{-1} \cdot \tilde{\boldsymbol{C}}^J \cdot \mathrm{dg}\boldsymbol{J} \\ \boldsymbol{R}^J = (\mathrm{dg}\boldsymbol{J})^{-1} \cdot \tilde{\boldsymbol{R}}^J \cdot \mathrm{dg}\boldsymbol{p} & \boldsymbol{R}^S = (\mathrm{dg}\boldsymbol{S}^{\mathrm{st}})^{-1} \cdot \tilde{\boldsymbol{R}}^S \cdot \mathrm{dg}\boldsymbol{p} \cdot \\ \boldsymbol{\varepsilon} = (\mathrm{dg}\boldsymbol{v})^{-1} \cdot \tilde{\boldsymbol{\varepsilon}} \cdot \mathrm{dg}\boldsymbol{S}^{\mathrm{st}} & \boldsymbol{\pi} = (\mathrm{dg}\boldsymbol{v})^{-1} \cdot \tilde{\boldsymbol{\pi}} \cdot \mathrm{dg}\boldsymbol{p} \end{array} \tag{2.120}$$

The symbol "dg" stands for the diagonal matrix, e.g., for a system with three reaction holds

$$\mathrm{dg}\boldsymbol{J} = \begin{pmatrix} J_1 & 0 & 0 \\ 0 & J_2 & 0 \\ 0 & 0 & J_3 \end{pmatrix}.$$

2.3.2.6 The Theorems of Metabolic Control Theory

Let us assume that we are interested in calculating the control coefficients for a system under investigation. Usually, the steady-state fluxes or concentrations cannot be expressed explicitly as function of the reaction rates. Therefore, flux and concentration control coefficients cannot simply be determined by taking the respective derivatives, as we did for the elasticity coefficients in Example 2.12.

Fortunately, the work with control coefficients is eased by of a set of theorems. The first type of theorems, the *summation theorems,* makes a statement about the total control over a flux or a steady-state concentration. The second type of theorems, the *connectivity theorems,* relates the control coefficients to the elasticity coefficients. Both types of theorems together with network information encoded in the stoichiometric matrix contain enough information to calculate all control coefficients.

Here, we will first introduce the theorems. Then, we will present a hypothetical perturbation experiment (as introduced by Kacser and Burns) to illustrate the summation theorem. Finally, the theorems will be derived mathematically.

2.3.2.7 The Summation Theorems

The summation theorems make a statement about the total control over a certain steady-state flux or concentration. The flux control coefficients and concentration control coefficients fulfill, respectively,

$$\sum_{k=1}^{r} C_{v_k}^{J_j} = 1 \quad \text{and} \quad \sum_{k=1}^{r} C_{v_k}^{S_i} = 0, \tag{2.121}$$

for any flux J_j and any steady-state concentration S_i^{st}. The quantity r is the number of reactions. The flux control coefficients of a metabolic network for one steady-state flux sum up to one. This means that all enzymatic reactions can share the control over this flux. The control coefficients of a metabolic network for one steady-state concentration are balanced. This means again that the enzymatic reactions can share the control over this concentration, but some of them exert a negative control while others exert a positive control. Both relations can also be expressed in matrix formulation. We get

$$C^J \cdot \mathbf{1} = \mathbf{1} \quad \text{and} \quad C^S \cdot \mathbf{1} = \mathbf{0}. \tag{2.122}$$

The symbols $\mathbf{1}$ and $\mathbf{0}$ denote column vectors with r rows containing as entries only ones or zeros, respectively. The summation theorems for the nonnormalized control coefficients read

$$\tilde{C}^J \cdot K = K \quad \text{and} \quad \tilde{C}^S \cdot K = \mathbf{0}, \tag{2.123}$$

where K is the matrix satisfying $N \cdot K = \mathbf{0}$ (see Section 2.2). A more intuitive derivation of the summation theorems is given in the following example according to Kacser and Burns [33].

Example 2.14

The summation theorem for flux control coefficients can be derived using a thought experiment.

Consider the following unbranched pathway with fixed concentrations of the external metabolites, S_0 and S_3:

$$S_0 \overset{v_1}{\leftrightarrow} S_1 \overset{v_2}{\leftrightarrow} S_2 \overset{v_3}{\leftrightarrow} S_3 \tag{2.124}$$

What happens to steady-state fluxes and metabolite concentrations, if we perform an experimental manipulation of all three reactions leading to the same fractional change α of all three rates?

$$\frac{\delta v_1}{v_1} = \frac{\delta v_2}{v_2} = \frac{\delta v_3}{v_3} = \alpha. \tag{2.125}$$

The flux must increase to the same extent, $\delta J/J = \alpha$, but, since rates of producing and degrading reactions increase to the same amount, the concentrations of the metabolites remain constant $\delta S_1/S_1 = \delta S_2/S_2 = 0$.

The combined effect of all changes in local rates on the system variables S_1^{st}, S_2^{st}, and J can be written as the sum of all individual effects caused by the local rate changes. For the flux holds

$$\frac{\delta J}{J} = C_1^J \frac{\delta v_1}{v_1} + C_2^J \frac{\delta v_2}{v_2} + C_3^J \frac{\delta v_3}{v_3}. \tag{2.126}$$

It follows

$$\alpha = \alpha(C_1^J + C_2^J + C_3^J) \quad \text{or} \quad 1 = C_1^J + C_2^J + C_3^J. \tag{2.127}$$

This is just a special case of Eq. (2.121). In the same way, for the change of concentration S_1^{st}, we obtain

$$\frac{\delta S_1^{st}}{S_1^{st}} = C_1^{S_1} \frac{\delta v_1}{v_1} + C_2^{S_1} \frac{\delta v_2}{v_2} + C_3^{S_1} \frac{\delta v_3}{v_3}. \tag{2.128}$$

Finally, we get

$$0 = C_1^{S_1} + C_2^{S_1} + C_3^{S_1} \quad \text{as well as} \quad 0 = C_1^{S_2} + C_2^{S_2} + C_3^{S_2}. \tag{2.129}$$

Although shown here only for a special case, these properties hold in general for systems without conservation relations. The general derivation is given in Section 2.3.2.9.

2.3.2.8 The Connectivity Theorems

Flux control coefficients and elasticity coefficients are related by the expression

$$\sum_{k=1}^{r} C_{v_k}^{J_j} \varepsilon_{S_i}^{v_k} = 0. \tag{2.130}$$

Note that the sum runs over all rates v_k for any flux J_j. Considering the concentration S_i of a specific metabolite and a certain flux J_j, each term contains the elasticity $\varepsilon_{S_i}^{v_k}$ describing the direct influence of a change of S_i on the rates v_k and the control coefficient expressing the control of v_k over J_j.

The connectivity theorem between concentration control coefficients and elasticity coefficients reads

$$\sum_{k=1}^{r} C_{v_k}^{S_h} \varepsilon_{S_i}^{v_k} = -\delta_{hi}. \tag{2.131}$$

Again, the sum runs over all rates v_k, while S_h and S_i are the concentrations of two fixed metabolites. The symbol $\delta_{hi} = \begin{cases} 0, & \text{if} \quad h \neq i \\ 1, & \text{if} \quad h = i \end{cases}$ is the so-called Kronecker symbol.

In matrix formulation, the connectivity theorems read

$$\boldsymbol{C}^J \cdot \boldsymbol{\varepsilon} = \boldsymbol{0} \quad \text{and} \quad \boldsymbol{C}^S \cdot \boldsymbol{\varepsilon} = -\boldsymbol{I}, \tag{2.132}$$

where $\boldsymbol{I}$ denotes the identity matrix of size $n \times n$. For nonnormalized coefficients, it holds

$$\tilde{\boldsymbol{C}}^J \cdot \tilde{\boldsymbol{\varepsilon}} \cdot \boldsymbol{L} = 0 \quad \text{and} \quad \tilde{\boldsymbol{C}}^S \cdot \tilde{\boldsymbol{\varepsilon}} \cdot \boldsymbol{L} = -\boldsymbol{L}, \tag{2.133}$$

where $\boldsymbol{L}$ is the link matrix that expresses the relation between independent and dependent rows in the stoichiometric matrix (Eq. (2.75)) A comprehensive representation of both summation and connectivity theorems for nonnormalized coefficients is given by the following equation:

$$\begin{pmatrix} \tilde{\boldsymbol{C}}^J \\ \tilde{\boldsymbol{C}}^S \end{pmatrix} \cdot \begin{pmatrix} \boldsymbol{K} & \tilde{\boldsymbol{\varepsilon}}\boldsymbol{L} \end{pmatrix} = \begin{pmatrix} \boldsymbol{K} & 0 \\ 0 & -\boldsymbol{L} \end{pmatrix}. \tag{2.134}$$

The summation and connectivity theorem together with the structural information of the stoichiometric matrix are sufficient to calculate the control coefficients for a metabolic network. This shall be illustrated for a small network in the next example.

Example 2.15

To calculate the control coefficients, we study the following reaction system:

$$P_0 \overset{v_1}{\leftrightarrow} S \overset{v_2}{\leftrightarrow} P_2 \tag{2.135}$$

The flux control coefficients obey the theorems

$$C_1^J + C_2^J = 1 \quad \text{and} \quad C_1^J \varepsilon_S^1 + C_2^J \varepsilon_S^2 = 0, \tag{2.136}$$

which can be solved for the control coefficients to yield

$$C_1^J = \frac{\varepsilon_S^2}{\varepsilon_S^2 - \varepsilon_S^1} \quad \text{and} \quad C_2^J = \frac{-\varepsilon_S^1}{\varepsilon_S^2 - \varepsilon_S^1}. \tag{2.137}$$

Since usually $\varepsilon_S^1 < 0$ and $\varepsilon_S^2 > 0$ (see Example 2.13), both control coefficients assume positive values $C_1^J > 0$ and $C_2^J > 0$. This means that both reactions exert a positive control over the steady-state flux, and acceleration of any of them leads to increase of J, which is in accordance with common intuition.

The concentration control coefficients fulfil

$$C_1^S + C_2^S = 0 \quad \text{and} \quad C_1^S \varepsilon_S^1 + C_2^S \varepsilon_S^2 = -1, \tag{2.138}$$

which yields

$$C_1^S = \frac{1}{\varepsilon_S^2 - \varepsilon_S^1} \quad \text{and} \quad C_2^S = \frac{-1}{\varepsilon_S^2 - \varepsilon_S^1}. \tag{2.139}$$

With $\varepsilon_S^1 < 0$ and $\varepsilon_S^2 > 0$, we get $C_1^S > 0$ and $C_2^S < 0$, i.e., increase of the first reaction causes a raise in the steady-state concentration of S while acceleration of the second reaction leads to the opposite effect.

2.3.2.9 Derivation of Matrix Expressions for Control Coefficients

After having introduced the theorems of MCA, we will derive expressions for the control coefficients in matrix form. These expressions are suited for calculating the coefficients even for large-scale models. We start from the steady-state condition

$$\boldsymbol{N}\boldsymbol{v}(\boldsymbol{S}^{\mathrm{st}}(\boldsymbol{p}), \boldsymbol{p}) = \boldsymbol{0}. \tag{2.140}$$

Implicit differentiation with respect to the parameter vector $\boldsymbol{p}$ yields

$$\boldsymbol{N}\frac{\partial \boldsymbol{v}}{\partial \boldsymbol{S}}\frac{\partial \boldsymbol{S}^{\mathrm{st}}}{\partial \boldsymbol{p}} + \boldsymbol{N}\frac{\partial \boldsymbol{v}}{\partial \boldsymbol{p}} = \boldsymbol{0}. \tag{2.141}$$

Since we have chosen reaction-specific parameters for perturbation, the matrix of nonnormalized parameter elasticities contains nonzero entries in the main diagonal and zeros elsewhere (compare Eq. (2.115)).

$$\frac{\partial \boldsymbol{v}}{\partial \boldsymbol{p}} = \begin{pmatrix} \frac{\partial v_1}{\partial p_1} & 0 & & 0 \\ 0 & \frac{\partial v_2}{\partial p_2} & & 0 \\ & & \cdots & \\ 0 & 0 & & \frac{\partial v_r}{\partial p_r} \end{pmatrix}. \tag{2.142}$$

Therefore, this matrix is regular and has an inverse. Furthermore, we consider the Jacobian matrix

$$\boldsymbol{M} = \boldsymbol{N}\frac{\partial \boldsymbol{v}}{\partial \boldsymbol{S}} = \boldsymbol{N}\tilde{\boldsymbol{\varepsilon}}. \tag{2.143}$$

The Jacobian $\boldsymbol{M}$ is a regular matrix if the system is asymptotically stable and contains no conservation relations. The case with conservation relations is considered below. Here, we may premultiply Eq. (2.141) by the inverse of $\boldsymbol{M}$ and rearrange to get

$$\frac{\partial \boldsymbol{S}^{\text{st}}}{\partial \boldsymbol{p}} = -\left(\boldsymbol{N}\frac{\partial \boldsymbol{v}}{\partial \boldsymbol{S}}\right)^{-1}\boldsymbol{N}\frac{\partial \boldsymbol{v}}{\partial \boldsymbol{p}} = -\boldsymbol{M}^{-1}\boldsymbol{N}\frac{\partial \boldsymbol{v}}{\partial \boldsymbol{p}} \equiv \tilde{\boldsymbol{R}}^{S}. \tag{2.144}$$

As indicated, $\partial \boldsymbol{S}^{\text{st}}/\partial \boldsymbol{p}$ is the matrix of nonnormalized response coefficients for concentrations. Postmultiplication by the inverse of the nonnormalized parameter elasticity matrix gives

$$\frac{\partial \boldsymbol{S}^{\text{st}}}{\partial \boldsymbol{p}}\left(\frac{\partial \boldsymbol{v}}{\partial \boldsymbol{p}}\right)^{-1} = -\left(\boldsymbol{N}\frac{\partial \boldsymbol{v}}{\partial \boldsymbol{S}}\right)^{-1}\boldsymbol{N} = \tilde{\boldsymbol{C}}^{S}. \tag{2.145}$$

This is the matrix of nonnormalized concentration control coefficients. The right (middle) site contains no parameters. This means, that the control coefficients do not depend on the particular choice of parameters to exert the perturbation as long as Eq. (2.115) is fulfilled. The control coefficients are only dependent on the structure of the network represented by the stoichiometric matrix $\boldsymbol{N}$, and on the kinetics of the individual reactions, represented by the nonnormalized elasticity matrix $\tilde{\boldsymbol{\varepsilon}} = \partial \boldsymbol{v}/\partial \boldsymbol{S}$.

The implicit differentiation of

$$\boldsymbol{J} = \boldsymbol{v}(\boldsymbol{S}^{\text{st}}(\boldsymbol{p}), \boldsymbol{p}), \tag{2.146}$$

with respect to the parameter vector $\boldsymbol{p}$ leads to

$$\frac{\partial \boldsymbol{J}}{\partial \boldsymbol{p}} = \frac{\partial \boldsymbol{v}}{\partial \boldsymbol{p}} + \frac{\partial \boldsymbol{v}}{\partial \boldsymbol{S}}\frac{\partial \boldsymbol{S}^{\text{st}}}{\partial \boldsymbol{p}} = \left(\boldsymbol{I} - \frac{\partial \boldsymbol{v}}{\partial \boldsymbol{S}}\left(\boldsymbol{N}\frac{\partial \boldsymbol{v}}{\partial \boldsymbol{S}}\right)^{-1}\boldsymbol{N}\right)\frac{\partial \boldsymbol{v}}{\partial \boldsymbol{p}} \equiv \tilde{\boldsymbol{R}}^{J}. \tag{2.147}$$

This yields, after some rearrangement, an expression for the nonnormalized flux control coefficients:

$$\frac{\partial \boldsymbol{J}}{\partial \boldsymbol{p}}\left(\frac{\partial \boldsymbol{v}}{\partial \boldsymbol{p}}\right)^{-1} = \boldsymbol{I} - \frac{\partial \boldsymbol{v}}{\partial \boldsymbol{S}}\left(\boldsymbol{N}\frac{\partial \boldsymbol{v}}{\partial \boldsymbol{S}}\right)^{-1}\boldsymbol{N} = \tilde{\boldsymbol{C}}^{J}. \tag{2.148}$$

The normalized control coefficients are (by use of Eq. (2.120))

$$C^J = I - (\mathrm{dg}J)^{-1}\left(\frac{\partial v}{\partial S}\left(N\frac{\partial v}{\partial S}\right)^{-1}N\right)(\mathrm{dg}J) \quad \text{and}$$
$$C^S = -(\mathrm{dg}S^{\mathrm{st}})^{-1}\left(\left(N\frac{\partial v}{\partial S}\right)^{-1}N\right)(\mathrm{dg}J). \tag{2.149}$$

These equations can easily be implemented for numerical calculation of control coefficients or used for analytical computation. They are also suited for derivation of the theorems of MCA. The summation theorems for the control coefficients follow from Eq. (2.149) by postmultiplication with the vector $\mathbf{1}$ (the row vector containing only 1s), and consideration of the relations $(\mathrm{dg}J)\cdot\mathbf{1} = J$ and $NJ = \mathbf{0}$. The connectivity theorems result from postmultiplication of Eq. (2.149) with the elasticity matrix $\varepsilon = (\mathrm{dg}J)^{-1}\cdot(\partial v/\partial S)\cdot \mathrm{dg}S^{\mathrm{st}}$, and using that multiplication of a matrix with its inverse yields the identity matrix I of respective type.

If the reaction system involves conservation relations, we eliminate dependent variables as explained in Section 1.2.4. In this case, the nonnormalized coefficients read

$$\tilde{C}^J = I - \frac{\partial v}{\partial S}L\left(N_R\frac{\partial v}{\partial S}\right)^{-1}N_R \quad \text{and} \quad \tilde{C}^S = -L\left(N_R\frac{\partial v}{\partial S}\right)^{-1}N_R \tag{2.150}$$

and the normalized control coefficients are obtained by applying Eq. (2.120).

An example for calculation of flux control coefficients can be found in the web material.

To investigate the implications of control distribution, we will now analyze the control pattern in an unbranched pathway:

$$\mathrm{S}_0 \xrightarrow{v_1} \mathrm{S}_1 \xrightarrow{v_2} \mathrm{S}_2 \cdots \mathrm{S}_{r-1} \overset{v_r}{\leftrightarrow} \mathrm{S}_r \tag{2.151}$$

with linear kinetics $v_i = k_i S_{i-1} - k_{-i} S_i$, the equilibrium constants $q_i = k_i/k_{-i}$ and fixed concentrations of the external metabolites, S_0 and S_r. In this case, one can calculate an analytical expression for the steady-state flux,

$$J = \frac{S_0 \prod_{j=1}^{r} q_j - S_r}{\sum_{l=1}^{r} \frac{1}{k_l} \prod_{m=l}^{r} q_m} \tag{2.152}$$

as well as an analytical expression for the flux control coefficients

$$C_i^J = \left(\frac{1}{k_i}\prod_{j=i}^{r} q_j\right)\cdot\left(\sum_{l=1}^{r}\frac{1}{k_l}\prod_{m=l}^{r} q_m\right)^{-1}. \tag{2.153}$$

Let us consider two very general cases. First assume that all reactions have the same individual kinetics, $k_i = k_+$, $k_{-i} = k_-$ for $i = 1, \ldots, r$ and that the equilibrium constants, which are also equal, satisfy $q = k_+/k_- > 1$. In this case, the ratio of two subsequent flux control coefficients is

$$\frac{C_i^J}{C_{i+1}^J} = \frac{k_{i+1}}{k_i} q_i = q > 1. \tag{2.154}$$

Hence, the control coefficients of the preceding reactions are larger than the control coefficients of the succeeding reactions and flux control coefficients are higher in the beginning of a chain than in the end. This is in agreement with the frequent observation that flux control is strongest in the upper part of an unbranched reaction pathway.

Now assume that the individual rate constants might be different, but that all equilibrium constants are equal to one, $q_i = 1$ for $i = 1, \ldots, r$. This implies $k_i = k_{-i}$. Equation (2.153) simplifies to

$$C_i^J = \frac{1}{k_i} \cdot \left(\sum_{l=1}^{r} \frac{1}{k_l} \right)^{-1}. \tag{2.155}$$

Consider now the relaxation time $\tau_i = 1/(k_i + k_{-i})$ (see Section 4.3) as a measure for the rate of an enzyme. The flux control coefficient reads

$$C_i^J = \frac{\tau_i}{\tau_1 + \tau_2 + \cdots + \tau_r}. \tag{2.156}$$

This expression helps to elucidate two aspects of metabolic control. First, all enzymes participate in the control since all enzymes have a positive relaxation time. There is no enzyme that has all control, i.e., determines the flux through the pathway alone. Second, slow enzymes with a higher relaxation time exert in general more control than fast enzymes with a short relaxation time.

The predictive power of flux control coefficients for directed changes of flux is illustrated in the following example.

Example 2.16

Assume that we can manipulate the pathway shown in Figure 2.12 by changing the enzyme concentration in a predefined way. We would like to explore the effect of the perturbation of the individual enzymes. For a linear pathway (see Eqs. (2.151)–(2.153)) consisting of four consecutive reactions, we calculate the flux control coefficients. For $i = 1, \ldots, 4$, it shall hold that (i) all enzyme concentrations $E_i = 1$, (ii) the rate constants be $k_i = 2$, $k_{-i} = 1$, and (iii) the concentrations of the external reactants be $S_0 = S_4 = 1$. The resulting flux is $J = 1$ and the flux control coefficients are $\mathbf{C}^J = (0.533 \quad 0.267 \quad 0.133 \quad 0.067)^T$ according to Eq. (2.149).

If we now perturb slightly the first enzyme, lets say perform a percentage change of its concentration, i.e., $E_1 \to E_1 + 1\%$, then Eq. (2.105) implies that the flux increases as $J \to J + C_1^J \cdot 1\%$. In fact, the flux in the new steady state is $J^{E_1 \to 1.01 \cdot E_1} = 1.00531$. Increasing E_2, E_3, or E_4 by 1% leads to flux values of 1.00265, 1.00132, and 1.00066, respectively. A strong perturbation would not yield similar effects. This is illustrated in Figure 2.12.

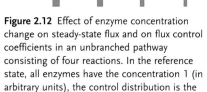

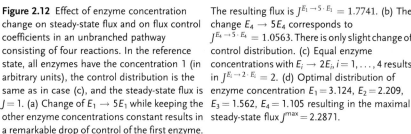

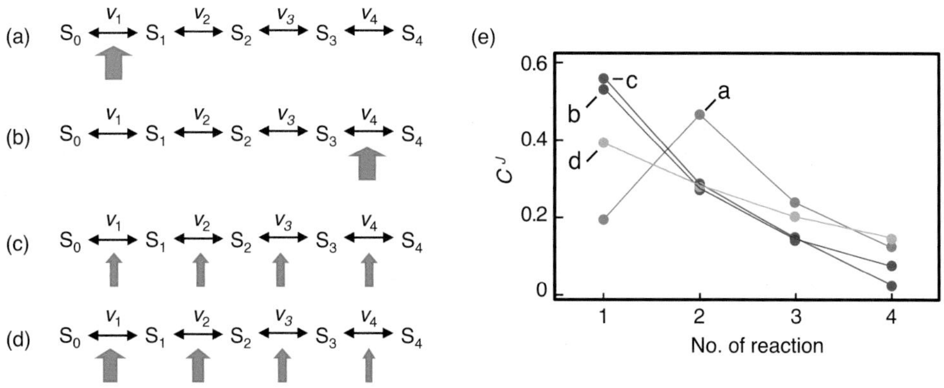

Figure 2.12 Effect of enzyme concentration change on steady-state flux and on flux control coefficients in an unbranched pathway consisting of four reactions. In the reference state, all enzymes have the concentration 1 (in arbitrary units), the control distribution is the same as in case (c), and the steady-state flux is $J = 1$. (a) Change of $E_1 \rightarrow 5E_1$ while keeping the other enzyme concentrations constant results in a remarkable drop of control of the first enzyme. The resulting flux is $J^{E_1 \rightarrow 5 \cdot E_1} = 1.7741$. (b) The change $E_4 \rightarrow 5E_4$ corresponds to $J^{E_4 \rightarrow 5 \cdot E_4} = 1.0563$. There is only slight change of control distribution. (c) Equal enzyme concentrations with $E_i \rightarrow 2E_i, i = 1, \ldots, 4$ results in $J^{E_i \rightarrow 2 \cdot E_i} = 2$. (d) Optimal distribution of enzyme concentration $E_1 = 3.124$, $E_2 = 2.209$, $E_3 = 1.562$, $E_4 = 1.105$ resulting in the maximal steady-state flux $J^{max} = 2.2871$.

2.4 Tools and Data Formats for Modeling

Summary

This section gives an overview about different simulation techniques and introduces tools, resources, and standard formats used in systems biology. Modeling and simulation functionalities of the tools are presented and common data formats used by these tools and in general in systems biology are introduced. Furthermore, model databases and databases of cellular and biochemical reaction networks are discussed.

The development of models of biological and in particular cellular systems starts by the collection of the model components and its interactions. Usually, in the first step, one formulates the biochemical reaction equations that define the topological structure of the reaction network and the reaction stoichiometries. For this purpose, it is often also useful to draw a diagram that illustrates the network structure either of the whole model or of a particular part. Once the reaction network and its stoichiometry are defined, a more detailed mathematical model can be constructed. For this purpose, often systems of ODEs are applied. Usually, this requires very detailed information about the kinetics of the individual reactions or appropriate assumptions have to be made.

In this section, databases are presented that provide information on the network structure of cellular processes such as metabolic pathways and signal transduction pathways. Moreover, data formats used for the structural, mathematical, and graphical description of biochemical reaction networks are introduced. We will start this section with an overview of simulation techniques and of software tools that support the user by the development of models.

2.4.1 Simulation Techniques

In systems biology, different simulation techniques are used such as systems of ODEs, stochastic methods, Petri nets, π-calculus, PDEs, cellular automata (CA) methods, agent-based systems, and hybrid approaches. The use of ODEs in biological modeling is widespread and by far the most common simulation approach in computational systems biology [39, 40]. The description of a biological model by a system of ODEs has already been discussed in the earlier sections. Some ODEs are simple enough to be solved analytically and have an exact solution. More complex ODE systems, as they are occurring in most systems biology simulations, must be solved numerically by appropriate algorithms. A first method for the numerical solution of ODEs was derived by Newton and Gauss. Methods that provide more improved computational accuracy are, for instance, Runge–Kutta algorithms and implicit methods that can also handle so-called stiff differential equations. Simulation tools for systems biology have to cope with systems of multiple reactants and multiple reactions. For the numerical integration of such complex ODE systems, they usually make use of more advanced programs such as LSODA [41, 42], CVODE [43], or LIMEX [44]. In the following, Petri nets and CA are described in more detail.

2.4.1.1 Petri Nets

An alternative to ODEs for the simulation of time-dependent processes are Petri nets. A Petri net is a graphical and mathematical modeling tool for discrete and parallel systems. The mathematical concept was developed in the early 1960s by Carl Adam Petri. The basic elements of a Petri net are places, transitions and arcs that connect places and transitions. When represented graphically, places are shown as circles and transitions as rectangles. Places represent objects (e.g., molecules, cars, and machine parts) and transitions describe if and how individual objects are interconverted. Places can contain zero or more tokens, indicating the number of objects that currently exist. If a transition can take place (can fire) or not depends on the places that are connected to the transition by incoming arcs, to contain enough tokens. If this condition is fulfilled, the transition fires and changes the state of the system by removing tokens from the input places and adding tokens to the output places. The number of tokens that are removed and added depends on the weights of the arcs.

Petri nets are not only an optically pleasing representation of a system but can also be described mathematically in terms of integer arithmetic. For simple types of Petri nets, certain properties can thus be calculated analytically, but often the net has to be run to study the long-term system properties. Over the years many, extensions to the basic Petri net model have been developed for the different simulation purposes [45].

1. Hybrid Petri nets that add the possibility to have places that contain a continuous token number instead of discrete values.
2. Timed Petri nets extend transitions to allow for a specific time delay between the moment when a transition is enabled and the actual firing.
3. Stochastic Petri nets that go one step further and allow a random time delay drawn from a probability distribution.
4. Hierarchical Petri nets, in which modularity is introduced by representing whole nets as a single place or transition of a larger net.
5. Colored Petri nets that introduce different types (colors) or tokens and more complicated firing rules for transitions.

With these extensions, Petri nets are powerful enough to be used for models in systems biology. Biochemical pathways can be modeled with places representing metabolites, transitions representing reactions and stoichiometric coefficients are encoded as different weights of input and output arcs. Consequently, Petri nets have been used to model metabolic networks [46, 47] and signal transduction pathways [48]. Many free and commercial tools are available to explore the behavior of Petri nets. The *Petri Nets World* webpage (http://www.informatik.uni-hamburg.de/TGI/PetriNets/) is an excellent starting point for this purpose.

2.4.1.2 **Cellular Automata**

Cellular Automata (CA) are tools for the simulation of temporal or spatiotemporal processes using discrete time and/or spatial steps (see Section 3.4.1.3). A cellular automaton consists of a regular grid or lattice of nearly identical components, called cells, where each cell has a certain state of a finite number of states. The states of the cells evolve synchronously in discrete time steps according to a set of rules. Each particular state of cell is determined by the previous states of its neighbors. CA were invented in the late 1940s by von Neumann and Ulam. A well-known CA simulation is Conway's Game of Life [49].

2.4.2 Simulation Tools

In the following, three different simulation tools are presented that essentially make use of ODE systems for simulation, and come along with further functionalities important for modeling, such as graphical visualization of the reaction network, advanced analysis techniques, and interfaces to external model and pathway databases. Further modeling and simulation tools are presented in Chapter 17. Modeling and simulations tools have also been reviewed by Alves *et al.* [50], Klipp *et al.* [51], Materi and Wishart [52], and Wierling *et al.* [53].

Modeling systems have to accomplish several requirements. They must have a well-defined internal structure for the representation of model components and reactions, and optionally functionalities for the storage of a model in a well-defined structure, standardized format, or database. Further desired aspects are a user-friendly interface for model development, a graphical representation of reaction networks, a detailed description of the mathematical model, integrated simulation engines, e.g., for deterministic or stochastic simulation, along with graphical representations of those simulation results, and functionalities for model analysis and model refinement. This is a very broad spectrum of functionalities. Existing tools cover different aspects of these functionalities. In the following, systems biology tools will be introduced that already accomplish several of the desired aspects. CellDesigner is one of those widely used in the systems biology community [51]. It has a user-friendly process diagram editor, uses the Systems Biology Markup Language (SBML; see Section 2.4.3.1) for model representation and exchange, and provides fundamental simulation and modeling functions. Another program with similar functionalities is COPASI. COPASI has an interface for the model definition and representation and provides several methods for simulation, model analysis, and refinement such as parameter scanning, MCA, optimization, or parameter estimation. Similarly, also PyBioS has rich functionalities for model design, simulation, and analysis. In contrast to the stand-alone programs CellDesigner and Copasi, PyBioS is a web application. A particular feature of PyBioS is its interfaces to pathway databases, like Reactome or KEGG, which can directly be used for model generation.

2.4.2.1 **CellDesigner**

CellDesigner provides an advanced graphical model representation along with an easy to use user-interface and an integrated simulation engine [54]. The current version of CellDesigner is 4.0.1. The process diagram editor of CellDesigner supports a rich set of graphical elements for the description of biochemical and gene-regulatory networks. Networks can be constructed from compartments, species, and reactions. CellDesigner comes with a large number of predefined shapes that can be used for different types of molecules, such as proteins, receptors, ion channels, small metabolites, etc. It is also possible to modify the symbols to indicate phosphorylations or other modifications. The program also provides several icons for special reaction types like catalysis, transport, inhibition, and activation. For version 4.0, it is announced that the graphical elements are compliant with the Systems Biology Graphical Notation (SBGN; see Section 2.4.3.3).

Reading and writing of the models is SBML-based (see Section 2.4.3.1 for more details on SBML) and the models written by CellDesigner pass the online validation at http://sbml.org/tools/htdocs/sbmltools.php and thus are conform with the SBML standard. A nice feature in this respect is the ability to display the SBML model structure as a tree (Figure 2.13, left side). A click on a species or reaction in this tree highlights the corresponding elements in the graphics canvas and in the matching tab on the right side showing further details. This tab is also the place where initial

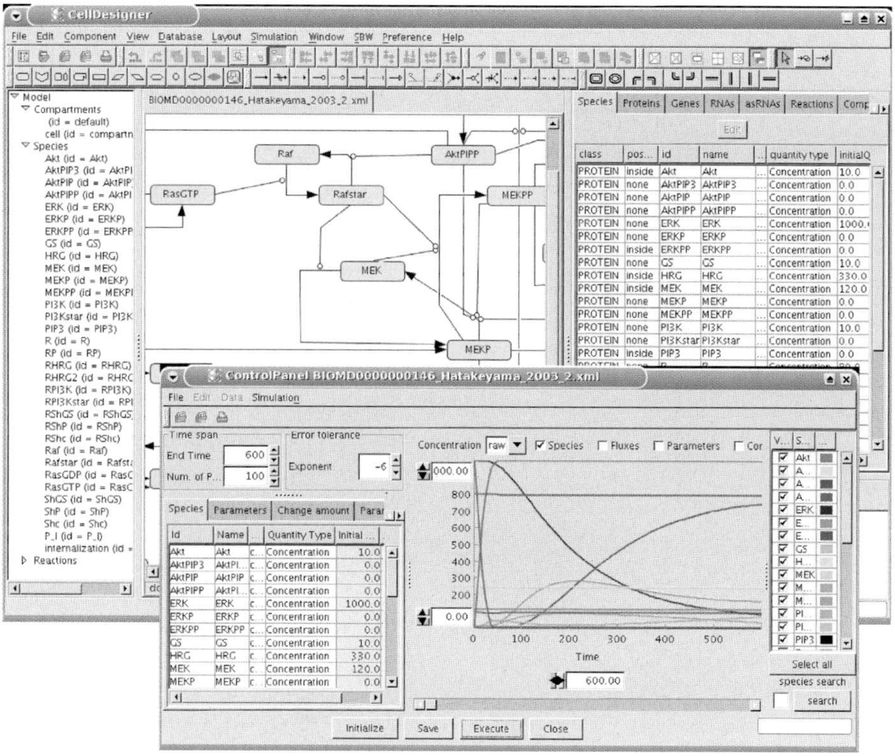

(a)

(b)

Figure 2.13 CellDesigner's process diagram editor (a) supports a rich set of graphical elements for different cellular species and reaction types. Simulations can be performed in CellDesigner using its integrated simulation engine (b).

concentrations and reaction details are entered. CellDesigner allows entering arbitrary kinetic equations, but has unfortunately no list of standard kinetics (mass action or Michaelis–Menten) that could be applied. For each reaction, the rate law has to be typed in by hand. A connection to the Systems Biology Workbench (SBW, see Section 17.4) is realized via the SBW menu and provides an interface to communicate with other SBW-compliant programs. For a further introduction to CellDesigner, a tutorial can be obtained at its website (http://www.celldesigner.org/). A movie introducing the usage of CellDesigner is availabe from the website of this book.

2.4.2.2 **COPASI**

Another platform-independent and user-friendly biochemical simulator that offers several unique features is COPASI [55]. COPASI is the successor to Gepasi [56, 57]. Its current version is 4.4 (http://www.copasi.org/). COPASI does not have such a rich visualization of the reaction network as CellDesigner, but it provides advanced functionalities for model simulation and analysis. In contrast to many other tools, it can switch between stochastic and deterministic simulation methods and supports hybrid deterministic-stochastic methods.

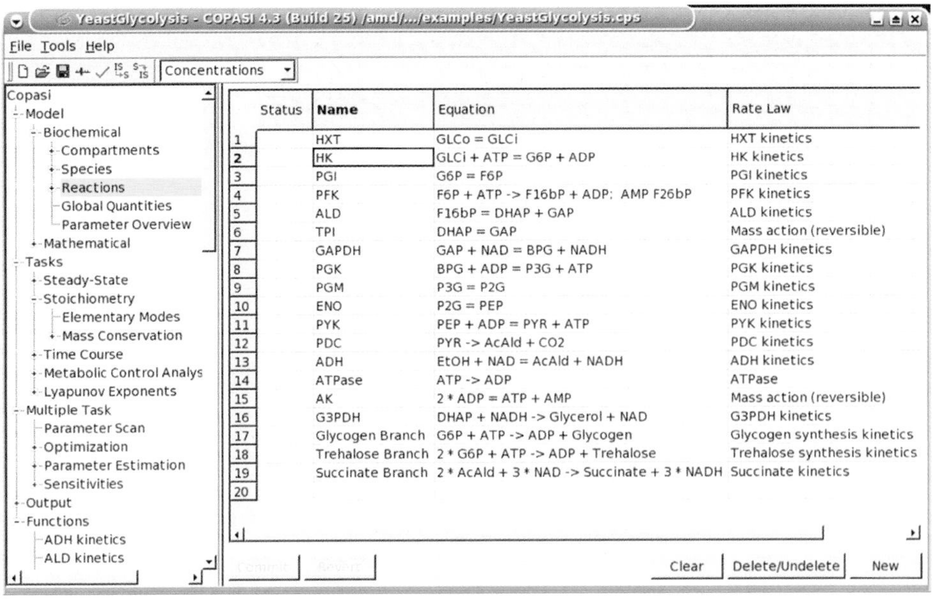

Figure 2.14 The different functionalities of COPASI are arranged in a hierarchical menu at left-hand side of its user interface. Details about the individual methods are listed in the right panel.

The user interface has a hierarchical menu (Figure 2.14, left side) that provides access to all the different functionalities of the tool. The biochemical model can be browsed according to its compartments, metabolites, and reactions including detailed list of the initial concentrations and kinetic parameters of the model. COPASI has a comprehensive set of standard methodologies for model analysis. It comprises the computation of steady states and their stability, supports the analysis of the stoichiometric network, e.g., the computation of elementary modes [25], supports MCA, and has methods for the optimization and parameter estimation. For compatibility with other tools, COPASI also supports the import and export of SBML-based models. For the definition of the kinetics, COPASI provides a copious set of predefined kinetic laws to choose from. A movie that is introducing the usage of COPASI is available from the website of this book.

2.4.2.3 **PyBioS**

Similarly as CellDesigner and Copasi, also PyBioS is designed for applications in systems biology and supports modeling and simulation [53]. PyBioS is a web-based environment (http://pybios.molgen.mpg.de/) that provides a framework for the conduction of kinetic models of various sizes and levels of granularity. The tool is a modeling platform for editing and analyzing biochemical models in order to predict the time-dependent behavior of the models. The platform has interfaces to external pathway databases (e.g., Reactome and KEGG) that can directly be used during model development for the definition of the structure of the reaction system. Figure 2.15

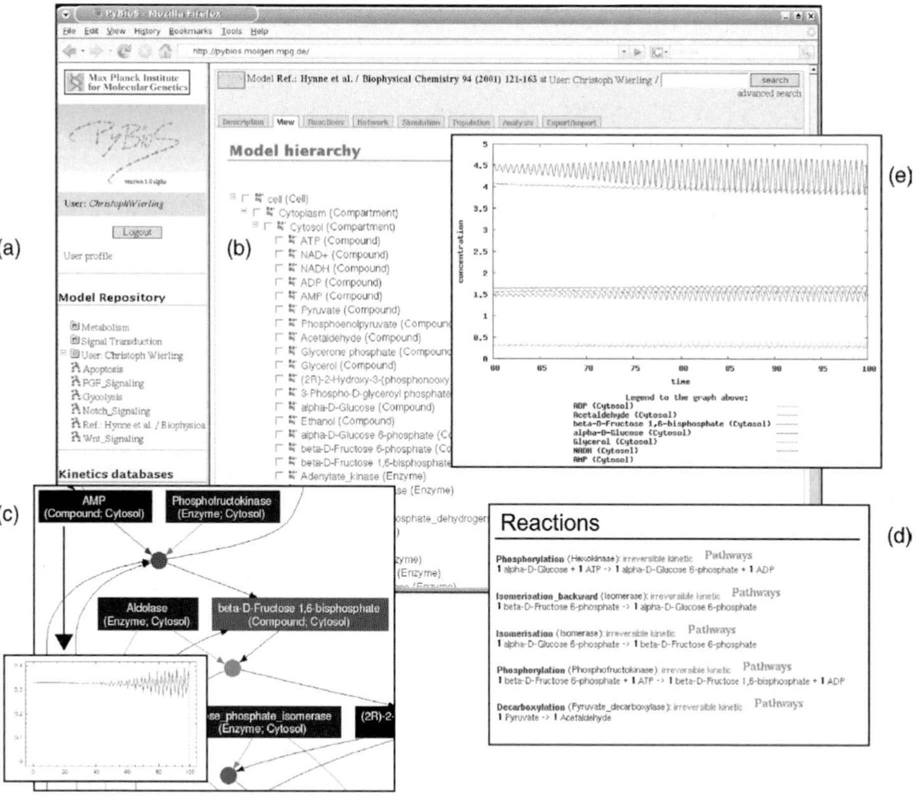

Figure 2.15 The PyBioS simulation environment. A particular model can be selected from the model repository (a) and its hierarchical model structure can be inspected via the View-tab at the top of the browser-window (b). A graphical representation of the model is provided by an automatically generated network diagram (accessible via the Network-tab), for example (c) shows the forward and reverse reaction of the isomerization of glucose-phosphate to fructose-phosphate of a glycolysis model. The Reactions-tab offers an overview of all reactions of the model (d). Simulations can be performed via the Simulation-tab (e). A simulation is based on an automatically generated mathematical model derived from the corresponding object-oriented model that comprises the network of all reactions and their respective kinetics.

shows screenshots of the PyBioS modeling and simulation environment. PyBioS defines a set of object classes (e.g., cell, compartment, compound, protein, complex, gene) for the definition of hierarchical models. Models are stored in a model repository. Support for the export and import of SBML-based models makes the platform compatible with other systems biology tools. Besides time course simulation, PyBioS also provides analysis methods, e.g., for the identification of steady states and their stability or for sensitivity analysis, such as the analysis of the steady-state behavior versus a varying parameter value or the computation of metabolic control coefficients. The reaction network of a model or individual parts of it can be visualized by network diagrams of the model components and their reactions that are connected via edges. Time course results of simulation experiments can be plotted into the network graphs and used for the interpretation of the model behavior.

2.4.3
Data Formats

The documentation and exchange of models need to be done in a defined way. In the easiest way – as usually found in publications – the biochemical reactions and the mathematical equations that are describing the model can be listed, using common formalism for the representation of biochemical and mathematical equations. These conventions provide a good standard for the documentation and exchange in publications. However, these formats are suitable for humans but not for the direct processing by a computer. This gave rise to the development of standards for the description of models. During the last years, the eXtensible Markup Language (XML, http://www.w3.org/XML) has been proved to be a flexible tool for the definition of standard formats. In the following text, a brief introduction to XML as well as a description of SBML, a standard for model description that is based on XML, is given. Moreover, BioPAX, a standard for the description cellular reaction systems, and SBGN, a standard for the graphical representation of reaction networks, will be described.

2.4.3.1 Systems Biology Markup Language

The Systems Biology Markup Language (SBML, http://www.sbml.org) is a free and open format for the representation of models common to research in many areas of computational biology, including cell signaling pathways, metabolic pathways, gene regulation, and others [58]. It is already supported by many software tools [59]. In January 2009, the SBML homepage listed more than 110 software systems supporting SBML. Currently, there are two SBML specifications denoted Level 1 and Level 2. Level 2 is the most recent specification and therefore it is described in the following text.

SBML is defined as an XML compliant format. XML documents are written as plain text and have a very clear and simple syntax that can easily be read by both humans and computer programs; however, it is generally intended to be written and read by computers, not humans. In XML, information is associated with tags indicating the type or formatting of the information. Tags are used to delimit and denote parts of the document or to add further information to the document structure. Using miscellaneous start tags (e.g., `<tag>`) and end tags (e.g., `</tag>`), information can be structured as text blocks in a hierarchical manner.

Example 2.17

The following example of the phosphorylation reaction of aspartate catalyzed by the aspartate kinase illustrates the general structure of an SBML file.

$$\text{Aspartate} + \text{ATP} \xrightarrow{\text{Aspartate kinase}} \text{Aspartyl phosphate} + \text{ADP}$$

```
(1) <?xml version="1.0" encoding="UTF-8"?>
(2)  <sbml level="2" version="1" xmlns="http://www.
sbml.org/sbml/level2">
(3)  <model id="AK_reaction">
(4)   <listOfUnitDefinitions>
(5)    <unitDefinition id="mmol">
(6)     <listOfUnits>
(7)      <unit kind="mole" scale="-3" />
(8)     </listOfUnits>
(9)    </unitDefinition>
(10)    <unitDefinition id="mmol_per_litre_per_sec">
(11)     <listOfUnits>
(12)      <unit kind="mole" scale="-3" />
(13)      <unit kind="litre" exponent="-1" />
(14)      <unit kind="second" exponent="-1" />
(15)     </listOfUnits>
(16)    </unitDefinition>
(17)   </listOfUnitDefinitions>
(18)   <listOfCompartments>
(19)      <compartment id="cell" name="Cell" size="1"
units="volume" />
(20)   </listOfCompartments>
(21)   <listOfSpecies>
(22)      <species id="asp" name="Aspartate"
compartment="cell" initialConcentration="2"
substanceUnits="mmol" />
(23)      <species id="aspp" name="Aspartyl phosphate"
compartment="cell" initialConcentration="0"
substanceUnits="mmol" />
(24)   <species id="atp" name="ATP" compartment="cell"
initialConcentration="0" substanceUnits="mmol" />
(25)   <species id="adp" name="ADP" compartment="cell"
initialConcentration="0" substanceUnits="mmol" />
(26)   </listOfSpecies>
(27)   <listOfReactions>
(28)    <reaction id="AK" reversible="false">
(29)     <listOfReactants>
(30)      <speciesReference species="asp"
stoichiometry="1" />
(31)      <speciesReference species="atp"
stoichiometry="1" />
(32)     </listOfReactants>
(33)     <listOfProducts>
(34)      <speciesReference species="aspp"
stoichiometry="1" />
```

```
(35)        <speciesReference species="adp" stoichiometry="1" />
(36)       </listOfProducts>
(37)       <kineticLaw>
(38)        <math xmlns="http://www.w3.org/1998/Math/MathML">
(39)          <apply>
(40)           <times />
(41)            <ci> k </ci>
(42)            <ci> asp </ci>
(43)            <ci> atp </ci>
(44)            <ci> cell </ci> <ci> cell </ci>
(45)          </apply>
(46)        </math>
(47)        <listOfParameters>
(48)       <parameter id="k" value="2.25" units="per_mM_and_min" />
(49)        </listOfParameters>
(50)       </kineticLaw>
(51)      </reaction>
(52)    </listOfReactions>
(53)  </model>
(54) </sbml>
```

Line 1 in the above example defines the document as a XML document. The SBML model is coded in lines 2–54. It is structured into several lists that define different properties of the model. Most important lists that are usually used are the definition of units (lines 4–17), of compartments (lines 18–20), of species (lines 21–26), and finally of the reactions themselves (lines 27–52). Most entries in SBML have one required attribute, id, to give the instance a unique identifier by which other parts of the SBML model definition can refer to it. Some base units, like gram, meter, liter, mole, second, etc., are already predefined in SBML. More complex units derived from the base units are defined in the list of units. For instance, mM/s that is equal to $\mathrm{mmol}\cdot\mathrm{l}^{-1}\,\mathrm{sec}^{-1}$ can be defined as shown in lines 10–16 and used by its id in the subsequent definition of parameters and initial concentrations. Compartments are used in SBML as a construct for the grouping of model species. They are defined in the list of compartments (lines 18–20) and can be used not only for the definition of cellular compartments but also for grouping in general. Each compartment can have a name attribute and defines a compartment size. Model species are defined in the list of species. Each species has a recommended id attribute that can be used to refer it and can define its name and initial value with its respective unit. Species identifiers are used in the list of reactions (lines 27–52) for the definition of the individual biochemical reactions. Reversibility of a reaction is indicated by an attribute of the reaction tag (lines 28). Reactants and products of a specific reaction along with their respective stoichiometry are specified in separate lists (lines 29–36).

The kinetic law of an individual reaction (lines 37–50) is specified in MathML for SBML Level 2. MathML is an XML-based markup language especially created for the representation of complicated mathematical expressions. In the above example, the rate law reads $k \cdot [\mathrm{asp}] \cdot [\mathrm{atp}] \cdot \mathrm{cell}^2$, where k is a kinetic parameter [asp] and [atp] are the concentrations of aspartate and ATP, respectively, and cell is the volume of the cell. The consideration of the cell volume is needed, since rate laws in SBML are expressed in terms of amount of substance abundance per time instead of the traditional expression in terms of amount of substance concentration per time. The formulation of the rate law in the traditional way embodies the tacit assumption that the participating reaction species are located in the same, constant volume. This is done because attempting to describe reactions between species located in different compartments that differ in volume by the expression in terms of concentration per time quickly leads to difficulties.

2.4.3.2 BioPAX

Another standard format that is used in systems biology and designed for handling information on pathways and topologies of biochemical reaction networks is BioPAX (http://www.biopax.org). While SBML is tuned toward the simulation of models of molecular pathways, BioPAX is a more general and expressive format for the description of biological reaction systems even it is lacking definitions for the representation of dynamic data such as kinetic laws and parameters. BioPAX is defined by the BioPAX working group (http://www.biopax.org/). The BioPax Ontology defines a large set of classes for the description of pathways, interactions, and biological entities as well as their relations. Reaction networks described by BioPAX can be represented by the use XML. Many systems biology tools and databases make use of BioPAX for the exchange of data.

2.4.3.3 Systems Biology Graphical Notation

Graphical representations of reaction networks prove as very helpful tools for the work in systems biology. The graphical representation of a reaction system is not only helpful during the design of a new model and as a representation of the model topology, it is also helpful for the analysis and interpretation for instance of simulation results. Traditionally, diagrams of interacting enzymes and compounds have been written in an informal manner of simple unconstrained shapes and arrows. Several diagrammatic notations have been proposed for the graphical representation (e.g., [60–64]). As a consequence of the different proposals, the Systems Biology Graphical Notation (SBGN) has been set up recently. It provides a common graphical notation for the representation of biochemical and cellular reaction networks. SBGN defines a comprehensive set of symbols, with precise semantics, together with detailed syntactic rules defining their usage. Furthermore, SBGN defines how such graphical information is represented in a machine-readable form to ensure its proper storage, exchange, and reproduction of the graphical representation.

SBGN defines three different diagram types: (i) State Transition diagrams that are depicting all molecular interactions taking place, (ii) Activity Flow diagrams that are representing only the flux of information going from one entity to another, and (iii) Entity Relationship diagrams that are representing the relationships between different molecular species. In a State Transition diagram, each node represents a given state of a species, and therefore a given species may appear multiple times. State Transition diagrams are suitable for following the temporal process of interactions. A drawback of State Transition diagrams, however, is that the representation of each individual state of a species results quickly in very large diagram and due to this, it becomes difficult to understand what interactions actually exist for the species in question. In such a case, an Entity Relation diagram is more suitable. In an Entity Relation diagram, a biological entity appears only once.

SBGN defines several kinds of symbols, whereas two types of symbols are distinguished: nodes and arcs. There are different kinds of nodes defined. Reacting state or entity nodes represent, e.g., macromolecules, such as protein, RNA, DNA, polysaccharide, or simple chemicals, such as a radical, an ion, or a small molecule. Container nodes are defined for the representation of a complex, compartment, or module. Different transition nodes are defined for the representation of transitions like biochemical reactions, associations, like protein-complex formation, or dissociations, like the dissociation of a protein complex. The influence of a node onto another is visualized by different types of arcs representing, e.g., consumption, production, modulation, stimulation, catalysis, inhibition, or trigger effect. Not all node and arc symbols are defined for each of the three diagram types. A detailed description of the different nodes, arcs, and the syntax of their usage by the different diagram types is given in the specification of SBGN (see http://sbgn.org/).

Examples of a State Transition and an Entity Relationship diagram is given in Figure 2.16.

2.4.3.4 Standards for Systems Biology

With the increasing amount of data in modern biology the requirement of standards used for data integration became more and more important. For example, in the course of a microarray experiment, a lot of different information accumulates, as information about the samples, the type of microarray that is used, the experimental procedure including the hybridization experiment, the data normalization, and the expression data itself. It turns out that an important part of systems biology is data integration. This requires a conceptual design and the development of common standards.

The development of a standard involves four steps: an informal design of a conceptual model, a formalization, the development of a data exchange format, and the implementation of supporting tools [65]. For micorarray experiments, a conceptual model about the minimum information that is required for the description of such an experiment is specified by MIAME (Minimum Information About a Microarray Experiment [65]). Similar specifications have also been done for, e.g., proteomics data with MIAPE (Minimum Information About a Proteomics Experiment [66]), or systems biology models with MIRIAM (Minimum information

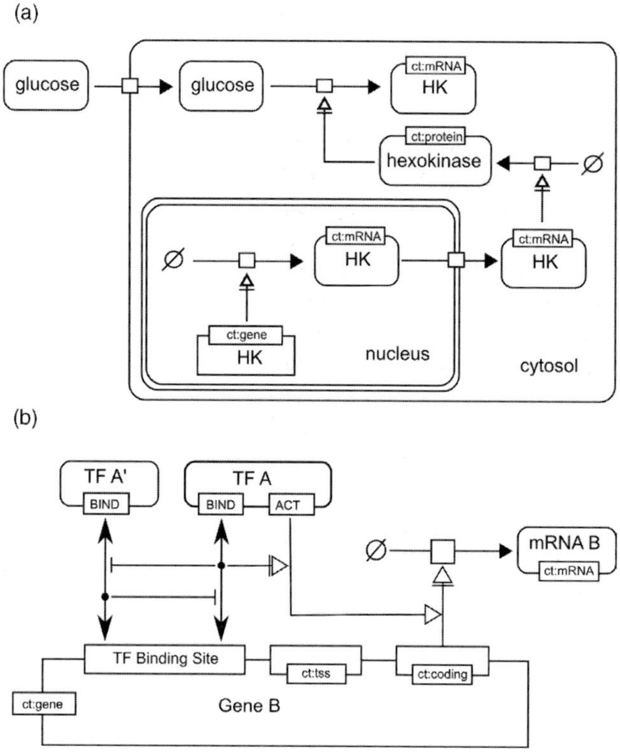

Figure 2.16 Systems Biology Graphical Notation (SBGN). (a) State transition diagram. (b) Entity relation diagram describing gene regulation and transcription of a gene. The two transcription factors TF A and TF A′ compete for the same transcription factor-binding site. If one of the transcription factors is bound, the binding site is blocked for the other one, but only TF A can activate the transcription of the gene. The abbreviation "ct" indicates conceptual types of the respective entity.

requested in the annotation of biochemical models). MIRIAM specifies a set of rules for curating quantitative models of biological systems that define procedures for encoding and annotating models represented in machine-readable form [67].

2.4.4 Data Resources

The development of models of biological systems requires diverse kind of data. This is, for instance, information about the different model components (e.g., metabolites, proteins, and genes) and their different functions and interactions. Such information can be extracted from literature or dedicated data resources, like pathway databases. Two pathway databases that are well known are KEGG und Reactome. Both are described below in more detail. Another important data for modeling are information about reaction kinetics. Database dealing with such data are described in more detail in Sections 2.4.4.2 and 3.1. Further information about databases providing primary data is given in Chapter 16.

2.4.4.1 Pathway Databases

Kyoto Enzyclopedia of Genes and Genomes Kyoto Enzyclopedia of Genes and Genomes (KEGG; http://www.genome.ad.jp/kegg/) is a reference knowledge base offering information about genes and proteins, biochemical compounds and reactions, and pathways. The data is organized in three parts: the gene universe (consisting of the GENES, SSDB, and KO database), the chemical universe (with the COMPOUND, GLYCAN, REACTION, and ENZYME databases which are merged as LIGAND database), and the protein network consisting of the PATHWAY database [68]. Besides this, the KEGG database is hierarchically classified into categories and subcategories at four levels. The five topmost categories are metabolism, genetic information processing, environmental information processing, cellular processes, and human diseases. Subcategories of metabolism are, e.g., carbohydrate, energy, lipid, nucleotide, or amino acid metabolism. These are subdivided into the different pathways, like glycolysis, citrate cycle, purine metabolism, etc. Finally, the fourth level corresponds to the KO (KEGG Orthology) entries. A KO entry (internally identified by a K number, e.g., K00001 for the alcohol dehydrogenase) corresponds to a group of orthologous genes that have identical functions.

The gene universe offers information about genes and proteins generated by genome sequencing projects. Information about individual genes is stored in the GENES database, which is semiautomatically generated from the submissions to GenBank, the NCBI RefSeq database, the EMBL database, and other publicly available organism-specific databases. K numbers are further assigned to entries of the GENES database. The SSDB database contains information about amino acid sequence similarities between protein-coding genes computationally generated from the GENES database. This is carried out for many complete genomes and results in a huge graph depicting protein similarities with clusters of orthologous and paralogous genes.

The chemical universe offers information about chemical compounds and reactions relevant to cellular processes. It includes more than 11,000 compounds (internally represented by C numbers, e.g., C00001 denotes water), a separate database for carbohydrates (nearly 11,000 entries; represented by a number preceded by G, e.g., G10481 for cellulose), more than 6000 reactions (with R numbers, e.g., R00275 for the reaction of the superoxide radical into hydrogen peroxide), and more than 4000 enzymes (denoted by EC numbers as well as K numbers for orthologous entries). All these data are merged as LIGAND database [69]. Thus, the chemical universe offers comprehensive information about metabolites with their respective chemical structures and biochemical reactions.

KEGG's protein network provides information about protein interactions comprising pathways and protein complexes. The 235 KEGG reference pathway diagrams (maps), offered on the website, give clear overviews of important pathways. Organism-specific pathway maps are automatically generated by coloring of organism-specific genes in the reference pathways.

The KEGG database can be queried via the web interface, e.g., for genes, proteins, compounds, etc. Access to the data via FTP (http://www.genome.ad.jp/anonftp) as well as access to it via a SOAP server (http://www.genome.ad.jp/kegg/soap) is possible for academic users, too.

Reactome Reactome (formerly known as Genome Knowledgebase [70–72]) is an open, online database of fundamental human biological processes. The Reactome project is managed as a collaboration of the Cold Spring Harbor Laboratory, the European Bioinformatics Institute (EBI), and the Gene Ontology Consortium. The database is divided into several modules of fundamental biological processes that are thought to operate in humans. Each module of the database has one or more primary authors and is further peer reviewed by experts of the specific field. Each module can also be referenced by its revision date and thus can be cited like a publication.

On one hand, the Reactome database is intended to offer valuable information for the wet-lab scientist, who wants to know, e.g., more about a specific gene product she or he is unfamiliar with. On the other hand, the Reactome database can be used by the computational biologist to draw conclusions from large data sets like expression data gained by cDNA chip experiments.

Another tool offered by Reactome is the "Pathfinder." This utility enables the user to find the shortest path between two physical entities, e.g., the shortest path between the metabolites D-fructose and pyruvate, or the steps from the primary mRNA to its processed form. The computed path can be shown graphically. The pathfinder offers also the possibility to exclude specific entities, like the metabolites ATP or NADH that show high connectivity and thus their input might lead to a path that is not the one intended to be found.

Data from Reactome can be exported in various formats upon which are SBML and BioPAX.

2.4.4.2 Databases of Kinetic Data

High-throughput projects, such as the international genome sequencing efforts, accumulate large amounts of data at an amazing rate. These data are essential for the reconstruction of phylogenetic trees and gene-finding projects. However, for kinetic modeling, which is at the heart of systems biology, kinetic data of proteins and enzymes are needed. Unfortunately, this type of data is notoriously difficult and time-consuming to obtain since proteins often need individually tuned purification and reaction conditions. Furthermore, the results of such studies are published in a large variety of journals from different fields. In this situation, the databases BRENDA and SABIO-RK aim to be comprehensive resources of kinetic data. They are discussed in more detail in Section 4.1.1.

2.4.4.3 Model Databases

A lot of different mathematical models of biological systems have already been developed in the past and are described in the literature. However, these models are usually not available in a computer-amenable format. During the last years, big efforts have been done on the gathering and implementation of existing models in databases. Two well-known databases on this are BioModels and JWS, which are described in more detail in the following.

BioModels The BioModels.net project (http://biomodels.net) is an international effort to (i) define agreed-upon standards for model curation, (ii) define agreed-upon vocabularies for annotating models with connections to biological data resources, and (iii) provide a free, centralized, publicly accessible database of annotated, computational models in SBML, and other structured formats. The ninth release of the databases has 192 models, of which 150 are in the curated and 42 are in the noncurated branch. Models can be browsed in the web interface, online simulations can be performed via the external simulation engine of JWS online (see below), or they can be exported in several prominent file formats (e.g., SBML, CellML, BioPAX) for external usage by other programs.

JWS Another model repository that is providing kinetic models of biochemical systems is JWS online [73]. As of February 2008, this model repository provides 84 models (http://jjj.biochem.sun.ac.za). Models in JWS online can be interactively run and interrogated over the internet.

Exercises and Problems

1. A canonical view of the upper part of glycolysis starts with glucose and comprises the following reactions (in brackets: possible abbreviations): The enzyme hexokinase (HK, E_1) phosphorylates glucose (Gluc, S_1) to glucose-6-phosphate (G6P, S_2) under consumption of ATP (S_5) and production of ADP (S_6). The enzyme phosphoglucoisomerase (PGI, E_2) converts glucose-6-phosphate to fructose-6-phosphate (F6P, S_3). The enzyme phosphofructokinase (PFK, E_3) phosphorylates F6P a second time to yield fructose-1,6-bisphosphate (F1,6,BP, S_4). The enzyme fructosebisphosphatase catalyzes the reverse reaction (E_4).

   (a) Sketch the reaction network and formulate a set of differential equations (without specifying the kinetics of the individual reactions).
   (b) Formulate the stoichiometric matrix $\boldsymbol{N}$. What is the rank of $\boldsymbol{N}$?
   (c) Calculate steady-state fluxes (matrix $\boldsymbol{K}$) and conservation relations (matrix $\boldsymbol{G}$).
   (d) Compare your results with Example 2.6.

2. (a) Write down the sets of differential equations for the networks N1–N6 given in Table 2.4 without specifying their kinetics.
   (b) Determine the rank of the stoichiometric matrices, independent steady-state fluxes, and conservation relations.
   Do all systems have a (nontrivial) steady state?

3. Inspect networks N3 and N4 in Table 2.4. Can you find elementary flux modes? Use an available tool (e.g., Metatool) to check out.

4. Assign the following kinetics to network N3 in Table 2.4: $v_1 = k_1$, $v_2 = (V_{max2} \cdot S_1)/(K_{m2} + S_1)$, $v_3 = (V_{max3} \cdot S_1)/(K_{m3} + S_1)$ with $k_1 = 10$, $V_{max2} = 3$, $K_{m2} = 0.2$, V_{max2} 5, and $K_{m2} = 0.4$. Compute the steady-state concentration of S_1 and calculate the flux control coefficients.

5. For the reaction system $A \xrightarrow{v_1} B$, $B \xrightarrow{v_2} C$, $C \xrightarrow{v_3} A$ with $v_1 = k_1 \cdot A$, $v_2 = k_2 \cdot B$, $v_3 = k_3 \cdot C$, and $k_1 = 2$, $k_2 = 2$, $k_3 = 1$, write down the set of systems equations.

   (a) Compute the Jacobian $\mathbf{J}$!
   (b) Determine the eigenvalues and eigenvectors of the Jacobian $\mathbf{J}$!
   (c) What is the general solution of the ODE system?
   (d) Compute the solution with the initial condition $A(0) = 1$, $B(0) = 1$, $C(0) = 0$!

6. The Jacobian $\mathbf{A}_a$ of the following ODE system depends on the parameter a:

$$\frac{d}{dt}\begin{pmatrix} x \\ y \end{pmatrix} = \begin{pmatrix} 0 & -1 \\ 10+a & a \end{pmatrix}\begin{pmatrix} x \\ y \end{pmatrix}$$

   (a) To every specific choice of parameter a belongs a point ($\text{Tr}\,\mathbf{A}_a$, $\text{Det}\,\mathbf{A}_a$) in the plane spaned by trace and determinate of $\mathbf{A}_a$. Draw the curve ($\text{Tr}\,\mathbf{A}_a$, $\text{Det}\,\mathbf{A}_a$) in this space for a as a changing parameter.
   (b) For which values of a is $(x,y) = (0,0)$ a saddle point, node or focus?

7. What is the use of standards important for the development of new systems biology tools?

References

1 Guldberg, C.M. and Waage, P. (1879) Über die chemische Affinität. *Journal fur Praktische Chemie*, **19**, 69.

2 Guldberg, C.M. and Waage, P. (1867) *Études sur les affinités chimiques*, Christiana.

3 Waage, P. and Guldberg, C.M. (1864) *Studies concerning affinity*, Forhandlinger: Videnskabs-Selskabet, Christiana, pp 35.

4 Brown, A.J. (1902) Enzyme action. *Journal of the Chemical Society*, **81**, 373–386.

5 Michaelis, L. and Menten, M.L. (1913) Kinetik der invertinwirkung. *Biochemistry Zeitung*, **49**, 333–369.

6 Briggs, G.E. and Haldane, J.B.S. (1925) A note on the kinetics of enzyme action. *The Biochemical Journal*, **19**, 338–339.

7 Lineweaver, H. and Burk, D. (1934) The determination of enzyme dissocation constants. *Journal of the American Chemical Society*, **56**, 658–660.

8 Eadie, G.S. (1942) The inhibition of cholinesterase by physostigmine and prostigmine. *The Journal of Biological Chemistry*, **146**, 85–93.

9 Hanes, C.S. (1932) Studies on plant amylases. I. The effect of starch concentratio upon the velocity of hydrolysis by the amylase of germinated barley. *The Biochemical Journal*, **26**, 1406–1421.

10 Haldane, J.B.S. (1930) *Enzymes*, Longmans, Green and Co., London.

11 Schellenberger, A. (1989) *Enzymkatalyse*, Fischer Verlag, Jena.

12 Wegscheider, R. (1902) Über simultane Gleichgewichte und die Beziehungen

zwischen Thermodynamik und Reaktionskinetik homogener Systeme. *Zeitschrift für Physikalische Chemie*, **39**, 257–303.
13 Hill, A.V. (1910) The possible effects of the aggregation of the molecules of hemoglobin on its dissociation curves. *The Journal of Physiology*, **40**, iv–vii.
14 Hill, A.V. (1913) The combinations of hemoglobin with oxygen and with carbon monoxide. *The Biochemical Journal*, **7**, 471–480.
15 Monod, J. *et al.* (1965) On the nature of allosteric transitions: A plausible model. *Journal of Molecular Biology*, **12**, 88–118.
16 Savageau, M. (1985) Mathematics of organizationally complex systems. *Biomed Biochim Acta*, **44**, 839–884.
17 Heijnen, J.J. (2005) Approximative kinetic formats used in metabolic network modelling. *Biotechnology and Bioengineering*, **91**, 534–545.
18 Liebermeister, W. and Klipp, E. (2006) Bringing metabolic networks to life: convenience rate law and thermodynamic constraints. *Theoretical Biology and Medical Modelling*, **3**, 42.
19 Glansdorff, P. and Prigogine, I. (1971) *Thermodynamic Theory of Structure, Stability and Fluctuations*, Wiley-Interscience, London.
20 Reder, C. (1988) Metabolic control theory: a structural approach. *Journal of Theoretical Biology*, **135**, 175–201.
21 Heinrich, R. and Schuster, S. (1996) *The Regulation of Cellular Systems*, Chapman & Hall, New York.
22 Michal, G. (1999) *Biochemical Pathways*, Spektrum Akademischer, Heidelberg.
23 Pfeiffer, T. *et al.* (1999) METATOOL: for studying metabolic networks. *Bioinformatics (Oxford, England)*, **15**, 251–257.
24 Schilling, C.H. *et al.* (1999) Metabolic pathway analysis: basic concepts and scientific applications in the post-genomic era. *Biotechnology Progress*, **15**, 296–303.
25 Schuster, S. *et al.* (1999) Detection of elementary flux modes in biochemical networks: a promising tool for pathway analysis and metabolic engineering. *Trends in Biotechnology*, **17**, 53–60.
26 Schuster, S. *et al.* (2000) A general definition of metabolic pathways useful for systematic organization and analysis of complex metabolic networks. *Nature Biotechnology*, **18**, 326–332.
27 Schuster, S. *et al.* (2002) Reaction routes in biochemical reaction systems: algebraic properties, validated calculation procedure and example from nucleotide metabolism. *Journal of Mathematical Biology*, **45**, 153–181.
28 Schilling, C.H. and Palsson, B.O. (2000) Assessment of the metabolic capabilities of *Haemophilus influenzae* Rd through a genome-scale pathway analysis. *Journal of Theoretical Biology*, **203**, 249–283.
29 Schilling, C.H. *et al.* (2000) Theory for the systemic definition of metabolic pathways and their use in interpreting metabolic function from a pathway-oriented perspective. *Journal of Theoretical Biology*, **203**, 229–248.
30 Wiback, S.J. and Palsson, B.O. (2002) Extreme pathway analysis of human red blood cell metabolism. *Biophysical Journal*, **83**, 808–818.
31 Bronstein, I.N. and Semendjajew, K.A. (1987) Taschenbuch der Mathematik, 23rd edition, Nauka, Moscow.
32 Heinrich, R. and Rapoport, T.A. (1974) A linear steady-state treatment of enzymatic chains. General properties, control and effector strength. *European Journal of Biochemistry*, **42**, 89–95.
33 Kacser, H. and Burns, J.A. (1973) The control of flux. *Symposia of the Society for Experimental Biology*, **27**, 65–104.
34 Bruggeman, F.J. *et al.* (2002) Modular response analysis of cellular regulatory networks. *Journal of Theoretical Biology*, **218**, 507–520.
35 Hofmeyr J.H. and Westerhoff, H.V. (2001) Building the cellular puzzle: control in multi-level reaction networks. *Journal of Theoretical Biology*, **208**, 261–285.
36 Kholodenko, B.N. *et al.* (2000) Diffusion control of protein phosphorylation in

signal transduction pathways. *The Biochemical Journal*, **350** (Pt 3), 901–907.

37 Liebermeister, W. *et al.* (2004) A theory of optimal differential gene expression. *Bio Systems*, **76**, 261–278.

38 Westerhoff, H.V. *et al.* (2002) ECA: control in ecosystems. *Molecular Biology Reports*, **29**, 113–117.

39 de Jong, H. (2002) Modeling and simulation of genetic regulatory systems: a literature review. *Journal of Computational Biology: A Journal of Computational Molecular Cell Biology*, **9**, 67–103.

40 Kitano, H. (2002) Computational systems biology. *Nature*, **420**, 206–210.

41 Hindmarsh, A.C. (1983) ODEPACK, A systematized collection of ODE solvers, in *Scientific Computing* (eds R.S. Stepleman *et al.*) North-Holland, Amsterdam, pp. 55–64.

42 Petzold, L. (1983) Automatic selection of methods for solving stiff and nonstiff systems of ordinary differential equations. *SIAM Journal on Scientific and Statistical Computing*, **4**, 136–148.

43 Cohen, S.D. and Hindmarsh, A.C. (1996) CVODE, a stiff/nonstiff ODE solver in C. *Computers in Physics*, **10**, 138–143.

44 Deuflhard, P. and Nowak, U. (1987) Extrapolation integrators for quasilinear implicit ODEs, in *Large Scale Scientific Computing* (eds P. Deuflhard and B. Engquist) Birkkäuser, Basel, pp. 37–50.

45 Bernardinello, L. and de Cindio, F. (1992) *A Survey of Basic Net Models and Modular Net Classes*, Springer, Berlin.

46 Küffner, R. *et al.* (2000) Pathway analysis in metabolic databases via differential metabolic display (DMD). *Bioinformatics*, **16**, 825–836.

47 Reddy, V.N. *et al.* (1996) Qualitative analysis of biochemical reaction systems. *Computers in Biology and Medicine*, **26**, 9–24.

48 Matsuno, H. *et al.* (2003) Biopathways representation and simulation on hybrid functional Petri net. *In Silico Biology*, **3**, 389–404.

49 Gardner, M. (1970) Mathematical games. *Scientific American*, **223**, 120–123.

50 Alves, R. *et al.* (2006) Tools for kinetic modeling of biochemical networks. *Nature Biotechnology*, **24**, 667–672.

51 Klipp, E. *et al.* (2007b) Systems biology standards – the community speaks. *Nature Biotechnology*, **25**, 390–391.

52 Materi, W. and Wishart, D.S. (2007) Computational systems biology in drug discovery and development: methods and applications. *Drug Discovery Today*, **12**, 295–303.

53 Wierling, C. *et al.* (2007) Resources, standards and tools for systems biology. *Briefings in Functional Genomics and Proteomics*, **6**, 240–251.

54 Funahashi, A. *et al.* (2003) CellDesigner: a process diagram editor for gene-regulatory and biochemical networks. *Biosilico*, **1**, 159–162.

55 Hoops, S. *et al.* (2006) COPASI – a COmplex PAthway SImulator. *Bioinformatics*, **22**, 3067–3074.

56 Mendes, P. (1993) GEPASI: a software package for modelling the dynamics steady states and control of biochemical and other systems. *Computer Applications in the Biosciences*, **9**, 563–571.

57 Mendes, P. (1997) Biochemistry by numbers: simulation of biochemical pathways with Gepasi 3. *Trends in Biochemical Sciences*, **22**, 361–363.

58 Hucka, M. *et al.* (2003) The systems biology markup language (SBML): a medium for representation and exchange of biochemical network models. *Bioinformatics*, **19**, 524–531.

59 Hucka, M. *et al.* (2004) Evolving a lingua franca and associated software infrastructure for computational systems biology: the Systems Biology Markup Language (SBML) project. *Systematic Biology (Stevenage)*, **1**, 41–53.

60 Kitano, H. (2003) A graphical notation for biochemical networks. *BIOSILICO*, **1**, 169–176.

61 Kitano, H. *et al.* (2005) Using process diagrams for the graphical representation of biological networks. *Nature Biotechnology*, **23**, 961–966.

62 Kohn, K.W. (1999) Molecular interaction map of the mammalian cell cycle control and DNA repair systems. *Molecular Biology of the Cell*, **10**, 2703–2734.

63 Moodie, S.L. *et al.* (2006) A graphical notation to describe the logical interactions of biological pathways. *Journal of Integrative Bioinformatics*, **3**, 36.

64 Pirson, I. *et al.* (2000) The visual display of regulatory information and networks. *Trends in Cell Biology*, **10**, 404–408.

65 Brazma, A. *et al.* (2001) Minimum information about a microarray experiment (MIAME)-toward standards for microarray data. *Nature Genetics*, **29**, 365–371.

66 Taylor, C.F. *et al.* (2007) The minimum information about a proteomics experiment (MIAPE). *Nature Biotechnology*, **25**, 887–893.

67 Le Novere, N. *et al.* (2005) Minimum information requested in the annotation of biochemical models (MIRIAM). *Nature Biotechnology*, **23**, 1509–1515.

68 Kanehisa, M. *et al.* (2004) The KEGG resource for deciphering the genome. *Nucleic Acids Research*, **32**, D277–D280.

69 Goto, S. *et al.* (2002) LIGAND: database of chemical compounds and reactions in biological pathways. *Nucleic Acids Research*, **30**, 402–404.

70 Joshi-Tope, G. *et al.* (2003) The genome knowledgebase: a resource for biologists and bioinformaticists. *Cold Spring Harbor Symposia on Quantitative Biology*, **68**, 237–243.

71 Joshi-Tope, G. *et al.* (2005) Reactome: a knowledgebase of biological pathways. *Nucleic Acids Research*, **33**, D428–D432.

72 Vastrik, I. *et al.* (2007) Reactome: a knowledge base of biologic pathways and processes. *Genome Biology*, **8**, R39.

73 Olivier, B.G. and Snoep, J.L. (2004) Web-based kinetic modelling using JWS Online. *Bioinformatics*, **20**, 2143–2144.

3
Specific Biochemical Systems

Systems biology aims to understand structure, function, regulation, or development of biological systems by combining experimental and computational approaches. It is important to understand that different parts of cellular organization are studied and understood in different ways and to different extent. This is related to diverse experimental techniques that can be used to measure the abundance of metabolites, proteins, mRNA, or other types of compounds. For example, enzyme kinetic measurements are performed for more than a century, while mRNA measurements (e.g., as microarray data) or protein measurements (e.g., as mass spectrometry analysis) have been developed more recently. Not all data can be provided with the same accuracy and reproducibility. These and other complications in studying life caused a nonuniform progress in modeling different parts of cellular life. Moreover, the diversity of scientific questions and the availability of computational tools to tackle them led to the development of very different types of models for different biological processes. In this chapter, we will introduce a number of classical and more recent areas of systems biological research. In the following, we discuss modeling of metabolic systems, signaling pathways, cell cycle regulation, and development and differentiation, primarily with ODE systems, as well as spatial modeling of biochemical systems. In the web-material, we introduce approaches to synthetic biology, population dynamics, aging, and pharmacokinetics.

3.1
Metabolic Systems

Summary

Living cells require energy and material for building membranes, storing molecules, turnover of enzymes, replication and repair of DNA, movement, and many other processes. Through metabolism, cells acquire energy and use it to build new cells. Metabolism is the means by which cells survive and reproduce. Metabolism is the general term for two kinds of reactions: (1) catabolic reactions (breakdown of complex compounds to get energy and building blocks) and (2) anabolic reactions

Systems Biology: A Textbook. Edda Klipp, Wolfram Liebermeister, Christoph Wierling, Axel Kowald, Hans Lehrach, and Ralf Herwig

ISBN: 978-3-527-31874-2

(construction of complex compounds used in cellular functioning). Metabolism is a highly organized process. It involves hundreds or thousands of reactions that are catalyzed by enzymes.

Metabolic networks consist of reactions transforming molecules of one type into molecules of another type. In modeling terms, the concentrations of the molecules and their rates of change are of special interest. In Chapter 2, we explained how to study such networks on three levels of abstraction:

1. Enzyme kinetics investigates the dynamic properties of the individual reactions in isolation.
2. The network character of metabolism is studied with stoichiometric analysis considering the balance of compound production and degradation.
3. Metabolic control analysis quantifies the effect of perturbations in the network employing the dynamics of individual concentration changes and their integration in the network.

Here, we will illustrate the theoretical concepts by applying them to a number of examples. We will specifically discuss cellular energy metabolism focusing on glycolysis and the threonine pathway as an example of amino acid synthesis. You may find the complete models and many other models also in modeling databases such as JWS online [1].

3.1.1
Basic Elements of Metabolic Modeling

Metabolic networks are defined by the enzymes converting substrates into products in a reversible or irreversible manner. Without enzymes, those reactions are essentially impossible or too slow. But networks are also characterized by the metabolites that are converted by the various enzymes. Biochemical studies have revealed a number of important catabolic pathways and pathways of the energy metabolism such as glycolysis, the pentose-phosphate pathway, the tricarboxylic acid (TCA) cycle, and oxidative phosphorylation. Among the known anabolic pathways are gluconeogenesis, amino acid synthesis pathways, and synthesis of fatty acids and nucleic acids. Databases such as the Kyoto Encyclopedia of Genes and Genomes Pathway (KEGG, http://http://www.genome.jp/kegg/pathway.html) provide a comprehensive overview of pathways in various organisms.

Here, we will focus on pathway characteristics, which are essential for modeling. Figure 3.1 provides a summary of the first steps to build a model. First, we can sketch the metabolites and the converting reactions in a cartoon to get an overview and an intuitive understanding. Based on that cartoon and on further information, we must set the limits of our model. That means, we must consider what kind of question we want to answer with our model, what information in terms of qualitative and quantitative data is available, and how we can make the model as simple as possible but as comprehensive as necessary. Then, for every compound, which is part of the system, we formulate the balance equations (see also Section 2.2) summing up all reaction that produce the compound (with a positive

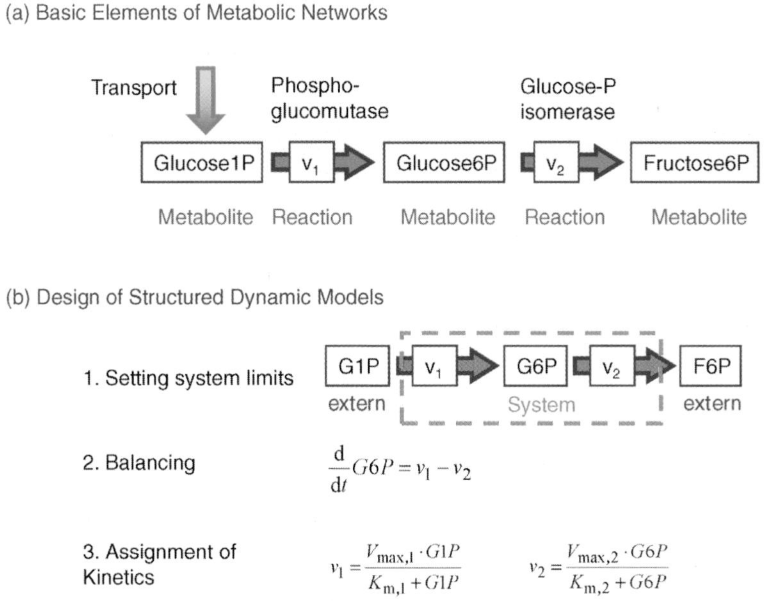

Figure 3.1 Designing metabolic models. (a) Basic elements of metabolic networks and (b) basic steps for designing structured dynamic models (see the text for further explanation).

sign) and all reaction that degrade the compound (with a negative sign). At this stage, the model is suited for a network analysis such as stoichiometric analysis (Section 2.2) or, with some additional information, flux balance analysis (Section 9.1). In order to study the dynamics of the system, we must add kinetic descriptions to the individual reactions. Keep in mind that the reaction kinetics may depend on

- the concentrations of substrates and products (here G1P and G6P),
- specific parameters such as K_m-values,
- the amount and activity of the catalyzing enzyme (here hidden in the V_{max} values, see Section 2.1), and
- the activity of modifiers, which are not shown in the example in Figure 3.1.

In the following, we will discuss in more detail models for three pathways: the upper glycolysis, the full glycolysis, and the threonine synthesis.

3.1.2 Toy Model of Upper Glycolysis

A first model of the upper part of glycolysis is depicted in Figure 3.2. It comprises six reactions and six metabolites. Note that we neglect the formation of phosphate P_i here. The ODE system reads

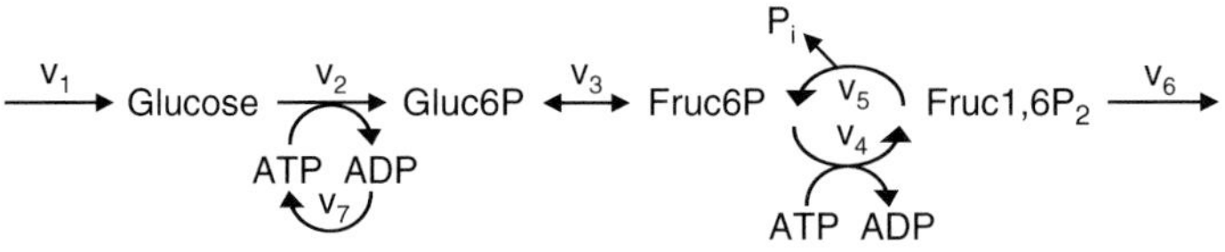

Figure 3.2 Toy model of the upper glycolysis. The model involves the reactions glucose uptake (v_1), the phosphorylation of glucose under conversion of ATP to ADP by the enzyme hexokinase (v_2), intramolecular rearrangments by the enzyme phosphoglucoisomerase (v_3), a second phosphorylation (and ATP/ADP conversion) by phosphofructokinase (v_4), dephosphorylation without involvement of ATP/ADP by fructose-bisphosphatase (v_5), and splitting of the hexose (6-C-sugar) into two trioses (3-C-sugars) by aldolase (v_6). Abbreviations: Gluc-6P – glucose-6-phosphate, Fruc-6P – fructose-6-phosphate, Fruc-1,6P$_2$ – fructose-1,6-bisphosphate.

$$\begin{aligned}
&\frac{\mathrm{d}}{\mathrm{d}t}Glucose = v_1 - v_2\\
&\frac{\mathrm{d}}{\mathrm{d}t}Gluc6P = v_2 - v_3\\
&\frac{\mathrm{d}}{\mathrm{d}t}Fruc6P = v_3 - v_4 + v_5\\
&\frac{\mathrm{d}}{\mathrm{d}t}Fruc1,6P_2 = v_4 - v_5 - v_6\\
&\frac{\mathrm{d}}{\mathrm{d}t}ATP = -\frac{\mathrm{d}}{\mathrm{d}t}ADP = -v_2 - v_4 + v_7.
\end{aligned} \tag{3.1}$$

With mass action kinetics, the rate equations read $v_1 = \text{const.} = k_1$, $v_2 = k_2 \cdot Glucose \cdot ATP$, $v_3 = k_3 \cdot Gluc6P - k_{-3} \cdot Fruc6P$, $v_4 = k_4 \cdot Fruc6P \cdot ATP$, $v_5 = k_5 \cdot Fruc1{,}6P_2$, $v_6 = k_6 \cdot Fruc1{,}6P_2$, and $v_7 = k_7 \cdot ADP$. Given the values of the parameters k_i, $i = 1, \ldots, 7$ and the initial concentrations, one may simulate the time behavior of the network as depicted in Figure 3.3.

We see that starting with zero concentrations of all hexoses (here glucose, fructose, and their phosphorylated versions), they accumulate until production and degradation are balanced. Finally, they approach a steady state. ATP rises and then decreases in the same way as ADP decreases and rises, while their sum remains constant. This is due to the conservation of adenine nucleotides, which could be revealed by stoichiometric analysis (Section 2.2).

For this upper glycolysis model, the concentration vector is $\boldsymbol{S} = (Glucose, Gluc6P, Fruc6P, Fruc1{,}6P_2, ATP, ADP)^{\mathrm{T}}$, the vector of reaction rates is $\mathbf{v} = (v_1, v_2, \ldots, v_7)^{\mathrm{T}}$, and the stoichiometric matrix reads

$$\boldsymbol{N} = \begin{pmatrix} 1 & -1 & 0 & 0 & 0 & 0 & 0\\ 0 & 1 & -1 & 0 & 0 & 0 & 0\\ 0 & 0 & 1 & -1 & 1 & 0 & 0\\ 0 & 0 & 0 & 1 & -1 & -1 & 0\\ 0 & -1 & 0 & -1 & 0 & 0 & 1\\ 0 & 1 & 0 & 1 & 0 & 0 & -1 \end{pmatrix}. \tag{3.2}$$

It comprises $r = 7$ reactions and has Rank $\boldsymbol{N} = 5$. Thus, the kernel matrix (see Section 2.2.2) has two linear independent columns. A possible representation is

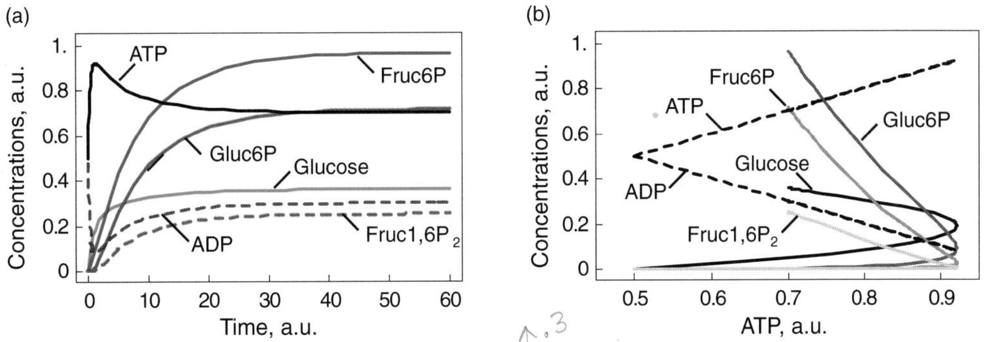

Figure 3.3 Dynamic behavior of the upper glycolysis model (Figure 3.2 and Eq. (3.1)). Initial conditions at $t = 0$: $Glucose(0) = Gluc\text{-}6P(0) = Fruc\text{-}6P(0) = Fruc\text{-}1{,}6P_2(0) = 0$ and $ATP(0) = ADP(0) = 0.5$ (arbitrary units). Parameters: $k_1 = 0.25, k_2 = 1, k_3 = 1, k_{-3} = 1, k_4 = 1, k_5 = 1, k_6 = 1$, and $k_7 = 2.5$. The steady-state concentrations are $Glucose^{st} = 0.357$, $Gluc\text{-}6P^{st} = 0.714$, $Fruc\text{-}6P^{st} = 0.964$, $Fruc\text{-}1{,}6P_2{}^{st} = 0.2$, and $ATP^{st} = 0.7$, and $ADP^{st} = 0.25$. The steady-state fluxes are $J_1 = J_2 = J_3 = J_5 = J_6 = 0.25, J_4 = 0.5$, and $J_7 = 0.75$. (a) Time-course plots (concentration versus time), (b) phase-plane plot (concentrations versus concentration of ATP with varying time); all curves start at $ATP = 0.5$ for $t = 0$.

$$\boldsymbol{K} = (\boldsymbol{k}_1 \quad \boldsymbol{k}_2) \quad \text{with} \quad \begin{aligned} \boldsymbol{k}_1 &= (0 \quad 0 \quad 0 \quad 1 \quad 1 \quad 0 \quad 1)^{\mathrm{T}}, \\ \boldsymbol{k}_2 &= (1 \quad 1 \quad 1 \quad -1 \quad -2 \quad 1 \quad 0)^{\mathrm{T}}. \end{aligned} \tag{3.3}$$

Figure 3.4 shows the flux and concentration control coefficients (see Section 2.3.2) for the model of upper glycolysis in gray scale (see scaling bar). Reaction v_1 has a

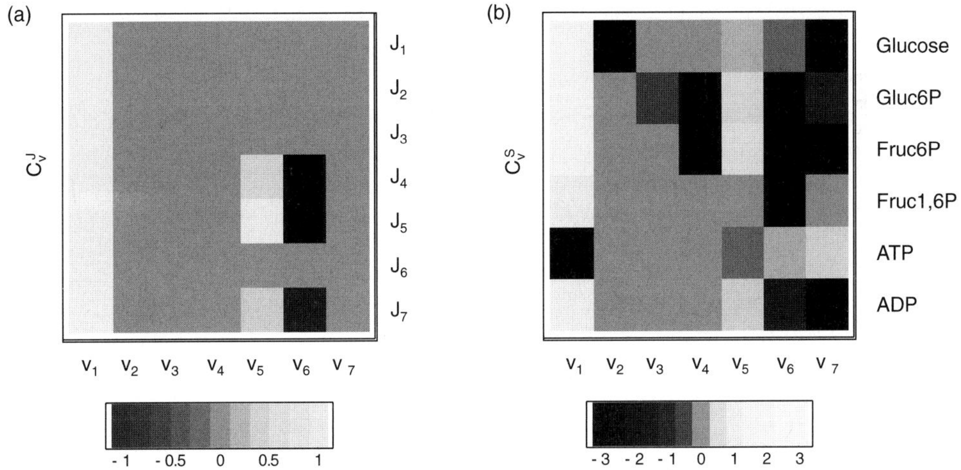

Figure 3.4 Flux and concentration control coefficients for the glycolysis model in Figure 3.2 with the parameters given in the legend of Figure 3.3. Values of the coefficients are indicated in gray-scale: gray means zero control, white or light gray indicates positive control, dark gray or black negative control, respectively.

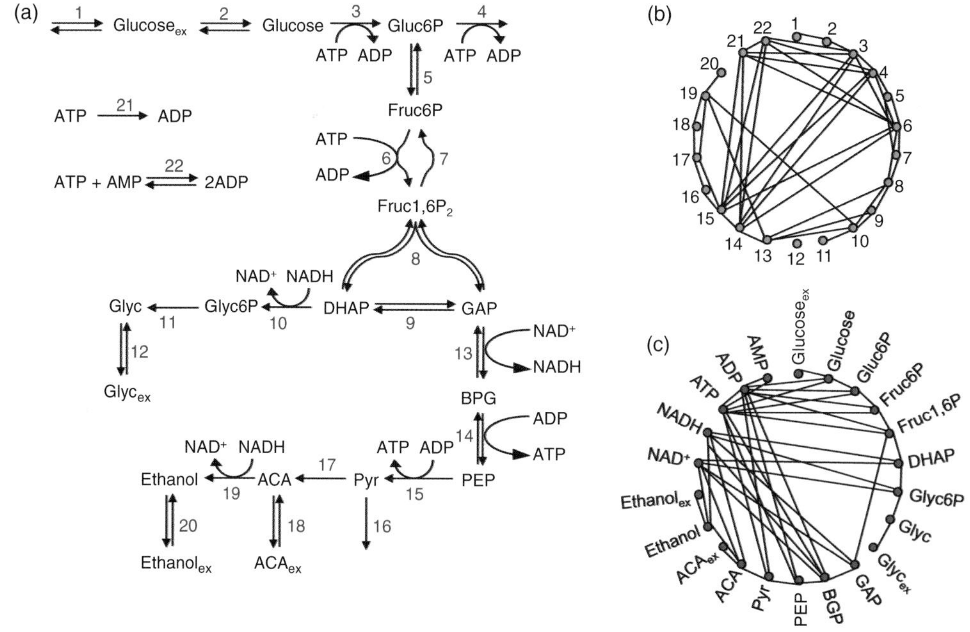

Figure 3.5 Full glycolysis models. (a) Main reactions and metabolites, (b) network of reactions connected by common metabolites, (c) network of metabolites connected by common reactions.

flux control of 1 over all steady-state fluxes, reactions v_2, v_3, v_4, and v_7 have no control over fluxes; they are dominated by v_1. Reactions v_5 and v_6 have positive or negative control over J_4, J_5, and J_7, respectively, since they control the turnover of fructose phosphates.

The concentration control shows a more interesting pattern. As a rule of thumb, it holds that producing reactions have a positive control and degrading reactions have a negative control, such as v_1 and v_2 for glucose. But also distant reactions can exert concentration control, such as v_4 to v_6 over Gluc6P.

More comprehensive models of glycolysis can be used to study details of the dynamics, such as the occurrence of oscillations or the effect of perturbations. Examples are the models of Hynne and colleagues [2] or the Reuss group [3, 4]. An overview of the most important reactions in glycolysis is given in Figure 3.5.

3.1.3
Threonine Synthesis Pathway Model

Threonine is an amino acid, which is essential for birds and mammals. The synthesis pathway from aspartate involves five steps (Figure 3.6). It is known for a long time and has attracted some interest with respect to its economic industrial production for a variety of uses. The kinetics of all the five enzymes from *Escherichia coli* have been

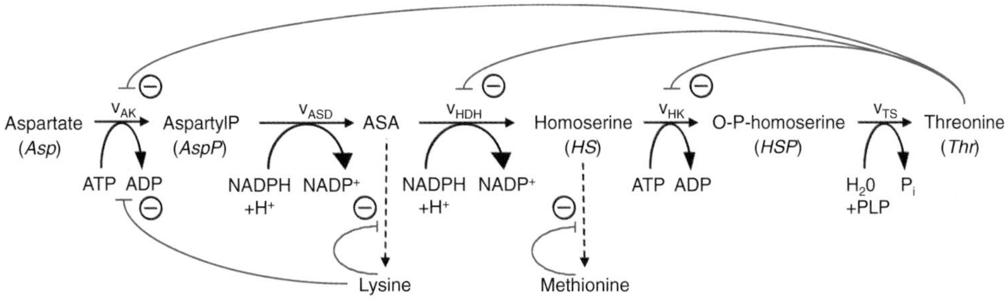

Figure 3.6 Model of the threonine pathway. Aspartate is converted into threonine in five steps. Threonine exerts negative feedback on its producing reactions. The pathway consumes ATP and NADPH.

studied extensively; the complete genome sequence of this organism is now known and there is an extensive range of genetic tools available. The intensive study and the availability of kinetic information make it a good example for metabolic modeling of the pathway.

The reaction system can be described with the following set of differential equations:

$$\begin{aligned}
\frac{\mathrm{d}}{\mathrm{d}t}Asp &= -v_{\mathrm{AKI}} - v_{\mathrm{AKIII}} \\
\frac{\mathrm{d}}{\mathrm{d}t}AspP &= v_{\mathrm{AKI}} + v_{\mathrm{AKIII}} - v_{\mathrm{ASD}} \\
\frac{\mathrm{d}}{\mathrm{d}t}ASA &= v_{\mathrm{ASD}} - v_{\mathrm{HDH}} \\
\frac{\mathrm{d}}{\mathrm{d}t}HS &= v_{\mathrm{HDH}} - v_{\mathrm{HK}} \\
\frac{\mathrm{d}}{\mathrm{d}t}HSP &= v_{\mathrm{HK}} - v_{\mathrm{TS}} \\
\frac{\mathrm{d}}{\mathrm{d}t}Thr &= v_{\mathrm{TS}},
\end{aligned} \tag{3.4}$$

with

$$v_{\mathrm{AKI}} = \frac{V_{\mathrm{AKI}} \cdot \left(Asp \cdot ATP - \frac{AspP \cdot ADP}{K_{\mathrm{eq,AK}}}\right)}{\left(K_{\mathrm{Asp,AKI}} \cdot \frac{1 + \left(\frac{Thr}{K_{\mathrm{iThr,AKI}}}\right)^{h_1}}{1 + \left(\frac{Thr}{\alpha_{\mathrm{AKI}} \cdot K_{\mathrm{iThr,AKI}}}\right)^{h_1}} + AspP \cdot \frac{K_{\mathrm{Asp,AKI}}}{K_{\mathrm{AspP,AKI}}} + Asp\right) \cdot \left(K_{\mathrm{ATP,AKI}} \cdot \left(1 + \frac{ADP}{K_{\mathrm{ADP,AKI}}}\right) + ATP\right)}$$

$K_{\mathrm{eq,AK}} = 6.4 \times 10^{-4}$, $K_{\mathrm{Asp,AKI}} = 0.97 \pm 0.48\,\mathrm{mM}$, $K_{\mathrm{ATP,AKI}} = 0.98 \pm 0.5\,\mathrm{mM}$, $K_{\mathrm{AspP,AKI}} = 0.017 \pm 0.004\,\mathrm{mM}$, $K_{\mathrm{ADP,AKI}} = 0.25\,\mathrm{mM}$, $K_{\mathrm{iThr,AKI}} = 0.167 \pm 0.003\,\mathrm{mM}$, $h_1 = 4.09 \pm 0.26$,

$\alpha_{AKI} = 2.47 \pm 0.17,$

$$v_{AK\,III} = \frac{V_{AK\,III} \cdot \left(Asp \cdot ATP - \frac{AspP \cdot ADP}{K_{eq,\,AK}}\right)}{\left(1 + \left(\frac{Lys}{K_{1\,Lys}}\right)^{h_{Lys}}\right)\left(K_{Asp,\,AK\,III}\left(1 + \frac{AspP}{K_{AspP,\,AK\,III}}\right) + Asp\right) \cdot \left(K_{ATP,\,AK\,III}\left(1 + \frac{ADP}{K_{ADP,\,AK\,III}}\right) + ATP\right)}$$

$K_{eq,AK} = 6.4 \times 10^{-4}$, $K_{Asp,AK\,III} = 0.32 \pm 0.08$ mM, $K_{ATP,AK\,III} = 0.22 \pm 0.02$ mM $K_{AspP,AK\,III} = 0.017 \pm 0.004$ mM, $K_{ADP,AK\,III} = 0.25$ mM, $K_{iLys} = 0.391 \pm 0.08$ mM, $h_{Lys} = 2.8 \pm 1.4$,

$$v_{ASD} = \frac{V_{ASD} \cdot \left(AspP \cdot NADPH - \frac{ASA \cdot NADP^+ \cdot P_i}{K_{eq,\,ASD}}\right)}{\left(K_{AspP,\,ASD}\left(1 + \frac{ASA}{K_{ASA,\,ASD}}\right) \cdot \left(1 + \frac{P_i}{K_{P_i}}\right) + AspP\right) \cdot \left(K_{NAPDH}\left(1 + \frac{NADP^+}{K_{NADP^+}}\right) + NADPH\right)}$$

$K_{eq,ASD} = 2.84 \times 10^5$, $K_{AspP,ASD} = 0.022 \pm 0.001$ mM, $K_{NADPH,ASD} = 0.029 \pm 0.002$ mM, $K_{ASA,ASD} = 0.11 \pm 0.008$ mM, $K_{NADP^+,ASD} = 0.144 \pm 0.02$ mM, $K_{P_i} = 10.2 \pm 1.4$ mM,

$$v_{HDH} = \frac{V_{HDH} \cdot \left(ASA \cdot NADPH - \frac{HS \cdot NADP^+}{K_{eq,HDH}}\right)}{\left(\frac{1 + \left(\frac{Thr}{K_{iThr,2}}\right)^{h_2}}{1 + \left(\frac{Thr}{\alpha_2 \cdot K_{iThr,2}}\right)^{h_2}}\right)\left(K_{ASA,HDH}\left(1 + \frac{HS}{K_{HS,HDH}}\right) + ASA\right) \cdot \left(K_{NADPH,HDH}\left(1 + \frac{NADP^+}{K_{NADP^+,AKIII}}\right) + NADPH\right)}$$

$K_{eq,HDH} = 1 \times 10^{11}\ M^{-1}$, $K_{ASA,HDH} = 0.24 \pm 0.03$ mM, $K_{NADPH,HDH} = 0.037 \pm 0.006$ mM, $K_{hs,HDH} = 3.39 \pm 0.33$ mM, $K_{NADP^+,HDH} = 0.067 \pm 0.006$ mM, $K_{iThr,2} = 0.097$ mM, $h_2 = 1.41$, $\alpha_2 = 3.93$,

$$v_{HK} = \frac{V_{HK} \cdot hs \cdot ATP}{\left(K_{HS,HK}\left(1 + \frac{ATP}{K_{iATP,HK}}\right) \cdot \left(1 + \frac{Thr}{K_{iThr,HK}}\right) + hs\right) \cdot \left(K_{ATP,HK}\left(1 + \frac{hs}{K_{iHS,HK}}\right) + ATP\right) \cdot \left(1 + \frac{Lys}{K_{iLys,HK}}\right)}$$

$K_{HS,HK} = 0.11$ mM, $K_{ATP,HK} = 0.072$ mM, $K_{iThr,HK} = 1.09$ mM, $K_{iLys,HK} = 9.45$ mM, $K_{iHS,HK} = 4.7$ mM, $K_{iATP,HK} = 4.35$ mM

$$v_{TS} = \frac{V_{TS} \cdot HSP}{K_{HSP,TS} + HSP}$$

$K_{HSP,TS} = 0.31 \pm 0.03$ mM.

This system has no nontrivial steady state, i.e., no steady state with nonzero flux, since aspartate is always degraded, while threonine is only produced. The same imbalance holds for the couples ATP/ADP and $NADPH + H^+/NADP^+$. The dynamics is shown in Figure 3.7.

Threonine exerts feedback inhibition on the pathway producing it. This is illustrated in Figure 3.8. The higher the threonine concentration, the lower the

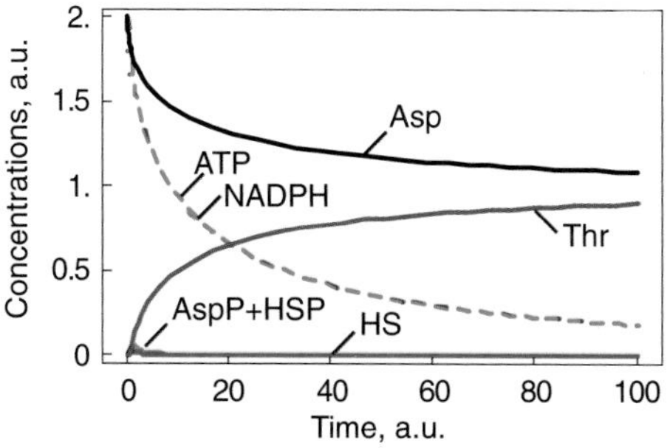

Figure 3.7 Dynamics of the threonine pathway model (Figure 3.6, Eq. (3.4)). The parameters are given in the text.

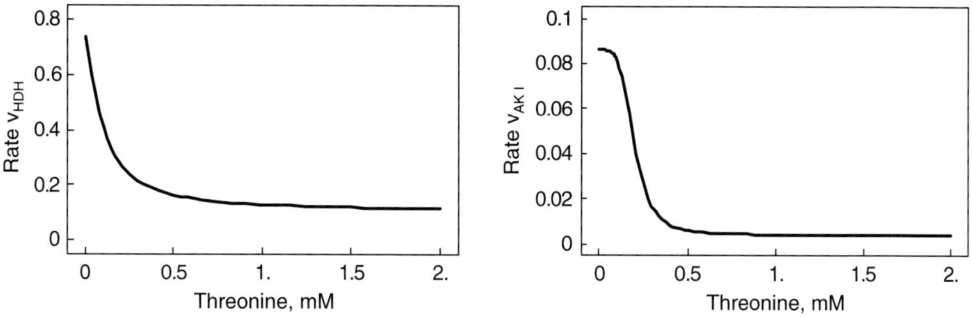

Figure 3.8 Effect of feedback inhibition in the model depicted in Figure 3.6.

rates of inhibited reactions. The effect is that production of threonine is downregulated as long as its level is sufficient, thereby saving aspartate and energy.

3.2 Signaling Pathways

Summary

This section introduces the structure of different cellular signaling pathways and their typical constituents such as receptors, G proteins, MAP kinase cascades, or phosphorelay systems. Different modeling approaches and various specific models are discussed. We analyze how the structure of pathways encoded in respective model assumptions determines the steady states and dynamic properties of signaling pathways. To describe the dynamic properties of signaling pathways, quantitative measures are used to assess the amplitude and duration of a signal or the crosstalk between distinct signaling pathways.

3.2.1 Introduction

Upon intercellular communication or cellular stress response, the cell senses extracellular signals. They are transformed into intracellular signals and sequences of reactions. Different external changes or events may stimulate signaling. Typical stimuli are hormones, pheromones, heat, cold, light, osmotic pressure, appearance, or concentration change of substances like glucose or K^+, Ca^+, or cAMP.

On a molecular level, signaling involves the same type of processes as metabolism: production or degradation of substances, molecular modifications (mainly phosphorylation, but also methylation, acetylation), and activation or inhibition of reactions. From a modeling point of view, there are some important differences between signaling and metabolism. First, signaling pathways serve for information processing and transfer of information, while metabolism provides mainly mass transfer. Second, the metabolic network is determined by the present set of enzymes catalyzing the reactions. Signaling pathways involve compounds of different types; they may form highly organized complexes and may assemble dynamically upon occurrence of the signal. Third, the quantity of converted material is high in metabolism (amounts are usually given in concentrations on the order of μM or mM) compared to the number of molecules involved in signaling processes (typical abundance of proteins in signal cascades is on the order of $10–10^4$ molecules per cell). Finally, different amounts of components have an effect on the concentration ratio of catalysts and substrates. In metabolism, this ratio is usually low, i.e., the enzyme concentration is much lower than the substrate concentration, which gives rise to the quasi-steady state assumption used in Michaelis–Menten kinetics (Section 2.1). In signaling processes, amounts of catalysts and their substrates are frequently in the same order of magnitude.

Modeling of the dynamic behavior of signaling pathways is often not straightforward. Knowledge about components of the pathway and their interactions is still limited and incomplete. The interpretation of experimental data is context- and knowledge-dependent. Furthermore, the effect of a signal often changes the state of the whole cell, and this implies difficulties for determination of system limits. But in many cases, we may apply the same tools as introduced in Chapter 2.

3.2.2 Function and Structure of Intra- and Intercellular Communication

Cells have a broad spectrum of molecular "facilities" to receive and process signals; not all of them can be considered here. A typical sequence of events in signaling pathways is shown in Figure 3.9 and proceeds as follows.

The "signal" (a substance acting as ligand or a physical stimulus) approaches the cell surface and is bound or sensed by a transmembrane receptor. The receptor changes its state from susceptible to active and stimulates an internal signaling cascade. This cascade frequently includes a series of changes of protein phosphorylation states. Activated proteins may cross the nuclear membrane and, eventually, transcription factors are activated or deactivated. Such a transcription factor

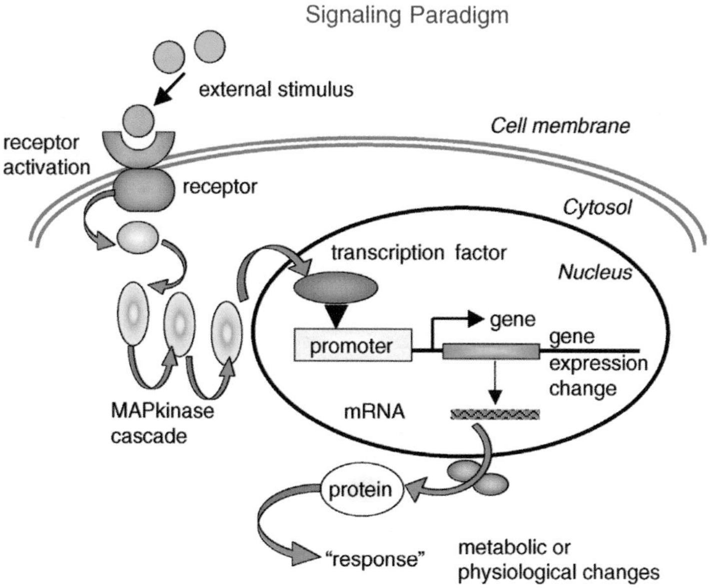

Figure 3.9 Visualization of the signaling paradigm (for description see the text). The receptor is stimulated by a ligand or another kind of signal, and it changes its own state from susceptible to active. The active receptor initiates the internal signaling cascade including a series of protein phosphorylation state changes. Subsequently, transcription factors are activated or deactivated. The transcription factors regulate the transcription rate of a set of genes. The absolute amount or the relative changes in protein concentrations alter the state of the cell and trigger the actual response to the signal.

changes its binding properties to regulatory regions on the DNA upstream of a set of genes; the transcription rate of these genes is altered (typically increased). Either newly produced proteins or the changes in protein concentration cause the actual response of the cell to the signal. In addition to this downstream program, signaling pathways are regulated by a number of control mechanisms including feedback and feed-forward activation or inhibition. Fast tracks of signal transduction work without changes in gene expression by changing binding properties or activity pattern of proteins (e.g., binding of Ste5 to $G\beta\gamma$ or regulation of Fps1 by $Hog1P_2$).

This is the typical picture; however, many pathways may work in completely different manner. As example, an overview on signaling pathways that are stimulated in yeast stress response is given in Figure 3.10.

3.2.3
Receptor–Ligand Interactions

Many receptors are transmembrane proteins; they receive the signal and transmit it. Upon signal sensing, they change their conformation. In the active form, they are able to initiate a downstream process within the cell (Figure 3.11).

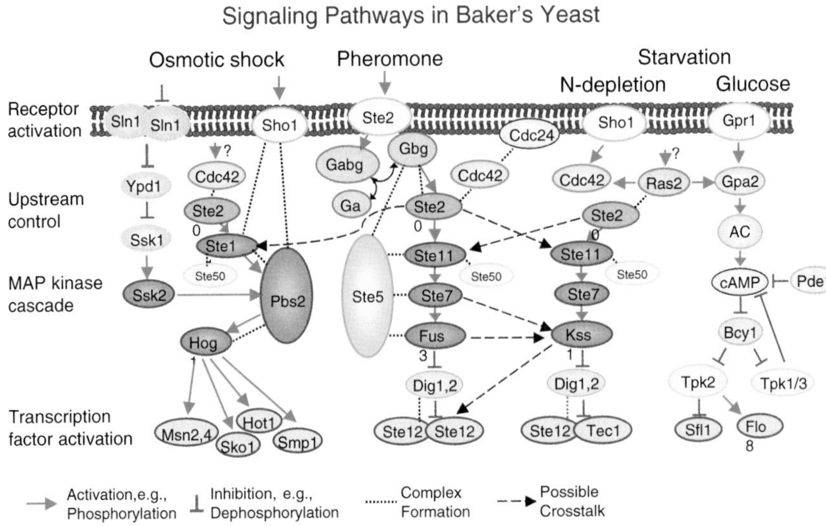

Figure 3.10 Overview on signaling pathways in yeast: HOG pathway activated by osmotic shock, pheromone pathway activated by a pheromone from cells of opposite mating type, and pseudohyphal growth pathway stimulated by starvation conditions. In each case, the signal interacts with the receptor. The receptor activates a cascade of intracellular processes including complex formations, phosphorylations, and transport steps. A MAP kinase cascade is a particular part of many signaling pathways; their components are indicated by bold border. Eventually, transcription factors are activated that regulate the expression of a set of genes. Beside the indicated connections, further interactions of components are possible. For example, crosstalk may occur, that is the activation of the downstream part of one pathway by a component of another pathway. This is supported by the frequent incidence of some proteins like Ste11 in the scheme.

The simplest concept of the interaction between receptor R and ligand L is reversible binding to form the active complex LR:

$$L + R \leftrightarrow LR. \quad (3.5)$$

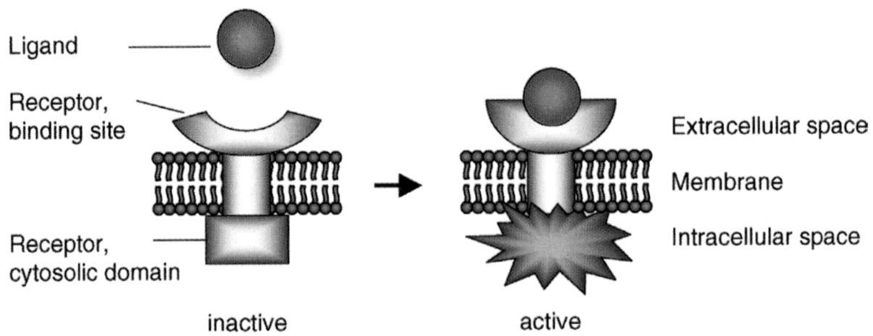

Figure 3.11 Schematic representation of receptor activation.

The dissociation constant is calculated as

$$K_D = \frac{L \cdot R}{LR}. \tag{3.6}$$

Typical values for K_D are 10^{-12}–10^{-6} M.

Cells have the ability to regulate the number and the activity of specific receptors, for example, in order to weaken the signal transmission during long-term stimulation. Balancing production and degradation regulates the number of receptors. Phosphorylation of serine/threonine or tyrosine residues of the cytosolic domain by protein kinases mainly regulates the activity. Hence, a more realistic scenario for ligand–receptor interaction is depicted in Figure 3.12(a).

For a more detailed model, we assume that the receptor is present in an inactive state R_i or in a susceptible state R_s. The susceptible form can interact with the ligand to form the active state R_a. The inactive or the susceptible forms are produced from precursors (v_{pi}, v_{ps}); all three forms may be degraded (v_{di}, v_{ds}, v_{da}). The rates of production and degradation processes as well as the equilibria between different states might be influenced by the cell's state, for example, by the cell-cycle stage. In general, the dynamics of this scenario can be described by the following set of differential equations:

$$\begin{aligned} \frac{d}{dt} R_i &= v_{pi} - v_{di} - v_{is} + v_{si} + v_{ai} \\ \frac{d}{dt} R_s &= v_{ps} - v_{ds} + v_{is} - v_{si} - v_{sa} + v_{as} \\ \frac{d}{dt} R_a &= -v_{da} + v_{sa} - v_{as} - v_{ai}. \end{aligned} \tag{3.7}$$

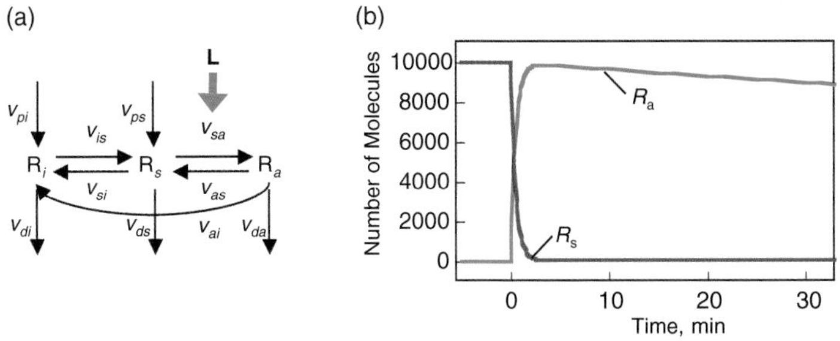

Figure 3.12 Receptor activation by ligand. (a) Schematic representation: L – ligand, R_i – inactive receptor, R_s – susceptible receptor, R_a – active receptor. v_{p*} – production steps, v_{d*} – degradation steps, other steps – transition between inactive, susceptible, and active state of receptor. (b) Time course of active (red line) and susceptible (blue line) receptor after stimulation with 1 μM α-factor at $t = 0$. The total number of receptors is 10,000. The concentration of the active receptor increases immediately and then declines slowly while the susceptible receptor is effectively reduced to zero.

For the production terms, we may either assume constant values or (as mentioned above) rates that depend on the current cell state. The degradation terms might be assumed to be linearly dependent on the concentration of their substrates ($v_{d^*} = k_{d^*} \cdot R_*$). This may also be a first guess for the state changes of the receptor (e.g., $v_{is} = k_{is} \cdot R_i$). The receptor activation is dependent on the ligand concentration (or any other value related to the signal). A linear approximation of the respective rate is $v_{sa} = k_{sa} \cdot R_s \cdot L$. If the receptor is a dimer or oligomer, it might be sensible to include this information into the rate expression for receptor activation as $v_{sa} = k_{sa} \cdot R_s \cdot K_B^n \cdot L^n/(1 + K_B^n \cdot L^n)$, where K_B denotes the binding constant to the monomer and n the Hill coefficient (Section 2.1, Eq. (2.44)).

Example 3.1

An experimentally confirmed example for the activation of receptor and G protein of the pheromone pathway has been presented by Yi and colleagues [5] for the binding of the pheromone α-factor to the receptor Ste2 in yeast. Concerning the receptor activation dynamics, they report a susceptible and an active form of the receptor, but no inactive form ($R_i = 0$, $v_{*i} = v_{i^*} = 0$). The remaining rates are determined as follows:

$$\begin{aligned} v_{ps} &= k_{ps} \\ v_{ds} &= k_{ds} \cdot R_s \\ v_{da} &= k_{da} \cdot R_a \\ v_{sa} &= k_{sa} \cdot R_s \cdot L \\ v_{as} &= k_{as} \cdot R_a, \end{aligned} \tag{3.8}$$

with the following values for the rate constants: $k_{ps} = 4$ molecules per cell per second, $k_{ds} = 4 \times 10^{-4}\,s^{-1}$, $k_{da} = 4 \times 10^{-3}\,s^{-1}$, $k_{sa} = 2 \times 10^6\,M^{-1}\,s^{-1}$, and $k_{as} = 1 \times 10^{-2}\,s^{-1}$. The time course of receptor activation is depicted in Figure 3.12.

3.2.4 Structural Components of Signaling Pathways

Signaling pathways may constitute highly complex networks, but it has been discovered that they are frequently composed of typical building blocks. These components include Ras proteins, G protein cycles, phosphorelay systems, and MAP kinase cascades. In this section, we will discuss their general composition and function as well as modeling approaches.

3.2.4.1 G proteins

G proteins are essential parts of many signaling pathways. The reason for their name is that they bind the guanine nucleotides GDP and GTP. They are heterotrimers, i.e., they consist of three different subunits. Note the difference to small G proteins consisting of one monomer, which are discussed below. G proteins are associated to cell surface receptors with a heptahelical transmembrane structure, the G protein-coupled receptors (GPCR). Signal transduction cascades involving (i) such a transmembrane surface receptor, (ii) an associated G protein, and (iii) an intracellular effector that produces a second messenger play an important role in cellular communication and are well-studied [6, 7]. In humans, GPCR mediate responses to light, flavors, odors, numerous hormones, neurotransmitters, and other signals [8–10]. In unicellular eukaryotes, receptors of this type mediate signals that affect such basic processes as cell division, cell–cell fusion (mating), morphogenesis, and chemotaxis [8, 11–13].

The cycle of G protein activation and inactivation is shown in Figure 3.13. When GDP is bound, the G protein α subunit (Gα) is associated with the G protein $\beta\gamma$ heterodimer (G$\beta\gamma$) and is inactive. Ligand binding to a receptor promotes guanine nucleotide exchange; Gα releases GDP, binds GTP, and dissociates from G$\beta\gamma$. The dissociated subunits Gα or G$\beta\gamma$, or both, are then free to activate target proteins (downstream effectors), which initiates signaling. When GTP is hydrolyzed, the subunits are able to reassociate. G$\beta\gamma$ antagonizes receptor action by inhibiting guanine nucleotide exchange. Regulator of G protein signaling (RGS) proteins bind to Gα, stimulate GTP hydrolysis, and thereby reverse G protein activation. This general scheme also holds for the regulation of small monomeric Ras-like GTPases, such as Rho. In this case, the receptor, G$\beta\gamma$, and RGS are replaced by GEF and GAP (see below).

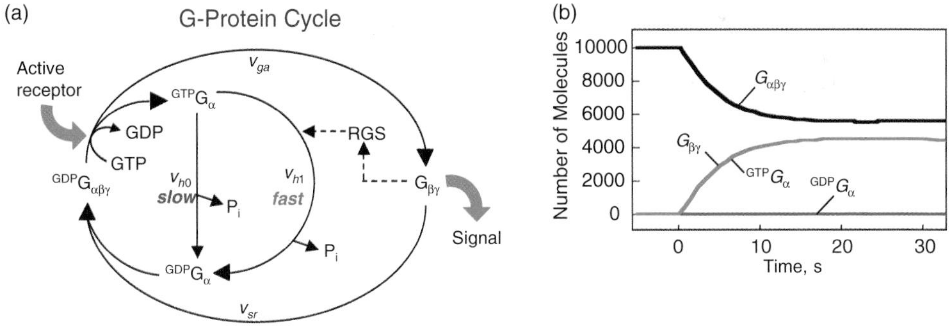

Figure 3.13 Activation cycle of G protein. (a) Without activation, the heterotrimeric G protein is bound to GPD. Upon activation by the activated receptor, an exchange of GDP with GTP occurs and the G protein is divided into GTP-bound Gα and the heterodimer G$\beta\gamma$. Gα-bound GTP is hydrolyzed, either slowly in reaction v_{h0} or fast in reaction v_{h1} supported by the RGS protein. GDP-bound Gα can reassociate with G$\beta\gamma$ (reaction v_{sr}). (b) Time course of G protein activation. The total number of molecules is 10,000. The concentration of GDP-bound Gα is low for the whole period due to fast complex formation with the heterodimer G$\beta\gamma$.

Direct targets include different types of effectors, such as adenylyl cyclase, phospholipase C, exchange factors for small GTPases, some calcium and potassium channels, plasma membrane Na^+/H^+ exchangers, and certain protein kinases [6, 14–16]. Typically, these effectors produce second messengers or other biochemical changes that lead to stimulation of a protein kinase or a protein kinase cascade (or, as mentioned, are themselves a protein kinase). Signaling persists until GTP is hydrolyzed to GDP and the Gα and Gβγ subunits reassociate, completing the cycle of activation. The strength of the G protein–initiated signal depends on (i) the rate of nucleotide exchange, (ii) the rate of spontaneous GTP hydrolysis, (iii) the rate of RGS-supported GTP hydrolysis, and (iv) the rate of subunit reassociation. RGS proteins act as GTPase-activating proteins (GAPs) for a variety of different Gα classes. Thereby, they shorten the lifetime of the activated state of a G protein, and contribute to signal cessation. Furthermore, they may contain additional modular domains with signaling functions and contribute to diversity and complexity of the cellular signaling networks [17–20].

Example 3.2

The model of the heterotrimeric G protein cycle of the yeast pheromone pathway was already mentioned in Example 3.1 and it is linked to the receptor activation model via the concentration of the active receptor. The G protein cycle model comprises two ODEs and two algebraic equations for the mass conservation of the subunits Gα and Gβγ:

$$
\begin{aligned}
\frac{d}{dt}G_{\alpha\beta\gamma} &= -v_{ga} + v_{sr} \\
\frac{d}{dt}G_{\alpha}GTP &= v_{ga} - v_{h0} - v_{h1} \\
G_{total\alpha} &= G_{\alpha\beta\gamma} + G_{\alpha}GTP + G_{\alpha}GDP \\
G_{total\beta\gamma} &= G_{\alpha\beta\gamma} + G_{\beta\gamma}.
\end{aligned}
\tag{3.9}
$$

The rate equations for the G protein activation, v_{ga}, the hydrolysis of $G_{\alpha}GTP$, v_{h0} and v_{h1}, and the subunit reassociation, v_{sr}, follow simple mass action kinetics:

$$
\begin{aligned}
v_{ga} &= k_{ga} \cdot R_a \cdot G_{\alpha\beta\gamma} \\
v_{hi} &= k_{hi} \cdot G_{\alpha}GTP, \quad i = 0, 1 \\
v_{sr} &= k_{sr} \cdot G_{\beta\gamma} \cdot G_{\alpha}GDP.
\end{aligned}
\tag{3.10}
$$

The parameters are $k_{ga} = 1 \times 10^{-5}$ (molecule per cell)$^{-1}$ s^{-1}, $k_{h0} = 0.004\,s^{-1}$, $k_{h1} = 0.11\,s^{-1}$, and $k_{sr} = 1$(molecule per cell)$^{-1}$ s^{-1}. Note that in the original work, two different yeast strains have been considered. For the strains with a constantly active RGS (*SST2*$^+$) or with a deletion of RGS (*sst2Δ*), the rate constants k_{h1} and k_{h0} have been set to zero, respectively. The time courses are shown in Figure 3.13.

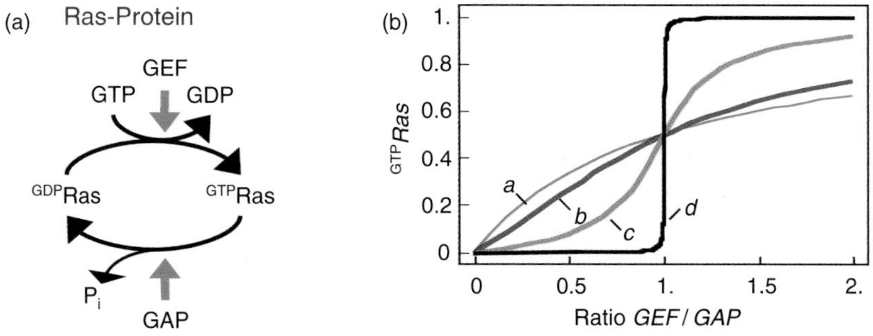

Figure 3.14 The Ras activation cycle. (a) Wiring diagram: GEF supports the transition form GDP-bound to GTP-bound states to activate Ras, while GAP induces hydrolysis of the bound GTP resulting in Ras deactivation. (b) Steady states of active Ras depending on the concentration ratio of its activator GEF and the inhibitor GAP. We compare the behavior for a model with mass action kinetics (curve a) with the behavior obtained with Michaelis–Menten kinetics for decreasing values of the K_m-value (curves b–d). The smaller the K_m-value, the more sigmoidal the response curve, leading to an almost steplike shape in the case of very low K_m-values. Parameters: $Ras_{total} = RasGTP + RasGDP = 1$, $k_1 = k_2 = 1$ (all curves), (b) $K_{m1} = K_{m2} = 1$, (c) $K_{m1} = K_{m2} = 0.1$, (d) $K_{m1} = K_{m2} = 0.001$.

3.2.4.2 **Small G proteins**

Small G proteins are monomeric G proteins with molecular weight of 20–40 kDa. Like heterotrimeric G proteins, their activity depends on the binding of GTP. More than a hundred small G proteins have been identified. They belong to five families: Ras, Rho, Rab, Ran, and Arf. They regulate a wide variety of cell functions as biological timers that initiate and terminate specific cell functions and determine the periods of time [21].

Ras proteins cycle between active and inactive states (Figure 3.14). The transition from GDP-bound to GTP-bound states is catalyzed by a guanine nucleotide exchange factor (GEF), which induces exchange between the bound GDP and the cellular GTP. The reverse process is facilitated by a GAP, which induces hydrolysis of the bound GTP. Its dynamics can be described with the following equation with appropriate choice of the rates ν_{GEF} and ν_{GAP}:

$$\frac{d}{dt}RasGTP = -\frac{d}{dt}RasGDP = \nu_{GEF} - \nu_{GAP}$$
$$\nu_{GEF} = \frac{k_1 \cdot GEF \cdot RasGDP}{(K_{m1} + RasGDP)} \quad \text{and} \quad \nu_{GAP} = \frac{k_2 \cdot GAP \cdot RasGTP}{(K_{m2} + RasGTP)}. \tag{3.11}$$

Figure 3.14 illustrates the wiring of a Ras protein and the dependence of its activity on the concentration ratio of the activating GEF and the deactivating GAP.

Mutations of the *Ras* protooncogenes (H-*Ras*, N-*Ras*, K-*Ras*) are found in many human tumors. Most of these mutations result in the abolishment of normal GTPase activity of *Ras*. The Ras mutants can still bind to GAP, but cannot catalyze GTP hydrolysis. Therefore, they stay active for a long time.

3.2.4.3 **Phosphorelay Systems**

Most phosphorylation events in signaling pathways take place under repeated consumption of ATP. Phosphorelay (also called phosphotransfer) systems employ another mechanism: after an initial phosphorylation using ATP (or another phosphate donor), the phosphate group is transferred directly from one protein to the next without further consumption of ATP (or external donation of phosphate). Examples are the bacterial phosphoenolpyruvate:carbohydrate phosphotransferase [22–25], the two-component system of *E. coli* (see also Section 6.4 on robustness) or the Sln1 pathway involved in osmoresponse of yeast [26].

Figure 3.15 shows a scheme of a phosphorelay system from the high osmolarity glycerol (HOG) signaling pathway in yeast as well as a schematic representation of a phosphorelay system.

The phosphorelay system in the yeast HOG pathway is organized as follows [27]. It involves the transmembrane protein Sln1, which is present as a dimer. Under normal conditions, the pathway is active, since Sln1 continuously autophosphorylates at a histidine residue, Sln1H-P, under consumption of ATP. Subsequently, this phosphate group is transferred to an aspartate residue of Sln1 (resulting in Sln1A-P), then to a histidine residue of Ypd1, and finally to an aspartate residue of Ssk1. Ssk1 is continuously dephosphorylated by a phosphatase. Without stress, the proteins are mainly present in their phosphorylated form. The pathway is blocked by an increase in the external osmolarity and a concomitant loss of turgor pressure in the cell. The phosphorylation of Sln1 stops, the pathway runs out of transferable phosphate groups, and the concentration of unphosphorylated Ssk1 rises. This is the signal for the next part of the pathway. The temporal behavior of a generalized

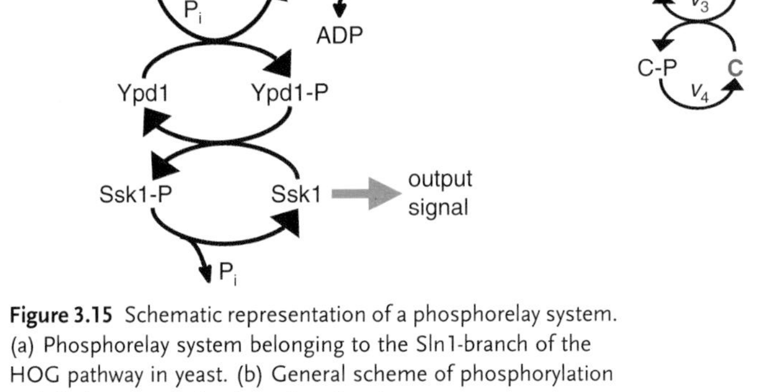

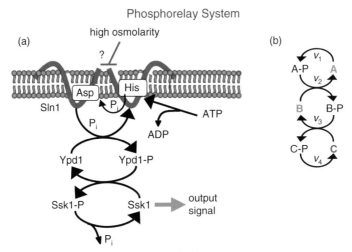

Figure 3.15 Schematic representation of a phosphorelay system. (a) Phosphorelay system belonging to the Sln1-branch of the HOG pathway in yeast. (b) General scheme of phosphorylation and dephosphorylation in a phosphorelay.

phosphorelay system (Figure 3.15) can be described with the following set of ODEs:

$$\begin{aligned}\frac{d}{dt}A &= -k_1 \cdot A + k_2 \cdot AP \cdot B\\ \frac{d}{dt}B &= -k_2 \cdot AP \cdot B + k_3 \cdot BP \cdot C\\ \frac{d}{dt}C &= -k_3 \cdot BP \cdot C + k_4 \cdot CP.\end{aligned} \tag{3.12}$$

For the ODE system in Eq. (3.12), the following conservation relations hold:

$$\begin{aligned}A_{\text{total}} &= A + AP\\ B_{\text{total}} &= B + BP\\ C_{\text{total}} &= C + CP.\end{aligned} \tag{3.13}$$

The existence of conservation relations is in agreement with the assumption that production and degradation of the proteins occurs on a larger time scale than the phosphorylation events.

The temporal behavior of a phosphorelay system upon external stimulation (here, setting the value of k_1 transiently to zero) is shown in Figure 3.16. Before the stimulus, the concentrations of A, B, and C assume low, but nonzero, levels due to continuous flow of phosphate groups through the network. During stimulation, they increase one after the other up to a maximal level that is determined by the total concentration of each protein. After removal of stimulus, all three concentrations return quickly to their initial values.

Figure 3.16(b) illustrates how the sensitivity of the phosphorelay system depends on the value of the terminal dephosphorylation of CP. For a low value of the rate constant k_4, e.g., $k_4 < 0.001$, the concentration C is low (almost) independent of the value of k_1, while for high k_4, e.g., $k_4 > 10$, the concentration C is (almost always) maximal. Changing of k_1 leads to a change of C-levels only in the range $0.001 < k_4 < 10$.

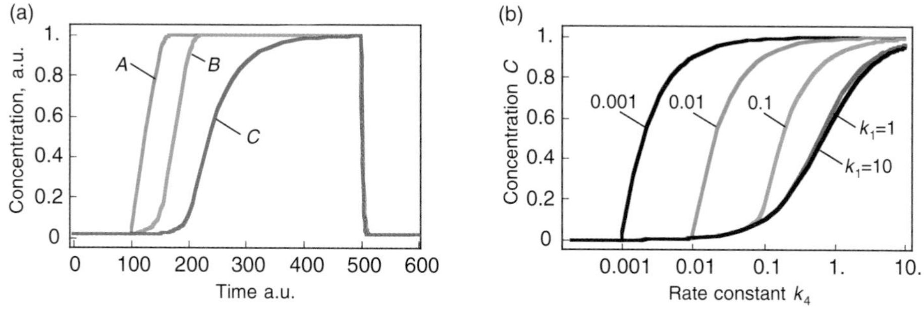

Figure 3.16 Dynamics of the phosphorelay system. (a) Time courses after stimulation from time 100 to time 500 (a.u.) by decreasing k_1 to zero. (b) Dependence of steady-state level of the phosphorelay output, C, on the cascade activation strength, k_1, and the terminal dephosphorylation, k_4. Parameter values: $k_1 = k_2 = k_3 = 1$, $k_4 = 0.02$, $A_{\text{total}} = B_{\text{total}} = C_{\text{total}} = 1$.

This system is an example for a case where we can draw preliminary conclusions about feasible parameter values just from the network structure and the task of the module. Another example for a phosphorelay system is discussed in Section 7.4.

3.2.4.4 MAP Kinase Cascades

Mitogen-activated protein kinases (MAPKs) are a family of serine/threonine kinases that transduce biochemical signals from the cell membrane to the nucleus in response to a wide range of stimuli. Independent or coupled kinase cascades participate in many different intracellular signaling pathways that control a spectrum of cellular processes, including cell growth, differentiation, transformation, and apoptosis. MAPK cascades are widely involved in eukaryotic signal transduction, and MAP kinase pathways are conserved from yeast to mammals.

A general scheme of a MAPK cascade is depicted in Figure 3.17. This pathway consists of several levels (usually three to four), where the activated kinase at each level phosphorylates the kinase at the next level down the cascade. The MAP kinase (MAPK) is at the terminal level of the cascade. It is activated by the MAPK kinase (MAPKK) by phosphorylation of two sites, conserved threonine and tyrosine residues. The MAPKK is itself phosphorylated at serine and threonine residues by the MAPKK kinase

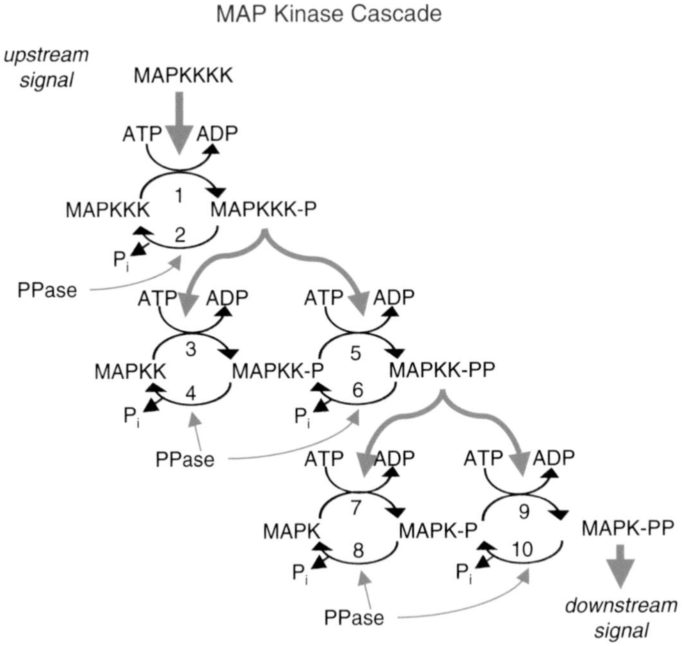

Figure 3.17 Schematic representation of the MAP kinase cascade. An upstream signal (often by a further kinase called MAP kinase kinase kinase kinase) causes phosphorylation of the MAPKKK. The phosphorylated MAPKKK in turn phosphorylates the protein at the next level. Dephosphorylation is assumed to occur continuously by phosphatases or autodephosphorylation.

Table 3.1 Names of the components of MAP kinase pathways in different organisms and different pathways.

Organism	Budding yeast		Xensopus oocytes	Human, cell cycle regulation		
	HOG pathway	Pheromone pathway			p38 pathway	JNK pathway
MAPKKK	Ssk2/Ssk22	Ste11	Mos	Rafs (c-, A- and B-),	Tak1	MEKKs
MAPKK	Pbs2	Ste7	MEK1	MEK1/2	MKK3/6	MKK4/7
MAPK	Hog1	Fus3	p42 MAPK	ERK1/2	p38	JNK1/2

(MAPKKK). Several mechanisms are known to activate MAPKKKs by phosphorylation of a tyrosine residue. In some cases, the upstream kinase may be considered as a MAPKKK kinase (MAPKKKK). Dephosphorylation of either residue is thought to inactivate the kinases, and mutants lacking either residue are almost inactive. At each cascade level, protein phosphatases can inactivate the kinase, although it is in some cases a matter of debate whether this dephosphorylation is performed by an independent protein or by the kinase itself as autodephosphorylation. Also ubiquitin-dependent degradation of phosphorylated proteins has been reported.

Although they are highly conserved throughout different species, elements of the MAPK cascade got different names in various studied systems. Some examples are listed in. Table 3.1 (see also [28]).

In the following, we will present typical modeling approaches for MAPK cascades and then discuss their functional properties. Their dynamics may be represented by the following ODE system:

$$
\begin{aligned}
&\frac{\mathrm{d}}{\mathrm{d}t} MAPKKK = -v_1 + v_2 \\
&\frac{\mathrm{d}}{\mathrm{d}t} MAPKKK\text{-}P = v_1 - v_2
\end{aligned}
\tag{3.14}
$$

$$
\begin{aligned}
&\frac{\mathrm{d}}{\mathrm{d}t} MAPKK = -v_3 + v_4 \\
&\frac{\mathrm{d}}{\mathrm{d}t} MAPKK\text{-}P = v_3 - v_4 - v_5 + v_6 \\
&\frac{\mathrm{d}}{\mathrm{d}t} MAPKK\text{-}P_2 = v_5 - v_6.
\end{aligned}
\tag{3.15}
$$

$$
\begin{aligned}
&\frac{\mathrm{d}}{\mathrm{d}t} MAPK = -v_7 + v_8 \\
&\frac{\mathrm{d}}{\mathrm{d}t} MAPK\text{-}P = v_7 - v_8 - v_9 + v_{10} \\
&\frac{\mathrm{d}}{\mathrm{d}t} MAPK\text{-}P_2 = v_9 - v_{10}.
\end{aligned}
\tag{3.16}
$$

The variables in the ODE system fulfill a set of moiety conservation relations, irrespective of the concrete choice of expression for the rates $v_1, \ldots, v_{10}$. It holds,

$$\begin{aligned} MAPKKK_{\text{total}} &= MAPKKK + MAPKKK\text{-}P \\ MAPKK_{\text{total}} &= MAPKK + MAPKK\text{-}P + MAPKK\text{-}P_2 \\ MAPK_{\text{total}} &= MAPK + MAPK\text{-}P + MAPK\text{-}P_2. \end{aligned} \tag{3.17}$$

The conservation relations reflect the fact that we do not consider production or degradation of the involved proteins in this model. This is justified by the supposition that protein production and degradation take place on a different time scale than signal transduction.

The choice of the expressions for the rates is a matter of elaborateness of experimental knowledge and of modeling taste. We will discuss here different possibilities. First, assuming only mass action results in linear and bilinear expression such as

$$\begin{aligned} v_1 &= k_{\text{kinase}} \cdot MAPKKK \cdot MAPKKKK \\ v_2 &= k_{\text{phosphatase}} \cdot MAPKKK\text{-}P. \end{aligned} \tag{3.18}$$

The kinetic constants k_{kinase} and $k_{\text{phosphatase}}$ are first- and second-order rate constants, respectively. In these expressions, the concentrations of the donor and acceptor of the transferred phosphate group, ATP and ADP, are assumed to be constant and included in the rate constants. Considering ATP and ADP explicitly results in

$$\begin{aligned} v_1 &= k_{\text{kinase}^*} \cdot MAPKKK \cdot MAPKKKK \cdot ATP \\ v_2 &= k_{\text{phosphatase}} \cdot MAPKKK\text{-}P. \end{aligned} \tag{3.19}$$

In this case, we have to care about the ATP–ADP balance and add three more differential equations

$$\begin{aligned} \frac{\mathrm{d}}{\mathrm{d}t} ATP &= -\frac{\mathrm{d}}{\mathrm{d}t} ADP = -\sum_{i \text{ odd}} v_i \\ \frac{\mathrm{d}}{\mathrm{d}t} P_i &= \sum_{i \text{ even}} v_i. \end{aligned} \tag{3.20}$$

Here we find two more conservation relations, the conservation of adenine nucleotides, $ATP + ADP = \text{const.}$ and the conservation of phosphate groups

$$\begin{aligned} &MAPKKK\text{-}P + MAPKK\text{-}P + 2 \cdot MAPKK\text{-}P_2 + MAPK\text{-}P \\ &\quad + 2 \cdot MAPK\text{-}P_2 + 3 \cdot ATP + 2 \cdot ADP + P = \text{const.} \end{aligned} \tag{3.21}$$

Second, one may assume that the kinases catalyzing the phosphorylation of the next kinase behave like saturable enzymes (e.g., [29]) and, therefore, consider Michaelis–Menten kinetics for the individual steps (e.g., [30]). Taking again the first and second reaction as examples for kinase and phosphatase steps, we get

$$\begin{aligned} v_1 &= k_1 \cdot MAPKKKK \frac{MAPKKK}{K_{m1} + MAPKKK} \\ v_2 &= \frac{V_{\max 2} \cdot MAPKKK\text{-}P}{K_{m2} + MAPKKK\text{-}P}, \end{aligned} \tag{3.22}$$

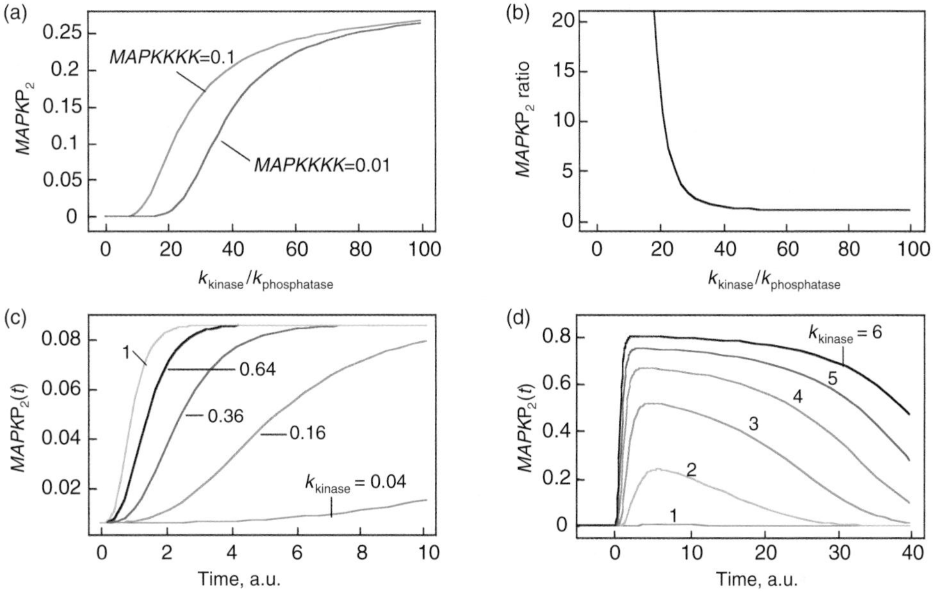

Figure 3.18 Parameter dependence of MAPK cascade performance. Steady-state simulations for changing values of rate constants for kinases, k_{kinase}, and phosphatases, $k_{phosphatase}$, are shown (in arbitrary units). (a) Absolute values of the output signal *MAPK*-PP depending on the input signal (high *MAPKKKK* = 0.1, or low *MAPKKKK* = 0.01) for varying ratio of $k_{kinase}/k_{phosphatase}$. (b) Ratio of the output signal for high versus low input signal (*MAPKKKK* = 0.1 or *MAPKKKK* = 0.01) for varying ratio of $k_{kinase}/k_{phosphatase}$. (c) Time course of MAPK activation for different values of k_{kinase} and a ratio $k_{kinase}/k_{phosphatase} = 20$. (d) Time course of MAPK activation for different values of k_{kinase} and fixed $k_{phosphatase} = 1$.

where k_1 is a first-order rate constant, K_{m1} and K_{m2} are Michaelis constants, and V_{max2} denotes a maximal enzyme rate. Reported values for Michaelis constants are 15 nM [30], 46 and 159 nM [31], and 300 nM [29]. For maximal rates, values of about $0.75\ \text{nM} \cdot \text{s}^{-1}$ [30] are used in models.

The performance of MAPK cascades, i.e., their ability to amplify the signal, to enhance the concentration of the double phophorylated MAPK notably, and the speed of activation, depends crucially on the kinetic constants of the kinases, k_{kinase}, and phosphatases, $k_{phosphatase}$ (Eq. (3.19)), and, moreover, on their ratio (see Figure 3.18). If the ratio $k_{kinase}/k_{phosphatase}$ is low (phosphatases stronger than kinases), then the amplification is high, but at very low absolute concentrations of phosphorylated MAPK. High values of $k_{kinase}/k_{phosphatase}$ ensure high absolute concentrations of MAPK-P_2, but with negligible amplification. High values of both k_{kinase} and $k_{phosphatase}$ ensure fast activation of downstream targets.

Frequently, the proteins of MAPK cascades interact with scaffold proteins. Binding to scaffold proteins can bring the kinases together in the correct spatial order or can reduce their diffusion through the cytosol or provide an anchor to the plasma membrane. This way, they contribute to the regulation of the efficiency, specificity, and localization of the signaling pathway.

3.2.4.5 Jak/Stat Pathways

Jak–Stat pathways play an important role in regulating immune responses and cellular homeostasis in human health and disease [32, 33]. They are activated by cytokines, a large family of extracellular ligands. The whole family of structurally and functionally conserved receptors comprises four Jaks and seven Stats. As is the case for many types of receptor families, downstream signaling entails tyrosine phosphorylation. Stat stands for "signal transducer and activator of transcription," because these proteins function both as signal transducer and transcription activator. They are inactive as monomers. Activation involves phosphorylation and dimerization.

A mathematical model of the Jak–Stat pathway presented by Swamaye and colleagues (2003) presupposes the binding of the ligand (here the hormone Epo) to the receptor (EpoR) that results in phosphorylation of Jak2 and of the cytoplasmatic domain of EpoR. The model involves the recruitment of monomeric Stat5 ($x_1 = Stat5$) to phosphorylated and thereby activated receptor, $EpoR_A$. Upon receptor recruitment, monomeric Stat5 is tyrosine phosphorylated ($x_2 = Stat5\text{-}P$). It dimerizes in a second step to yield x_3, and migrates in the third step to the nucleus (x_4), where it binds to the promoter of target genes. After it has fulfilled its task, it is dephosphorylated and exported to the cytoplasm (fourth step). Using simple mass action kinetics for the four steps indicated in Figure 3.19, the respective ODE system reads

$$\begin{aligned}
\frac{dx_1(t)}{dt} &= -k_1 \cdot x_1(t) \cdot EpoR_A + 2 \cdot k_4 \cdot x_3(t-\tau) \\
\frac{dx_2(t)}{dt} &= -k_2 \cdot x_2^2(t) + k_1 \cdot x_1(t) \cdot EpoR_A \\
\frac{dx_3(t)}{dt} &= -k_3 \cdot x_3(t) + \frac{1}{2} k_2 \cdot x_2^2(t) \\
\frac{dx_4(t)}{dt} &= -k_4 \cdot x_3(t-\tau) + k_3 \cdot x_3(t).
\end{aligned} \tag{3.23}$$

The parameter τ represents the delay time that Stat5 molecules have to reside in the nucleus. This model has been used to show that recycling of Stat5 molecules is an important event in the activation cycle and necessary to explain experimental data.

In the web material, we present a model of the human Erbk signaling network consisting of a receptor and several signaling pathways including a MAPK pathway, which shows interesting feedback and crosstalk phenomena.

3.2.5
Signaling – Dynamic and Regulatory Features

Signaling pathways can exhibit interesting dynamic and regulatory features. Representative pathway structures that form the basis for characteristic dynamic behaviors

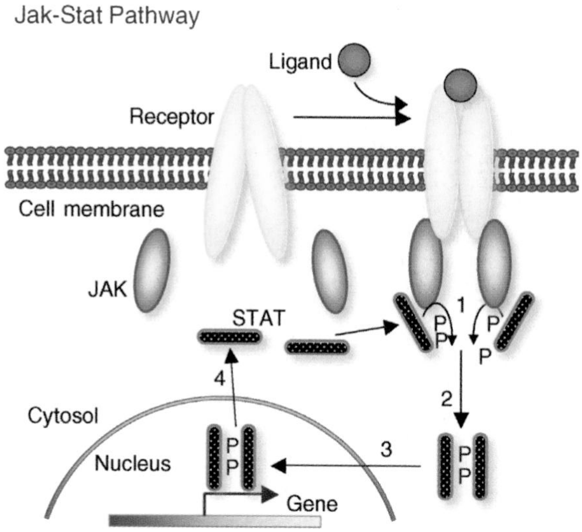

Figure 3.19 The Jak–Stat signaling pathway. Upon binding ligand, receptor-associated Jaks become activated and mediate phosphorylation of specific receptor tyrosine residues. This leads to the recruitment of specific Stats, which are then also tyrosine-phosphorylated. Activated Stats are released from the receptor, dimerize, translocate to the nucleus, and bind to enhancers.

(so-called dynamic motifs) are discussed in detail in Section 8.2. Among the various regulatory features of signaling pathways, negative feedback has attracted outstanding interest. It also plays an important role in metabolic pathways, for example, in amino acid synthesis pathways, where a negative feedback signal from the amino acid at the end to the precursors at the beginning of the pathway prevents an overproduction of this amino acid. The implementation of feedback and the respective dynamic behavior show a wide variation. Feedback can bring about limit cycle type oscillations, for instance, in cell cycle models [34]. In signaling pathways, negative feedback may cause an adjustment of the response or damped oscillations.

3.2.5.1 Quantitative Measures for Properties of Signaling Pathways

The dynamic behavior of signaling pathways can be quantitatively characterized by a number of measures [35]. Let $P_i(t)$ be the time-dependent concentration of the kinase i (or another interesting compound). The signaling time τ_i describes the average time to activate the kinase i. The signal duration ϑ_i gives the average time during which the kinase i remains activated. The signal amplitude S_i is a measure for the average concentration of activated kinase i. The following definitions have been introduced. The quantity

$$I_i = \int_0^\infty P_i(t)\mathrm{d}t \tag{3.24}$$

measures the total of active kinase i generated during the signaling period, i.e., the integrated response of X_i (the area covered by a plot $P_i(t)$ versus time). Further measures are

$$T_i = \int_0^\infty t \cdot P_i(t)\mathrm{d}t \quad \text{and} \quad Q_i = \int_0^\infty t^2 \cdot P_i(t)\mathrm{d}t. \tag{3.25}$$

The signaling time can now be defined as

$$\tau_i = \frac{T_i}{I_i}, \tag{3.26}$$

i.e., as the average of time, analogous to a center of time, or to the mean value of a statistical distribution. The signal duration

$$\vartheta_i = \sqrt{Q_i/I_i - \tau_i^2} \tag{3.27}$$

gives a measure of how the signaling response extends around the mean time (compatible to standard deviation). The signal amplitude is defined as

$$A_i = \frac{I_i}{2\vartheta_i}. \tag{3.28}$$

In a geometric representation, this is the height of a rectangle whose length is $2\vartheta_i$ and whose area equals the area under the curve $P_i(t)$. Note that this measure might be different from the maximal value P_i^{max} that $P_i(t)$ assumes during the time course.

Figure 3.20 shows a signaling pathway with successive activation of compounds and the respective time courses. The characteristic quantities are given in Table 3.2 and for $P_1(t)$ shown in the figure.

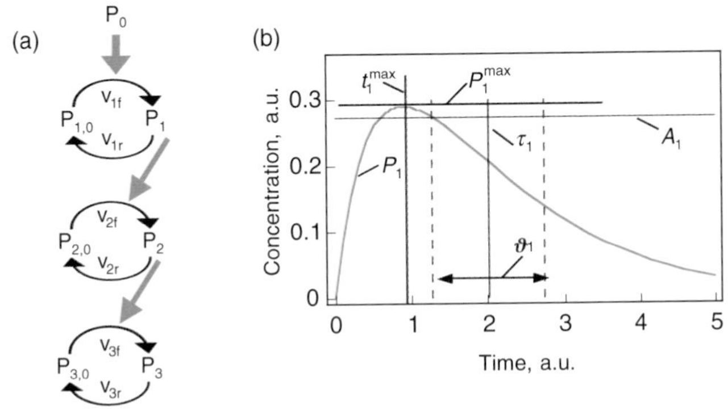

Figure 3.20 Characteristic measures for dynamic variables. (a) Wiring of an example signaling cascade with $v_{if} = k_{if} \cdot P_{i-1}(t) \cdot (1 - P_i(t))$, $v_{ir} = k_{ir} \cdot P_i(t)$, $k_{if} = k_{ir} = 1$, $dP_0(t)/dt = -P_0(t)$, $P_0(0) = 1$, $P_i(0) = 0$ for $i = 1, \ldots, 3$. (b) Time courses of X_i. The horizontal lines indicate the concentration measures for X_1, i.e., the calculated signal amplitude A_1 and P_1^{max}, and vertical lines indicate time measures for P_1, i.e., the time t_1^{max} of P_1^{max}, the characteristic time τ_1, and the dotted vertical lines cover the signaling time ϑ_1.

Table 3.2 Dynamic characteristics of the signaling cascade shown in Figure 3.15.

Compound	Integral, I_i	Maximum, X_i^{max}	Time (X_i^{max}), t_i^{max}	Characteristic time, τ_i	Signal duration, ϑ_i	Signal amplitude, A_i
X_1	0.797	0.288	0.904	2.008	1.458	0.273
X_2	0.695	0.180	1.871	3.015	1.811	0.192
X_3	0.629	0.133	2.855	4.020	2.109	0.149

3.2.5.2 Crosstalk in Signaling Pathways

Signal transmission in cellular context is often not as precise as in electric circuits in the sense that an activated protein has a high specificity for just one target. Instead, there might be crosstalk, i.e., proteins of one signaling pathway interact with proteins assigned to another pathway. Strictly speaking, the assignment of proteins to one pathway is often arbitrary and may result, for example, from the history of their function discovery. Frequently, protein interactions form a network with various binding, activation, and inhibition events, such as illustrated in Figure 3.10.

In order to introduce quantitative measures for crosstalk, let us consider the simplified scheme in Figure 3.21: external signal α binds to receptor R_A, which activates target T_A via a series of interactions. In the same way, external signal β binds to receptor R_B, which activates target T_B. In addition, there are processes that mediate an effect of receptor R_B on target T_A.

Let us concentrate on pathway A and define all measures from its perspective. Signaling from α via R_A to T_A shall be called intrinsic, while signals from β to T_A are extrinsic. Further, in order to quantify crosstalk, we need a quantitative measure for the effect of an external stimulus on the target. We have different choices: if we are interested in the level of activation, such a measure might be the integral over the time course of T_A (Eq. (3.24)), its maximal value, or its amplitude (Eq. (3.28)). If we are interested in the response timing, we can consider the time of the maximal value or the characteristic time (for an overview on measures, see Table 3.2). Whatever measure we chose, it shall be denoted by X in the following.

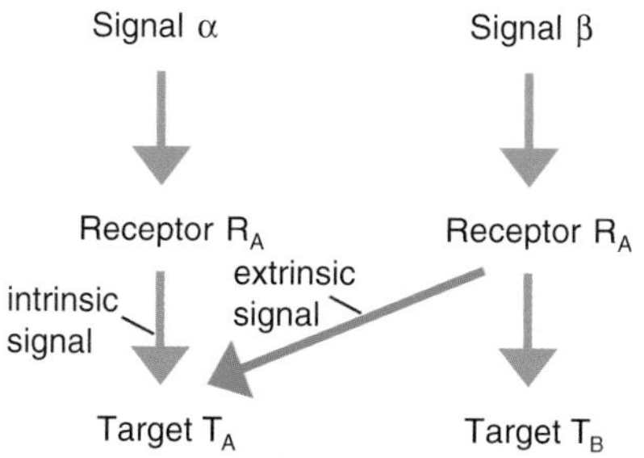

Figure 3.21 Crosstalk of signaling pathways.

Table 3.3 Effect of crosstalk on signaling.

	$S_e > 1$	$S_e < 1$
$S_i > 1$	Mutual signal inhibition	Dominance of intrinsic signal
$S_i < 1$	Dominance of extrinsic signal	Mutual signal amplification

The crosstalk measure C is the activation of pathway A by the extrinsic stimulus β relative to the intrinsic stimulus α

$$C = \frac{X_{\text{extrinsic}}}{X_{\text{intrinsic}}} = \frac{X_{T_A}(\beta)}{X_{T_A}(\alpha)}. \tag{3.29}$$

The fidelity F [36] is defined as output due to the intrinsic signal divided by the output in response to the extrinsic signal and reads in our notation:

$$F = \frac{X_{T_A}(\alpha)/X_{R_A}(\alpha)}{X_{T_A}(\alpha)/X_{R_B}(\beta)}. \tag{3.30}$$

In addition, the intrinsic sensitivity S_i expresses how an extrinsic signal modifies the intrinsic signal when acting in parallel, while the extrinsic sensitivity S_e quantifies the effect of the intrinsic signal on the extrinsic signal [37]:

$$S_i(A) = \frac{X_{T_A}(\alpha)}{X_{T_A}(\alpha,\beta)} \quad \text{and} \quad S_e(A) = \frac{X_{T_A}(\beta)}{X_{T_A}(\alpha,\beta)}. \tag{3.31}$$

Table 3.3 shows how different specificity values can be interpreted.

Example 3.3

Consider the coupling of a faster and a slower signaling pathway as depicted in Figure 3.21, described with rate equations used in Figure 3.22 with the exception $v_{3Af} = k_{3Af} \cdot (P_{2A}(t) + P_{2B}(t)) \cdot (1 - P_{3A}(t))$. Let A be the slower pathway (all $k_{iAf} = k_{iAr} = 1$) and B the faster pathway (all $k_{iBf} = k_{iBr} = 10$). The pathways are activated by setting either $P_{0A}(0)$ or $P_{0B}(0)$ or both from zero to one, respectively. The time courses show that crosstalk from pathway B to pathway A affects the pathway output $P_{3A}(t)$. Concomitant activation of A by α and B by β leads to faster activation of $P_{3A}(t)$ than α alone. Activation by β alone leads to drastically reduced $P_{3A}(t)$. Table 3.4. reports the quantitative crosstalk measures. We note mutual signal amplification in terms of integrated response (I_{3A}) and maximal response ($\text{Max}(P_{3A})$), but dominance of the intrinsic signal on the level of signal timing (here $t_{P_{3A}}^{max}$).

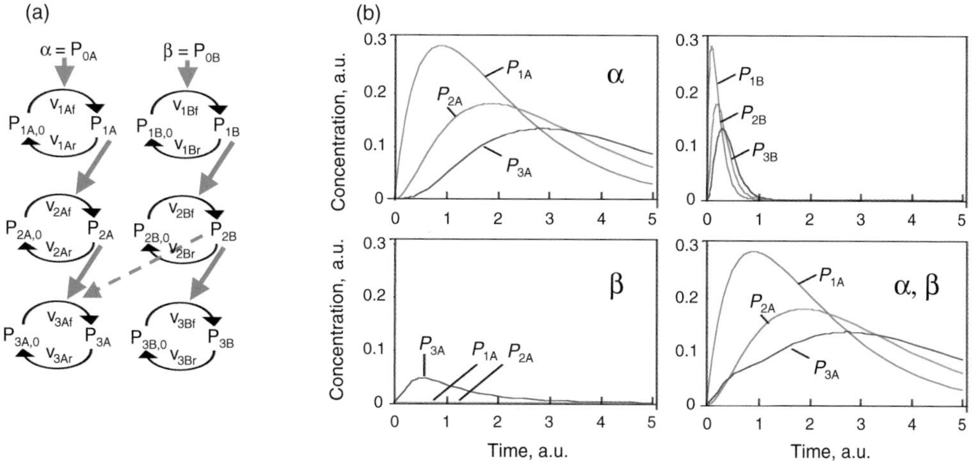

Figure 3.22 Crosstalk of MAP kinase pathways. (a) Pathway A leads to activation of P_{3A} upon stimulation by α, pathway B transmits signal from β to P_{3B}. Crosstalk occurs through signaling from P_{2B}. (b) Dynamics of pathways A and B upon stimulation by α, β, or both (as indicated).

3.3
The Cell Cycle

Summary

The cell cycle is a fundamental cellular process that dominates many aspects of cellular biochemistry. In this section, different phases of the mitotic cell cycle are introduced. The regulatory mechanisms that control the periodic process are discussed and mathematical models of different complexity that describe the oscillatory process are introduced.

Growth and reproduction are major characteristics of life. Crucial for these is the cell division by which one cell divides into two and all parts of the mother cell are distributed to the daughter cells. This also requires that the genome has to be

Table 3.4 Crosstalk measures for the pathway in Example 3.3.

	$X_A(\alpha)$	$X_A(\beta)$	$X_A(\alpha,\beta)$	$S_i(A)=\frac{X_A(\alpha)}{X_A(\alpha,\beta)}$	$S_e(A)=\frac{X_A(\beta)}{X_A(\alpha,\beta)}$	$C=\frac{X_A(\beta)}{X_A(\alpha)}$
$I_3=\int_0^\infty P_{3A}(t)dt$	0.628748	0.067494	0.688995	0.912557	0.09796	0.107347
$t_{P_{3A}}^{max}$	2.85456	0.538455	2.73227	1.04476	0.197072	0.18863
$Max(P_{3A})$	0.132878	0.0459428	0.136802	0.971314	0.335833	0.345752

duplicated in advance, which is performed by the DNA polymerase, an enzyme that utilizes desoxynucleotide triphosphates (dNTPs) for the synthesis of two identical DNA double strands from one parent double strand. In this case, each single strand acts as template for one of the new double strands. Several types of DNA polymerases have been found in prokaryotic and eukaryotic cells, but all of them synthesize DNA only in $5' \rightarrow 3'$ direction. In addition to DNA polymerase, several further proteins are involved in DNA replication: proteins responsible for the unwinding and opening of the mother strand (template double strand), proteins that bind the opened single stranded DNA and prevent it from rewinding during synthesis, an enzyme called primase that is responsible for the synthesis of short RNA primers that are required by the DNA polymerase for the initialization of DNA polymerization, and a DNA ligase responsible for linkage of DNA fragments that are synthesized discontinuously on one of the two template strands because of the limitation to $5' \rightarrow 3'$ synthesis. Like the DNA, also other cellular organelles have to be doubled, such as the centrosome involved in the organization of the mitotic spindle.

The cell cycle is divided into two major phases: the interphase and the M phase (Figure 3.23). The interphase is often a relatively long period between two subsequent cell divisions. Cell division itself takes place during M phase and consists of two steps: first, the nuclear division in which the duplicated genome is separated into two parts, and second, the cytoplasmatic division or cytokinesis, where the cell divides into two cells. The latter not only distributes the two separated genomes between each of the newly developing cells, but also divides up cytoplasmatic organelles and substances between them. Finally, the centrosome is replicated and divided between both cells as well.

DNA replication takes place during interphase in the so-called S phase (S = synthesis) of the cell cycle (Figure 3.23). This phase is usually preceded by a gap phase, G_1, and followed by another gap phase, G_2. From G_1 phase, cells can also leave the cell cycle and enter a rest phase, G_0. The interphase normally represents 90% of the cell cycle. During interphase, the chromosomes are dispersed as chromatin in the nucleus. Cell division occurs during M phase, which follows the G_2 phase, and consists of mitosis and cytokinesis. Mitosis is divided into different stages. During the first stage – the prophase – chromosomes condense into their compact form and the two centrosomes of a cell begin recruiting microtubles for the formation of the mitotic spindle. In later stages of mitosis, this spindle is used for the equal segregation of the chromatides of each chromosome to opposite cellular poles. During the following prometaphase, the nuclear envelope dissolves and the microtubles of the mitotic spindle attach to protein structures, called kinetochores, at the centromeres of each chromosome. In the following metaphase, all chromosomes line up in the middle of the spindle and form the metaphase plate. Now, during anaphase, the proteins holding together both sister chromatids are degraded and each chromatid of a chromosome segregate into opposite directions. Finally, during telophase, new nuclear envelopes are recreated around the separated genetic materials and form two new nuclei. The chromosomes unfold again into chromatin. The mitotic reaction is often followed by a cytokinesis where the cellular

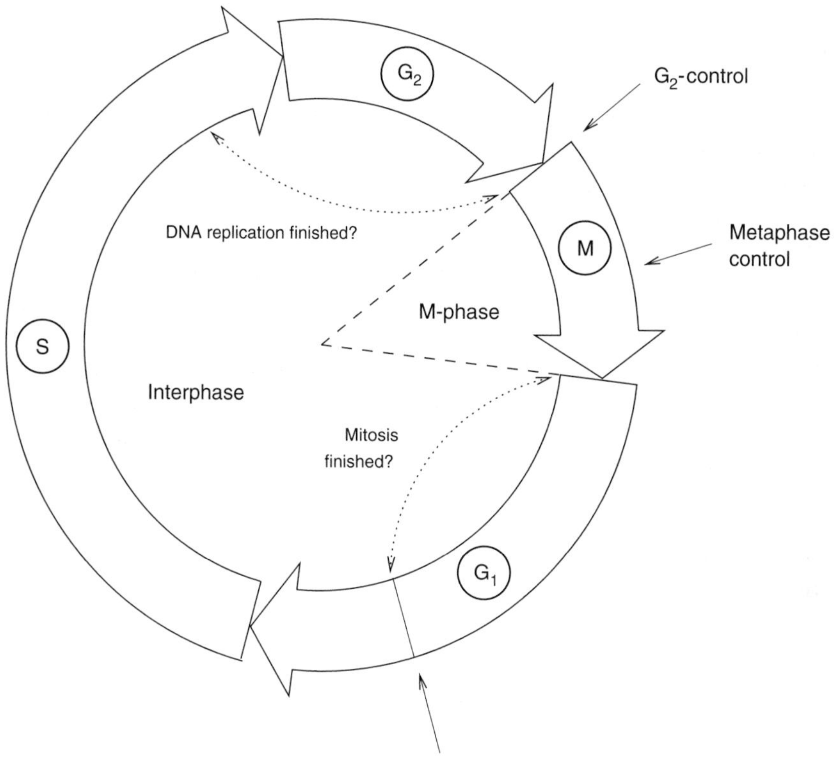

Figure 3.23 The cell cycle is divided into the interphase, which is the period between two subsequent cell divisions, and the M phase, during which one cell separates into two. Major control points of the cell cycle are indicated by arrows. More details are given in the text.

membrane pinches off between the two newly separated nuclei and two new cells are formed.

The cell cycle is strictly controlled by specific proteins. When a certain checkpoint, the restriction point, in the G_1 phase is passed, this leads to a series of specific steps that end up in cell division. At this point, the cell checks whether it has achieved a sufficient size and the external conditions are suitable for reproduction. The control system ensures that a new phase of the cycle is only entered if the preceding phase has been finished successfully. For instance, to enter a new M phase, it has to be assured that DNA replication during S phase has correctly been brought to an end. Similarly, entering in S phase requires a preceding mitosis.

Passage through the eukaryotic cell cycle is strictly regulated by the periodic synthesis and destruction of cyclins that bind and activate cyclin-dependent kinases (CDKs). The term "kinase" expresses that their function is phosphorylation of proteins with controlling functions. A contrary function is carried out by a "phosphatase." Its function is to dephosphorylate a previously phosphorylated protein and by this toggle its activity. Cyclin-dependent kinase inhibitors (CKI) also play important roles in cell cycle control by coordinating internal and external signals and impeding proliferation at several key checkpoints.

The general scheme of the cell cycle is conserved from yeast to mammals. The levels of cyclins rise and fall during the stages of the cell cycle. The levels of CDKs appear to remain constant during cell cycle, but the individual molecules are either unbound or bound to cyclins. In budding yeast, one CDK (Cdc28) and nine different cyclins (Cln1–Cln3, Clb1–Clb6) that seem to be at least partially redundant are found. In contrast, mammals employ a variety of different cyclins and CDKs. Cyclins include a G1 cyclin (cyclin D), S phase cyclins (A and E), and mitotic cyclins (A and B). Mammals have nine different CDKs (referred to as CDK1-9) that are important in different phases of the cell cycle. The anaphase-promoting complex (APC) triggers the events leading to destruction of the cohesions, thus allowing the sister chromatids to separate and degrades the mitotic cyclins.

3.3.1 Steps in the Cycle

Let us take a course through the mammalian cell cycle starting in G1 phase. As the level of G_1 cyclins rises, they bind to their CDKs and signal the cell to prepare the chromosomes for replication. When the level of S phase promoting factor (SPF) rises, which includes cyclin A bound to CDK2, it enters the nucleus and prepares the cell to duplicate its DNA (and its centrosomes). As DNA replication continues, cyclin E is destroyed, and the level of mitotic cyclins begins to increase (in G_2). The M phase-promoting factor (the complex of mitotic cyclins with the M-phase CDK) initiates (i) assembly of the mitotic spindle, (ii) breakdown of the nuclear envelope, and (iii) condensation of the chromosomes. These events take the cell to metaphase of mitosis. At this point, the M phase-promoting factor activates the APC, which allows the sister chromatids at the metaphase plate to separate and move to the poles (anaphase), thereby completing mitosis. APC destroys the mitotic cyclins by coupling them to ubiquitin, which targets them for destruction by proteasomes. APC turns on the synthesis of G_1 cyclin for the next turn of the cycle and it degrades geminin, a protein that has kept the freshly synthesized DNA in S phase from being re-replicated before mitosis.

A number of checkpoints ensure that all processes connected with cell cycle progression, DNA doubling and separation, and cell division occur correctly. At these checkpoints, the cell cycle can be aborted or arrested. They involve checks on completion of S phase, on DNA damage, and on failure of spindle behavior. If the damage is irreparable, apoptosis is triggered. An important checkpoint in G_1 has been identified in both yeast and mammalian cells. Referred to as "Start" in yeast and as "restriction point" in mammalian cells, this is the point at which the cell becomes committed to DNA replication and completing a cell cycle [38–41]. All the checkpoints require the services of complexes of proteins. Mutations in the genes encoding some of these proteins have been associated with cancer. These genes are regarded as oncogenes. Failures in checkpoints permit the cell to continue dividing despite damage to its integrity. Understanding how the proteins interact to regulate the cell cycle has become increasingly important to researchers and clinicians when it was discovered that many of the genes that encode cell cycle regulatory activities are targets for alterations that underlie the development of cancer. Several therapeutic agents, such as DNA-damaging drugs, microtubule inhibitors, antimetabolites, and topoisomerase inhibitors, take advantage of this disruption in normal cell cycle regulation to target checkpoint controls and ultimately induce growth arrest or apoptosis of neoplastic cells.

For the presentation of modeling approaches, we will focus on the yeast cell cycle since intensive experimental and computational studies have been carried out using different types of yeast as model organisms. Mathematical models of the cell cycle can be used to tackle, for example, the following relevant problems:

- The cell seems to monitor the volume ratio of nucleus and cytoplasm and to trigger cell division at a characteristic ratio. During oogenesis, this ratio is abnormally small (the cells accumulate maternal cytoplasm), while after fertilization cells divide without cell growth. How is the dependence on the ratio regulated?
- Cancer cells have a failure in cell cycle regulation. Which proteins or protein complexes are essential for checkpoint examination?
- What causes the oscillatory behavior of the compounds involved in the cell cycle?

3.3.2
Minimal Cascade Model of a Mitotic Oscillator

One of the first genes to be identified as being an important regulator of the cell cycle in yeast was *cdc2/cdc28* [42], where *cdc2* refers to fission yeast and *cdc28* to budding yeast. Activation of the *cdc2/cdc28* kinase requires association with a regulatory subunit referred to as a cyclin.

A minimal model for the mitotic oscillator involving a cyclin and the Cdc2 kinase has been presented by Goldbeter [43]. It covers the cascade of posttranslational modifications that modulate the activity of Cdc2 kinase during cell cycle. In the first cycle of the bicyclic cascade model, the cyclin promotes the activation of the Cdc2 kinase by reversible dephosphorylation, and in the second cycle, the Cdc2 kinase activates a cyclin protease by reversible phosphorylation. The model was used to test the hypothesis that cell cycle oscillations may arise from a negative feedback loop, i.e., the cyclin activates the Cdc2 kinase, while the Cdc2 kinase triggers the degradation of the cyclin.

The minimal cascade model is represented in Figure 3.24. It involves only two main actors, cyclin and CDK. Cyclin is synthesized at constant rate, v_i, and triggers the transformation of inactive (M+) into active (M) Cdc2 kinase by enhancing the rate of a phosphatase, v_1. A kinase with rate v_2 reverts this modification. In the lower cycle, the Cdc2 kinase phosphorylates a protease (v_3) shifting it from the inactive (X+) to the active (X) form. The activation of the cyclin protease is reverted by a

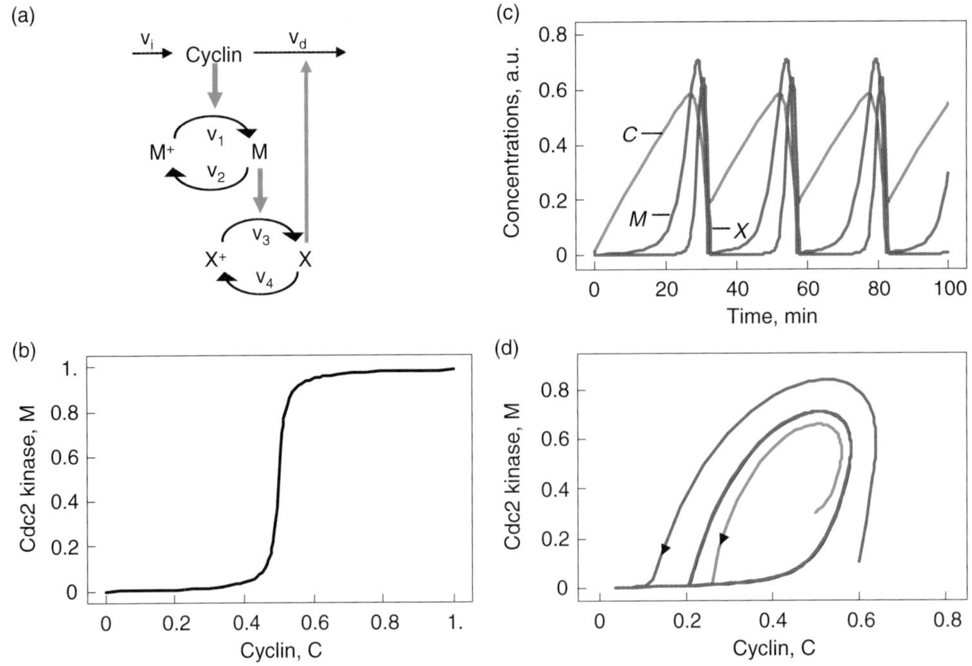

Figure 3.24 Goldbeter's minimal model of the mitotic oscillator. (a) Illustration of the model comprising cyclin production and degradation, phosphorylation and dephosphorylation of Cdc2 kinase, and phosphorylation and dephosphorylation of the cyclin protease (see text). (b) Threshold-type dependence of the fractional concentration of active Cdc2 kinase on the cyclin concentration. (c) Time courses of cyclin (C), active Cdc2 kinase (M), and active cyclin protease (X) exhibiting oscillations according to Equation system in Eq. (3.1). (d) Limit cycle behavior, represented for the variables C and M. Parameter values: $K_{mi} = 0.05$ ($i = 1, \ldots, 4$), $K_{mc} = 0.5$, $k_d = 0.01$, $v_i = 0.025$, $v_d = 0.25$, $V_{m1} = 3$, $V_{m2} = 1.5$, $V_{m3} = 1$, $V_{m4} = 0.5$. Initial conditions in (b) are $C(0) = M(0) = X(0) = 0.01$, and in (c) are $X(0) = 0.01$. Units: μM and min^{-1}.

further phosphatase with rate v_4. The dynamics is governed by the following ODE system:

$$\frac{dC}{dt} = v_i - v_d \frac{X \cdot C}{K_{md} + C} - k_d C$$
$$\frac{dM}{dt} = \frac{V_{m1} \cdot (1-M)}{K_{m1} + (1-M)} - \frac{V_{m2} \cdot M}{K_{m2} + M} \qquad (3.32)$$
$$\frac{dX}{dt} = \frac{V_{m3} \cdot (1-X)}{K_{m3} + (1-X)} - \frac{V_{m4} \cdot X}{K_{m4} + X},$$

where C denotes the cyclin concentration; M and X represent the fractional concentrations of active Cdc2 kinase and active cyclin protease, while $(1 - M)$ and $(1 - X)$ are the fractions of inactive kinase and phosphatase, respectively. K_m values are Michaelis constants. $V_{m1} = V_1 C/(K_{mc} + C)$ and $V_{m3} = V_3 \cdot M$ are effective maximal rates. Note that the differential equations for the changes of M and X are modeled with the so-called Goldbeter–Koshland switch.

This model involves only Michaelis–Menten type kinetics, but no form of positive cooperativity. It can be used to test whether oscillations can arise solely as a result of the negative feedback provided by the Cdc2-induced cyclin degradation and of the threshold and time delay involved in the cascade. The time delay is implemented by considering posttranslational modifications (phosphorylation/dephosphorylation cycles v_1/v_2 and v_3/v_4). For certain parameters, they lead to a threshold in the dependence of steady-state values for M on C and for X on M (Figure 3.24(b)). Provided that this threshold exists, the evolution of the bicyclic cascade proceeds in a periodic manner (Figure 3.24(c)). Starting from low initial cyclin concentration, this value accumulates at constant rate, while M and X stay low. As soon as C crosses the activation threshold, M rises. If M crosses the threshold, X starts to increase sharply. X in turn accelerates cyclin degradation and consequently, C, M, and X drop rapidly. The resulting oscillations are of the limit cycle type. The respective limit cycle is shown in phase plane representation in Figure 3.24(d).

3.3.3 Models of Budding Yeast Cell Cycle

Tyson, Novak, and colleagues have developed a series of models describing the cell cycle of budding yeast in very detail [45–48]. These comprehensive models employ a set of assumptions that are summarized in the following.

The cell cycle is an alternating sequence of the transition from G_1 phase to S/M phase, called "Start" (in mammalian cells, it is called "restriction point"), and the transition from S/M to G_1, called "Finish." An overview is given in Figure 3.25.

The CDK (Cdc28) forms complexes with the cyclins Cln1 to Cln3 and Clb1 to Clb6, and these complexes control the major cell cycle events in budding yeast cells. The complexes Cln1-2/Cdc28 control budding, the complex Cln3/Cdc28 governs the executing of the checkpoint "Start," Clb5-6/Cdc28 ensures timely DNA replication, Clb3-4/Cdc28 assists DNA replication and spindle formation, and Clb1-2/Cdc28 is necessary for completion of mitosis.

The cyclin–CDK complexes are in turn regulated by synthesis and degradation of cyclins and by the Clb-dependent kinase inhibitor (CKI) Sic1. The expression of the gene for Cln2 is controlled by the transcription factor SBF, the expression of the gene for Clb5 by the transcription factor MBF. Both the transcription factors are regulated by CDKs. All cyclins are degraded by proteasomes following ubiquitination. APC is one of the complexes triggering ubiquitination of cyclins.

For the implementation of these processes in a mathematical model, the following points are important. Activation of cyclins and CDKs occurs in principle by the negative feedback loop presented in Goldbeter's minimal model (see Figure 3.24). Furthermore, the cells exhibit exponential growth. For the dynamics of the cell, mass M holds $dM/dt = \mu M$. At the instance of cell division, M is replaced by $M/2$. In some

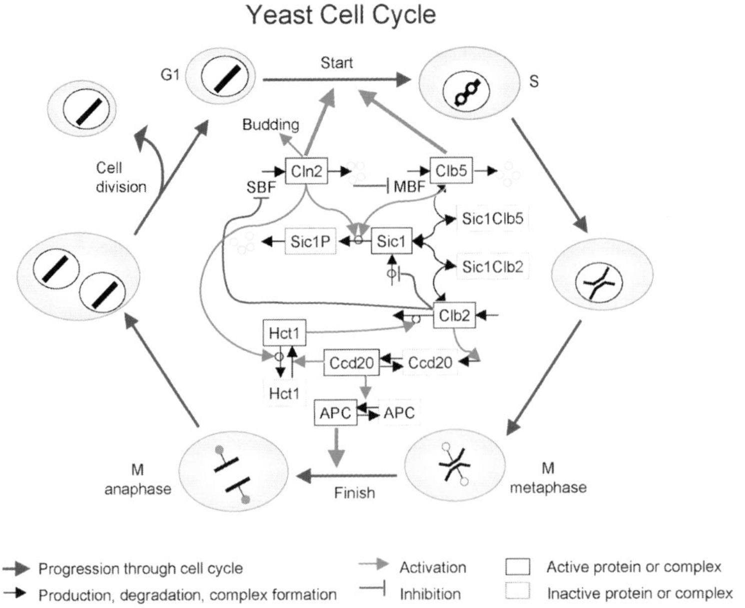

Figure 3.25 Schematic representation of the yeast cell cycle (inspired by Fall *et al.* [44]). The outer ring represents the cellular events. Beginning with cell division, it follows the G1 phase. The cells possess a single set of chromosomes (shown as one black line). At "Start," the cell goes into the S phase and replicates the DNA (two black lines). The sister chromatids are initially kept together by proteins. During M phase, they are aligned, attached to the spindle body, and segregated to different parts of the cell. The cycle closes with formation of two new daughter cells. The inner part represents main molecular events driving the cell cycle comprising (1) protein production and degradation, (2) phosphorylation and dephosphorylation, and (3) complex formation and disintegration. For the sake of clarity, CDK Cdc28 is not shown. The "Start" is initiated by activation of CDK by cyclins Cln2 and Clb5. The CDK activity is responsible for progression through S and M phase. At Finish, the proteolytic activity coordinated by APC destroys the cyclins and renders thereby the CDK inactive.

cases, uneven division is considered. Cell growth implies adaptation of the negative feedback model to growing cells.

The transitions "Start" and "Finish" characterize the wild-type cell cycle. At "Start," the transcription factor SBF is turned on and the levels of the cyclins Cln2 and Clb5 increase. They form complexes with Cdc28. The boost in Cln2/Cdc28 has three main consequences: it initiates bud formation, it phosphorylates the CKI Sic1 promoting its disappearance, and it inactivates Hct1, which in conjunction with APC was responsible for Clb2 degradation in G1 phase. Hence, DNA synthesis takes place and the bud emerges. Subsequently, the level of Clb2 increases and the spindle starts to form. Clb2/Cdc28 inactivates SBF and Cln2 decreases. Inactivation of MBF causes Clb5 to decrease. Clb2/Cdc28 induces progression through mitosis. Cdc20 and Hct1, which target proteins to APC for ubiquitination, regulate the metaphase–anaphase transition. Cdc20 has several tasks in the anaphase. Furthermore, it activates Hct,

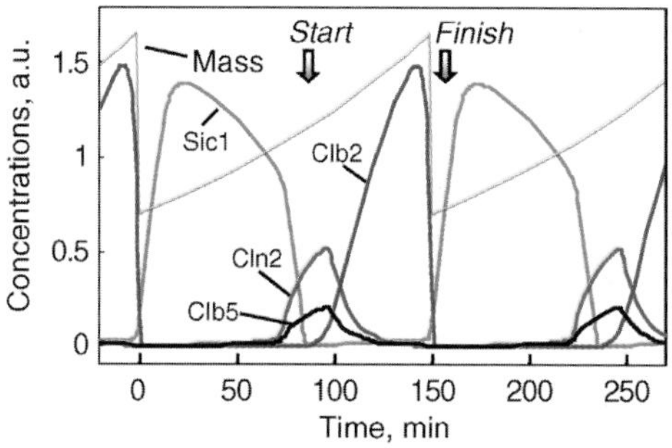

Figure 3.26 Temporal behavior of some key players during two successive rounds of yeast cell cycle. The dotted line indicates the cell mass that halves after every cell division. The levels of Cln2, $Clb2_{total}$, $Clb5_{total}$, and $Sic1_{total}$ are simulated according to the model presented by Chen *et al.* [47].

promoting degradation of Clb2, and it activates the transcription factor of Sic1. Thus, at "Finish," Clb2 is destroyed and Sic1 reappears.

The dynamics of some key players in cell cycle according to the model given in Chen *et al.* [47] is shown in Figure 3.26 for two successive cycles. At "Start," Cln2 and Clb5 levels rise and Sic1 is degraded, while at "Finish," Clb2 vanishes and Sic1 is newly produced.

3.3.4 Modeling Nucleo/Cytoplasmatic Compartmentalization

Compartmentalization is a major characteristic of eukaryotic cells. The partitioning of a cell by membranes results in a separation of functional units and in the formation of reaction spaces that might differ significantly in their molecular composition. This is due to a restricted permeability of the membranes and the controlled shuttling of molecules (e.g., mRNAs, proteins, protein-complexes) between compartments, e.g., between the cytosol and the nucleus. This compartmentalization has also regulatory aspects, e.g., for the cell cycle.

Barberis *et al.* [49] have set up a model of G_1/S transition of the budding yeast cell cycle that takes into account compartmentalization. The structure of the model is displayed in Figure 3.27. The model is composed of two compartments – the cytoplasm and the nucleus. The partitioning allows us to consider differences in the concentrations of same molecule species that are in different compartments. All proteins of the model have synthesis and degradation reactions. Protein synthesis takes place in the cytoplasm. Since the expression of the cyclins Cln1,2 and Clb5,6 is regulated by transcription factors of the mode (SBF, MBF), they are explicitly modeled by transcription events taking place in the nucleus, a transfer of the respective mRNAs into the cytoplasm, and their subsequent translation. Cln3 is the most upstream cyclin in the yeast cell cycle progression. In growing cells, the Cln3 protein enters the nucleus and forms a binary complex with Cdk1 (Cdk1–Cln3). Active nuclear Cdk1–Cln3 activates the transcription factors SBF and MBF. This

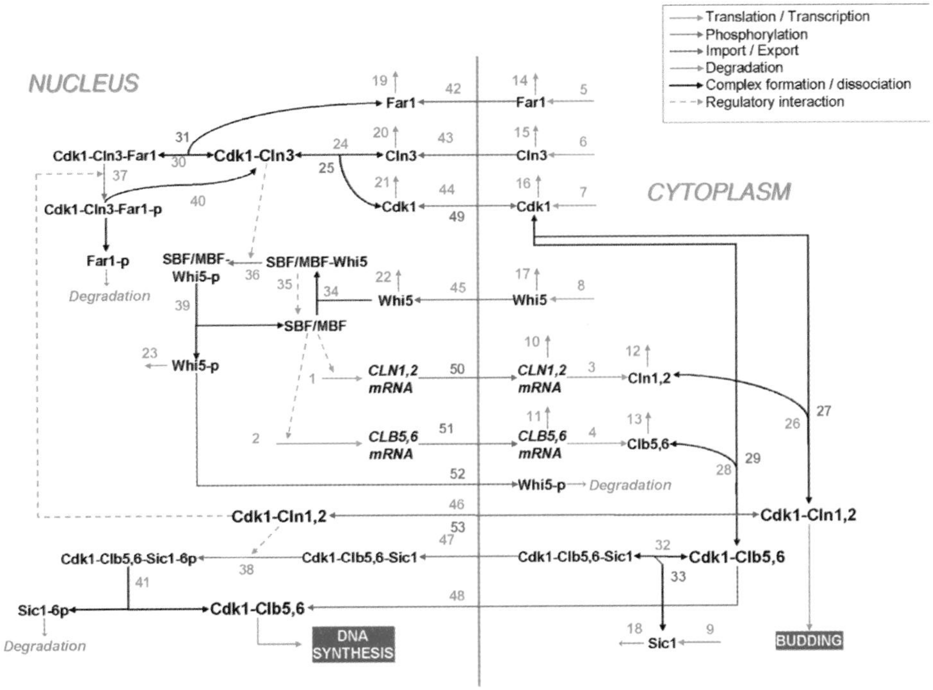

Figure 3.27 Processes regulating the G_1/S transition in budding yeast (this figure was kindly provided by M. Barberis [49]).

happens indirectly by Cdk1–Cln3 mediated phosphorylation of Whi5 and its subsequent dissociation from SBF and MBF. The activation of SBF and MBF commits a cell to DNA replication and budding. This happens due to SBF-mediated transcription of Cln1,2. Similarly, the transcription factor MBF activates Clb5,6 transcription. This activation cascade is modulated by the Cdk inhibitor protein Far1. Far1 is largely enriched in newborn cells and forms a ternary complex with Cdk1–Cln3. Given the presence of a substantial amount of Far1 in the cell, Far1 traps Cdk1–Cln3 in the inactive form. Growth-dependent accumulation of Cln3 allows it to overcome the threshold that is set by Far1. Furthermore, in the presence of Cdk1–Cln1,2, Far1 can be phosphorylated and hence primed for degradation. The degradation of Far1 yields in a substantial amount of active Cdk1–Cln3.

The newly expressed proteins Cln1 and Cln2 form a cytoplasmatic complex with Cdk1 that promotes the biochemical reactions relevant for budding. Moreover, Clb5 and Clb6 bind to Cdk1 and migrate into the nucleus where the Cdk1–Clb5,6 complex initiates DNA replication. Like Far1 is an inhibitor of Cdk1–Cln3 activity, Sic1 is an inhibitor of Cdk1–Clb5,6 activity. But in the same way as Far1 can be targeted for degradation by phosphorylation, also Sic1 can be phosphorylated by Cdk1–Cln1,2 and subsequently degraded.

The model defines two thresholds that subsequently have being overcome during the upstream events of "Start": (i) Cln3–Cdk1 has a threshold that is set by Far1 and

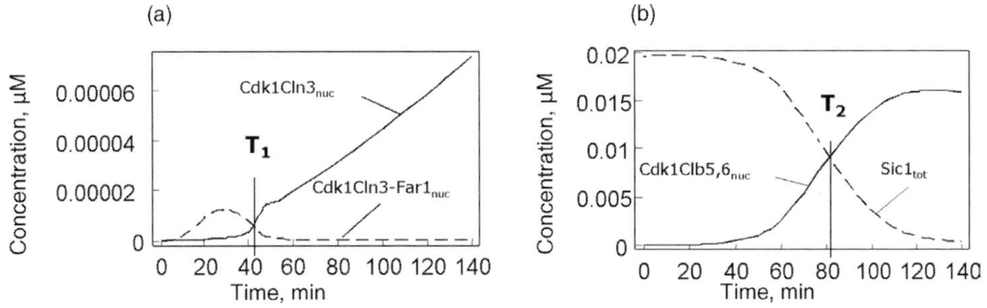

Figure 3.28 Simulation results of the G_1/S transition model. (a) Nuclear Cdk1-Cln3-Far1 complex reaches its maximal concentration after 30 min and becomes degraded upon overcoming Cln3/Far1 threshold (T_1). (b) The half-maximal concentration of nuclear Cdk1-Clb5,6 is reached at around 80 min, thereby setting the Clb5,6/Sic1 threshold (T_2) (this figure was kindly provided by Barberis [49]).

(ii) Cdk1–Clb5,6 has a threshold that is set by Sic1. The simulation results depicted in Figure 3.28 show these thresholds.

Compartmentalization as described by this model addresses the following regulatory issues:

1. Gene expression involves the migration of the mRNA from the nucleus to the cytosol, where proteins are synthesized.
2. Both import and export of proteins to or from the nucleus can be regulated independently.
3. Controlled partitioning affects binding equilibria by altering the actual concentration of a given protein available for binding to a given interactor within a subcellular compartment.

3.4 Spatial Models

Summary

Cells and organisms show complex spatial structures, which are vital for the processes of life. Biochemical reaction–diffusion systems can establish, maintain, and adapt spatial structures in a self-organized and robust manner. The body plan of animals, for instance, is shaped during embryonic development by spatial-temporal profiles of morphogen levels. Dynamic instabilities in such systems can give rise to spontaneous pattern formation. The spatiotemporal dynamics of substance concentrations can be modeled in different mathematical frameworks, including compartment models, reaction–diffusion equations, and stochastic simulations.

Cells, tissues, and organisms show complex spatial structures, and many biological processes involve spatiotemporal dynamics. Prominent examples are calcium waves within cells, neural activity in the brain, patterning during embryonic development, or the invasion of tissues by cancer cells. Such spatiotemporal processes can be modeled in different mathematical frameworks, including compartment and reaction–diffusion models [50]. Spatial simulation can increase the numerical cost quite drastically, but characteristic dynamic behavior like waves or pattern formation can already be studied in relatively simple models with one or two substances.

Spatial structures are vital for many processes in living cells. Organelles can contain different compositions of enzymes and provide suitable environments for different biochemical processes (e.g., presence of hydrolases and low pH in lysosomes); membranes allow to establish gradients of concentrations or chemical potential, e.g., proton gradients that provide an energy storage in bacteria and mitochondria. The localization of molecules also plays a role in signaling: in the Jak–Stat pathway, for instance, active Stat proteins accumulate in the nucleus to induce transcriptional changes. Besides the compartments, there is also structure on the microscopic scale: scaffold proteins can hold together protein complexes. By localizing several functions in close vicinity, they create a "critical mass" of enzymatic activity. In channeling, for instance, intermediates are directly passed from enzyme to enzyme, which increases the efficiency of enzymes.

3.4.1
Types of Spatial Models

How can spatial substance distributions be described in models? If molecules move freely and independently and if diffusion is much faster than chemical reactions, inhomogeneities will rapidly disappear, and substances may be described by their concentrations averaged over the cell. On the other hand, if molecules are not distributed homogeneously, e.g., because membranes slow down the diffusion of molecules, then spatial location and structure need to be modeled.

3.4.1.1 Compartment Models and Partial Differential Equations

One possibility is to describe substances by their concentrations in different compartments, e.g., organelles in the cell. Compartments are also used in pharmacokinetics, to model the distribution and degradation of substances in different organs [51, 52]. Compartment models are based on the assumption of fast diffusion within each compartment; if biological compartments resemble each other (e.g., the mitochondria in a cell) and rapid mixing between them would not make a difference, they can be treated as a single, effective compartment.

If diffusion is slow within compartments, it will not wear away the spatial inhomogeneities in substance concentrations: on the contrary, coupling between diffusion and chemical reactions may generate dynamic patterns (e.g., waves) out of homogeneous substance distributions. The dynamics of such patterns can be described by *reaction–diffusion systems,* which describe substance concentrations in continuous space and time. The partial differential equations can be solved numerically by splitting the space in question into *finite elements*, small volume elements which formally resemble compartments, but are chosen according to numerical requirements.

3.4.1.2 Stochastic Models

Partial differential equation models assume that concentrations are smooth functions in space – which only holds on a spatial scale much larger than the average distance between molecules. If a substance is present in small amounts, the behavior of individual molecules – thermal movement and chemical reactions – can be simulated by stochastic models. A stochastic simulation may track each individual particle, describing its diffusion by a random walk. If molecules are in close vicinity, they may participate in a chemical reactions and be transformed into product molecules. The numerical effort for such simulations is high, especially if many particles are modeled. Instead of tracking the histories of individual particles, we can also split the cell into subvolumes and simulate the particle numbers within subvolumes by a random process describing reaction and diffusion (see Section 7.1.3 and Chapter 14).

3.4.1.3 Cellular Automata

In *cellular automata* models [53], space is represented by a discrete array of nodes, so-called cells. Each cell can show different discrete states, which are updated in discrete time steps; the new state can be chosen deterministically or stochastically and depends typically on the current states of the cell and its neighbors. A prominent example of a cellular automaton is Conway's *game of life* [54]. In this model, cells form a square lattice and can assume two different states, "dead" (or 0) and "live" (or 1). The states are updated synchronously according to the following rules: (i) a live cell with fewer than 2 or more than 3 neighbors dies; a live cell with 2 or 3 neighbors remains alive. (ii) If a dead cell has exactly three neighbors, it comes to life, otherwise it remains dead. These simple rules give rise to a surprisingly rich dynamic behavior (see exercise 4). More complicated models can be used to simulate the proliferation of cells and organisms in space.

3.4.2 Compartment Models

In compartment models, we assume that concentrations are homogeneous within each compartment. Transport between compartments –, e.g., diffusion across membranes –, is modeled by transport reactions. Passive exchange through membranes or pores, for instance, may be described as diffusion with a rate

$$v^*(s_1, s_2) = AP(s_1 - s_2), \tag{3.33}$$

where the permeability P (in $\mathrm{m \cdot s^{-1}}$) depends on the physicochemical properties of membrane, channels, and molecules, and A denotes the membrane area; the indices 1 and 2 refer to the compartments. Active transport by transporter proteins may be modeled by a saturable rate law, for instance, irreversible Michaelis–Menten kinetics. Importantly, transport rates are measured as *amounts* per time (in $\mathrm{mol \cdot s^{-1}}$), but for physical reasons, their values depend on compound *concentrations* in mM (e.g., the difference $s_1 - s_2$ in Eq. (3.33)).

So, although compartment models are not very different from usual kinetic models, we need to pay some attention to the correct conversion between substance amounts, concentrations, and compartment volumes. It is practical to start with the amounts a_i (where the subscript i indicates a substance located in a compartment). With the reaction velocities v^* (in mol $\cdot$ s^{-1}), we obtain the rate equation

$$\frac{da_i}{dt} = \sum_l n_{il} v_l^*(s), \tag{3.34}$$

where the n_{il} are the stoichiometric coefficients. Each amount a_i is defined in a compartment with index $k(i)$ and a volume $V_{k(i)}$ (in m^3). After introducing the concentrations $s_i = a_i / V_{k(i)}$, we can rewrite the time derivative in Eq. (3.34) as

$$\frac{da_i}{dt} = \frac{d}{dt}(V_{k(i)} s_i) = V_{k(i)} \frac{ds_i}{dt} + \frac{dV_{k(i)}}{dt} s_i. \tag{3.35}$$

By combining Eqs. (3.34) and (3.35), we obtain the rate equation for concentrations

$$\frac{ds_i}{dt} = \sum_l \frac{n_{il}}{V_{k(i)}} v_l^*(s) - \frac{dV_{k(i)}/dt}{V_{k(i)}} s_i. \tag{3.36}$$

It shows that concentration changes can be caused by chemical reactions (first term) and volume changes (second term). If all compartments in Eq. (3.36) have the same time-independent volume, we can replace $v_l^* / V_{k(i)}$ by the usual reaction velocity v_l in mM $\cdot$ s^{-1}; the second term vanishes, so we obtain the usual form of kinetic models. But we can also consider the transport of a substance between two compartments (1 and 2) of different volume. If the volume sizes are constant in time, the second term vanishes and we obtain, for this reaction alone,

$$V_1 \frac{ds_1}{dt} = -V_2 \frac{ds_2}{dt}. \tag{3.37}$$

The minus sign stems from the stoichiometric coefficients. The volumes play an important role in transport between cells and the external medium: intra- and extracellular concentration changes are converted to each other by the volume ratio V_{cell}/V_{ext}, where V_{cell} is the volume of a single cell and V_{ext} denotes the extracellular volume divided by the number of cells.

The second term in Eq. (3.36) describes the effect of temporal volume changes: substances in growing cells are diluted, so their concentration will decrease even if they are not consumed by chemical reactions. If a cell population grows at a rate $\mu(t)$, the total cell volume V increases according to

$$\frac{dV}{dt} = \mu(t) V(t), \tag{3.38}$$

so the prefactor in the second term in Eq. (3.36) is just the growth rate $\mu(t)$. Dilution of molecules in a growing cell population formally resembles linear degradation, with the cell growth rate μ appearing as an effective degradation constant.

3.4.3 Reaction–Diffusion Systems

3.4.3.1 The Diffusion Equation

The diffusion equation describes the space- and time-dependent concentration $s(\boldsymbol{r}, t)$ of a diffusing substance, where $\boldsymbol{r}$ is a position in space, and t is a moment in time. In spatial models, positions are generally represented by three-dimensional vectors $\boldsymbol{r} = (x, y, z)^{\mathrm{T}}$, but in the following, we will sometimes consider a single space dimension only. This simplification is justified if we model a long, thin compartment or if we assume homogeneity along two space directions. The flow of a substance can be described by a vectorial flow field $\boldsymbol{j}(\boldsymbol{r}, t)$; we can interpret the flow as a product $\boldsymbol{j}(\boldsymbol{r}, t) = s(\boldsymbol{r}, t)\, \boldsymbol{w}(\boldsymbol{r}, t)$, where $\boldsymbol{w}(\boldsymbol{r}, t)$ is the locally averaged particle velocity. If a substance is conserved (no production or degradation by chemical reactions), its concentration obeys the continuity equation

$$\frac{\partial s(\boldsymbol{r}, t)}{\partial t} = -\nabla \cdot \boldsymbol{j}(\boldsymbol{r}, t). \tag{3.39}$$

Fick's law states that a small concentration gradient in a homogeneous, isotropic medium will evoke a flow

$$\boldsymbol{j}(\boldsymbol{r}, t) = -D\, \nabla s(\boldsymbol{r}, t), \tag{3.40}$$

with a *diffusion constant* D. By inserting Eq. (3.40) into the continuity equation (3.39), we obtain the diffusion equation

$$\frac{\partial s(\boldsymbol{r}, t)}{\partial t} = D\, \nabla^2 s(\boldsymbol{r}, t), \tag{3.41}$$

with the *Laplace operator*

$$\nabla^2 s = \frac{\partial^2 s}{\partial x^2} + \frac{\partial^2 s}{\partial y^2} + \frac{\partial^2 s}{\partial z^2}. \tag{3.42}$$

In one space dimension, the Laplace operator simply reads $\nabla^2 s(r, t) = \partial^2 s/\partial r^2$. The diffusion equation (3.41) for concentrations corresponds to the Fokker–Planck equation for Brownian random motion of individual particles (see Chapter 14).

To solve it in a region in space, we need to specify initial conditions (a concentration field $s(\boldsymbol{r}, 0)$ at time $t = 0$) and boundary conditions for all points $\boldsymbol{r}_0$ on the boundary. It is common to fix concentrations $s(\boldsymbol{r}_0, t)$ on the boundary (a *Dirichlet boundary condition*) or to assume that the boundary is impermeable, i.e., the flow orthogonal to the boundary vanishes. As the flow points along the concentration gradient, this is an example of a *von Neumann boundary condition*, which in general sets the values of $\nabla s(\boldsymbol{r}_0)\cdot \boldsymbol{n}(\boldsymbol{r}_0)$, where $\boldsymbol{n}$ is a unit vector orthogonal to the surface. In one space dimension, an impermeable boundary implies that $\partial s(r, t)/\partial r|_{r=r_0} = 0$, so the slope of the concentration is always zero at the boundary. The diffusion equation, together with proper initial and boundary conditions, determines the time-dependent concentration field $s(\boldsymbol{r}, t)$ at times $t \geq 0$.

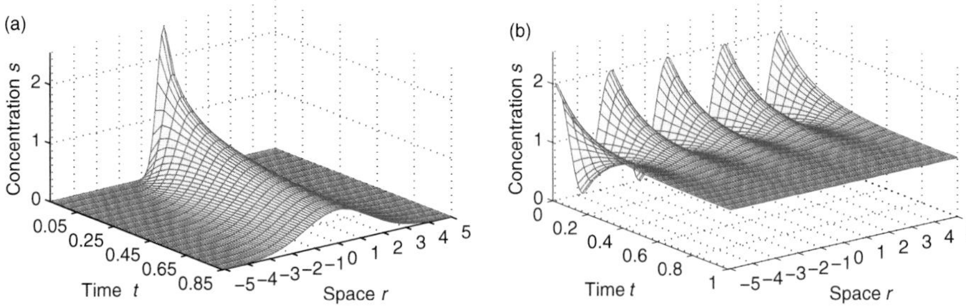

Figure 3.29 Diffusion tends to blur spatial concentration patterns. (a) A localized substance amount leads to a Gaussian-like cloud of increasing width. Parameters $a = 2$, $D = 1$. Time, space, and concentration in arbitrary units. (b) An initial cosine wave pattern keeps its shape, but its amplitude decreases exponentially in time. Parameters $s_0 = 1$, $D = 1$, $k = 2\pi/(5/2)$, base line concentration 1.

3.4.3.2 Solutions of the Diffusion Equation

Diffusion tends to remove spatial heterogeneity: local concentration maxima (with negative curvature $\nabla^2 s$) will shrink and local minima are filled. This is illustrated by some special solutions of the diffusion equation in one space dimension.

1. Stationary concentration profiles in one space dimension have vanishing curvature. If concentrations at the boundaries $r = 0$ and $r = \mathrm{L}$ are fixed, one obtains a linear stationary profile $s^{\mathrm{st}}(r)$ in which substance flows down the concentration gradient. For impermeable boundaries, the stationary solution is a homogeneous, constant profile $s^{\mathrm{st}}(r) = \mathrm{const}$ corresponding to a thermodynamic equilibrium.

2. If a substance amount a is initially concentrated in the point $r = 0$ and if we impose the boundary condition $s(r, t) \to 0$ for $r \to \pm\infty$, diffusion will lead to a Gaussian-shaped concentration profile (see Figure 3.29(a))

$$s(r,t) = \frac{a}{\sqrt{2\pi(2Dt)}} e^{-\frac{r^2}{2(2Dt)}}. \tag{3.43}$$

   The width $\sqrt{2Dt}$ increases with the square root of diffusion constant D and time t.

3. Now we consider a finite region $0 \leq r \leq L$ with impermeable boundaries, i.e., $\partial s/\partial r = 0$ at both $r = 0$ and $r = \mathrm{L}$ and choose, as initial condition, a cosine pattern, i.e. an eigenmode of the diffusion operator. Under diffusion, the pattern will keep its shape, but the amplitude decreases exponentially (Figure 3.29(b)):

$$s(r,t) = s_0\, e^{-\lambda(k)t} \cos(k\, r). \tag{3.44}$$

   To ensure positive concentration values, a base line concentration can be added. Due to the boundary conditions, the possible wave numbers k are restricted to values $k = n\pi/L$ with integer n. The time constant λ is given by the dispersion relation $\lambda(k) = -D\,k^2$, so narrow-spaced cosine patterns (with large wave numbers k) are smoothed out faster than broad patterns.

As the diffusion equation is linear, general solutions can be obtained by convolution integrals or linear combinations of the profiles (3.43) or (3.44).

3.4.3.3 Reaction–Diffusion Equation

A reaction–diffusion system consists of several substances that diffuse and participate in chemical reactions. By combining a kinetic model for the chemical reactions with the diffusion equation (3.41), we obtain a reaction–diffusion equation

$$\frac{\partial s_i(\mathbf{r},t)}{\partial t} = \sum_l n_{il}\, v_l(\mathbf{s}(\mathbf{r},t)) + D_i \nabla^2 s_i(\mathbf{r},t) \tag{3.45}$$

for the concentrations s_i. The first term represents local chemical reactions, while the second term describes diffusion with substance-specific diffusion constants D_i. As the rate laws $v_l(\mathbf{s})$ are usually nonlinear, most reaction–diffusion models can only be solved numerically, e.g., by finite-element methods. Reaction–diffusion equations can show various kinds of dynamic behavior including pattern formation, traveling and spiraling waves, or chaos, some of which is also observed in biological systems (Figure 3.30). For instance, traveling waves arising from

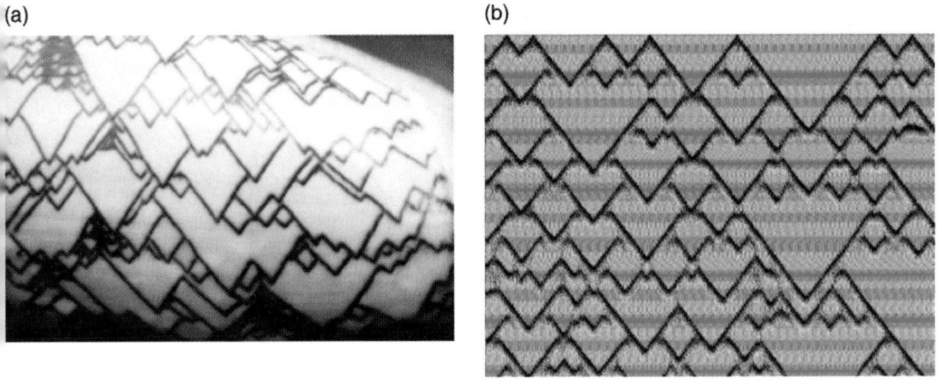

Figure 3.30 Patterns on sea shells arising from a reaction–diffusion system. (a) Color patterns on the shell of *Oliva porphyria* are formed as more material is added to the growing edge of the shell, so the vertical direction in the picture can be interpreted as a time axis. The patterns are preformed by a chemical reaction–diffusion system: in this case traveling waves lead to diagonal lines. (b) The patterns can be simulated by an activator-inhibitor system (black and red) with an additional global signaling substance (green) that counteracts the pairwise annihilation of waves [55, 56]. The vertical axis represents time from top to bottom (Courtesy of H. Meinhardt).

simple reaction–diffusion systems have been used to model the patterns on sea shells [55, 56].

3.4.4
Pattern Formation in Tissue Development

The body plan of multicellular organisms is established in embryonic development by coordinated growth and differentiation of cells. Organisms can develop very specific shapes in a robust manner, which we can see from the similarity between twins and the symmetry of our bodies.

The development process is organized by spatial patterns of *morphogens*, which act as a coordinate system in the developing tissue. If a morphogen level shows a gradient along the anterior–posterior axis of the embryo, cells can sense their positions on this axis and differentiate accordingly [57]. Morphogen fields follow a spatiotemporal dynamics, which arises from its interactions with the growing tissue and is implicitly determined by the way cells sense and produce the morphogens.

Comparable forms of cell communication and collective dynamics also appear in bacteria (in quorum sensing) or in colonies of the social amoeba *Dictyostelium discoideum*, which can turn temporarily into a multicellular organism. Another example is the hydra, a multicellular animal that can regrow its main organs, foot and head, after it is cut into halves, and which can even re-associate from individual cells. The spontaneous development of a new body axis in the hydra by biochemical pattern formation has been described qualitatively by mathematical models [58, 59].

The fly *Drosophila melanogaster* is a prominent model organism for embryonic development: its anterior–posterior body axis is established in early oocyte stage by a gradient of a morphogen protein called Bicoid. Bicoid is produced from mRNA that is attached to microtubules at the anterior end of the unfertilized egg; it then forms a gradient that marks the anterior part of the embryo and serves as a reference for further patterning processes (see Figure 3.31(a)). To compute a stationary Bicoid profile in a simple model, we assume a steady-state balance of production, diffusion, and linear degradation. The concentration $s(r,t)$ in one dimension (pointing along the anterior–posterior axis) can be described by the reaction–diffusion equation

$$\frac{\partial s(r,t)}{\partial t} = D\nabla^2 s(r,t) - \kappa s(r,t), \tag{3.46}$$

with diffusion constant D and degradation constant κ. The stationary profile $s^{st}(r)$ has to satisfy the steady-state condition

$$0 = D\nabla^2 s^{st}(r) - \kappa s^{st}(r), \tag{3.47}$$

which can be solved by a sum of exponential profiles

$$s^{st}(r) = a_1 e^{-r/L_0} + a_2 e^{r/L_0}, \tag{3.48}$$

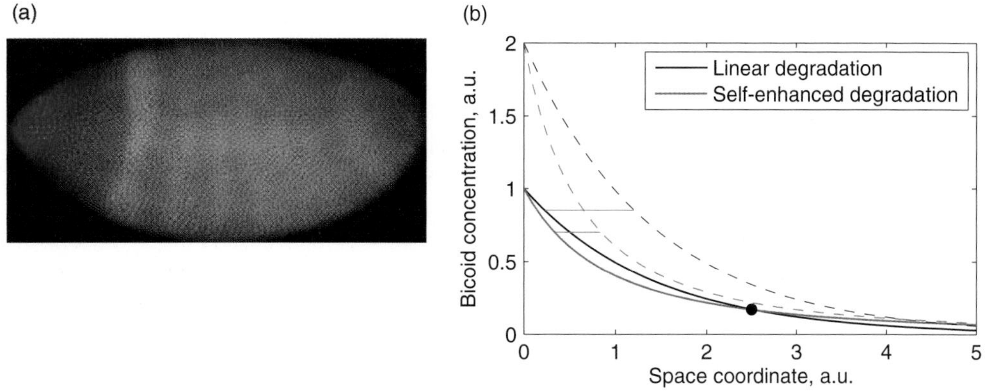

Figure 3.31 Spatial pattern of the morphogen Bicoid. (a) Microscope image [60] showing expression patterns of the genes *even-skipped* (red), *caudal* (green), and *bicoid* (blue). From the FlyEx database [61]. (b) Model results. Solid curves show simulated profiles obtained from models with linear degradation (black) or self-enhanced degradation (blue) and parameters $D = 0.01$, $\kappa = 0.02$, $s_0 = 1$. The Bicoid concentrations in both models coincide at $r = 0$ and $r \approx 2.5$ (dot). The broken curves show profiles that would result from an increased concentration $s_0 = 2$ at the anterior end. The change of this boundary condition shifts profiles to the right by a constant amount (shift sizes marked by red lines).

with the characteristic degradation length $L_0 = \sqrt{D/\kappa}$. The coefficients a_1 and a_2 need to be chosen according to the boundary conditions. We describe Bicoid production by fixing a constant concentration $s(r = 0) = s_0$ at the anterior boundary of the cell; s_0 is proportional to the protein production rate and therefore to the amount of mRNA. On the posterior end, Bicoid cannot leave the cell, so we set $\mathrm{d}s^{\mathrm{st}}/\mathrm{d}r|_{r=L} = 0$. With these boundary conditions, the coefficients in Eq. (3.48) read

$$a_1 = \frac{\beta^2 s_0}{1+\beta^2} \quad a_2 = \frac{s_0}{1+\beta^2}, \tag{3.49}$$

with the abbreviation $\beta = \exp(L/L_0)$. If the characteristic length L_0 is much shorter than the length L of the embryo, we can also use the boundary condition $\lim_{r\to\infty} s^{\mathrm{st}}(r) = 0$ as an approximation. In this case, the second term in Eq. (3.48) vanishes, and we obtain the exponential profile

$$s^{\mathrm{st}}(r) = s_0\, e^{-r/L_0}. \tag{3.50}$$

In an alternative model [62], Bicoid is assumed to catalyze its own degradation, which leads to a steeper profile near the source; with a degradation rate $\kappa s^2(r, t)$ instead of $\kappa s(r, t)$ and boundary conditions as above, the steady-state profile reads (see exercise 6)

$$s^{\mathrm{st}}(r) = \frac{6D/\kappa}{\left(r + \sqrt{6D/(\kappa s_0)}\right)^2}. \tag{3.51}$$

This pattern combines two properties that are favorable for reliable patterning [62]. The amounts of mRNA, and therefore morphogen production, may vary from embryo to embryo: an increased production, for example, will shift the emerging pattern to the right (see Figure 3.31(b)). This effect can only be suppressed by a steep initial decrease around $r=0$. However, in the exponential profile (3.50), a steep decrease would automatically lead to small Bicoid levels along the embryo, which could easily be distorted by noise. The profile implemented by Eq. (3.51), on the other hand, combines a steep decrease near the source with relatively high levels along the embryo. In Figure 3.31(b), for instance, both profiles show the same Bicoid level at the center of the embryo, but model (3.51) shows a much smaller shift after overexpression of Bicoid.

3.4.5 Spontaneous Pattern Formation

Some color patterns, e.g,. on the furs of zebras and leopards, are thought to arise from a self-organized pattern formation. Even if the identity of the biological morphogens and the biochemical interactions in these cases remain elusive, the geometries of these patterns can be well reproduced by simple reaction–diffusion models [63]. Figure 3.32 shows, as an example, the formation of spots in the Gierer–Meinhardt model

$$\begin{aligned}\frac{\partial a}{\partial t} &= \frac{\rho a^2}{b(1+\kappa a^2)} - \mu_a a + D_a \nabla^2 a \\ \frac{\partial b}{\partial t} &= \rho a^2 - \mu_b b + D_b \nabla^2 b.\end{aligned} \tag{3.52}$$

with parameters ρ and κ (for production), μ_a and μ_b (for degradation), and D_a and D_b (for diffusion). The concentrations a and b correspond, respectively, to an activator (which has a positive influence on both production terms) and an inhibitor (which

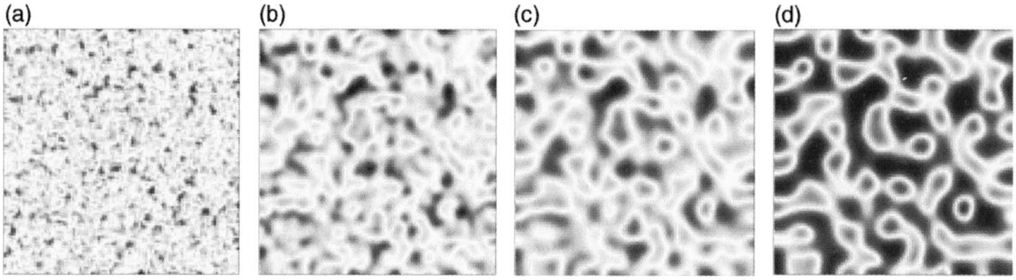

Figure 3.32 Stripe formation in the Gierer–Meinhardt model. The pictures show snapshots (activator concentration) from a simulation at time points $t=50$ (a), $t=200$ (b), $t=50$ (c), $t=200$ (d). A stripe pattern emerges spontaneously from a noisy initial concentration profile (uniform random values from the interval [0.1, 1]. Parameters $D_a=0.002$, $D_b=0.2$, $r=1$, $\mu_a=0.01$, $\mu_b=0.015$, $\kappa=0.1$, discretization $\Delta x=0.2$, $\Delta t=1$ (arbitrary units).

inhibits production of the activator). Variants of this model with different parameter sets can lead to spots, stripes, and gradients. The pattern in Figure 3.32 has a typical length scale (distance between spots), which depends on the reaction and diffusion parameters, but not on the size of the tissue. The exact shape is random and depends on the initial random fluctuations.

In reaction–diffusion systems, spatial patterns can emerge spontaneously from an almost homogeneous distribution – a paramount example of spontaneous symmetry breaking. Similar patterns arise in clouds or sand ripples. Although the underlying physical systems are completely different, their ability to form patterns relies on the same general mechanism called *Turing instability* [64]. For spontaneous pattern formation, the system must have a homogeneous steady state. This steady state must be stable against homogeneous concentration changes, but unstable against spatial variation. Fluctuations of a certain finite wavelength must be amplified more strongly than fluctuations of smaller or larger wavelength.

These conditions can be fulfilled in simple reaction–diffusion systems [58] with two substances called "activator" and "inhibitor" as shown in Figure 3.33(a). If the homogeneous steady state of the system is unstable against local fluctuations, even smallest fluctuations will be amplified and lead to a stable pattern with separated regions (typically spots or stripes) of high or low activator levels. Even if the full nonlinear behavior of reaction–diffusion systems may be complicated, the necessary conditions for pattern formation can be obtained from a linear stability analysis (see web supplement). Pattern formation in activator–inhibitor systems requires that the inhibitor diffuses faster than the activator, so whereas pure diffusion removes patterns, diffusion is necessary for pattern formation in this case. Propagating waves (as shown in Figure 3.30), in contrast, require that the inhibitor has a longer life-time and that it diffuses more slowly than the activator.

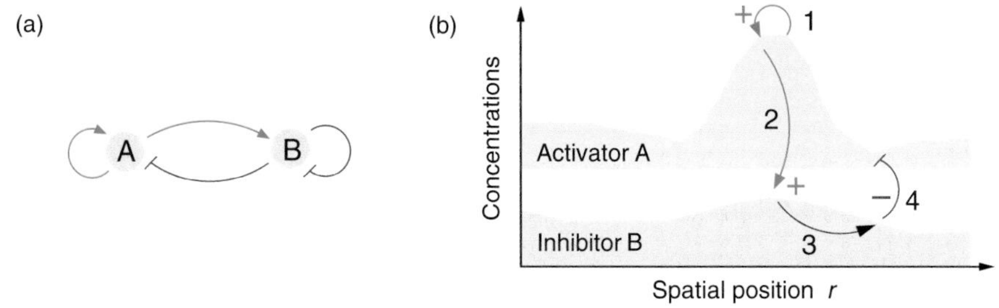

Figure 3.33 Activator–inhibitor system. (a) High levels of A (the activator) locally increase both concentrations, while B (the inhibitor) decreases them. In a nonspatial model, this system is assumed to have a stable steady state. (b) A reaction-diffusion mechanism can amplify existing local inhomogeneities: a local elevation of A catalyzes its own further increase (1). In addition, it increases the level of B (2), which diffuses faster than A (3) and represses the level of A in a distance (4). By the same mechanism, the resulting valley will further increase the original elevation and create another concentration peak nearby.

3.5 Apoptosis

Summary

Similarly as cells always divide, damaged or excess cells can be removed by a kind of cell suicide called *programmed cell death*. Apoptosis, a well-studied form of programmed cell death, can be elicited by extracellular or intracellular signals. Both extracellular signals of death receptors or intracellular signals, e.g., due to DNA damage or oxidative stress activate a signaling cascade. Extracellular or intracellular signals activate initiator caspases, which vice versa activate executioner caspases that finally lead to the death of the cell. The activation of the apoptotic program is an irreversible process – once the "point of no return" has been passed, the process cannot be reverted. The mathematical modeling of the apoptotic signaling cascade can be used for the identification of potential therapeutic targets. Furthermore, the model can be used for the analysis of certain characteristics of the apoptotic signaling cascade, such as bistability and irreversibility.

Multicellular organisms begin their life as a single cell that develops into a fully formed individual. This developmental process is controlled by a precise execution of the organism's genetic program. Although it is obvious that developmental processes require cell division and differentiation, it turned out that a specific and coordinated cell death is essential, too. The crucial role of cell death usually continues into adulthood. As well as our cells permanently proliferate, billions of cells die each day by a suicide program that is precisely coordinated and known as programmed cell death. Cells dying by apoptosis, the most common and best-understood form of programmed cell death, undergo characteristic morphological changes. The cells shrink, their cytoskeleton collapses, the nuclear envelope disassembles, the chromatin breaks up into fragments, and finally, they form so-called apoptotic bodies, which have a chemically altered surface and are usually rapidly engulfed by neighboring cells or macrophages. In contrast to cells dying accidentally by necrosis, apoptosis does not elicit an inflammatory response. Apoptosis plays an important role during development; e.g., the removal of specific cells during embryogenesis helps to sculpt the fingers of the hand, or during frog's metamorphosis it is causative for the degeneration of the tadpole's tail. Moreover, apoptosis functions as a quality control, eliminating abnormal or nonfunctional cells.

3.5.1 Molecular Biology of Apoptosis

Apoptosis depends on an intracellular proteolytic cascade mediated by caspases, a family of proteases with a cystein at their active site, which cleave their target proteins at specific aspartic acids. Caspases are synthesized in the cell as inactive precursors, or procaspases, which then become activated by proteolytic cleavage. Caspases involved in apoptosis are classified as initiator caspases (caspases 2, 8, 9, 10) and executioner caspases (caspases 3, 6, 7). Initiator caspases act at the start of the proteolytic cascade and activate downstream executioner procaspases. Executioner caspases conduct the cell death by, e.g., activating other executioner procaspases, cleavage of nuclear lamins that results in the breakdown of the nuclear lamina, cleavage of DNA-endonuclease inhibitors that results in the fragmentation of the genomic DNA, and the cleavage of components of the cytoskeleton and cell–cell adhesion. Initiator caspases can be activated either by intracellular or extracellular signals. Figure 3.34 gives an overview of the apoptotic signaling cascade. The extracellular or extrinsic apoptotic pathway is mediated by so-called death receptors and can be induced, e.g., by immune cells that display an appropriate ligand able to

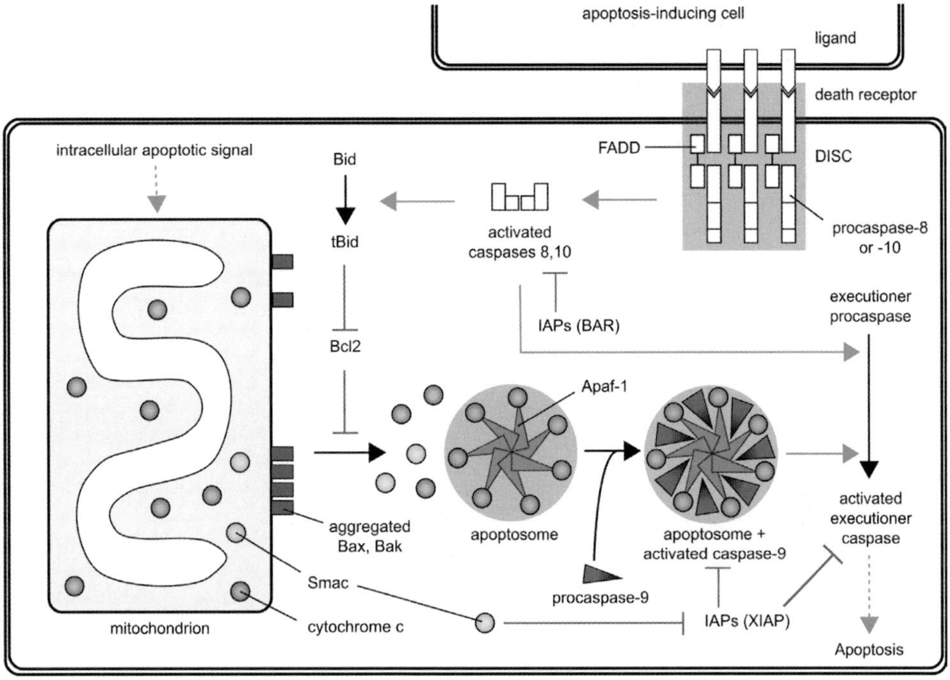

Figure 3.34 Molecular processes of the apoptotic signaling cascade. Apoptosis can be activated via extrinsic or intrinsic signals. The extrinsic apoptotic pathway is initiated by ligands binding to the death receptor, the formation of the DISC complex and the subsequent activation of the initiator caspase-8 or caspase-10. Intracellular signals, such as stress or DNA damage, can lead to an aggregation of Bax or Bak proteins on the surface of the mitochondrial membrane and initiate the release of cytochrome c from the mitochondrial intermembrane space into the cytosol. Together with Apaf-1, cytochrome c can form the apoptosome, which can bind and activate caspase-9. Both, caspases 8 and 10 of the extrinsic pathway and caspase-9 of the intrinsic pathway can cleave and activate executioner procaspases (caspases 3, 6, 7) that subsequently mediate cell death. Intrinsic apoptosis can also be activated by the extrinsic pathway by the truncation of Bid and formation of active tBid. tBid is an inhibitor of Bcl-2, which, under normal condition, binds Bax or Bak and inhibits their aggregation.

bind to its respective death receptor. Death receptor ligands are members of the tumor necrosis factor (TNF) protein family such as TNF-α, TRAIL, or the Fas ligand (FasL). Death receptors belong to the TNF receptor family, which includes a receptor for TNF itself and the Fas receptor (FasR). Binding of a ligand to a respective death receptor induces in the target cell the formation of a complex termed DISC (death-inducing signaling complex). DISC consists of the activated death receptor, the protein FADD (Fas-associated death domain protein), and one of the initiator procaspases (caspase-8 or caspase-10). This complex triggers the self-cleavage of the procaspase and thereby the formation of the respective activated initiator caspase, which in turn activates executioner caspases that finally lead to the progression of apoptosis.

On the other hand, the intracellular or intrinsic apoptotic pathway can be initiated by intracellular signals such as DNA damage or the lack of oxygen, nutrients, or extracellular survival signals. Intracellular apoptotic signals can lead to the aggregation of the pro-apoptotic proteins Bax and Bak, which mediate the release of cytochrome c and Smac from the mitochondrial intermembrane space into the cytosol. Cytochrome c is a water-soluble protein that is usually involved in the mitochondrial electron-transport chain. In the cytosol, cytochrome c binds a procaspase-activating adaptor protein called Apaf1 (apoptotic protease activating factor-1) and leads to the formation of a wheel-like heptamer called apoptosome. The apoptosome recruits the initiator procaspase-9, which then gets activated and subsequently leads to the downstream activation of the executioner procaspases.

Via a crosstalk between the extrinsic and the intrinsic pathway, an extracellular apoptotic signal can be amplified. Activated initiator caspases of the extrinsic pathway cleave the protein Bid. The truncated Bid protein, tBid, acts as a pro-apoptotic protein that is able to inhibit antiapoptotic proteins, such as Bcl2 or Bcl-X_L. Under non-apoptotic conditions, these antiapoptotic proteins oppose the aggregation of Bax or Bak and thereby suppress the onset of apoptosis.

Apoptosis cannot only be inhibited by antiapoptotic proteins belonging to the Bcl2-like protein family, but also by proteins that specifically inhibit active caspases. These proteins are called inhibitors of apoptosis (IAPs). One of the most potent IAP is the X-linked inhibitor of apoptosis protein (XIAP), which is known to inhibit the initiator caspase caspase-9 and the executioner caspases 3 and 7. The function of XIAP in turn can be inhibited by interaction with Smac.

Another protein that has a major effect on the regulation of apoptosis is the protein p53 (sometimes also termed Trp53 in mice or TP53 in humans). Often, p53 is also called a tumor suppressor gene, since it is able to cause cell cycle arrest or apoptosis. It has been shown that several DNA-damaging agents, such as X-rays, ultraviolet radiation, or certain drugs, increases the p53 protein level. p53 can hold the cell cycle and provide the cell with time to repair the DNA damage before the cell cycle proceeds. If the DNA damage cannot be repaired, an increasing amount of p53 acting as a transcription factor can lead to the expression of pro-apoptotic regulators of the Bcl2-family, such as Bax, and initiate by this intrinsic apoptosis.

Once apoptosis is initialized, essential structures of the cell become destructed. This implies that apoptosis should show an irreversible all-or-none behavior, since, e.g., already a partial destruction of the genomic DNA would introduce irreparable damage to the cell. The existence of an all-or-none behavior, i.e., of a bistability, implies a nonlinear behavior of the system.

Dysregulation of apoptosis is associated with various pathological conditions, such as cancer and neurodegenerative disorders. Dysregulation of apoptosis might be due to an overexpression or dysfunction of its regulatory proteins. For example, an overexpression of XIAP that is inhibiting caspase-9 leads to a decrease of the amount of pro-apoptotic proteins and thus shifts the balance between antiapoptotic and pro-apototic proteins in favor of the former and would lead to a survival of cells that are devoted to die. This can be a reason for the onset of cancer. On the other hand, an overexpression of pro-apoptotic proteins or the dysfunction of antiapoptotic proteins due to mutations could result in an unintended apoptosis leading to, e.g., neurodegenerative disorders such as Alzheimer's disease or Parkinson's disease.

3.5.2
Modeling of Apoptosis

Several mathematical models describing different parts and aspects of apoptosis have been developed. A large-scale model of intrinsic and extrinsic apoptosis has been proposed by Fussenegger *et al.* [65]. The model was used to investigate the impact of the overexpression or mutation of several key components of the apoptosis signaling cascade. Using the mathematical model, they analyzed the impact of different combined therapies on simultaneous extrinsic- and intrinsic-induced apoptosis. Table 3.5. shows predicted effects of such combined therapies. This table indicates therapies that are expected to decrease the executioner caspase activation during simultaneous extrinsic- and intrinsic-induced apoptosis. It turned out that no single therapy (results in the diagonal of Table 3.5.), with the exception of IAPs overexpression, is able to block executioner caspase activation. Some combinations of overexpression/disruption or mutation also show an effect, but several combinations

Table 3.5 Predicted effects of combined therapies based on simultaneous extrinsic- and intrinsic-induced apoptosis[a].

	Overexpression				Disruption or mutation	
	$Bcl\text{-}2/Bcl\text{-}X_L$	Bax/Bad/Bik	FLIPs	IAPs	FADD	P53
$Bcl\text{-}2/Bcl\text{-}X_L$	−	−	+	+	+	−
Bax/Bad/Bik	−	−	−	+	−	−
FLIPs	+	−	−	+	−	+
IAPs	+	+	+	+	+	+
FADD	+	−	−	+	−	+
P53	−	−	−	+	+	−

[a]Entries in the diagonal denote therapies with a single target; others are combinations of potential therapies. A plus sign (+) denotes therapies with decreased activation of executioner caspase, and the minus sign (−) denotes the opposite [65].

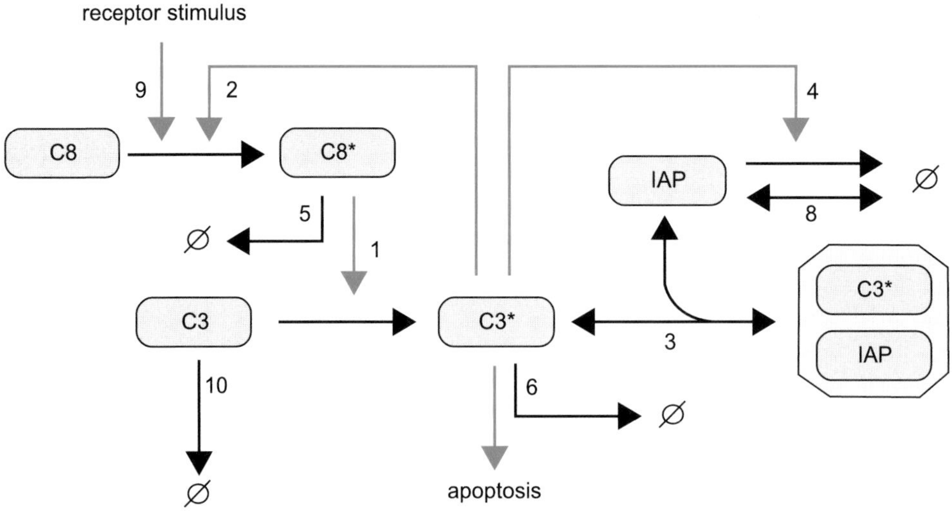

Figure 3.35 Outline of the apoptotic model developed by Eissing *et al.* [66]. It comprises the components of the extrinsic pathway of apoptosis. The asterisk (*) denotes the activated form of a caspase.

do not, because they target only a single activation route. For example, the over-expression of several antiapoptotic members of the Bcl-2 protein family does not block receptor-mediated activation and thus apoptosis can proceed. Similarly, a disruption or mutation of FADD does not block the stress-induced activation of apoptosis via the intrinsic pathway.

Another model describing the extrinsic pathway of apoptosis was developed by Eissing *et al.* [66]. The reaction schema of the model is depicted in Figure 3.35. The model is described by a system of eight ordinary differential equations.

$$\begin{aligned}
\frac{\mathrm{d}[C8]}{\mathrm{d}t} &= -v_2 - v_9 \\
\frac{\mathrm{d}[C8^*]}{\mathrm{d}t} &= v_2 - v_5(-v_{11}) \\
\frac{\mathrm{d}[C3]}{\mathrm{d}t} &= -v_1 - v_{10} \\
\frac{\mathrm{d}[C3^*]}{\mathrm{d}t} &= v_1 - v_3 - v_6 \\
\frac{\mathrm{d}[IAP]}{\mathrm{d}t} &= -v_3 - v_4 - v_8 \\
\frac{\mathrm{d}[C3^* \sim IAP]}{\mathrm{d}t} &= -v_2 - v_9 \\
\frac{\mathrm{d}[BAR]}{\mathrm{d}t} &= -v_{11} - v_{12} \\
\frac{\mathrm{d}[C8^* \sim BAR]}{\mathrm{d}t} &= -v_{11} - v_{13}.
\end{aligned} \tag{3.53}$$

The rate equations read as follows:

$$
\begin{aligned}
v_1 &= k_1 \cdot [C8^*] \cdot [C3] \\
v_2 &= k_2 \cdot [C3^*] \cdot [C8] \\
v_3 &= k_3 \cdot [C3^*] \cdot [IAP] - k_{-3} \cdot [C3^* \sim IAP] \\
v_4 &= k_4 \cdot [C3^*] \cdot [IAP] \\
v_5 &= k_5 \cdot [C8^*] \\
v_6 &= k_6 \cdot [C3^*] \\
v_7 &= k_7 \cdot [C3^* \sim IAP] \\
v_8 &= k_8 \cdot [IAP] - k_{-8} \\
v_9 &= k_9 \cdot [C8] - k_{-9} \\
v_{10} &= k_{10} \cdot [C3] - k_{-10} \\
v_{11} &= k_{11} \cdot [C8^*] \cdot [BAR] - k_{-11} \cdot [C8^* \sim BAR] \\
v_{12} &= k_{12} \cdot [BAR] - k_{-12} \\
v_{13} &= k_{13} \cdot [C8^* \sim BAR].
\end{aligned}
\qquad (3.54)
$$

In this model, procaspase-8 ($C8$, denoting initiator procaspases 8 and 10) is activated by an extracellular signal mediated by death receptors. Activated caspase-8 ($C8^*$) subsequently cleaves and activates procaspase-3 ($C3$, representing the executioner caspases in general, e.g., caspases 3, 6, 7) by forming active caspase-3 ($C3^*$). Caspase-3 leads to apoptosis and acts in terms of a positive feedback loop onto procaspase-8. The caspase inhibitor IAP can bind caspase-3 reversibly by forming the complex $C3^* \sim IAP$. Activated caspases as well as $C3^* \sim IAP$ are continuously degraded. Furthermore, IAP degradation is mediated by caspase 3. In addition to this, an inhibitor of $C8^*$ called BAR [67] was introduced by Eissing *et al.* [66].

The model was used for the study of the bistable switch from the status "alive" into the apoptotic state. Therefore, simulations were performed by Eissing *et al.* [66] using the following initial concentrations and parameter values. Concentrations of the model components are given as molecules per cell. With an estimated cell volume of 1 pl, one can easily transform these values into more common units. Initial concentrations for caspase-8 and -3 are 130,000 and 21,000 molecules/cell, respectively. The initial concentrations of active caspase-3 and the complexes $C3^* \sim IAP$ and $C8^* \sim BAR$ are assumed to be 0 molecules/cell. Concentrations of the inhibitors IAP and BAR are assumed to be 40,000 molecules/cell at the beginning. The initial amount of activated caspase-8 ($C8^*$) represents the input signal of the signaling cascade. In the example displayed here, it varies between 0 and 3000 molecules/cell. The kinetic parameters of the model as elaborated by Eissing *et al.* [66] mostly from literature are displayed in Table 3.6.

As outlined above, apoptosis should display a bistable behavior, but the status "alive" must be stable and resistant toward minor accidental trigger signals, i.e., noise. However, once the apoptotic signal is beyond a certain threshold, the cell must irreversibly enter apoptosis.

Simulations of the model, using the parameters shown in Table 3.6, show a bistable behavior (Figure 3.36). The simulation results, with varying input signals between 0 and 3000 molecules/cell of activated caspase-8, show a low amount of active caspase-3

Table 3.6 Parameter values of the model described by Eissing *et al.* [66].

Parameter	Value	Reverse parameter	Value
k_1	$5.8\times10^{-5}\,\text{cell}\,\text{min}^{-1}\,\text{mo}^{-1}$	K_{-1}	0
k_2	$10^{-5}\,\text{cell}\,\text{min}^{-1}\,\text{mo}^{-1}$	k_{-2}	0
k_3	$5\times10^{-4}\,\text{cell}\,\text{min}^{-1}\,\text{mo}^{-1}$	k_{-3}	$0.21\,\text{min}^{-1}$
k_4	$3\times10^{-4}\,\text{cell}\,\text{min}^{-1}\,\text{mo}^{-1}$	k_{-4}	0
k_5	$5.8\times10^{-3}\,\text{min}^{-1}$	k_{-5}	0
k_6	$5.8\times10^{-3}\,\text{min}^{-1}$	k_{-6}	0
k_7	$1.73\times10^{-2}\,\text{min}^{-1}$	K_{-7}	0
k_8	$1.16\times10^{-2}\,\text{min}^{-1}$	k_{-8}	$464\,\text{mo}\,\text{cell}^{-1}\,\text{min}^{-1}$
k_9	$3.9\times10^{-3}\,\text{min}^{-1}$	k_{-9}	$507\,\text{mo}\,\text{cell}^{-1}\,\text{min}^{-1}$
k_{10}	$3.9\times10^{-3}\,\text{min}^{-1}$	k_{-10}	$81.9\,\text{mo}\,\text{cell}^{-1}\,\text{min}^{-1}$
k_{11}	$5\times10^{-4}\,\text{min}^{-1}$	k_{-11}	$0.21\,\text{min}^{-1}$
k_{12}	$10^{-3}\,\text{min}^{-1}$	k_{-12}	$40\,\text{mo}\,\text{cell}^{-1}\,\text{min}^{-1}$
k_{13}	$1.16\times10^{-2}\,\text{min}^{-1}$	k_{-13}	0

until the concentration of active caspase-8 exceeds a threshold. Then the model switches from the status "alive" into the apoptotic state indicated by a steep rise in the amount of active caspase-3. The apoptotic state is reached with a time delay that is inversely proportional to the initial input signal. Both the states ("alive" and apoptotic)

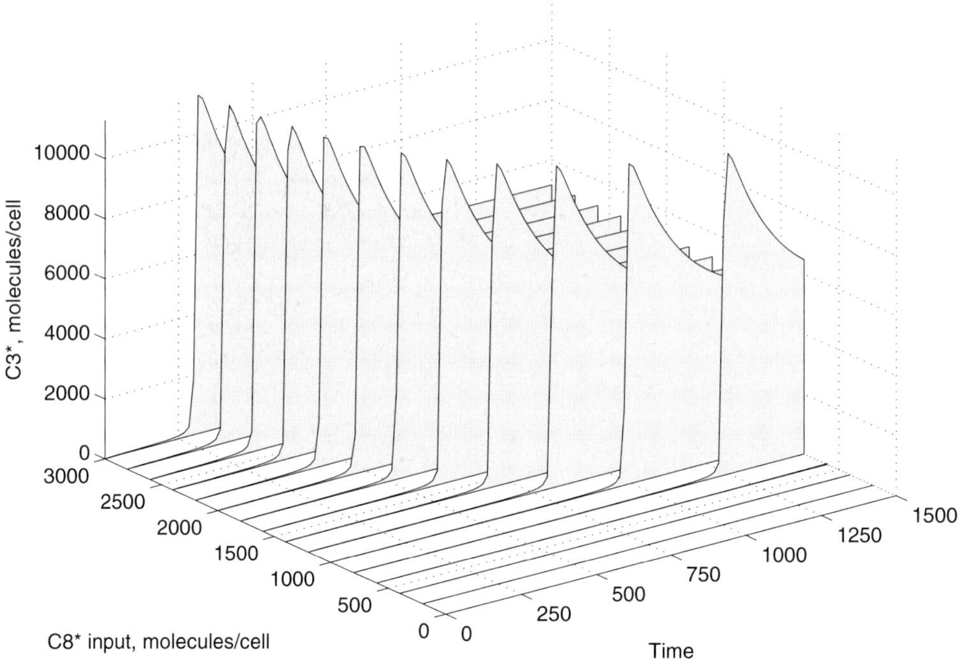

Figure 3.36 Bistable behavior of the extrinsic apoptosis model versus varying input signals. The input signal is modeled by the initial concentration of the activated caspase-8 [66].

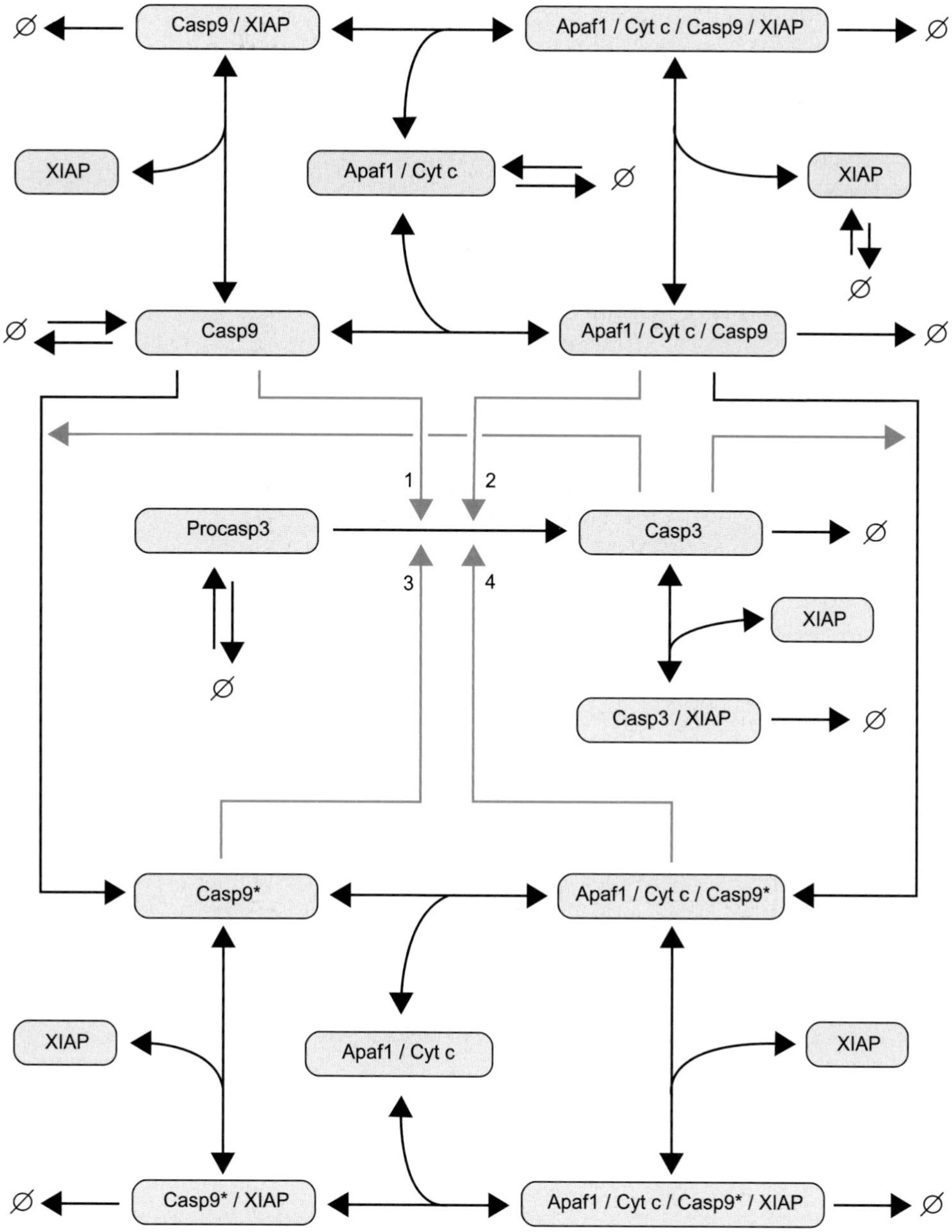

Figure 3.37 Schematic representation of central components of the intrinsic apoptotic signaling pathway developed by Legewie *et al.* [68]. Casp9 denotes the autoproteolytically processed form of caspase-9 that is cleaved at Asp^{315}, and $Casp9^{*}$ is the form processed by caspase-3 at Asp^{330}.

are stable states with the used parameter values for this model. Eissing *et al.* [66] showed that the same model without the inhibition of activated caspase-8 by BAR ("single inhibition model") also shows a bistable behavior, but with an unstable life steady state within the used kinetic parameter space.

Legewie *et al.* [68] developed a model of a central part of the intrinsic apoptotic pathway that describes the activation of caspase-3 by active caspase-9 (Figure 3.37). Caspase-9 can be activated in two different ways (Figure 3.38). First of all recruited by the apoptosome, it can be autoproteolytically processed at amino acid Asp^{315} that results into the formation of the two subunits p35/p12. Furthermore, caspase-9 can also be activated by active caspase-3 through proteolysis at Asp^{330} that results in the formation of the two subunits p37 and p10. The activation of caspase-9 by caspase-3 results in a positive feedback activation and signal amplification. The stimulation of intrinsic apoptosis is given in this model by the amount of the apoptosomes (Apaf1/Cyt c). It is assumed that caspase-9, which is associated with the apoptosome, cleaves procaspase-3 much more efficiently (70 times) than free caspase-9. Furthermore, caspase-9 that was processed by caspase-3 at Asp^{330} is 10 times more efficient than caspase-9 that was processed autocatalytically at Asp^{315}. Both caspase-3 and caspase-9 can be inhibited by XIAP (and other IAPs that are not explicitly modeled). Legewie *et al.* [68] have demonstrated that the inhibition of caspase-3 and caspase-9 by XIAP results in an implicit positive feedback. Cleaved caspase-3 augments its own activation by sequestering the inhibitor XIAP away from caspase-9. This implicit positive feedback brings about bistability, which is an essential claim on apoptosis. Furthermore, the authors show that this positive feedback cooperates with caspase-3-mediated feedback cleavage of caspase-9 to generate irreversibility in the caspase activation.

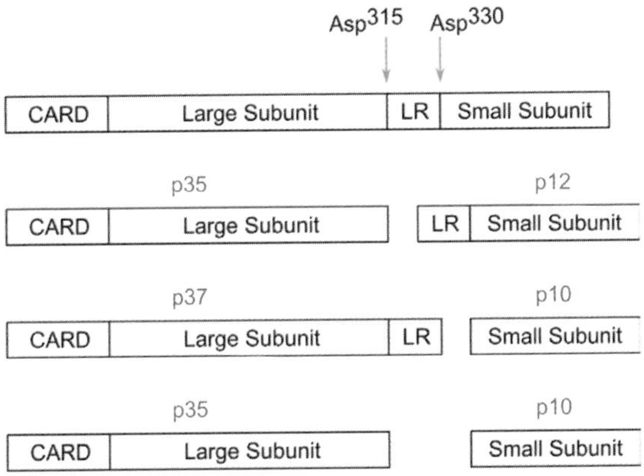

Figure 3.38 Diagram of procaspase-9 and its proteolytic products by caspase-9-mediated cleavage at Asp^{315}, caspase-3-mediated cleavage at Asp^{330}, or both [69].

Exercises and Problems

1. Calculate the flux control coefficients for the model of the threonine synthesis pathway. If required, use a computational tool providing the necessary functions.

2. Consider the Ras activation cycle shown in Figure 3.14 with the parameters given there. The concentration of GAP be 0.1. GEF gets activated according to $\mathrm{GEF} = \begin{cases} 0, & t < 0 \\ e^{-0.2t}, & t \geq 0 \end{cases}$. Calculate the signaling time $\tau_{Ras_{GTP}}$ and the signal duration $\vartheta_{Ras_{GTP}}$ (Eqs. (3.26) and (3.27)).

3. MAP kinase cascades comprise kinases and phosphatases. How would such a cascade behave if there were no phosphatases?

4. Game of Life. (a) Invent two initial configurations that remain unchanged under the updating rules of the game of life. (b) Simulate the following patterns (called "glider" and "lightweight spaceship") with paper and pencil. The surrounding cells are supposed to be empty ("dead"). (c) Implement the game of life as a computer program and play with random initial configurations.

(1) 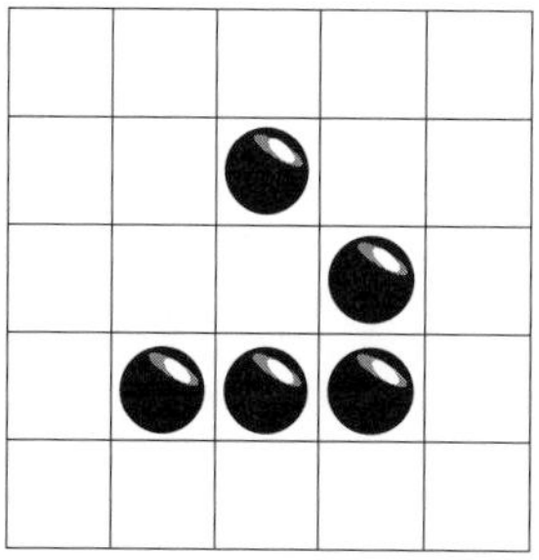

(2) 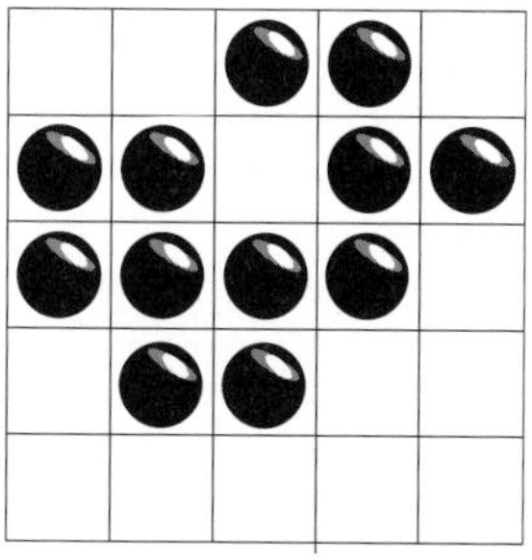

5. Show that the diffusion equation is solved by spatial cosine profiles with temporally decreasing amplitude

$$s(x,t) = s_o\, e^{-\lambda(k)t} \cos(kx)$$

and compute the dispersion relation $\lambda(k)$.

6. Show that the stationary profile

$$s^{st}(x) = \frac{6D/\kappa}{(x + \sqrt{6D/(\kappa s_o)})^2} = \frac{6D/\kappa}{(x + (2Da/j(0))^{1/3})^2}$$

where $a = 6D/\kappa$ is a solution of the Bicoid reaction–diffusion system with autocatalytic degradation term $-\kappa \cdot s(x,t)^2$ (see Section 3.4.4). Hint: use the ansatz $s^{st}(x) = a/(x+b)^2$.

7. The pair-rule gene *eve* is expressed in seven stripes in the blastoderm of the fruit fly *Drosophila melanogaster*. The stripes do not arise from spontaneous pattern formation, but from a response to existing patterns of the regulatory proteins *Krüppel*, *Bicoid*, *Giant*, and *Hunchback*. The response is hard-coded in the regulatory region of the *eve* gene. Speculate in broad terms about advantages and disadvantages of spontaneous and "hardwired" pattern formation.

8. Describe the different phases of the eukaryotic cell cycle. What are the three most important regulatory cell-cycle checkpoints?

9. Describe the crosslink between the intrinsic and the extrinsic apoptotic pathway.

10. How can a mathematical model of, e.g., apoptosis be used for the identification of potential drug targets?

References

1 Snoep, J.L. and Olivier, B.G. (2002) Java Web Simulation (JWS); a web-based database of kinetic models. *Molecular Biology Reports*, **29**, 259–263.

2 Hynne, F. *et al.* (2001) Full-scale model of glycolysis in *Saccharomyces cerevisiae*. *Biophysical Chemistry*, **94**, 121–163.

3 Rizzi, M. *et al.* (1997) *In vivo* analysis of metabolic dynamics in *Saccharomyces cerevisiae*: II. Mathematical model. *Biotechnology and Bioengineering*, **55**, 592–608.

4 Theobald, U. *et al.* (1997) *In vivo* analysis of metabolic dynamics in *Saccharomyces cerevisiae*: I. Experimental observations. *Biotechnology and Bioengineering*, **55**, 305–316.

5 Yi, T.M. *et al.* (2003) A quantitative characterization of the yeast heterotrimeric G protein cycle. *Proceedings of the National Academy of Sciences of the United States of America*, **100**, 10764–10769.

6 Neer, E.J. (1995) Heterotrimeric G proteins: organizers of transmembrane signals. *Cell*, **80**, 249–257.

7 Dohlman, H.G. (2002) G proteins and pheromone signaling. *Annual Review of Physiology*, **64**, 129–152.

8 Blumer, K.J. and Thorner, J. (1991) Receptor-G protein signaling in yeast. *Annual Review of Physiology*, **53**, 37–57.

9 Dohlman, H.G. *et al.* (1991) Model systems for the study of seven-transmembrane-segment receptors. *Annual Review of Biochemistry*, **60**, 653–688.

10 Buck, L.B. (2000) The molecular architecture of odor and pheromone sensing in mammals. *Cell*, **100**, 611–618.

11 Banuett, F. (1998) Signalling in the yeasts: an informational cascade with links to the filamentous fungi. *Microbiology and Molecular Biology Reviews*, **62**, 249–274.

12 Dohlman, H.G. *et al.* (1998) Regulation of G protein signalling in yeast. *Seminars in Cell & Developmental Biology*, **9**, 135–141.

13 Wang, P. and Heitman, J. (1999) Signal transduction cascades regulating mating, filamentation, and virulence in *Cryptococcus neoformans*. *Current Opinion in Microbiology*, **2**, 358–362.

14 Offermanns, S. (2000) Mammalian G-protein function *in vivo*: new insights through altered gene expression. *Reviews of Physiology, Biochemistry and Pharmacology*, **140**, 63–133.

15 Dohlman, H.G. and Thorner, J.W. (2001) Regulation of G protein-initiated signal

transduction in yeast: paradigms and principles. *Annual Review of Biochemistry*, **70**, 703–754.

16 Meigs, T.E. *et al.* (2001) Interaction of Galpha 12 and Galpha 13 with the cytoplasmic domain of cadherin provides a mechanism for beta-catenin release. *Proceedings of the National Academy of Sciences of the United States of America*, **98**, 519–524.

17 Dohlman, H.G. and Thorner, J. (1997) RGS proteins and signaling by heterotrimeric G proteins. *The Journal of Biological Chemistry*, **272**, 3871–3874.

18 Siderovski, D.P. *et al.* (1999) Whither goest the RGS proteins? *Critical Reviews in Biochemistry and Molecular Biology*, **34**, 215–251.

19 Burchett, S.A. (2000) Regulators of G protein signaling: a bestiary of modular protein binding domains. *Journal of Neurochemistry*, **75**, 1335–1351.

20 Ross, E.M. and Wilkie, T.M. (2000) GTPase-activating proteins for heterotrimeric G proteins: regulators of G protein signaling (RGS) and RGS-like proteins. *Annual Review of Biochemistry*, **69**, 795–827.

21 Takai, Y. *et al.* (2001) Small GTP-binding proteins. *Physiological Reviews*, **81**, 153–208.

22 Postma, P.W. *et al.* (1989) The role of the PEP: carbohydrate phosphotransferase system in the regulation of bacterial metabolism. *FEMS Microbiology Reviews*, **5**, 69–80.

23 Postma, P.W. *et al.* (1993) Phosphoenolpyruvate: carbohydrate phosphotransferase systems of bacteria. *Microbiological Reviews*, **57**, 543–594.

24 Rohwer, J.M. *et al.* (2000) Understanding glucose transport by the bacterial phosphoenolpyruvate: glycose phosphotransferase system on the basis of kinetic measurements *in vitro*. *The Journal of Biological Chemistry*, **275**, 34909–34921.

25 Francke, C. *et al.* (2003) Why the phosphotransferase system of *Escherichia coli* escapes diffusion limitation. *Biophysical Journal*, **85**, 612–622.

26 Klipp, E. *et al.* (2005) Integrative model of the response of yeast to osmotic shock. *Nature Biotechnology*, **23**, 975–982.

27 Hohmann, S. (2002) Osmotic stress signaling and osmoadaptation in yeasts. *Microbiology and Molecular Biology Reviews*, **66**, 300–372.

28 Wilkinson, M.G. and Millar, J.B. (2000) Control of the eukaryotic cell cycle by MAP kinase signaling pathways. *The FASEB Journal*, **14**, 2147–2157.

29 Huang, C.Y. and Ferrell, J.E. Jr (1996) Ultrasensitivity in the mitogen-activated protein kinase cascade. *Proceedings of the National Academy of Sciences of the United States of America*, **93**, 10078–10083.

30 Kholodenko, B.N. (2000) Negative feedback and ultrasensitivity can bring about oscillations in the mitogen-activated protein kinase cascades. *European Journal of Biochemistry*, **267**, 1583–1588.

31 Force, T. *et al.* (1994) Enzymatic characteristics of the c-Raf-1 protein kinase. *Proceedings of the National Academy of Sciences of the United States of America*, **91**, 1270–1274.

32 Kisseleva, T. *et al.* (2002) Signaling through the JAK/STAT pathway, recent advances and future challenges. *Gene*, **285**, 1–24.

33 Schindler, C.W. (2002) Series introduction. JAK–STAT signaling in human disease. *The Journal of Clinical Investigation*, **109**, 1133–1137.

34 Goldbeter, A. (1991b) A minimal cascade model for the mitotic oscillator involving cyclin and cdc2 kinase. *Proceedings of the National Academy of Sciences of the United States of America*, **88**, 9107–9111.

35 Heinrich, R. *et al.* (2002) Mathematical models of protein kinase signal transduction. *Molecular Cell*, **9**, 957–970.

36 Komarova, N.L. *et al.* (2005) A theoretical framework for specificity in cell signalling. *Molecular Systems Biology* 1:2005.0023.

37 Schaber, J. *et al.* (2006) A modelling approach to quantify dynamic crosstalk between the pheromone and the starvation pathway in baker's yeast. *FEBS Journal*, **273**, 3520–3533.

38 Hartwell, L.H. (1974) *Saccharomyces cerevisiae* cell cycle. *Bacteriological Reviews*, **38**, 164–198.

39 Hartwell, L.H. *et al.* (1974) Genetic control of the cell division cycle in yeast. *Science*, **183**, 46–51.

40 Pardee, A.B. (1974) A restriction point for control of normal animal cell proliferation. *Proceedings of the National Academy of Sciences of the United States of America*, **71**, 1286–1290.

41 Nurse, P. (1975) Genetic control of cell size at cell division in yeast. *Nature*, **256**, 547–551.

42 Nurse, P. and Bissett, Y. (1981) Gene required in G1 for commitment to cell cycle and in G2 for control of mitosis in fission yeast. *Nature*, **292**, 558–560.

43 Goldbeter, A. (1991a) A minimal cascade model for the mitotic oscillator involving cyclin and cdc2 kinase. *Proceedings of the National Academy of Sciences of the United States of America*, **88**, 9107–9111.

44 Fall, C.P. *et al.* (2002) *Computational Cell Biology*, Springer, New York.

45 Tyson, J.J. *et al.* (1996) Chemical kinetic theory: understanding cell-cycle regulation. *Trends in Biochemical Sciences*, **21**, 89–96.

46 Novák, B. *et al.* (1999) Finishing the cell cycle. *Journal of Theoretical Biology*, **199**, 223–233.

47 Chen, K.C. *et al.* (2000) Kinetic analysis of a molecular model of the budding yeast cell cycle. *Molecular Biology of the Cell*, **11**, 369–391.

48 Chen, K.C. *et al.* (2004) Integrative analysis of cell cycle control in budding yeast. *Molecular Biology of the Cell*, **15**, 3841–3862.

49 Barberis, M. *et al.* (2007) Cell size at S phase initiation: an emergent property of the G1/S network. *PLoS Computational Biology*, **3**, e64.

50 Murray, J.D. (2003) *Mathematical Biology. II: Spatial Models and Biomedical Applications*, Springer, Berlin.

51 Poulin, P. and Theil, F. (2002) Prediction of pharmacokinetics prior to *in vivo* studies. II. Generic physiologically based pharmacokinetic models of drug disposition. *Journal of Pharmaceutical Sciences*, **91** (5), 1358–1370.

52 Theil, F., Guentert, T.W., Haddad, S. and Poulin, P. (2003) Utility of physiologically based pharmacokinetic models to drug development and rational drug discovery candidate selection. *Toxicology Letters*, **138**, 29–49.

53 Deutsch, A. and Dormann, S. (2004) *Cellular Automaton Modeling and Biological Pattern Formation*, Birkhäuser Verlag AG, Basel.

54 Gardner, M. (1970) Mathematical games: The fantastic combinations of John Conway's new solitaire game "Life". *Scientific American*, **223**, 120–123.

55 Meinhardt, H. and Klingler, M. (1987) A model for pattern formation on the shells of molluscs. *Journal of Theoretical Biology*, **126**, 63–69.

56 Meinhardt, H. (2003) *The Algorithmic Beauty of Sea Shells*, Springer, Heidelberg, New York.

57 Gurdon, J.B. and Bourillot, P.-Y. (2001) Morphogen gradient interpretation. *Nature*, **413**, 797–803.

58 Meinhardt, H. and Gierer, A. (1974) Applications of a theory of biological pattern formation based on lateral inhibition. *Journal of Cell Science*, **15**, 321–346.

59 Meinhardt, H. (1993) A model for pattern formation of hypostome, tentacles, and foot in hydra: how to form structures close to each other, how to form them at a distance. *Developmental Biology*, **157**, 321–333.

60 Kosman, D., Small, S. and Reinitz, J. (1998) Rapid preparation of a panel of polyclonal antibodies to Drosophila segmentation proteins. *Development Genes and Evolution*, **208**, 290–294.

61 Poustelnikova, E., Pisarev, A., Blagov, M., Samsonova, M. and Reinitz, J. (2004) A database for management of gene expression data *in situ*. *Bioinformatics*, **20**, 2212–2221.

62 Eldar, A., Rosin, D., Shilo, B.Z. and Barkai, N. (2003) Self-enhanced ligand degradation underlies robustness of morphogen gradients. *Developmental Cell*, **5**, 635–646.

63 Gierer, A. and Meinhardt, H. (1972) A theory of biological pattern formation. *Kybernetik*, **12**, 30–39.

64 Turing, A.M. (1952) The chemical basis of morphogenesis. *Philosophical Transactions of the Royal Society of London*, **237** (641), 37–72.

65 Fussenegger, M. *et al.* (2000) A mathematical model of caspase function in apoptosis. *Nature Biotechnology*, **18**, 768–774.

66 Eissing, T. *et al.* (2004) Bistability analyses of a caspase activation model for receptor-induced apoptosis. *The Journal of Biological Chemistry*, **279**, 36892–36897.

67 Stegh, A.H. *et al.* (2002) Inactivation of caspase-8 on mitochondria of Bcl-xL-expressing MCF7-Fas cells: role for the bifunctional apoptosis regulator protein. *The Journal of Biological Chemistry*, **277**, 4351–4360.

68 Legewie, S. *et al.* (2006) Mathematical modeling identifies inhibitors of apoptosis as mediators of positive feedback and bistability. *PLoS Computational Biology*, **2**, e120.

69 Zou, H. *et al.* (2003) Regulation of the Apaf-1/caspase-9 apoptosome by caspase-3 and XIAP. *The Journal of Biological Chemistry*, **278**, 8091–8098.

4
Model Fitting

4.1
Data for Small Metabolic and Signaling Systems

Summary

The mathematical equations that are used to develop kinetic models of biochemical systems are so complex that, except for the most simple cases, it is impossible to solve them analytically. Therefore, numerical simulations are required to predict how concentrations develop over time and when and if the system will reach a steady state. But numerical simulations need numerical data to assign specific values to a large number of molecule properties. Among these properties are Michaelis–Menten constants, K_m, and maximal velocities, $V_{max,}$ (for enzymes), but also biological half-lives, binding constants, molecule concentrations, and diffusion rates. In the early days of mathematical modeling, it was very difficult to obtain enough data of sufficient quality to make reliable model predictions. In such a situation, only qualitative models can be constructed that investigate the question if a certain behavior is at all possible or not. Although such a model provides valuable information about a system of biochemical reactions, most models today aim to be quantitative. This means that the model should agree well with measured concentrations and also predictions regarding changes of molecule concentrations are given as specific numbers instead of a qualitative up or down statement. To develop quantitative models, it is therefore essential to obtain a large number of reliable data for the model parameters. One source are specialized databases, which will be discussed in this section. But the process of filling these databases is currently very time-consuming, since most kinetic data have to be extracted by hand from the existing literature. Recently developed experimental techniques aim to improve the situation by enabling researchers to measure large numbers of kinetic data with high accuracy. Some of these techniques will be described at the end of chapter 4.1.

Systems Biology: A Textbook. Edda Klipp, Wolfram Liebermeister, Christoph Wierling, Axel Kowald, Hans Lehrach, and Ralf Herwig

ISBN: 978-3-527-31874-2

4.1.1
Databases for Kinetic Modeling

BRENDA is a database that aims to be a comprehensive enzyme information system (http://www.brenda-enzymes.info). BRENDA is a curated database that contains a large number of functional data for individual enzymes (Figure 4.1). These data are gathered from the literature and made available via a web interface. Table 4.1 gives an overview of the types of information that is collected and the number of entries for the different information fields (as of November 2007). For instance, enzymes representing 4762 different EC numbers and almost 80,000 different K_m values exist in the database.

One of BRENDA's strengths is the multitude of ways the database can be searched. It is easy to find all enzymes that are above a specific molecular weight, belong to *C. elegans*, or have a temperature optimum above 30 °C. If desired, the list of results can then be downloaded as a tab separated text file for later inspection. Using the Advanced Search feature, it is possible to construct arbitrarily complex search queries involving the information fields shown in Table 4.1.

Sometimes it is desirable to search for all enzymes that are glycosylases without knowing the corresponding EC number, or to find all enzymes that are found in horses without knowing the exact scientific name. In this situation the ECTree

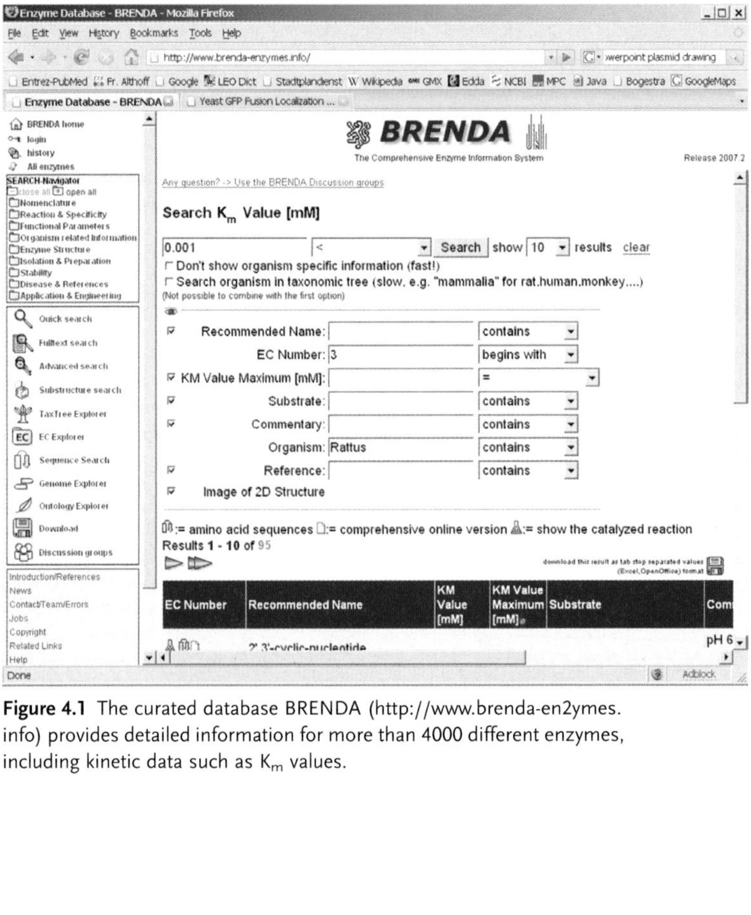

Figure 4.1 The curated database BRENDA (http://www.brenda-en2ymes.info) provides detailed information for more than 4000 different enzymes, including kinetic data such as K_m values.

Table 4.1 BRENDA collects many types of information regarding enzymes. Each information field can be used for search queries, which makes it possible to perform very complex and specific searches.

Information field	Entries	Information field	Entries
Enzyme nomenclature		*Functional parameters*	
EC number	4762	K_m value	79,435
Recommended name	4757	Turnover number	240,77
Systematic name	3650	Specific activity	30,420
Synonymes	53,396	pH range and optimum	6609/25,681
CAS Registry Number	4383	Temperature range and optimum	2186/12,319
Reaction	10,731	*Molecular properties*	
Reaction type	7783	pH stability	4650
Enzyme structure		Temperature stability	13,149
Molecular weight	24,424	General stability	6653
Subunits	22,750	Organic solvent stability	787
Sequence links	283,733	Oxidation stability	599
Posttranslational modifications	4687	Storage stability	9084
Crystallization	5105	Purification	25,927
3D-structure, PDB links	35,400	Cloned	16,303
Enzyme–ligand interactions		Engineering	23,235
Substrates/products	222,285	Renatured	625
Natural substrates	51,126	Application	4760
Cofactor	16,302	*Organism-related information*	
Activating compound	18,466	Organism	364,770
Metals/ions	27,668	Source tissue, organ	65,938
Inhibitors	11,2470	Localization	29,906
Bibliographic data			
References	30,0190		

browser and the TaxTree search are helpful by providing a browser like interface to search down the hierarchy of EC number descriptions or taxonomic names.

BRENDA is also well connected to other databases that can provide further information about a specific enzyme. Associated GO terms are directly linked to the AmiGO browser, substrates and products of the catalyzed reactions can be displayed as chemical structures, links to the taxonomic database NEWT (http://www.ebi.ac.uk/newt) exist for information on the organism, sequence data can be obtained form Swiss-Prot and if crystallographic data exist, a link to PDB (see Chapter 16) is provided. Finally, literature references (including PubMed IDs) are provided and the implemented web service allows programmatic access to the data via a SOAP (Simple Object Access Protocol) interface (http://www.brenda-enzymes.org/soap).

SABIO-RK (http://sabio.villa-bosch.de/SABIORK) is another web-based database for information about biochemical reactions, kinetic rate equations, and numerical values for kinetic parameters. The information contained in SABIO-RK is partly extracted from KEGG (see Chapter 16) and partly from the literature. Currently the database (version 20090312) is much smaller than BRENDA, containing for instance K_m values for 367 reactions of *E. coli*, 817 reactions of *H. sapiens*, or 128 reactions of *S. cerevisiae*. The main access to the data is via a search for reactions. Several constraints for the reaction like participating enzyme and reactants, biochemical pathway, organism and cellular location can be used to narrow down the search. The results page provides further information about the reaction (with links to EC information, UniProt, and PubMed) and available kinetic data. A potentially very useful feature of SABIO-RK is that the kinetic information for selected reactions can be exported as SBML format (see Section 6), which could considerably speed up the development in models for simulations. However, there are several points that need special consideration. It is advisable to search only reactions for which K_m, V_{max} and a rate law exists, otherwise the SBML file will contain no reaction and unknown parameters will be set to zero. For SBML export it is also important to select "export parameters normalized to SI base units" to ensure that always standard units are used. In addition the produced SBML file should be inspected manually to check the result. Finally, like BRENDA, the contents of SABIO-RK can be accessed via web services.

4.1.2
Measuring Promoter Activities Using GFP Reporter Genes

The kinetic data in BRENDA or SABIO-RK are extracted from the literature of the last decades. This is not only very time-consuming, but it also means that the data were obtained from a multitude of different organisms under different experimental conditions from different experimenters. Recently green fluorescent protein (GFP)-based high throughput techniques have been developed that have the potential to improve the situation considerably. GFP is a 27 kDa protein found in jellyfish [1], and is frequently used as reporter gene (see also Section 11.14). Work by [2] shows that kinetic parameters of *E. coli* promoters can be determined in parallel by using GFP reporter constructs to measure promoter activity with high accuracy and temporal resolution. For this purpose the promoter region of interest is cloned in front of a GFP gene and the whole construct is placed on a plasmid together with a selection marker and a low copy origin of replication (see also Section 11.2). The authors used this approach to study eight operons of the bacterial SOS repair system by measuring fluorescence and optical density (OD) every 3 min. From the resulting 99 data points per operon kinetic parameters of the promoters can be derived using a simple mathematical approach.

The activity of promoter *i*, X_i, is proportional to the number of GFP molecules synthesized per time interval per cell. Since degradation of GFP can be neglected, promoter activity is given by the derivative of the amount G_i of GFP, normalized by the optical density.

$$X_i(t) = \frac{dG_i(t)/dt}{OD_i(t)}.$$

A single transcription factor suppresses all operons of the SOS system without influence from other transcription factors. It is therefore reasonable to model the promoter activity by a Michaelis–Menten type kinetics, where $A(t)$ is the repressor concentration, β_i is the activity of the unrepressed promoter i, and K_i is the repressor concentration at half maximal repression.

$$X_i(t) = \frac{\beta_i}{1 + A(t)/K_i}.$$

All kinetic parameters as well as the time-dependent activities $A(t)$ of the repressor LexA were estimated by a least-squares fit. For the fitting, all time series $X_i(t)$ were normalized to the same maximal activity. The values of $A(t)$ and the K_i can only be determined up to a scaling factor because a rescaling $A \to \lambda A$, $K_i \to \lambda K_i$ does not affect the model predictions. As further constraints, it was required that $A(t) > 0$ (no negative concentrations) and $A(0) = 1$ (normalization). The following table shows the obtained values for the eight studied promoters. For six of the eight cases the mean error for the predicted promoter activity is below 22%, which is a very good quantitative prediction. The genes *uvrY* and *polB*, however, showed errors of 30–45%, indicating that these genes are possibly influenced by additional factors. This study shows that kinetic data can be obtained using an approach that can, in principle, be scaled up to the whole genome.

Gene	K	β	Error	Function
uvrA	0.09 ± 0.04	2800 ± 300	0.14	Nucleotide excision repair
lexA	0.15 ± 0.08	2200 ± 100	0.10	Transcriptional repressor
recA	0.16 ± 0.07	3300 ± 200	0.12	LexA autocleavage, replication fork blocking
umuD	0.19 ± 0.1	330 ± 30	0.21	Mutagenesis repair
polB	0.35 ± 0.15	70 ± 10	0.31	Translesion DNA synthesis, replication fork recovery
ruvA	0.37 ± 0.1	30 ± 2	0.22	Double strand break repair
uvrD	0.65 ± 0.3	170 ± 20	0.20	Nucleotide excision repair, recombination repair
uvrY	0.51 ± 0.25	300 ± 200	0.45	Unknown function

The use of GFP and its variants for measuring kinetic and other data has several advantages over traditional experimental techniques.

- It opens the possibility to obtain kinetic data in a high throughput approach.
- The measurements have a high time resolution (one data point every few minutes).
- The kinetic parameters are measured under *in vivo* conditions.
- Using high throughput flow cytometry and microscopy it is possible to perform single cell measurements (see also Section 11.14).
- The reproducibility of the measurements is very good (around 10% error).

These attractive features have led to a number of very interesting studies in recent years. One limitation of the algorithm used by [2] is that it cannot be applied to systems where more than one transcription factor controls the promoter activity.

For this it is necessary to have a quantitative understanding how the input signals of different transcription factors are combined into the output signal (promoter activity). Section 6.1. describes, in detail, how this has been achieved for the promoter of the *lac* operon of *E. coli.*

In another study, 52 promoters of *E. coli* amino acid biosynthesis pathways were investigated by placing the regulatory regions in front of a GFP gene [3]. Cells were shifted from a medium without any amino acids to a medium that contained a single amino acid and GFP expression was measured every 8 min for 8 h. The results showed that the promoters of enzymes early in unbranched pathways have the shortest response time and strongest activity. This design principle agree nicely with the results of a mathematical model that was optimized to achieve a flux goal with minimal enzyme production. The same group extended this GFP-based approach to a genomic scale by generating reporter strains for all intergenic regions in *E. coli* that are larger than 40 bp [4]. The resulting library of 2000 constructs was used in a diauxic shift experiment, where cells first feed on glucose and then switch to lactose once the glucose levels are depleted. This led to the discovery of 80 previously unknown promoters.

In another high throughput experiment, GFP constructs were used to provide genome wide information about protein localization in *S. cerevisiae* [5]. For each annotated ORF, a pair of oligonucleotides was synthesized with homologies to the desired chromosomal insertion site. After placing the GFP sequence between these short sequences, the whole construct was inserted at the C terminus of each ORF using homologous recombination. This resulted in 4156 fusion proteins (75% of the yeast proteome) with a C terminal GFP tag. The information regarding the cellular localization of these proteins is publicly available at http://yeastGFP.ucsf.edu. Together with the spatial information, the website also provides information about individual protein numbers per cell.

4.2
Parameter Estimation

Summary

Parameters in a model can be determined by fitting the model to experimental data. In the method of least squares, a common approach in parameter estimation, the sum of squared residuals between model predictions and data is minimized. For data with additive standard Gaussian errors, this method is equivalent to maximum likelihood estimation. The variability of parameter estimates due to noisy and insufficient data can be assessed by repeating the estimation with resampled data ("bootstrapping") and the quality of model predictions can be tested by cross-validation. In Bayesian parameter estimation, parameter sets are scored by how well they agree with both available data and with certain prior assumptions, which are expressed by probability distributions of the parameters. The parameter estimation often leads to minimization problems, which can be solved with a variety of local or global optimization algorithms. Local optimizers are relatively fast, but they may get stuck in suboptimal local optima. Global optimizers like simulated annealing or genetic algorithms can evade local minima, but they may be numerically demanding.

In modeling of biochemical systems, the mathematical structure of a model (e.g., the stoichiometric matrix and the kinetic laws) is often known, while the parameter values (e.g., kinetic constants or external concentrations) still need to be determined. Parameter values can be obtained by fitting the model outputs (e.g., concentration time series) to a set of experimental data. If a model is correct and the data are free of experimental errors, the parameters can be adjusted such that model outputs and data coincide. Moreover, if the model is structurally identifiable (a property that will be explained below) and if enough data are available, this procedure will allow us to determine exactly the true parameter set because for all other parameter sets, data and model output would differ.

In reality, however, experimental data are noisy. A common assumption is that the measured values (possibly on logarithmic scale) represent true values – which correspond to the model outputs – plus Gaussian-distributed random errors. Despite these errors, we can use such data to obtain *parameter estimates* that approximate the true parameter values. Statistical methods can help us to find good estimation procedures and to assess the uncertainty of the estimates [6]. Common modeling tools contain routines for parameter estimation [7]. For an example of parameter estimation and model selection, see [8].

4.2.1 Regression

Regression is a good example of parameter estimation. Here, we shall discuss regression problems to introduce concepts like estimators and likelihood. Later, in Section 4.4 on model selection, we shall apply the same concepts to dynamical models. In the linear regression problem shown in Figure 4.2, a number of data points (t_m, y_m) have to be approximated by a straight line $x = f(t, \theta) = \theta_1 t + \theta_2$. If the data points were already located on a straight line, we could choose a parameter vector $\theta = (\theta_1, \theta_2)^T$ such that $\forall i: y_m = f(t_m, \theta)$. In practice, experimental data points will rather be scattered around a line, so we require that the regression line should be as close as possible to the data points. The deviation between line and data can be quantified by the sum of squared residuals (SSR), $R(\theta) = \sum_m (y_m - f(t_m, \theta))^2$. With this choice, the regression problem leads to an optimization problem, namely, finding the minimum of the function $R(\theta)$.

4.2.2 Estimators

The use of the SSR as a distance measure can be justified by statistical arguments, assuming that the data have been generated by a known model with unknown

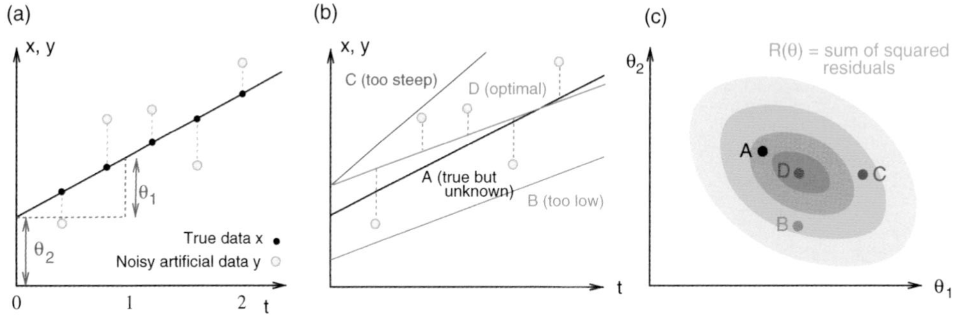

Figure 4.2 Linear regression leads to an optimization problem. (a) Artificial data points (t_m, y_m) (grey) are created by adding Gaussian noise to data points (black) from a model $x(t) = \theta_1(t) + \theta_2$ (straight line). Each possible line is characterized by two parameters, the slope θ_1 and the offset θ_2. The aim in linear regression is to reconstruct the unknown true parameters from noisy data (in this case, the artificial data set $\mathbf{y}$). (b) The distance between a possible line (four lines A, B, C, and D are shown) and the data points can be measured by the sum of squared residuals (SSR). The residuals are shown for line D (red dashed lines). (c) Each of the lines A, B, C, and D corresponds to a point (θ_1, θ_2) in parameter space. The SSR as a function $R(\theta)$ forms a landscape in parameter space (schematically shown by shades of pink, dark pink indicates small SSR). Line D minimizes the SSR value.

parameters. As an example, we consider a curve $f(t, \theta)$ with the independent variable t (e.g., time) and curve parameters $\theta_1, \ldots, \theta_N$. For a given number of values t_m, the model yields the output values $x_m = f(t_m, \theta)$, which form a vector $\mathbf{x} = \mathbf{x}(\theta)$. By adding random errors ξ_m, we obtain the noisy data

$$y_m = f(t_m, \theta) + \xi_m. \tag{4.1}$$

If the random errors are independent Gaussian with mean 0 and variance σ_m^2, then each of the data points y_m is a Gaussian-distributed random number with mean $f(t_m, \theta)$ and variance σ_m^2.

In parameter estimation, the process of data generation is inverted: we start with a model (given as a function $\mathbf{x}(\theta)$ and noise variances σ_m^2) and a set of noisy data $\mathbf{y}$ (a specific realization of the above random numbers) and try to infer approximately the unknown parameter set θ. This is done by an *estimator* $\hat{\theta}(\mathbf{y})$; a function of the data that is supposed to approximate the true parameter vector θ.

A practical and fairly simple estimator can be derived from the *principle of maximum likelihood*: given a generative model $\mathbf{y} = \mathbf{x}(\theta) + \xi$, the probability density for observing a data set y given the true parameter set θ is called $p(\mathbf{y}|\theta)$. If a certain data set $\mathbf{y}$ is given, this probability density, as a function of the parameter set θ, is called the *likelihood* function $L(\theta|\mathbf{y}) = p(\mathbf{y}|\theta)$. The maximum likelihood estimate $\hat{\theta}_{ML}(\mathbf{y})$ is defined as the parameter set that maximizes the likelihood:

$$\hat{\theta}_{ML}(\mathbf{y}) = \text{argmax}_\theta\, L(\theta|\mathbf{y}). \tag{4.2}$$

We assume here that there is a unique maximum point. If this is not the case, the model is not identifiable (see Section 4.2.3).

4.2.2.1 Method of Least Squares and Maximum-Likelihood Estimation

Let us now compute the likelihood function for the model (Eq. (4.1)) with additive Gaussian noise. If the model yields the true value x_m, a noisy value y_m will be observed with a probability density $p_\xi(y_m - x_m)$, where $p_\xi(\xi)$ is probability density of the error term. We assume that each ξ_m is independently Gaussian distributed with mean 0 and variance σ_m^2, so its density reads

$$p_{\xi_m}(\xi) = \frac{1}{\sqrt{2\pi}\sigma_m} e^{-\frac{\xi^2}{2\sigma_m^2}}. \tag{4.3}$$

From a single data point y_m, we would obtain the likelihood function

$$L(\theta|y_m) = p(y_m|\theta) = p_{\xi_m}(y_m - x_m(\theta)). \tag{4.4}$$

As the noise for different data points is supposed to be independent, the probability to observe an entire data set $\mathbf{y}$ is the product of the probabilities for the individual data points. Hence, the likelihood is given by

$$L(\theta|\mathbf{y}) = p(\mathbf{y}|\theta) = \prod_m p_{\xi_m}(y_m - x_m(\theta)). \tag{4.5}$$

By inserting the probability density (4.3) into Eq. (4.5) and taking the logarithm, we obtain

$$\ln L(\theta|\mathbf{y}) = \sum_m -\frac{(y_m - x_m(\theta))^2}{2\sigma_m^2} + \text{const.} \tag{4.6}$$

If we assume that the noise for all data points has the same variance σ^2, the logarithmic likelihood reads

$$\begin{aligned} \ln L(\theta|\mathbf{y}) &= -\frac{1}{2\sigma^2}\sum_m (y_m - x_m(\theta))^2 + \text{const.} \\ &= -R(\theta)/(2\sigma^2) + \text{const.}, \end{aligned} \tag{4.7}$$

where $R(\theta) = ||\mathbf{y} - \mathbf{x}(\theta)||^2$ is the sum of squared residuals. Thus, with the error model (4.3), maximizing the likelihood is equivalent to the principle of least squares.

The above argument also holds for data values on a logarithmic scale. The additive Gaussian errors for logarithmic data are equivalent to multiplicative log-normally distributed errors for the original, non-logarithmic data. By assuming the same variance σ^2 for all the logarithmic data, we imply that the non-logarithmic data have the same range of *relative errors*.

4.2.3 Identifiability

The likelihood function forms a landscape in parameter space (just like the SSR shown in Figure 4.2) and the maximum likelihood estimate $\hat{\theta}$ is the maximum point of this landscape – provided that it is indeed a single isolated point. In this case, the logarithmic likelihood function $\ln L(\theta|\mathbf{y})$ can be expanded to second order based on the local curvature matrix $\partial^2 \ln L(\theta|\mathbf{y})/\partial\theta_i\partial\theta_k$ and in a unique maximum point, the

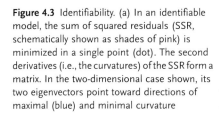

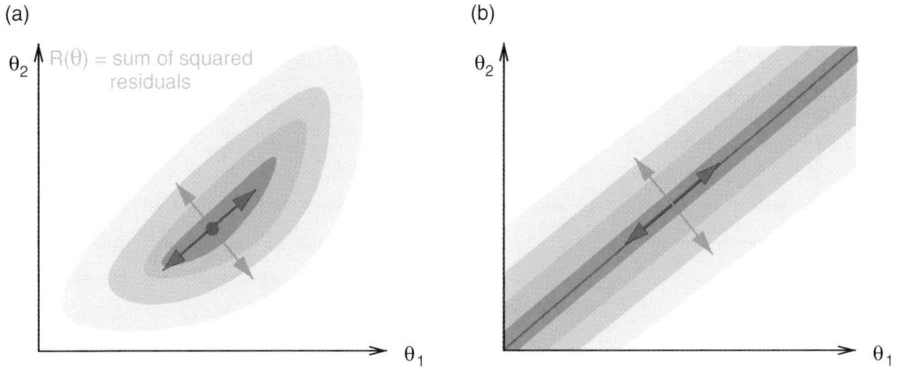

Figure 4.3 Identifiability. (a) In an identifiable model, the sum of squared residuals (SSR, schematically shown as shades of pink) is minimized in a single point (dot). The second derivatives (i.e., the curvatures) of the SSR form a matrix. In the two-dimensional case shown, its two eigenvectors point toward directions of maximal (blue) and minimal curvature (magenta), respectively. (b) In a nonidentifiable model, the SSR is minimal on a line (or in general, a manifold) in parameter space. Some linear combinations of parameters (magenta arrow) can be inferred from the data, while others (blue arrow) are nonidentifiable – accordingly, the curvature of the SSR vanishes in these directions.

curvatures are strictly negative. Directions with a small curvature correspond to parameter deviations that would only have little effect on the likelihood.

In parameter estimation, different parameter sets may happen to agree equally well with the data. In this case, the maximum likelihood criterion cannot be applied and the estimation problem is underdetermined (Figure 4.3). Often, the likelihood function becomes maximal on an entire curve or surface in parameter space rather than in a single point. Such cases of *non-identifiability* can have two reasons:

1. *Structural non-identifiability.* If two parameters θ_a and θ_b appear in a model only in the form of the product $c = \theta_a \theta_b$, then any choice $\theta'_a = \lambda\theta_a$ and $\theta'_b = \theta_b/\lambda$ would yield the same result $\theta'_a\theta'_b = \theta_a\theta_b$, leading to the same model predictions and to the same likelihood value. Thus, a maximum likelihood estimation (which compares model predictions to data) may suffice to determine the product $c = \theta_a\theta_b$, but not the individual parameter values θ_a and θ_b. In such cases, the model is called *structurally non-identifiable.* To resolve the problem in this example, we could replace the product $\theta_a\theta_b$ by a new, possibly identifiable parameter θ_c. Structural non-identifiability can arise from various kinds of formulas and may be difficult to detect and to resolve.

2. *Practical non-identifiability.* Even if a model is structurally identifiable, parameters may still be *practically non-identifiable* if the data are insufficient, i.e., either too few or the wrong kind of data are used for the estimation. In particular, if the number of parameters exceeds the number of data points, the parameters cannot be determined. Let us assume that each possible parameter set θ corresponds to a data set $\boldsymbol{x}(\theta)$ (no experimental noise) and that the function $\boldsymbol{x}(\theta)$ is continuous. If the dimensionality of θ is larger than the dimensionality of $\boldsymbol{x}$, it is certainly impossible to invert the function $\boldsymbol{x}(\theta)$ and to reconstruct the parameters from a

given data set. A rule for the minimum number of experimental data needed to reconstruct differential equation models is given in [9].

If a model is not identifiable, numerical parameter optimization with different starting points will lead to different estimates $\hat{\theta}$, which may all lie on the same manifold in parameter space. In the above example, for instance, the parameter estimates for θ_a and θ_b would be different every time, but they would always satisfy the relation $\ln\theta_a + \ln\theta_b = \ln c$ with the same value for c, so on a logarithmic scale, all estimates would lie on a straight line (provided that all other model parameters are identifiable).

The task of parameter identification from given data is often called an *inverse problem*. If the solution of an inverse problem is not unique, the problem is *ill-posed* and additional assumptions are required to pinpoint a unique solution. For instance, we may postulate that the sum of squares of all parameter values is supposed to be minimal. This additional requirement can help to determine a particular solution, a trick called "regularization".

4.2.4 Bootstrapping

A noisy data set $\mathbf{y} = \mathbf{x}(\theta) + \xi$ will not allow us to determine the true model parameters θ, but only an estimate $\hat{\theta}(\mathbf{y})$. Each time we repeat the estimation with different data sets, we deal with a different realization of the random error ξ and obtain a different estimate $\hat{\theta}$. Ideally, the mean value $\langle\hat{\theta}\rangle$ of these estimates should be identical to the true parameter value (in this case, the estimator is called "unbiased"), and their variance should be small. In practice, however, only a single data set is available, so we obtain a single point estimate $\hat{\theta}$ without knowing its distribution. *Bootstrapping* [10] provides a way to determine, at least approximately, the statistical properties of the estimator $\hat{\theta}$. First, hypothetical data sets (of the same size as the original data set) are generated from the original data by resampling with replacement (see Figure 4.4) and the estimate $\hat{\theta}$ is calculated for each of them. The empirical distribution of these estimates is then taken as an approximation of the true distribution of $\hat{\theta}$. The bootstrapping method is asymptotically consistent, that is, the approximation becomes exact as the size of the original data set goes to infinity. However, for finite data sets, it does not provide any guarantees.

Example 4.1: Bootstrapping applied to the estimation of mean values

Ten numbers $(x_1, \ldots, x_{10})$ are drawn from a random distribution. We use the empirical mean $\bar{x} = 1/10\sum_{m=1}^{10} x_m$ of this sample to estimate the true expected value $\langle x\rangle$ of the underlying random variable X. Our aim is to assess the mean and the variance of the estimator $\bar{x}$. In the bootstrapping method, we randomly draw numbers z from the given sample $(x_1, \ldots, x_{10})$. Using these random numbers, we form new tuples (bootstrap samples) $z^{(k)} = (z_1^{(k)}, \ldots, z_{10}^{(k)})$ and compute the empirical mean $\bar{z}^{(k)} = 1/10\sum_{i=1}^{10} z_i^{(k)}$ for each of them. A statistics of the values $\bar{z}^{(k)}$ is used as an approximation of the true distribution of $\bar{x}$.

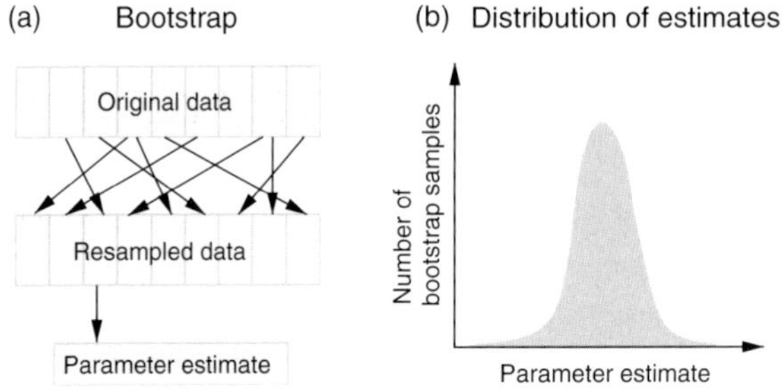

Figure 4.4 The bootstrapping method. (a) Hypothetical data sets are created by resampling data values from the original data set. Each resampled data set yields a parameter estimate $\hat{\theta}$. (b) The distribution of the parameter estimates, obtained from the bootstrap samples, approximates the true distribution of the estimator $\hat{\theta}$. A good approximation requires a large original data set.

4.2.5 Crossvalidation

There exists a fundamental difference between model fitting and prediction. If a model has been fitted to a given data set, it will probably show a better agreement with these *training data* than with new *test data* that have not been used for model fitting. The reason is that in model fitting, we enforce an agreement with the data. Therefore, a fitted model will often fit the data better than the true model itself, a phenomenon called *overfitting*. Despite its good fit, however, an overfitted model will not predict new data as reliably as the true model does. Moreover, the parameters of an overfitted model may differ strongly from the true parameter values. Therefore, strong overfitting should be avoided.

We have seen an example in Figure 4.2: the least-squares regression line yields a lower SSR than the true model itself – because it has been optimized for it. This apparent improvement is achieved by fitting the noise, i.e., by adjusting the line to this very specific realization of the random errors in the data. However, this adjustment does not help when it comes to predicting points from a new data set; here, the true model is likely to perform better.

How can we check how a model performs in prediction? In *crossvalidation* (see Figure 4.5), a given data set (size N) is split into two parts: a training set of size n and a test set consisting of all remaining data. The model is fitted to the training data and the prediction error is evaluated for the test data. Then, a different part of the data is chosen as the test set. By repeating this procedure for many choices of test sets, we can judge how well the model, after being fitted to n data points, will predict new data. The mean prediction error is an important quality measure of a model. It allows to reject models that are prone to overfitting (e.g., because they contain too many parameters, see Section 4.4.). However, crossvalidation – just like bootstrapping – is numerically demanding because of the repeated estimation runs.

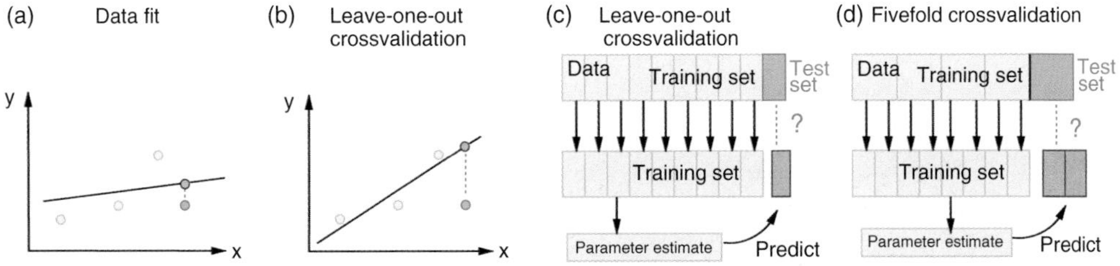

Figure 4.5 Crossvalidation can be used to detect overfitting. (a) In a linear regression, a straight line is fitted to four data points (grey and pink). The fitting error (dotted red line) is the distance between a data point (pink) and the corresponding value of the regression line (blue). The regression line is optimized for small fitting errors. (b) In leave-one-out crossvalidation, we pretend that a point (pink) is unknown and has to be predicted from the model. As the regression line is fitted to the remaining (grey) points, the deviation for the pink point (prediction error) will be larger than the fitting error shown in (a). (c) Scheme of leave-one-out crossvalidation. The model is fitted to all data points except for one ("training set") and the remaining data point ("test set") is predicted. This procedure is repeated for every data point to be predicted and yields an estimate of the average prediction error. (d) In *k*-fold crossvalidation, the data are split into *k* subsets. In every run, $k-1$ subsets serve as training data, while the remaining subset is used as test data.

4.2.6
Bayesian Parameter Estimation

In parameter estimation as explained above, we suppose that there exists a single true parameter set, which is fixed, but unknown. Bayesian parameter estimation, an alternative approach, is based on a completely different premise: The parameter set θ is not fixed, but described as a random variable. By choosing its probability distribution, called the *prior*, we can state which parameter sets we regard as most plausible in advance. For each possible parameter set θ, we assume that a specific data set $\mathbf{y}$ will be observed with a probability density (likelihood) $p(\tilde{\mathbf{y}}|\theta)$. Hence, parameters and data follow a joint probability distribution with density $p(\mathbf{y}, \theta) = p(\mathbf{y}|\theta)p(\theta)$ (see Figure 4.6).

From this joint distribution, we can also compute the conditional probabilities of parameters given the data. If a data vector $\mathbf{y}$ has been observed, the conditional probability of a parameter set given these data is called the *posterior probability*. With the Bayesian formula, the posterior probability density can be written as

$$p(\theta|\mathbf{y}) = \frac{p(\mathbf{y}|\theta)p(\theta)}{p(\mathbf{y})}. \tag{4.8}$$

It is proportional to the product of likelihood and prior density and represents a compromise between them. For a given data set $\mathbf{y}$, the denominator $p(\mathbf{y})$ is a fixed number, which appears only as a normalization term.

Bayesian parameter estimation and maximum likelihood estimation differ both in their interpretation and in their practical use. In maximum likelihood estimation, we ask "which hypothesis about the parameters would make the data look probable?", while in Bayesian estimation, we directly ask "which parameters appear most

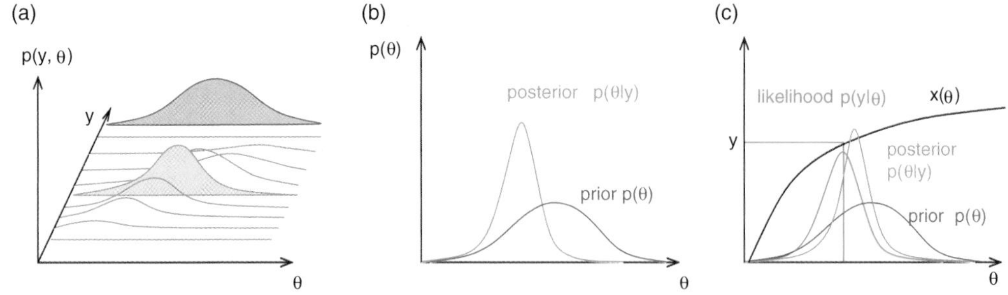

Figure 4.6 Bayesian parameter estimation. (a) In Bayesian estimation, the parameters θ and the data **y** follow a joint probability distribution with density $p(\mathbf{y}, \theta)$. The marginal probability density $p(\theta)$ of the parameters is called the prior (blue), while the conditional density $p(\theta|\mathbf{y})$ given a certain data set is called the posterior (magenta). (b) The posterior (magenta) is more narrow than the prior (blue), which reflects the information gained by considering the data. (c) Prior, likelihood and posterior. In a model, the data **y** are given by a mean prediction $\mathbf{x}(\theta)$ (black line) plus Gaussian noise. An observed value **y** gives rise to a likelihood function $L(\theta|\mathbf{y}) = p(\mathbf{y}|\theta)$ in parameter space. The posterior is proportional to the product of prior and likelihood function.

probable given the data?". Moreover, the aim in Bayesian statistics is usually not to choose a single parameter set, but to characterize the entire probability distribution (e.g., marginal distributions of individual parameters, probabilities for model predictions). For complicated problems, this is usually done by sampling parameter sets θ from the posterior $p(\theta|\mathbf{y})$, for instance, using the Metropolis–Hastings algorithm described below.

The prior in Bayesian parameter estimation is usually used to express general beliefs or previous knowledge about the parameter values. Besides this, it can also be used as a regularization term to make models identifiable. By taking the logarithm of Eq. (4.8), we obtain the logarithmic posterior

$$\ln p(\theta|\mathbf{y}) = \ln L(\theta|\mathbf{y}) + \ln p(\theta) + \text{const.} \tag{4.9}$$

If the logarithmic likelihood (the first term) does not have a unique maximum point in parameter space (for instance, as in Figure 4.3, right), the model will not be identifiable by maximum likelihood estimation. Nevertheless, if the logarithmic prior $\ln p(\theta|\mathbf{y})$ is added in Eq. (4.9), a unique maximum point can emerge at least for the posterior density.

4.2.7
Local and Global Optimization

Model fitting often leads to an optimization problem of the form

$$\min \stackrel{!}{=} f(\mathbf{x}), \tag{4.10}$$

where $\mathbf{x}$ is a vector and the function f is real and differentiable twice. In the method of least squares, for instance, $\mathbf{x}$ denotes the parameter vector θ and f is the sum of squared residuals (SSR). In addition to Eq. (4.10), we may restrict the allowed vectors $\mathbf{x}$ by constraints such as $x_i^{\min} \le x_i \le x_i^{\max}$. Global and local minima are defined as follows. A parameter set $\boldsymbol{x}^*$ is a global minimum point if no allowed parameter set $\boldsymbol{x}$ has a smaller value of the objective function. A parameter set $\boldsymbol{x}^*$ is a local minimum point if no other allowed parameter set $\boldsymbol{x}$ in a neighborhood around $\boldsymbol{x}^*$ has a smaller value of the objective function. To find such optimal points numerically, algorithms usually evaluate the objective function f (and possibly its derivatives) in a series of points $\boldsymbol{x}$ leading to better and better points until a convergence criterion is met.

4.2.7.1 Local Optimization

Local optimizers are used to find a local optimum point in the vicinity of a given starting point. Usually, they evaluate the local gradient and improve the objective function step be step until convergence. Simple *gradient descent* is based on the local gradient $\nabla f(\boldsymbol{x})$, a vector that indicates the direction of the strongest increase of f. A sufficiently small step in the opposite direction of the gradient will lead to lower function values. Thus for a sufficiently small coefficient c,

$$f(\boldsymbol{x}-c\nabla f(\boldsymbol{x}))<f(\boldsymbol{x}). \tag{4.11}$$

In gradient descent, we iteratively jump from the current point $\boldsymbol{x}^{(n)}$ to the new point by

$$\boldsymbol{x}^{(n+1)} = \boldsymbol{x}^{(n)}-c\nabla f(\boldsymbol{x}^{(n)}). \tag{4.12}$$

The coefficient c can be adapted in each step, e.g., by a numerical line search

$$c = \mathrm{argmin}_{c'} f(\boldsymbol{x}-c'\nabla f(\boldsymbol{x})). \tag{4.13}$$

Newton's method is based on a local second-order approximation of the objective function

$$f(\boldsymbol{x}+\Delta\boldsymbol{x}) \approx f(\boldsymbol{x}) + \nabla f(\boldsymbol{x})\Delta\boldsymbol{x} + \frac{1}{2}\Delta\boldsymbol{x}^{\mathrm{T}} H(\boldsymbol{x})\Delta\boldsymbol{x} \tag{4.14}$$

with the Hessian matrix $H_{ij}=\partial^2 f/\partial x_i\,\partial x_j$. If we disregard the approximation error in Eq. (4.14), a direct jump $\Delta\boldsymbol{x}$ to an extremum would require that

$$\nabla f(\boldsymbol{x}) + H(\boldsymbol{x})\Delta\boldsymbol{x} = 0. \tag{4.15}$$

In the iterative Newton method, we therefore jump from the current point $\boldsymbol{x}^{(n)}$ to the new point

$$\boldsymbol{x}^{(n+1)} = \boldsymbol{x}^{(n)} - H(\boldsymbol{x}^{(n)})^{-1}\nabla f(\boldsymbol{x}^{(n)}). \tag{4.16}$$

Again, the second term can be multiplied by a relaxation coefficient $0<c<1$ to make the iteration process more stable.

4.2.7.2 Global Optimization

Theoretically, a global optimum point could be found by scanning the entire parameter space using an arbitrarily fine grid. However, for a problem with n

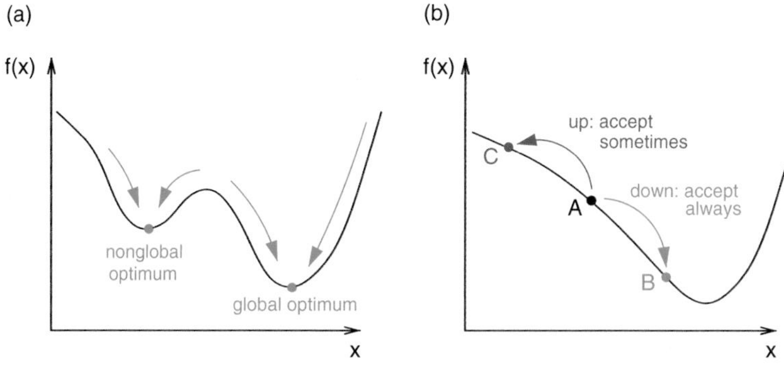

Figure 4.7 Global optimization. (a) In a local minimum point $\boldsymbol{x}$, the function f assumes a minimal value for a neighborhood around $\boldsymbol{x}$. A function may display different local minima with different function values. (b) The Metropolis–Hastings algorithm employs an iterative jump process in which points $\boldsymbol{x}$ are sampled with probabilities related to their function values $f(\boldsymbol{x})$. A jump that leads to lower f values (A → B) is always accepted, while an upward jump (A → C) is only accepted with probability $p = \exp(f(\boldsymbol{x}_A) - f(\boldsymbol{x}_C))$.

parameters and m values for each of them, this would require m^n function evaluations, which soon becomes intractable. In practice, most global optimization algorithms scan the parameter space by series of random jumps (Figure 4.7). Their objective is to find high quality solutions (preferably solutions very close to a global optimum or the global optimum itself as it usually happens) in short computation times (or in an affordable number of function evaluations). In order to be able to surmount basins of attraction containing local solutions, the algorithm may have to allow movements toward worse solutions in some stages of the search. There is a variety of global optimization algorithms [11, 12]. Examples of popular stochastic algorithms are *simulated annealing* and *genetic algorithms.*

Besides pure local and global methods, there are also hybrid methods [13, 14], which combine the robustness of global optimization algorithms with the efficiency of local methods. They work by applying a local search from a selection of points created in the global phase, which can accelerate the convergence to optimal solutions up to some orders of magnitude. Hybrid methods usually implement a set of filters to avoid local searches leading to optima that had been found previously.

4.2.7.3 **Sampling Methods**

Sampling methods like simulated annealing have been inspired by statistical thermodynamics. In a physical analogy, we consider a particle with position x (scalar or vectorial) that moves by stochastic jumps in an energy landscape $E(x)$. In a thermal equilibrium at temperature T, the particle position x follows the *Boltzmann distribution* with density

$$p(x) \sim \mathrm{e}^{-E(x)/(k_\mathrm{B}T)}, \tag{4.17}$$

where k_B is Boltzmann's constant. The Boltzmann distribution can be realized by the following random jump process ("Monte Carlo Markov chain") called *Metropolis–Hastings algorithm* [15, 16].

1. Given the current position $x^{(n)}$ with energy $E(x^{(n)})$, choose randomly a new potential position x^*.
2. If x^* has an equal or lower energy $E(x^*) \leq E(x^{(n)})$, the jump is accepted, and we set $x^{(n+1)} = x^*$.
3. If the new position has a higher energy $E(x^*) \geq E(x^{(n)})$, the jump is only accepted with a probability

$$p = \exp\left(\frac{E(x^{(n)}) - E(x^*)}{k_B T}\right).$$

To accept or reject a potential jump in the algorithm, we draw a uniform random number z between 0 and 1; if $z < p$, we accept the jump and set $x^{(n+1)} = x^*$. Otherwise, we keep the old position and set $x^{(n+1)} = x^{(n)}$.

Programming the Metropolis–Hastings algorithm is straightforward; an important restriction is that the potential jump in step 1 has to satisfy the following property: the probability for a potential jump from position x' to position x'' must be the same as for the potential jump from x'' to x'. Otherwise, the different probabilities need to be taken into account by a modified acceptance function in step 3. Problems can also arise if the potential jumps are too small. In this case, the particle will tend to stay close to its current position, so the distribution will converge only very slowly to the true Boltzmann distribution.

According to the Boltzmann distribution (4.17), the particle will spend more time – and will yield more samples – in positions with lower energies, and this effect becomes more pronounced if the temperature is low. At temperature $T = 0$, only jumps to lower or same energies will be accepted, so the particle ends up, possibly after a long time, in a global energy minimum. The Metropolis–Hastings algorithm can be used to (i) sample from given probability distributions and (ii) to minimize arbitrary objective functions $f(\mathbf{x})$, which replace the energy function $E(\mathbf{x})$.

1. The Metropolis–Hastings algorithm at fixed temperature can be used to sample the posterior distribution (4.8) in Bayesian statistics: we set $k_B T = 1$ and choose $E(\theta) = p(y|\theta)p(\theta)$, ignoring the constant factor $1/p(y)$. From the resulting samples, we can compute, for instance, the posterior mean values and variances of individual parameters θ_i.

2. For simulated annealing [17], $E(x)$ is replaced by a function to be minimized, the factor k_B is set to 1, and the temperature is varied during the optimization process. Simulated annealing starts with a high temperature, which is then continuously lowered during the sampling process. If the temperature decrease is slow enough, the system will end up in almost all cases (i.e., with probability 1) in a global optimum. In practice, the temperature has to be decreased faster, so convergence to a global optimum is not guaranteed.

4.2.7.4 Genetic Algorithms

Genetic algorithms like differential evolution [18] are inspired by the process of mutation and selection occurring in the evolution of species. Instead of improving a single possible solution (as in simulated annealing), genetic algorithms simulate an entire population of possible solutions (called "individuals") with subsequent generations. In each generation, the fitness of every individual is evaluated. Individuals with good scores (as compared to the other individuals in the population) can have offspring, which then forms the following generation. In addition, mutations (i.e., small random changes) or crossover (random exchange of properties between individuals) allow the population to explore larger regions of the parameter space. For problems with additional constraints, stochastic ranking [19] provides an efficient way to trade the objective function against the need to obey the constraints.

4.3 Reduction and Coupling of Models

Summary

The aim in model reduction is to simplify complex models, i.e., to capture their key dynamical properties with fewer equations and parameters. This facilitates understanding, numerical and analytical calculations, and model fitting. A reduced model has to emulate the behavior of relevant variables under relevant conditions and on the relevant time scale. To reduce a model, elements can be omitted, lumped, or replaced by effective descriptions, and global model behavior can be approximated by global modes or simplified black-box models. Important simplifying concepts like quasi-equilibrium or quasi-steady state can be justified by a distinction between fast and slow processes. Once models for parts of the cell have been established, they may be combined to form move complex models, which may show new emergent behavior.

Biochemical systems are complex, but in order to understand them, we can use simple mental pictures that neglect many details and show processes as if they happened in isolation. Simplicity is just a matter of perspective: if we average over many microscopic events, we will obtain a smooth behavior of macroscopic substance concentrations. If we observe a fast complex system over a long period of time, its effective average behavior may look simple. In computational models, we can choose a level of detail that suits our needs: we may consider smaller or larger pathways and simplify, lump, or disregard substances and reactions. We can do this either from the very beginning by *model assumptions*, or we can simplify an existing model by *model reduction*. If a model turns out to be too simple, we may zoom into the system and acknowledge details that we neglected before, or zoom out and include more parts of the environment into the model.

4.3.1 Model Simplification

Any biochemical model represents a compromise between biological complexity and practical simplicity. Its form will depend on data and biological knowledge available

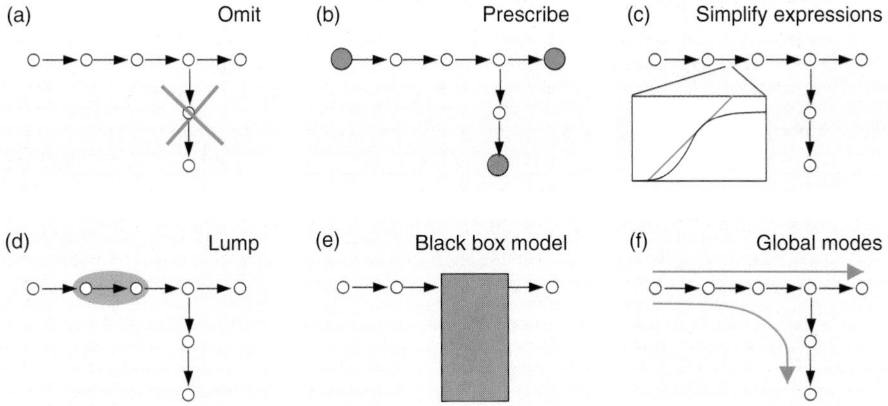

Figure 4.8 Simplifications in biochemical models. The scheme shows a branched pathway of metabolites (circles) and reactions (arrows). (a) Omitting substances or reactions. (b) Predefining the values of concentrations or fluxes or relations between them. (c) Simplifying the mathematical expressions (e.g., omitting terms in a kinetic law, using simplified kinetic laws [21], neglecting insensitive parameters [22]). (d) Lumping the substances, for instance, similar metabolites, protonation states of a metabolite, or metabolite concentrations in different compartments. Likewise, subsequent reactions in a pathway or elementary steps in a reaction can be replaced by a single reaction of the same velocity; for parallel reactions, like the action of isoenzymes, the velocities are summed up; for the two directions of a reaction, the velocities are subtracted. (e) Replacing the model parts by a dynamic black-box model that mimics the input–output behavior [23]. (f) Describing the dynamic behavior by global modes (e.g., elementary flux modes or eigenmodes of the Jacobian).

and on the questions to be answered. Small models provide several advantages: it is easier to understand them, the effort for simulations is lower, and with fewer parameters, model fitting is easier and more reliable.

Different ways to simplify a given model [20] are shown schematically in Figure 4.8. A basic rule for keeping models simple is to omit all elements that have little influence on the model predictions, for instance, reactions with very small rates. Often, elements cannot be omitted, but they can be described in a simplified or effective manner for conditions or time scales of interest. Examples are constant concentrations or flux ratios, effective kinetic laws fitted to measurements, or linearization of nonlinear kinetics that hold within the physiological range.

Such simplifications can speed up model building and simulations because fewer equations, variables, and parameters are needed, differential equations can be replaced by algebraic equations, and stiff differential equations can be avoided. All simplifications, though, have to be justified: a reduced model should yield a good approximation of the original model for certain quantities of interest, a certain time scale, and certain conditions (a range of parameter values, the vicinity of a certain steady state, or a certain qualitative behavior under study).

Even the most detailed biochemical model is still a simplified, reduced picture of a much more complex reality. Therefore, considerations about model reduction do not only help to simplify existing models, but also to justify common basic model assumptions and our use of mental models in general.

4.3.2 Tacit Model Assumptions

Mathematical models describe biological systems in two complementary ways: in a positive way, by how processes *are* modeled and in a negative way, by omission of processes, simplification of mechanisms, and the decision to treat certain quantities as constant. The positive facts about the system are stated explicitly, while the negative ones – which are just as important – remain hidden in the model assumptions. Arguably, the most important negative statement is that a system as a whole can be seen as a module, that is, its environment – e.g., the cell surrounding a pathway – can be neglected. Experiments test both kinds of statements at the same time, and they should be designed from the very beginning such that the simplifying model assumptions will later be justified.

Example 4.2: Stabilization by negative feedback

Consider a simple kinetic model [24]

$$\frac{ds}{dt} = \frac{a}{1 + s/K_I} - b\,s \qquad (4.18)$$

of self-inhibited protein production (with the protein level s, maximal production rate a, inhibition constant K_I, and degradation constant b). The model predicts that the protein level can be stabilized against noise by self-inhibition. Without inhibition ($K_I \to \infty$), the Jacobian of the system reads $\mathbf{A} = -b$; with inhibition, the Jacobian $\mathbf{A} = -aK_I/(K_I + s^{st})^2 - b$ has a larger negative value, so s becomes more stable against small random perturbations. Becskei and Serrano [24] have approved this stabilization effect in an experiment with synthetic genetic circuits.

However, the experiment does not only test the model (4.18) itself – the positive statements –, but also all kinds of simplifying assumptions made: (i) in the model, details of transcription and translation, as well as stochastic effects due to small particle numbers, are ignored; (ii) the behavior of the protein level s is entirely determined by s itself and interactions with other processes are neglected; (iii) the model parameters are assumed to be constant while in reality, they may depend on the cell state, be noisy or influenced by s itself, thus forming an additional feedback loop.

The model in Example 4.2 predicts stabilization for an isolated, deterministic system, but only the experiment can prove that an actual biochemical implementation of this loop, embedded in a living cell, shows the predicted behavior. Moreover, the successful prediction shows that the behavior is *robust* against typical perturbations that would occur in living cells. All this supports the working hypothesis that a subsystem can be modeled *at all* without considering the complexity of the surrounding cell.

4.3.3 Reduction of Fast Processes

If processes take place on different time scales (see Chapter 1), this may allow us to reduce the number of differential equations. In gene expression, for instance, binding and unbinding of transcription factors can happen on the order of microseconds, changes in transcription factor activity on the order of minutes, while the culture conditions may change on the order of hours. In a model, we may use a fast equilibrium or time averages for transcription factor binding, a dynamical model for signal transduction and gene expression, and constant values for the culture conditions.

The characteristic time scale of biochemical processes concerns both their internal dynamics (e.g., relaxation to steady state, periodic oscillations) and their susceptibility to external fluctuations. Cellular processes occur on a wide range of time scales from microseconds to hours, and also the time scale of enzymatic reactions can differ strongly due to the very different enzyme concentrations and kinetic constants.

4.3.3.1 Response Time

One way to define time constants is by observing how a system relaxes to steady state, like in the following example. We consider a substance that is produced at a rate v and linearly degraded with rate constant λ; its concentration s satisfies the rate equation

$$\frac{ds(t)}{dt} = v(t) - \lambda s(t). \tag{4.19}$$

If the production rate v is constant, then the concentration s will relax from an initial value $s(0) = s_0$ to its steady-state value $s^{st} = v/\lambda$ according to

$$s(t) = s^{st} + (s_0 - s^{st})e^{-\lambda t}. \tag{4.20}$$

We can define the response time $\tau = 1/\lambda$ as the time at which the initial deviation $\Delta s(t) = s^{st}$ from the steady state has decreased by a factor $1/e$. The response time is closely related to the response half time $\tau_{(1/2)} = \ln 2/\lambda$, at which half of the relaxation has been reached.

4.3.3.2 Time-Scale Separation

In numerical simulations, a single fast process, e.g., a rapid conversion between two substances $A \rightleftarrows B$ (as in Figure 4.9(b)), can force the numerical solver to use very small integration steps. If the same model also contains slow processes, simulations have to cover a long time scale, and the numerical effort can become enormous. However, fast reactions can be approximated rather easily because the concentration ratio s_B/s_A will always be close to the equilibrium constant. If we approximate this by an exact equilibrium in every moment in time, we can replace the reaction by the algebraic relation $s_B/s_A = K_{eq}$ and get rid of the stiff differential equation that caused the big numerical effort.

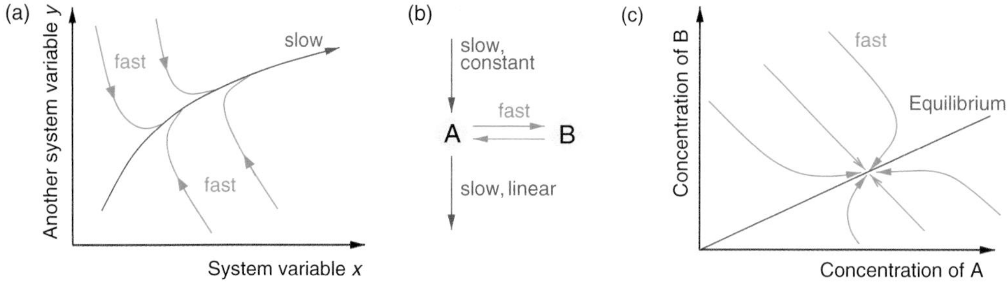

Figure 4.9 Time-scale separation. (a) The dynamics of a system can be illustrated by its trajectories in state space. If the system state is attracted by a submanifold (in the two-dimensional case, a curve), trajectories starting from any point (red) will rapidly approach this manifold (blue). Later, the system will move slowly on the manifold, satisfying an algebraic equation. (b) A small reaction system with different time scales. Fast conversion between metabolites A and B will keep their concentration ratio s_b/s_a close to the equilibrium constant K_{eq}, while slow production and degradation of A only changes the sum $s_a + s_b$. (c) Schematic trajectories for the system shown in (b). For any initial conditions, the concentrations s_A and s_B will rapidly approach the line $s_B/s_A = K_{eq}$ and then move slowly toward the steady state.

The mathematical justification for such an effective algebraic equation is illustrated in Figure 4.9: In state space, fast processes may rapidly move the system state toward a submanifold, on which certain relationships hold (e.g., an equilibrium between different concentrations). After an initial relaxation phase, the system state will change more slowly and remain close to this manifold. In the approximation, the system moves exactly within the manifold. In general, there may be a hierarchy of such manifolds which are related to different time scales [25].

Time-scale arguments can be used to justify various kinds of simplifications: (i) fast movements in molecular dynamics average out behind slow changes of the thermodynamic ensemble (e.g., fast jittering movements versus slow conformation changes in proteins). (ii) Fast diffusion leads to homogeneous concentrations, so spatial structure can be neglected. (iii) In a quasi-equilibrium as considered above, the ratios between substance concentrations are replaced by the equilibrium constant. (iv) In a quasi-steady state, the concentration of a substance may be determined by its production rate. The latter two approximations can be used, for instance, to justify the Michaelis–Menten rate law (see Section 2.1.3).

Example 4.3: Quasi-steady-state and quasi-equilibrium

We shall illustrate two types of approximation, quasi-steady state and quasi-equilibrium, with a simple model of upper glycolysis (see Section 3.1.2).

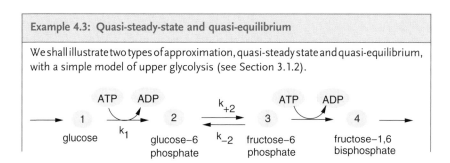

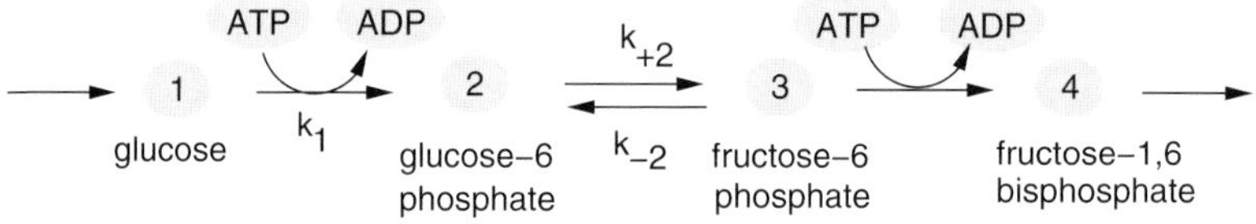

Glucose (GLC) is taken up at a rate ν_0 and converted subsequently into glucose-6-phosphate (G6P), fructose-6-phosphate (F6P), and fructose-1,6-bisphosphate (FBP), which is then consumed by the following steps of glycolysis. In this model, the cofactors ATP and ADP have fixed concentrations. With mass-action kinetics and a reversible reaction between G6P and F6P, the rate equations read:

$$\frac{ds_1}{dt} = \nu_0 - k_1\, s_A\, s_1 \tag{4.21}$$

$$\frac{ds_2}{dt} = k_1\, s_A\, s_1 - k_{+2}\, s_2 + k_{-2}\, s_3 \tag{4.22}$$

$$\frac{ds_3}{dt} = k_{+2}\, s_2 - k_{-2}\, s_3 - k_3\, s_A\, s_3 \tag{4.23}$$

$$\frac{ds_4}{dt} = k_3\, s_A\, s_3 - k_4\, s_4. \tag{4.24}$$

The numbers refer to the metabolites and reactions in the scheme and s_A denotes the constant ATP concentration. We first assume that all reactions take place on a similar time scale, setting $k_{+2} = 2$ and all other rate constants and the ATP concentration to a value of 1 (arbitrary units). Figure 4.10(a) shows simulated concentration curves of GLC, G6P, F6P, and FBP; the initial concentrations are chosen to be zero. For the first 5 time units, the influx has a value of $\nu_0 = 2$, and the intermediate levels rise one after the other. Then, the influx is reduced to $\nu_0 = 1$, and the levels decrease again.

How would the system behave if either the first or the second reaction was very fast? The two scenarios can be approximated, respectively, by a quasi-steady-state for glucose or a quasi-equilibrium between G6P and F6P.

If k_1 is increased to a value of 5 (Figure 4.10(b)), glucose is rapidly consumed, so its steady-state level will stay low; due to its high turnover, glucose will also adapt almost instantaneously to changes of the input flux. This behavior can be approximated by a quasi-steady-state approximation for the slow time scale: we replace the glucose concentration in each time point by the steady-state value $s_1^{st}(t) = \nu_0(t)/(k_1 s_A)$ based on the current value of $\nu_0(t)$. This algebraic equation replaces the differential equation (4.21) for s_1. Formally, we could obtain the same result by setting the left-hand side of the differential equation to zero.

Next, we assume a rapid and reversible conversion between the hexoses G6P and F6P. We increase both rate constants at the same time by a large factor ($k_{+2} = 10$ and $k_{-2} = 5$ in Figure 4.10(c)) while keeping their ratio $k_{eq} = k_{+2}/k_{-2}$ fixed: in the simulation, the ratio of F6P to G6P levels rapidly approaches the equilibrium constant $[F6P]/[G6P] = s_3/s_2 = K_{eq}$. In the quasi-equilibrium approximation, we assume that this ratio is exactly maintained in every moment. By adding Eqs. (4.22) and (4.23), we obtain the equation

$$\frac{ds_{2+3}}{dt} = \frac{d(s_2 + s_3)}{dt} = k_1\, s_A\, s_1 - k_3\, s_A\, s_3. \tag{4.25}$$

Given s_{2+3} and K_{eq}, we can substitute $s_3 = s_{2+3} K_{eq}/(1 + K_{eq})$ in Eq. (4.24) and obtain a simplified differential equation system in which the fast reaction does not appear any more. The two differential equations for s_2 or s_3 are replaced by a single differential equation (for the sum of the two variables) and an algebraic equation $s_3/s_2 = K_{eq}$ for the concentration ratio.

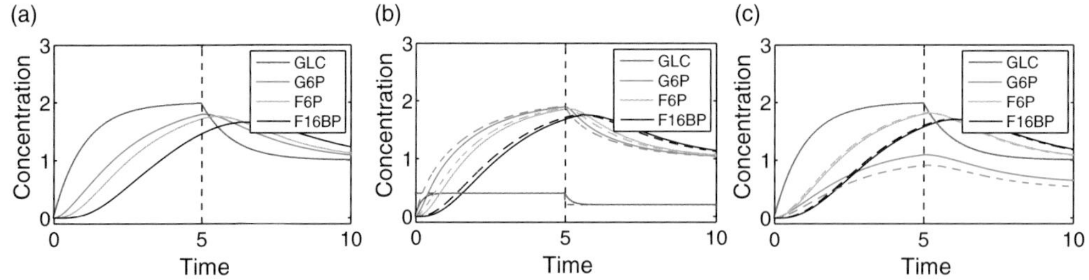

Figure 4.10 Simulation results for the model of upper glycolysis. (a) Results from the original model, showing levels of GLC, G6P, F6P, and FBP (abbreviations see text, time and concentrations measured in arbitrary units). (b) Results from the model with fast glucose turnover $k_1 = 5$ (solid lines) and the quasi-steady-state approximation (broken lines). (c) Results from the model with fast reversible conversion G6P ↔ F6P (solid lines), parameters $k_{+2} = 10$, $k_{-2} = 5$ and the quasi-equilibrium approximation (broken lines).

4.3.4 Global Model Reduction

If the state of a system is constrained to a submanifold in state space (as shown in Figure 4.9(a)), its movement on the manifold can be described by a smaller number of variables. Such constraints can, for instance, arise from linear conservation relations between metabolite concentrations (see Section 2.2.4): If rows of the stoichiometric matrix N are linearly dependent, the system state can be described by a number of independent metabolite concentrations (effective variables), from which all other concentrations could be computed by algebraic equations. The vector of metabolite concentrations is confined to a linear subspace. Other constraints may arise from fast processes that effectively lead to algebraic relationships, as we saw in the quasi-steady-state and quasi-equilibrium approximation.

The effective variables do not have to describe individual substances: For a general linear manifold, they may consist of linear combinations of all substance concentrations, representing global modes of the system's dynamics. Such global modes appear, for instance, in metabolic systems that are linearized around a steady state: Each mode will represent a pattern of metabolite levels (actually, their deviations from steady state), which follows a certain temporal dynamics (e.g., exponential relaxation). Such modes are comparable to harmonics on a guitar string, which display spatial patterns with a characteristic temporal behavior. Actual movements of the string can be obtained by linear superposition of these modes.

4.3.4.1 Linearized Biochemical Models

Most biochemical models are nonlinear; one way to simplify them is by linearizing them around a steady state. Consider a kinetic model (see Section 2.3.1)

$$\frac{\mathrm{d}v}{\mathrm{d}t} = N\, v(s, p) \tag{4.26}$$

with stoichiometric matrix $\boldsymbol{N}$, reaction velocity vector $\boldsymbol{v}$, and parameter vector $\boldsymbol{p}$. We assume that for given parameter sets $\boldsymbol{p}$, the system shows a stable steady state $s^{\mathrm{st}}(\boldsymbol{p})$. To linearize Eq. (4.26), we determine the steady state $s_0^{\mathrm{st}} = s^{\mathrm{st}}(\boldsymbol{p}_0)$ at a reference parameter vector $\boldsymbol{p}_0$ and compute the elasticity matrices $\tilde{\varepsilon} = \partial \boldsymbol{v}/\partial \boldsymbol{s}$ and $\tilde{\pi} = \partial \boldsymbol{v}/\partial \boldsymbol{p}$ (see Chapter 2). For small deviations of concentrations $\boldsymbol{x}(t) = \boldsymbol{s}(t) - \boldsymbol{s}_0^{\mathrm{st}}$ and parameters $\boldsymbol{u}(t) = \boldsymbol{p}(t) - \boldsymbol{p}_0$, linearizing Eq. (4.26) leads to

$$\frac{\mathrm{d}\boldsymbol{x}(t)}{\mathrm{d}t} = \boldsymbol{A}\boldsymbol{x}(t) + \boldsymbol{B}\,\boldsymbol{u}(t) \tag{4.27}$$

with the Jacobian $\boldsymbol{A} = \boldsymbol{N}\,\tilde{\varepsilon}$ and the matrix $\boldsymbol{B} = \boldsymbol{N}\,\tilde{\pi}$. In general, the approximation (4.27) holds only close to the expansion point, so for larger deviations $\boldsymbol{u}$ or $\boldsymbol{x}$, the accuracy decreases. In addition, linearized models may not be able to reproduce certain kinds of dynamic behavior, e.g., a stable limit cycle.

Biochemical systems show characteristic responses to external perturbations, so we can try to mimic complex models by linearized black-box models with the same input–output relation. An important special case are small perturbations of a stable system: if parameter perturbations are slow, the entire system will follow them in a quasi-steady-state. To linear order, the system's input–output relation $y(\boldsymbol{u})$ (for parameter deviations $\boldsymbol{u}$ and steady-state output variables like fluxes or concentrations) can be approximated by the linear response

$$\Delta y \approx \tilde{\boldsymbol{R}}_{\mathrm{p}}^{\mathrm{y}} \Delta \boldsymbol{u} \tag{4.28}$$

with the metabolic response matrix $\tilde{\boldsymbol{R}}_{\mathrm{p}}^{\mathrm{y}}$. The response to oscillating parameter perturbations [26, 27] and the response of transient behavior to stationary perturbations [28] can be treated accordingly.

4.3.4.2 Linear Relaxation Modes

With Eq. (4.27), we can express the model behavior as a superposition of global modes z_j, each corresponding to one of the eigenvectors of $\boldsymbol{A}$ (see Section 2.3.1). For constant system parameters ($\boldsymbol{u} = 0$), small deviations $\boldsymbol{x} = \boldsymbol{s} - \boldsymbol{s}_0^{\mathrm{st}}$ follow approximately

$$\frac{\mathrm{d}\boldsymbol{x}}{\mathrm{d}t} = \boldsymbol{A}\boldsymbol{x}. \tag{4.29}$$

In the following, we assume that the Jacobian is diagonalizable, $\boldsymbol{A} = \boldsymbol{Q}\Lambda\boldsymbol{Q}^{-1}$ with a diagonal matrix $\Lambda = \mathrm{Dg}(\lambda_i)$ and a transformation matrix $\boldsymbol{Q} = \{q_{ji}\}$. Furthermore, we assume that all its eigenvalues λ_i have negative (or, possibly, vanishing) real parts. We introduce the transformed vector $\boldsymbol{z} = \boldsymbol{Q}^{-1}\boldsymbol{x}$, which follows the equation

$$\frac{\mathrm{d}\boldsymbol{z}}{\mathrm{d}t} = \Lambda \boldsymbol{z}, \tag{4.30}$$

so whenever $\boldsymbol{A}$ is diagonalizable, we obtain an individual equation

$$\frac{\mathrm{d}}{\mathrm{d}t} z_j = \lambda_j z_j \tag{4.31}$$

for each global mode z_j. The behavior of the original variables x_i can be written as

$$x_i(t) = \sum_j q_{ij} z_j(t) = \sum_j q_{ij} z_j(0) \mathrm{e}^{-\gamma_j t} \tag{4.32}$$

with the initial value $z(0) = Q^{-1} x(0)$.

The different modes can be characterized by response times as introduced above. If the eigenvalue λ_i is a real number, z_j relaxes exponentially to the value 0 with a response time $\tau_j = 1/\lambda_j$. A pair of complex conjugated eigenvalues, in contrast, leads to a pair of oscillatory modes with time constant $\tau_i = 1/\mathrm{Re}(\lambda_i)$. An eigenvalue $\lambda_i = 0$ (corresponding to an infinitely slow mode) can arise, for instance, from linear conservation relations.

To simplify the system, we can neglect fast global modes (with small τ_j) in the sum (4.32), assuming that they will relax immediately. In metabolic network models, this will reduce the accuracy at fast time scales, but none of the metabolites or reactions will be omitted from the model. The system state is projected to the space of slow modes and the number of variables is effectively reduced.

Even if $\boldsymbol{A}$ cannot be diagonalized, the state space can still be split into subspaces related to fast and slow dynamics: by neglecting the fast subspace, the number of variables can then be reduced adaptively during computer simulations [29]. Powerful methods for linear model reduction like balanced truncation [23, 30] have been developed in control engineering (see the web supplement).

4.3.5 Coupled Systems and Emergent Behavior

All biological systems, from organisms down to cellular pathways, are embedded in larger environments that influence their dynamics. A metabolic pathway, for instance, is part of a larger network and coupled to a transcription network that adjusts its enzyme levels. For the dynamics of such a system, it can make a big difference if the environment's state is kept fixed or if both systems interact dynamically. In our terminology, a system is either studied *in isolation* (with fixed or controlled environment) or *coupled* to a dynamic environment. This fundamental distinction does not only hold for models, but also for experimental systems: in an *in vitro* enzyme assay, for instance, conditions like pH or the levels of cofactors can be experimentally controlled; in living cells, these values may be regulated dynamically, usually in an unknown manner.

When systems are coupled, new dynamic behavior can emerge. Single yeast cells, for instance, can communicate by the exchange of chemicals: Such interactions can lead, for instance, to synchronized glycolytic oscillations, which have been observed both in experiments and in models [31]. The following two examples illustrate the difference between isolated and coupled systems.

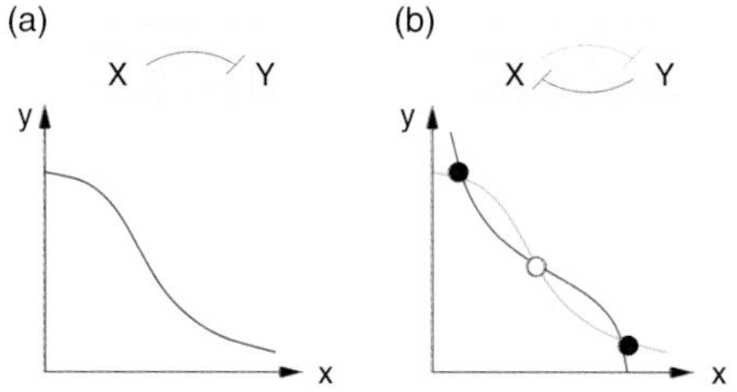

Figure 4.11 Bistability can emerge from mutual inhibition. (a) A gene level y is modeled in isolation with another gene level x acting as a regulatory input. The steady-state level y^{st} (blue) depends on the given value of x. (b) Two mutually interacting genes show bistability as an emergent property, with two stable fixed points (black dots) and one unstable fixed point (white dot) at the intersection of the two nullclines.

Example 4.4: Bistable switch

Let us consider two genes X and Y that mutually inhibit each other (Figure 4.11); we describe their levels x and y by the differential equation model

$$\frac{dx}{dt} = f(x, y)$$
$$\frac{dy}{dt} = g(x, y). \tag{4.33}$$

By setting the second equation to zero and solving for y, we obtain the steady-state value of y as a function of x. The curve $y^{st}(x)$ in Figure 4.11(a) is called the *nullcline* of y. Likewise, we obtain another nullcline $x^{st}(y)$ from the first equation. These nullclines represent response curves for the individual systems. When both systems are coupled, both steady-state requirements $y^{st} = f(x^{st})$ and $x^{st} = g(y^{st})$ have to be satisfied at the same time. We obtain three fixed points, two of which are stable, as indicated by the slopes of the nullclines. Due to the positive feedback loop, a bistable switch has emerged. The bistability is not a property of the individual genes X and Y – it is an systemic property which is only caused by their coupling.

Example 4.5: Reaction velocity and steady-state flux

Figure 4.12 shows two coupled chemical reactions. To study the first reaction in isolation, we fix the concentrations of substrate X and product Y. The reaction rate is given by the kinetic law $\nu_1(s_X, s_Y, E_1)$, and the response to a small increase of enzyme activity is described by the elasticity coefficient $\tilde{\pi}^{\nu_1}_{E_1} = \partial \nu_1 / \partial E_1$. As the enzyme activity increases, the reaction rate can be made arbitrarily large.

Alternatively, we can study the stationary flux in the two coupled reactions, with the levels of X and Z fixed and the level of Y determined by a steady-state requirement. Now the rate of the first reaction equals the steady-state flux $j(x, z, E_1, E_2)$ and the effect of an increased enzyme activity is given by a response coefficient $\tilde{R}^j_{E_1} = \partial j / \partial E_1$.

In this setting, the first enzyme will have a limited effect on the reaction rate: As its activity increases, the enzyme will lose its control and the reaction flux will be mostly controlled by the second enzyme.

The two approaches – whether isolated and coupled dynamics – are characteristic for two contrary views on complex systems. *Reductionism* studies the parts of a system in isolation and great detail. In this view, which is dominant in molecular biology and biochemistry, the global behavior of a system is explained in terms of interactions between the system's parts, and the dynamics is explained in terms of causal chains. *Holism,* on the contrary, emphasizes the fact that new dynamic behavior can emerge from the coupling of subsystems. Instead of tracing individual causal effects, it emphasizes how the global system dynamics responds to changes of external conditions.

4.3.6 Modeling of Coupled Systems

4.3.6.1 Bottom-Up and Top-Down Modeling

According to the concepts of reductionism and holism, there are two complementary modeling approaches, called bottom-up and top-down modeling; both proceed from simplicity to complexity, but in very different ways. In *bottom-up* modeling [32, 33], one studies elementary processes in isolation and aggregates them to a model. An example is the glycolysis model of Teusink et al. [32] that was built from kinetic rate laws measured *in vitro*. *In vitro* measurements of enzyme kinetics allow for an exact characterization and manipulation of quantitative parameters. A metabolic pathway model was constructed by merging the reactions. Without further tuning, it yielded a fairly plausible steady-state description of glycolysis. In *top-down* modeling, on the contrary, a model is built by refining a coarse-grained model of the entire system. If the model structure is biologically reasonable, such a model can be expected to yield fairly good data fits, but there is no general guarantee that it will remain valid as part of

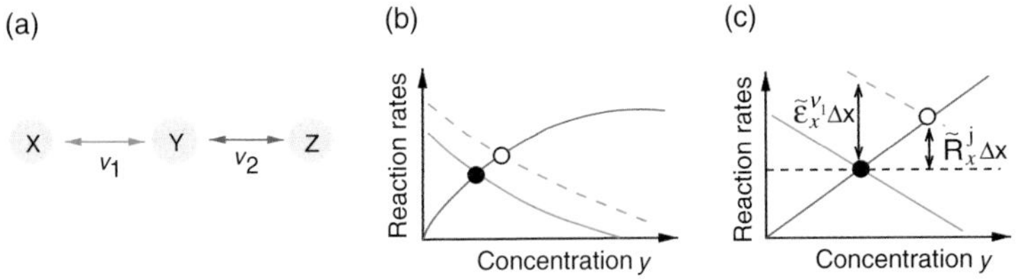

Figure 4.12 Elasticities and response coefficients describe local and global response to external changes. (a) Chain of two reactions with external metabolites X and Z and an intermediate Y. (b) The reaction rates v_1 (red) and v_2 (blue) depend on the intermediate level y. A steady state requires that both rates are identical (black dot). If v_1 is increased – e.g, by an increase of the external substrate X (broken red line), the steady-state flux and concentration are shifted (white dot). (c) The magnified scheme compares the direct increase of the reaction rate $\tilde{\varepsilon}^{v_1}_x \Delta x$ (depending on the reaction elasticity $\tilde{\varepsilon}^{v_1}_x$) to the steady-state flux increase $\tilde{R}^j_x \Delta x$ (depending on the response coefficient $\tilde{R}^j_x$).

a merged model. The two approaches pursue different goals: A bottom-up model is constructed to be locally correct (describing individual reactions by correct rate laws and parameters), while a top-down model, on the other hand, is optimized for a good global fit to *in vivo* behavior. In a model of limited size, it is unlikely that both requirements will be fulfilled at the same time.

4.3.6.2 **Modeling the System Boundary**

When building a biochemical model, we distinguish between a *system of interest* (which is explicitly modeled) and its *environment*, which is either not modeled or described only very roughly. Although this distinction is artificial, it cannot be avoided. The communicating quantities on the boundary may be external substance levels or fluxes, and their values have to be specified by model assumptions.

If the boundary variables of a system are kept fixed, the system is modeled as if it was in isolation. To ensure that this assumption is at least approximately justified, one should carefully choose the experimental system and the description of communicating variables. The system boundary should be chosen such that the interactions are weak, constant in time, or average out (because they are fast or random) and can thus be buried in the parameters. If the communicating variables are supposed to change in time, time series of the communicating variables can be obtained from experiments or from a separate environment model and be inserted into the model as given, time-dependent functions. Alternatively, the environment can be described as part of the model, either by effective algebraic relationships [34] or by simplified dynamic black-box models [23].

4.3.6.3 **Coupling of Submodels**

The coupling of several submodels (often called "modules") works quite similarly. The communicating variables *connect* the subsystems, but they also *shield* them from each other: If their temporal behavior was known, then the dynamics of each module could be computed without referring to the other modules. If the influences between modules form an acyclic graph, we can first simulate the dynamics of upstream modules, compute their outputs, and use them later as inputs for the downstream modules. If the coupling involves feedback loops, all modules need to be simulated together. We will come back to this point in Section 8.3.4.

An important consequence is that metabolic pathways can be driven by both supply and demand [35]. In a chain of chemical reactions, the steady-state flux depends on the concentration of the initial substrate. However, if the reactions are reversible or if enzyme activities are controlled by metabolite concentrations, also the end product may exert control on the flux. Supply–demand analysis [35] dissects metabolism into individual blocks, which are coupled by matching their supply and demand variables. The elasticities of supply and demand, which are experimentally measurable properties of the individual blocks, are then used to describe the behavior, control, and regulation of metabolism.

4.3.6.4 **Model Merging**

As more and more models become available (see Section 3.4.4), it is a tempting idea to build cell models by merging preexisting models of subsystems [36–39]. As the

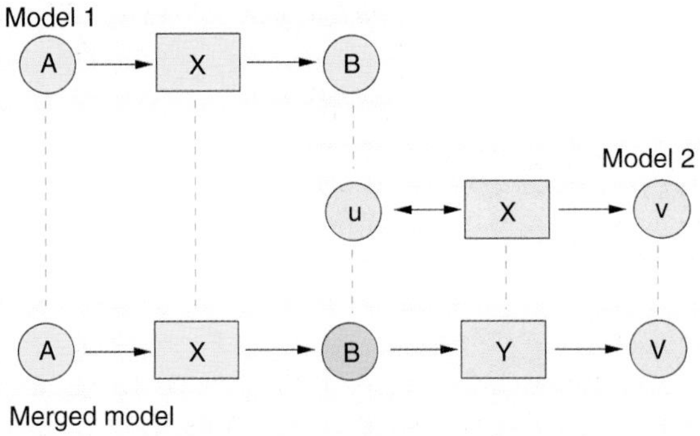

Figure 4.13 Merging of models. Two models (top and center) are merged to a single model (bottom) containing all model elements. Symbols represent model elements, for instance, substances and reactions. For merging, model elements are aligned (red dashed lines) according to their biological meaning as indicated by annotations (not shown). A simple name comparison would be unreliable because models can use different naming conventions.

models can overlap in their elements (e.g., substances or reactions described), elements from different models have to be matched to each other, as shown in Figure 4.13.

Model merging is based on the reductionist assumption that a mechanistic model will remain correct in different environments. However, both manual and computer-assisted merging (e.g., with SemanticSBML, see [38] and Chapter 17) pose various kinds of challenges [39]: (i) Model elements (variables, parameters, chemical reactions) have to be compared according to their biological meaning, which requires a clear description by (possibly computer-readable) annotations (e.g., MIRIAM-compliant RDF annotations [40]). (ii) Units must be compared and unified. (iii) Explicit conflicts between the models – e.g., different kinetics for the same reaction – have to be detected and resolved. (iv) Implicit conflicts may arise if the input models make contradicting assumptions or obey contradicting constraints (e.g., thermodynamic relationships between kinetic parameters). (v) If the model parameters have been determined by global fits, they possibly need to be refitted in the merged model. Some of these difficulties can be avoided if submodels are already designed with a common nomenclature and modeling framework. Model merging is greatly facilitated by standardization efforts for experiments and model building [41].

4.4 Model Selection

Summary

Mathematical models have to meet various requirements: they should fit experimental data, allow for prediction of biological behavior, represent complex biological mechanisms under study, and describe them in a simple, understandable form.

Systems biology models are often refined in iterative cycles until they agree with all relevant data. Alternative models may include different levels of detail or represent different biological hypotheses, and statistical model selection can help to choose between them. Complex models tend to overfit the data, so for choosing a reliable model, the number of free model parameters needs to be restricted, e.g., by likelihood ratio tests, by selection criteria like the Akaike criterion, or by Bayesian model selection.

One of the main issues in mathematical modeling is to choose between alternative model structures and to justify this choice. It is often arguable which biological elements need to be considered. Models may cover different cellular subsystems, different components or interactions within a subsystem (e.g., feedback interactions), different descriptions of the same process (e.g., different kinetic laws, fixed or variable concentrations), and different levels of detail (subprocesses or time scales). Alternative versions of model parts can lead to a combinatorial explosion of model variants, so we need to rule out models that are incorrect or too complicated [42, 43]. With limited and inaccurate data, we will not be able to pinpoint a single very detailed model, but statistical criteria can at least tell us which of the models are best supported by the data.

4.4.1 What is a Good Model?

A good model need not describe a biological system in all details. Borges writes in a story [44]: "In that empire, the art of cartography attained such perfection that the map of a single province occupied the entirety of a city, and the map of the empire, the entirety of a province. In time, those unconscionable maps no longer satisfied, and the cartographers guilds struck a map of the empire whose size was that of the empire, and which coincided point for point with it."

Systems biology models range from very simple to very complex maps of the cell, but just like usual maps, they never become an exact copy of the biological system. If they did, they would be almost as hard to understand as the biological system itself. Or, as George Box put it [45], "Essentially, all models are wrong, but some are useful." But – useful for what? As models are made for different purposes, they have to meet different requirements (see Figure 4.14):

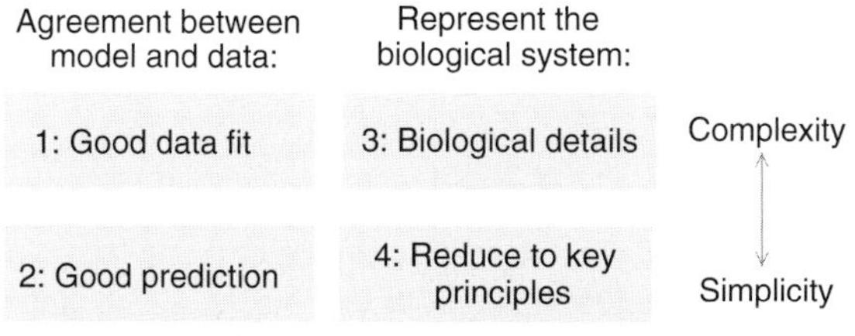

Figure 4.14 Possible requirements for a good model.

1. In *data fitting*, we aim to describe individual data points by a general mathematical function. Instead of storing many data pairs (x, y) that lie on a curve, we can store a few curve parameters (e.g., offset and slope for a straight line). If the points are not exactly on a curve, we may attribute the discrepancy between model and data to statistical errors in the measurement. Given a model structure, we can adjust the model parameters such as to optimize the fit, e.g., by minimizing the sum of squared residuals (SSR) (see Section 4.2). Fitting equally applies to dynamical models, which effectively define a mapping between parameters and data curves.

2. When used for *prediction*, a model is supposed to state general relationships between measured quantities that will also hold for future observations: In the language of statistical learning, the model should generalize well to new data.

3. A *detailed mechanistic model* is supposed to describe processes "as they happen in reality." Of course, the description of an entire cell will never be complete down to molecular or lower levels. In practice, mechanistic models will focus on parts of the cell only and use simplifying assumptions and model reduction to simplify them to a tractable level.

4. To emphasize the *key principles* of a biological process, a model needs to be *as simple as possible*. Simplicity is especially important if a model is supposed to serve as a didactic or prototypic example. This also holds for experimental model systems, e.g., the Lac operon as a model for microbial gene regulation.

These properties are partially interrelated. A good data fit supports the hypothesis that a model is biologically correct and covers the key features of a system. But – it does not prove it: a complex model – even with an implausible structure – may achieve better fits than a simpler, biologically plausible model. As a rule of thumb, a model with many free parameters may fit given data more easily ("With four parameters I can fit an elephant, and with five I can make him wiggle his trunk." J. von Neumann, quoted in [46]). But as the fit becomes better and better, the average amount of experimental information per parameter decreases, so the parameter estimates and predictions from the model become poorly determined. Such overfitting is a notorious problem when many free parameters are fitted to few data points or if a large number of possible models is prescreened for good data fits (Freedman's paradox [47]). It can be detected and avoided, though, by making proper use of statistics.

4.4.2
Statistical Tests and Model Selection

Let us suppose that a number of alternative models have been proposed for a biological process. We intend to choose between them based on experimental data, in particular, time series of substance concentrations.

Example 4.6: Reversible or irreversible reaction?

As a running example, we will consider two alternative models for a chemical reaction $S \leftrightarrow P$. The first model ("A") assumes mass-action kinetics with rate constants k_+ and k_- and a fixed product concentration c. The substrate concentration s follows the rate equation

$$\frac{ds}{dt} = -k_+ s + k_- c. \tag{4.34}$$

The second model ("B") assumes that the reaction is irreversible, i.e., the rate constant k_- vanishes. For the concentration of S, the two models predict a temporal behavior

$$\text{Model A}: \ s(t) = s^{st} + (s_0 - s^{st})\, e^{-k_+ t} \tag{4.35}$$

$$\text{Model B}: \ s(t) = s_0\, e^{-k_+ t} \tag{4.36}$$

with the initial concentration s_0 and the steady-state concentration $s^{st} = c\, k_-/k_+$ in model A. The solution of model A depends on the values of k_+, k_-, s_0, and c. However, the parameters k_- and c only appear in the form of a product $a = k_- c$, which means that they are not identifiable individually (see 4.2.3). For parameter estimation and model selection, we keep three model parameters, k_+, s_0, and a. Model B contains only two parameters, k_+ and s_0.

In model selection, we compare the two models to experimental data, e.g., to a concentration time series for S consisting of triples (t_i, y_i, σ_i) for the ith measurement, each containing a time point t_i, a measured concentration value y_i, and a standard error σ_i. By the approach of model selection, we aim to find out if there is a considerable backward flux from P to S.

We can choose between competing models by statistical tests and model selection criteria. In *statistical tests,* we compare a more complex model to a simpler background model. According to the null hypothesis, both models perform equally well. In the test, we favor the background model unless it statistically contradicts the observed data. In this case, we would conclude that the data support the more complex model. A test at a confidence level α will ensure that if the null hypothesis is correct, there is only an α% chance that we wrongly reject it.

Alternatively, several candidate models can be compared by a *selection criterion* [48–51]. Selection criteria are mathematical scoring functions that balance agreement with experimental data against model complexity. To compensate for the advantage of complex models in fitting large numbers of free parameters in the model are punished. Selection criteria can be used to rank the models, choose between them, and to weight them in averaging. In model selection, we choose between model structures just as we choose between parameter values in parameter fitting: In both cases, we intend to find a model that agrees with biological knowledge and that matches experimental data. The two tasks are interrelated:

In parameter estimation, parameter values are determined for a given model structure, while model selection often involves a parameter estimation run for each of the candidate models.

4.4.3
Maximum-Likelihood Estimation and χ^2-Test

We can judge the quality of a model by comparing its predictions to experimental data. The structure and parameters of a model can be scored by its *likelihood* (see Chapter 13), the probability that the model assigns to actual observations. Consider the model "Tomorrow, the sun will shine with 80% probability": If sunshine is observed, the model has a likelihood of 0.8. Mathematically, the likelihood for a model or parameter set θ is defined as $L(\theta|y) = p(y|\theta)$, that is, the conditional probability to observe the data y given the model.

To compute likelihood values for biochemical models, we need to relate the model predictions to experimental data. In a simple statistical model, we regard the experimental data y_i as a sum

$$y_i = x_i(\theta) + \xi_i \tag{4.37}$$

of the model results and measurement errors ξ_i, described by independent Gaussian random variables with mean 0 and width σ_i. The subscript i can refer to both substances and time points. The assumption of additive Gaussian errors greatly simplifies calculations, but it need not hold in all cases. With Eq. (4.37) and the probability density $p_{\xi i}(\xi)$, the likelihood $L(\theta|y)$ can be written as a function of the model parameters (see Eq. (4.5)). For further calculations, we consider the expression

$$-2\log L(\theta|y) = -2\log p(y|\theta) = -2\sum_{i=1}^{n} \log p_{\xi_i}(y_i(t) - x_i(\theta)). \tag{4.38}$$

By inserting the Gaussian probability density $p_\xi(\xi) \sim \exp(-\xi^2/(2\sigma^2))$, we obtain

$$-2\,\log L(\theta|y) = \sum_{i=1}^{n} \frac{(y_i - x_i(\theta))^2}{\sigma_i^2} + \text{const.} \tag{4.39}$$

The quality of the model (4.37) can be judged from the sum in expression (4.39), the weighted sum of squared residuals (wSSR). If our model is correct, the y_i will be independent Gaussian random variables with means x_i and variances σ_i^2, so the weighted SSR will follow a χ^2-distribution with n degrees of freedom. On the contrary, if the result of (4.39) for a given model and given data falls in the upper 5% quantile of the χ_n^2-distribution, the model can be rejected on a 5% confidence level. We would conclude in this case that the model is wrong. If parameters have been fitted before, the number of degrees of freedom in the χ^2-distribution should be reduced to account for possible overfitting. In *maximum-likelihood estimation*, we determine a parameter set $\hat{\theta}(y)$ that maximizes the likelihood

$p(y|\theta)$ for a given data set y (see 4.2.2.1): The resulting likelihood value measures the *goodness of fit*.

The likelihood can also be used to choose between different model structures. For instance, the above statement A, "Tomorrow, the sun will shine with 80% probability" can be compared to the statement B, "Tomorrow, the sun will shine with 50 percent probability". If sunshine has been observed, statement A will have a higher likelihood ($\text{Prob(data}|A) = 0.8$) than statement B, ($\text{Prob(data}|B) = 0.5$), and should be chosen if likelihood is used to select models. Biochemical models can be selected in the same manner, but only if their parameters have been fixed in advance, as we shall explain now.

4.4.4 Overfitting

If models were selected by their maximized likelihood (and not by the likelihood arising from predefined, fixed parameters) overfitting could severely distort the selection of models. Consider a statistical model with true parameters θ and data y: The maximum-likelihood estimator $\hat{\theta}(y)$ will lead to a higher likelihood $L(\hat{\theta}(y)|y) > L(\theta|y)$ than the true parameter set θ just because it was optimized for high likelihood for the observed data. The empirical (maximized) log-likelihood will exceed the log-likelihood of the true parameters, on average, by a certain amount $\Delta \log L$. This bias depends on how easily the model can fit the noise; usually, it increases with the number of free model parameters.

Before using real experimental data, it is often instructive to consider artificial data obtained from model simulations. If we generated the data ourselves, we can judge more easily if a model selection method is able to recover the original, supposedly true, model.

Example 4.7: Likelihood values

For our running example, we assume an original model of form A with parameters $k_{\pm} = 1$, $s_0 = 1$, $c = 0.1$. Figure 4.15 shows a simulation run of this model. Artificial noisy data were generated by adding Gaussian random numbers with a standard deviation of 25% of the true value. These data can now be compared to potential candidate models, using the wSSR, $\sum_{i=1}^{n} (y_i - x_i(\theta))^2/\sigma_i^2$ to measure the goodness of fit. For models A and B with predefined parameter values (see Figure 4.15(a)), the fit is rather poor. After maximum-likelihood parameter estimation (by minimizing the weighted SSR), we obtain a much closer match (Figure 4.15(b), numerical values in Table 4.2). In fact, both models fit the data even better than the original model does. This is a case of slight overfitting. As expected, model A (with 3 parameters) performs better than model B (with 2 parameters only). The question remains: which of them should we choose?

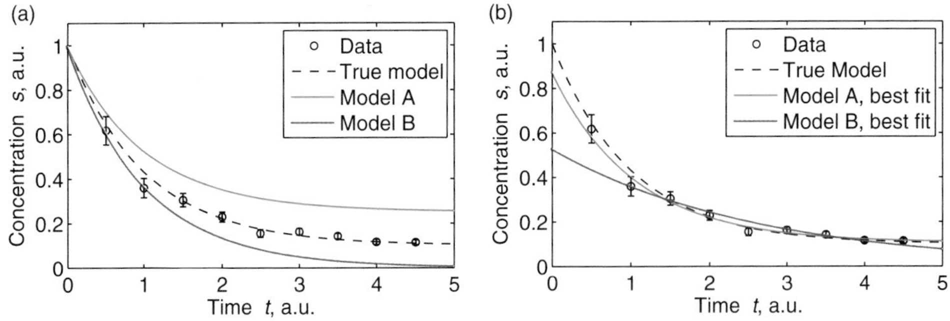

Figure 4.15 Fit of the example models. (a) Artificial data (a concentration time series, black dots) were generated by adding Gaussian noise to results of the true model (dashed line). Solid curves show simulations from model A (red) and B (blue) with fixed parameters. (b) After estimating the parameters of models A and B, a better fit is obtained.

4.4.5 Likelihood Ratio Test

A philosophical principle called *Ockham's razor* (*Entia non sunt multiplicanda praeter necessitatem*, entities should not be multiplied without necessity) states that a theory should not contain unnecessary elements. In statistical model selection, complexity in a model always needs to be supported by data. A good fit by itself will not suffice as a support if the same data have been used twice, for parameter estimation and model selection. To find models with reliable parameter estimates and good potential for predictions, we need to give all models equal chances. To correct for the advantage of complex models, we may apply the likelihood ratio test or selection criteria, which both favor models with few parameters.

The *likelihood ratio test* [52] compares two models A and B (with k_A and k_B free parameters, respectively) by their maximal likelihood values L_A and L_B. The two models have to be nested, that is, model B must be obtainable from model A by fixing a number of parameters in advance. In the test, the null hypothesis states that both models explain the data equally well. But even if model B is correct, model A will show a higher empirical likelihood because its additional parameters make it easier to fit the

Table 4.2 Parameter sets and goodness of fit for versions of the example model (compare Fig. 4.15)

	k_+	a	s_0	Weighted SSR
Original model	1	1	1	7.32
A, fixed parameters	1	0.25	1	102.59
B, fixed parameters	1	–	1	65.92
A, optimized parameters	0.8345	0.0921	0.6815	4.98
B, optimized parameters	0.3123	–	0.4373	6.13

[a]The last column shows the wSSR, $\sum_i (y_i - x_i)^2/\sigma_i^2$ describing the goodness of fit.

noise. The test accounts for this fact. For large numbers of data points and independent, Gaussian-distributed measurement errors, the expression $r = 2\ \ln(L_A/L_B)$ asymptotically follows a χ^2-distribution, with $k_A - k_B$ degrees of freedom. This distribution is used for the statistical test: if the empirical value of r is significantly high, we reject the null hypothesis and accept model A. Otherwise, we accept the simpler model B. The likelihood ratio test can also be applied sequentially to more than two models, provided that subsequent models are nested. For a practical example, see [53].

Example 4.8: Likelihood ratio test

In our running example, the test statistics has a value of $2\ \ln(L_A/L_B) \approx 6.13 - 4.98 = 1.15$. The 95% quantile for χ^2-distribution with $3 - 2 = 1$ degree of freedom is much higher, about 3.84. So according to the likelihood ratio test, we cannot reject model B. However, the likelihood values depend on the noise levels $\sigma_i(t)$ assumed in the likelihood function: With a smaller noise level (same artificial data, noise level corresponding to 10% of the original values), the weighted SSR for the two models read approximately 5.0 (model A) and 19.8 (model B). In this case, the test statistics has a value of $19.8 - 5.0 = 14.8$, which is highly significant, so the data would support model A.

4.4.6 Selection Criteria

We saw that the maximal likelihood contains a certain bias $\Delta \log L$, so for model selection, it would be better to score models by an unbiased estimator of the true likelihood $\Delta \log L(\hat{\theta}(y)|y) - \Delta L$. The value of $\Delta \log L$ is unknown in general, but mathematical expressions for it, so-called *selection criteria*, have been proposed for certain forms of models. By minimizing these objective functions (instead of the likelihood itself), we attempt to find a model that best explains the data, while taking into account the possibility of overfitting. The Akaike information criterion [54]

$$\mathrm{AIC} = -2 \log L(\hat{\theta}(y)|y) + 2k, \tag{4.40}$$

for instance, directly penalizes the number k of free parameters. If we assume additive Gaussian measurement noise of width 1, the term $-2 \log L(\theta|y)$ in Eq. (4.40) equals the sum of squared residuals $R(\theta)$ and we obtain

$$\mathrm{AIC} = R(\theta) + 2k \tag{4.41}$$

A correction for small sample sizes yields

$$\mathrm{AICc} = \mathrm{AIC} + \frac{2k(k+1)}{n-k-1} \tag{4.42}$$

where n is the number of data. The Schwarz criterion [55]

$$\mathrm{BIC} = -2 \log L(\theta|y) + k \log n \tag{4.43}$$

penalizes free parameters more strongly. In contrast to AIC, the BIC is consistent, i. e., as the number of data n goes to infinity, the true model will be selected with probability 1. The selection criteria allow to rank models and to choose between them, but there is no notion of significance for the result of such a model selection.

Example 4.9: Selection criteria

Table 4.3 shows the values of different model selection criteria for the running example 4.6. To produce the artificial data, the standard deviation for the noise in each data point was 25% of the true values. If we assume the same noise levels for the model selection procedure, all selection criteria favor the simpler model B. However, if we refit the models to the same artificial data, but assuming a smaller noise level in the model selection (corresponding to 10% of the original values), model A is favored because in this case, a good fit becomes more important.

In some cases, the selection criteria may suggest that none of the models is considerably better than all others. In this situation, we may decide not to select a single model and instead consider several models. For example, to estimate a model parameter, we may average over the parameter values obtained from different models. To assign higher weight to parameters from the more reliable models, weighting factors can be constructed from the selection criteria [54].

4.4.7 Bayesian Model Selection

Practical reasoning in everyday life is contrary to the logic of maximum likelihood. In real life, we would not ask: "Under which explanation would our observations seem most likely?", but rather: "What is the most plausible explanation for our observations?"

Table 4.3 Calculation of selection criteria for the running example.[a]

	σ large		σ small	
	Model A	**Model B**	**Model A**	**Model B**
n	3	2	–	
k	9	9		
$2k$	6	4	–	
$2k + \frac{2k(k+1)}{n-k-1}$	4.67	2.33		
$k \log n$	6.59	4.39		
Weighted SSR	4.98	6.13	4.99	19.81
AIC	10.98	10.13	10.99	23.81
AICc	9.64	8.46	9.66	22.14
BIC	11.57	10.52	11.58	24.20

[a] For each of the criteria (weighted sum of squared residuals (SSR), Akaike information criteria (AIC and AICc), and Schwarz criterion (BIC), the more favorable values are shown in red.

Imagine that you toss a coin and obtain heads. Now you have to choose between the statements A: "The coin always shows heads," B: "It shows heads and tails with equal probability." According to the maximum-likelihood criterion, you should choose A – which is counterintuitive, because you know that real coins will not always show heads. But how can such kind of prior knowledge – the probability of different explanations besides our current observations – be included in model selection?

Bayesian statistics is doing just that in a formalized way [56, 57]. Instead of considering distributions of parameter sets (as in Section 4.2.6), we now treat the model structure itself by a probability distribution. Before observing the data, all we know about the model (including its structure $\mathcal{M}$, its parameters θ, or both) is its marginal probability, the *prior* $p(\mathcal{M}, \theta)$. We can compute the posterior from Bayes' theorem about conditional probabilities:

$$p(\mathcal{M}, \theta|y) = \frac{p(y|\mathcal{M}, \theta)p(\mathcal{M}, \theta)}{p(y)}. \tag{4.44}$$

According to this formula, we obtain the posterior by multiplying the likelihood $L(\mathcal{M}, \theta|y) = p(y|\mathcal{M}, \theta)$ (stating how well the model explains the data) with the prior (describing how probable the model is in general). By taking the logarithm, we can rewrite Eq. (4.44) in the form of a sum

$$\ln p(\mathcal{M}, \theta|y) = \ln p(y|\mathcal{M}, \theta) + \ln p(\mathcal{M}, \theta) + \text{const.} \tag{4.45}$$

In practice, the posterior density (4.44) can often not be computed analytically. However, sampling methods like Monte Carlo Markov chains [56] allow to draw representative models and parameter sets from the posterior distribution and to extract all statistical information to arbitrary accuracy. The usual aim in Bayes estimation is not to select a single model, but to assign probabilities to different models. In addition, we can also obtain the marginal distribution of a certain parameter, probabilities for structural features that appear in several models, or probabilities for quantitative model predictions. By considering many possible models and weighting them according to their probabilities, we may obtain more reliable results than from a point estimate by maximum-likelihood estimation.

An application of Bayesian statistics is model selection by the *Bayes factor.* With equal priors $p(\mathcal{M}_1) = p(\mathcal{M}_2)$ for both model structures, the posterior ratio of two models $\mathcal{M}_1$ and $\mathcal{M}_2$, called the *Bayes factor,* reads

$$\frac{p(\mathcal{M}_2|y)}{p(\mathcal{M}_1|y)} = \frac{p(y|\mathcal{M}_2)}{p(y|\mathcal{M}_1)}. \tag{4.46}$$

In contrast to the likelihood ratio, the Bayes factor does not score a model based on a single optimized parameter set; instead, it is computed from weighted averages over all possible parameter vectors θ_1 and θ_2,

$$\frac{p(y|\mathcal{M}_2)}{p(y|\mathcal{M}_1)} = \frac{\int p(y|\theta_2, \mathcal{M}_2)p(\theta_2|\mathcal{M}_2)d\theta_2}{\int p(y|\theta_1, \mathcal{M}_1)p(\theta_1|\mathcal{M}_1)d\theta_1}. \tag{4.47}$$

For complex models, these integrals can be approximated by Monte Carlo sampling.

The prior probability can also be seen as a regularization term: if the data alone are insufficient to identify a parameter set or a model structure, model selection is an underdetermined (or *ill-posed*) problem; with the prior, a single solution can be selected, and model selection becomes well determined.

The posterior distribution depends strongly on how we choose the priors for model structures and parameter values. With a uniform prior (the same prior probability for each model $\mathcal{M}$), the posterior is proportional to the likelihood. The choice of the prior can reflect both our biological expectations and our demands for simplicity. This subjective choice forces modelers to state explicitly their assumptions about the system structure. Furthermore, a prior distribution can be used, like the above-mentioned selection criteria, to punish models with many parameters.

4.4.8 Cycle of Experiments and Modeling

Modeling in systems biology usually starts with literature studies and data collection. The first step toward a quantitative model is to develop hypotheses about the biological system. Which objects and processes (e.g. substances, chemical reactions, cell compartments) are relevant? Which mathematical framework is appropriate (continuous or discrete model, kinetic or stochastic, spatial or nonspatial)?

After the model parameters have been fixed tentatively, models (structure and parameters) can be judged by how well their results agree with experimental data. A correct model should explain or predict the data within their error range; a χ^2-test or a parametric bootstrap can be used to rule out models seem to be wrong. Then, different model variants are formulated and fitted to experimental data, and their dynamic behavior is studied (e.g. by bifurcation analysis or sensitivity analysis). In practice, modeling often involves several cycles of model generation, fitting, testing, and selection [42, 58].

Sometimes, model structures can be selected according to known qualitative properties: for instance, the chemotaxis system in bacteria is known to show precise adaptation to external stimuli and a model of it should account for this fact. In certain chemotaxis models, this robustness property follows from the network structure, and other model structure, which do not ensure precise adaptation, can be ruled out (see Section 7.4). Such requirements can also be stated in the form of model priors.

In the model selection process, a number of models may still perform equally well, and additional data are needed to choose between them. Optimal experimental design [59] is aimed to determine experiments that are most likely to yield the information needed to distinguish between the models; The resulting cycle of experiments and modeling can overcome many of the limitations of one-step model selection.

4.4.9 Models are Growing in Complexity

Systems biology modeling is usually intended to yield fairly plausible mechanistic models that include all relevant key processes for a biochemical system. In practice, models are selected for various aspects: Does the model reflect the basic biological facts about the system? Is it simple enough to be simulated and fitted? Does it explain the existing data and can it predict anything that was not known before? If data are limited – and they always are – there is a trade-off between these requirements, and statistical model selection can help to avoid overfitting.

As more data or more accurate data become available, models can resolve more and more details of biological reality. This is illustrated by the development of models during the last decades: With increasing amounts of data, models of metabolism, cell cycle, or signaling pathways have become more complex, more accurate, and more predictive. By the time, simple initial models are replaced by detailed biochemical models that account for many experimental observations and come closer and closer to biological reality.

Exercises and Problems

Problems

1. Use BRENDA to search for all hydrolases from *Rattus norvegicus* that have a K_m value below 0.001 mM.

2. What are the advantages of using GFP constructs for measuring the cellular response to perturbations compared to DNA microarrays?

3. Use http://yeastGFP.ucsf.edu to find out how many copies of the mitochondrial DNA polymerase catalytic subunit exist in a yeast cell. The gene name can be found with the help of http://www.yeastgenome.org.

4. *Linear regression*. A data set $\{(t_1,y_1),(t_2,y_2),\ldots\}$ has been obtained from a linear model

$$y(t) = \theta_1 t + \theta_2 + \xi_t$$

with random errors ξ_t. (a) Given the vectors $\mathbf{t} = (t_1, t_2, \ldots)^T$ and $\mathbf{y} = (y_1, y_2, \ldots)^T$, explain how to estimate the model parameters θ_1 and θ_2 by maximizing the likelihood. Assume that the errors ξ_t are independent Gaussian random variables with mean 0 and variance σ^2.

5. *Bootstrapping procedure for the empirical mean*. The expected value of a random number X can be estimated by the empirical mean value $\bar{x} = 1/n \sum_{m=1}^{n} x^{(m)}$ of n realizations $x^{(1)}, \ldots, x^{(n)}$. (a) Compute the mean and the variance of the estimator $\bar{x}$. (b) Choose a distribution of X and approximate the mean and the variance of $\bar{x}$ numerically, by repeatedly drawing samples $(x^{(1)}, \ldots, x^{(n)})$. (c) Implement a bootstrapping procedure and assess the distribution of the estimate $\bar{x}$ based on a single sample $(x^{(1)}, \ldots, x^{(n)})$. (d) Explain why these three results differ.

6. *One-norm and two-norm*. The method of least squares can be derived from the maximal likelihood estimator, assuming independent standard Gaussian errors. (a) Assume that the experimental noise ξ is not Gaussian, but follows an

exponential distribution with density $p(\xi) \sim \exp(-|\xi|/a)$. Find the minimization principle that would replace in this case the method of least squares. (b) Assume that a model is fitted to the same data set (i) by the principle of least squares or (ii) by the minimization principle derived in (a). What will be the qualitative difference between the two fitting results?

7. *Local and global optimization* (a) Why is it important in parameter estimation to find a global optimum rather than a suboptimal local one? Do local optimum points also have a relevance?

8. A substance appears in a kinetic model in two forms, either free or bound to proteins; only the free form participates in chemical reactions, and there is a fast conversion between both forms. Explain how the model could be modified in order to describe the substance by its total concentration.

9. (a) Discuss Aristotle's proposition "The whole is more than the sum of its parts" in the context of biochemical systems and mathematical models describing them. (b) Speculate about the advantages and disadvantages of reductionist and holistic approaches in systems biology.

10. Does the concept of a complete cell model make any sense at all? (a) Speculate about possible definitions. (b) Estimate roughly the number of variables and parameters in models of living cells. Consider the following types of model: (i) Kinetic model of the entire metabolism without spatial structure. (ii) Compartment model including organelles. (iii) Particle-based model describing single molecules and their complexes in different conformation states. (iv) Model with atomic resolution.

11. Discuss the phrase by George Box: "Essentially, all models are wrong, but some are useful." What do you think of it? Does it give any helpful advice for modeling?

12. A kinetic model has been fitted to an experimental concentrations time series. An additional data point can be measured in the time series, and you can choose the time point at which the measurement will take place. How would you choose the best point in time for the measurement, and what circumstances would influence your choice?

13. Three models A, B, C have been fitted to experimental data ($n = 10$ data points) by a maximum-likelihood parameter fit. The respective optimized likelihood values and the numbers k of free parameters are given below. (a) Calculate the selection criteria AIC, AICc, and BIC, and use the results to choose between the models. (b) Assume that the models are nested, that is, A is a submodel of B, and B is a submodel of C. Decide for one of the models by using the likelihood ratio test.

Model	A	B	C
k	2	3	4
$\ln L$	10.0	5.0	2.0

References

1 Tsien, R.Y. (1998) The green fluorescent protein. *Annu Rev Biochem*, **67**, 509–544.

2 Ronen, M. *et al.* (2002) Assigning numbers to the arrows: parameterizing a gene regulation network by using accurate expression kinetics. *Proc Natl Acad Sci USA*, **99**, 10555–10560.

3 Zaslaver, A. *et al.* (2004) Just-in-time transcription program in metabolic pathways. *Nat Genet*, **36**, 486–491.

4 Zaslaver, A. *et al.* (2006) A comprehensive library of fluorescent transcriptional reporters for *Escherichia coli*. *Nat Methods*, **3**, 623–628.

5 Huh, W.K. *et al.* (2003) Global analysis of protein localization in budding yeast. *Nature*, **425**, 686–691.

6 Seber, G.A.F. and Wild, C.J. (2005) *Nonlinear Regression*. Wiley-IEEE.

7 Hoops, S., Sahle, S., Gauges, R., Lee, C., Pahle, J., Simus, N., Singhal, M., Xu, L., Mendes, P. and Kummer, U. (2006) COPASI - a COmplex PAthway SImulator. *Bioinformatics*, **22**, 3067–3074.

8 Timmer, J., Müller, T.G., Swameye, I., Sandra, O. and Klingmüller, U. (2004) Modelling the nonlinear dynamics of cellular signal transduction. *Int. J. of Bifurcation and Chaos*, **14** (6), 2069–2079.

9 Sontag, E.D. (2002) For differential equations with r parameters, 2r + 1 experiments are enough for identification. *Journal of Nonlinear Science*, **12** (6), 553–583.

10 Efron, B. and Tibshirani, R. (1993) *An Introduction to the Bootstrap*, Chapman & Hall/CRC, London.

11 Mendes, P. and Kell, D.B. (1998) Non-linear optimization of biochemical pathways: application to metabolic engineering and parameter estimation. *Bioinformatics*, **14** (10), 869–883.

12 Moles, C.G., Mendes, P. and Banga, J.R. (2003) Parameter estimation in biochemical pathways: a comparison of global optimization methods. *Genome Research*, **13** (11), 2467–2474.

13 Rodriguez-Fernandeza, M., Mendes, P. and Banga, J.R. (2006) A hybrid approach for efficient and robust parameter estimation in biochemical pathways. *Biosystems*, **83** (2–3), 248–265.

14 Rodriguez-Fernandez, M., Egea, J.A. and Banga, J.R. (2006) Novel metaheuristic for parameter estimation in nonlinear dynamic biological systems. *BMC Bioinformatics*, **7** (483).

15 Rosenbluth, M.N., Teller, A.H., Metropolis, N., Rosenbluth, A.W., and Teller, E. (1953) Equations of state calculations by fast computing machines. *Journal of Chemical Physics*, **21** (6), 1087–1092.

16 Hastings, W.K. (1970) Monte Carlo sampling methods using Markov chains and their applications. *Biometrika*, **57** (1), 97–109.

17 Kirkpatrick, S., Gelatt, C.D. and Vecchi, M.P. (1983) Optimization by simulated annealing. *Science*, **220** (4598), 671–680.

18 Storn, R. and Price, K. (1997) Differential evolution – a simple and efficient heuristic for global optimization over continuous spaces. *Journal of Global Optimization*, **11**, 341–359.

19 Runarsson, T.P. and Yao, X. (2000) Stochastic ranking for constrained evolutionary optimization. *IEEE Transaction on Evolutionary Computation*, **4** (3), 284–294.

20 Okino, M.S. and Mavrovouniotis, M.L. (1998) Simplification of mathematical models of chemical reaction systems. *Chemical reviews*, **98** (2), 391–408.

21 Visser, D., Schmid, J.W., Mauch, K., Reuss, M. and Heijnen, J.J. (2004) Optimal re-design of primary metabolism in Escherichia coli using linlog kinetics. *Metab Eng*, **6** (4), 378–390.

22 Degenring, D., Frömel, C., Dikta, G. and Takors, R. (2004) Sensitivity analysis for the reduction of complex metabolism models. *J. Process Contr.*, **14**, 729–745.

23 Liebermeister, W., Baur, U. and Klipp, E. (2005) Biochemical network models simplified by balanced truncation. *FEBS Journal*, **272** (16), 4034–4043.

24 Becskei, A. and Serrano, L. (2000) Engineering stability in gene networks by autoregulation. *Nature*, **405**, 590–592.

25 Roussel, M.R. and Fraser, S.J. (2001) Invariant manifold methods for metabolic model reduction. *Chaos*, **11** (1), 196–206.

26 Ingalls, B.P. (2004) A frequency domain approach to sensitivity analysis of biochemical systems. *J Phys Chem B*, **108**, 1143–1152.

27 Liebermeister, W. (2005) Metabolic response to temporal parameter fluctuations in biochemical networks. *J Theor Biol*, **234** (3), 423–438.

28 Ingalls, B.P. and Sauro, H.M. (2003) Sensitivity analysis of stoichiometric networks: an extension of metabolic control analysis to non-steady state trajectories. *J Theor Biol*, **222** (1), 23–36.

29 Zobeley, J., Lebiedz, D., Ishmurzin, A. and Kummer, U. (2003) A new time-dependent complexity reduction method for biochemical systems. In *Transactions on Computational Systems Biology*, ed. C. Prami *et al.*, 90–110. Springer, LNCS 3380.

30 Moore, B.C. (1981) Principal component analysis in linear systems: Controllability, observability, and model reduction. *IEEE Trans AC*, AC-26, 17–32.

31 Wolf, J. and Heinrich, R. (2000) Effect of cellular interaction on glycolytic oscillations in yeast: a theoretical investigation. *Biochemical Journal*, **345**, 312–334.

32 Teusink, B., Passarge, J., Reijenga, C.A., Esgalhado, E., van der Weijden, C.C., Schepper, M., Walsh, M.C., Bakker, B.M., van Dam, K., Westerhoff, H.V. and Snoep, J.L. (2000) Can yeast glycolysis be understood in terms of *in vitro* kinetics of the constituent enzymes? Testing biochemistry. *European Journal of Biochemistry*, **267**, 5313–5329.

33 Chassagnole, C., Raïs, B., Quentin, E., Fell, D.A. and Mazat, J. (2001) An integrated study of threonine-pathway enzyme kinetics in *Escherichia coli*. *Biochem J*, **356**, 415–423.

34 Petersen, S., Lieres, E.v., de Graaf, A.A., Sahm, H. and Wiechert, W. (2004) *Metabolic engineering in the post genomic era*, chapter A multi-scale approach for the predictive modeling of metabolic regulation. Horizon Bioscience, UK.

35 Hofmeyr, J.-H.S. and Cornish-Bowden, A. (2000) Regulating the cellular economy of supply and demand. *FEBS Letters*, **476** (1–2), 47–51.

36 Bhalla, U.S. and Iyengar, R. (1999) Emergent properties of networks of biological signaling pathways. *Science*, **283** (5400), 381–387.

37 Snoep, J.L., Bruggeman, Frank, Olivier, B.G. and Westerhoff, H.V. (2006) Towards building the silicon cell: A modular approach. *Biosystems*, **83**, 207–216.

38 www.semanticsbml.org

39 Liebermeister, W. (2008) Validity and combination of biochemical models. *Proceedings of 3rd International ESCEC Workshop on Experimental, Standard Conditions on Enzyme Characterizations.*

40 Le Novère, N., Finney, A., Hucka, M., Bhalla, U.S., Campagne, F., Collado-Vides, J., Crampin, E.J., Halstead, M., Klipp, E., Mendes, P., Nielsen, P., Sauro, H., Shapiro, B., Snoep, J.L., Spence, H.D. and Wanner, B.L. (2005) Minimum information requested in the annotation of biochemical models (MIRIAM). *Nat Biotech.*, **23** (12), 1509–1515.

41 Klipp, E., Liebermeister, W., Helbig, A., Kowald, A. and Schaber, J. (2007) Systems biology standards - the community speaks. *Nature Biotech.*, **25**, 390–391.

42 Wiechert, W. (2004) Metabolic Engineering in the Post Genomic Era, chapter *Validation of Metabolic Models: Concepts, Tools, and Problems*, Chap 11, Horizon Bioscience.

43 Haunschild, M., Freisleben, B., Takors, R. and Wiechert, W. (2005) Investigating the dynamic behaviour of biochemical networks using model families. *Bioinformatics*, **21**, 1617–1625.

44 Borges, J.L. Suarez Miranda,Viajes de varones prudentes, Libro IV, Cap. XLV, Lerida, 1658, Jorge Luis Borges, Collected Fictions, Penguin.

45 Box, G.E.P. and Draper, N.R. (1987) *Empirical Model-Building and Response Surfaces*, Wiley, New York.

46 Dyson, F. (2004) A meeting with Enrico Fermi. *Nature*, **427**, 297.

47 Freedman, D.A. (1983) A Note on Screening Regression Equations. *The American Statistician*, **37** (2), 152–155.

48 Atkinson, A.C. (1981) Likelihood Ratios, Posterior Odds and Information Criteria. *Journal. of Econometrics*. **16**, 15–20.

49 Ghosh, J.K. and Samanta, T. (2001) Model selection - an overview. *Current science*, **80** (9), 1135.

50 Hansen, M.H. and Yu, B. (2001) Model selection and the principle of minimum description length. *Journal of the American Statistical Association*, **454**, 746–774.

51 Johnson Jerald B. and Omland Kristian S. (2004) Model selection in ecology and evolution. *Trends in Ecology & Evolution*, **19** (2), 101–108.

52 Vuong, Q.H. (1989) Likelihood ratio tests for model selection and non-nested hypotheses. *Econometrica*, **57** (2), 307–333.

53 Timmer, J. and Müller, T.G. (2004) Modeling the nonlinear dynamics of cellular signal transduction. *International Journal of Bifurcation and Chaos*, **14** (6), 2069–2079.

54 Akaike, H. (1974) A new look at the statistical model identification. *IEEE Transactions on Automatic Control*, **19** (6), 716–723.

55 Schwarz, G. (1978) Estimating the dimension of a model. *Annals of Statistics*, **6** (2), 461–464.

56 Gelman, A., Carlin, J.B., Stern, H.S. and Rubin, D.B. (1997) *Bayesian Data Analysis*, Chapman & Hall, New York.

57 Stewart, Warren E. and Henson, T.L. (1996) Model discrimination and criticism with single-response data. *AIChE Journal*, **42** (11), 3055.

58 Vanrolleghem, P.A. and Heijnen, J.J. (1998) A structured approach for selection among candidate metabolic network models and estimation of unknown stoichiometric coefficients. *Biotechnol Bioeng*, **58** (2–3), 133–138.

59 Takors, R., Wiechert, W. and Weuster-Botz, D. (1997) Experimental Design for the Identification of Macrokinetic Models and Model Discrimination. *Biotechnology and Bioengineering*, **56**, 564–567.

5
Analysis of High-Throughput Data

5.1
High-Throughput Experiments

Summary

The analysis of transcriptome data has become increasingly popular over the last decades due to the advent of new high-throughput technologies in genome research. Often, these data build the basis for defining the essential molecular read-outs for a particular disease, developmental state, or drug response being subject to computational modeling. In particular, DNA arrays have become the most prominent experimental technique to analyze gene expression data. A DNA array consists of a solid support that carries DNA sequences representing genes – the probes. In hybridization experiments with the target sample of labeled mRNAs and through subsequent data capture a numerical value, the signal intensity, is assigned to each probe. It is assumed that this signal intensity is proportional to the amount of molecules of the respective gene in the target sample. Changes in signal intensities are interpreted as concentration changes. Several experimental platforms are available that enable the genome-wide analysis of gene expression. Another recently emerging high-throughput technology is next generation sequencing. These new sequencing techniques provide in many cases flexible alternatives to DNA array techniques in identifying the abundance of specific sequences, providing information on transcript abundance or RNA processing events.

5.1.1
DNA Array Platforms

DNA array platforms date back to the late 80s when they were described for the first time as a tool to screen thousands of DNA sequences in parallel by a single hybridization experiment [1] and to use this, among other applications, to determine transcript levels for many genes in parallel. Since then, several array platforms have been developed and a vast amount of studies have been conducted. The principle of these techniques is the same: large amounts of probes are immobilized on a solid

Systems Biology: A Textbook. Edda Klipp, Wolfram Liebermeister, Christoph Wierling, Axel Kowald, Hans Lehrach, and Ralf Herwig

ISBN: 978-3-527-31874-2

surface and hybridization experiments with a complex pool of labeled RNAs are performed. After attaching to the reverse complementary sequence the amount of bound labeled material is quantified by a scanning device and transformed into a numerical value that reflects the abundance of the specific probe in the RNA pool. The different technologies differ in the material of the solid support, the labeling procedure, and the nature of the probes.

Historically, macroarrays were the first DNA array platform. This technique, developed in the late 80s [1–3] employs PCR products of cDNA clones that are immobilized on nylon filter membranes. The mRNA target material is labeled radioactively (^{32}P) by reverse transcription. cDNA macroarrays typically have a size of $8 \times 12\,cm^2$ to $22 \times 22\,cm^2$ and cover up to 80,000 different cDNAs. The bound radioactivity is detected using a phosphor imager. Multiple studies using this technique have been published [4–6].

Another platform consists in microarrays. Here, single-stranded cDNA sequences are immobilized on glass surfaces and hybridizations are carried out with fluorescently labeled target material. Chips are small, 1.8×1.8 cm, and allow the spotting of tens of thousands of different cDNA clones. cDNA microarrays are widely used in genome research [7–10]. A specific advantage of this technology is the fact that two RNA samples labeled with different dyes can be mixed within the same hybridization experiment. For example, the material of interest (tissue, time point, etc.) can be labeled with the Cy3-dye and control material (tissue pool, reference time point) can be labeled with the Cy5-dye. The labeled RNAs of both reverse transcription steps can be mixed and bind to the immobilized gene probes. Afterward, the fluorescence of bound mRNA is detected by two scanning procedures and two digital images are produced for the first dye- and second dye-labeling, respectively (Figure 5.1).

While the first two platforms are widely used in academic research most commercially available DNA arrays are oligonucleotide chips. Slides are typically small ($1.28 \times 1.28\,cm^2$) and the number of probes and lengths of oligonucleotides vary according to the producer. Target mRNA is labeled fluorescently and detection of the signals is performed with a scanning device. The most prominent oligonucleotide DNA array technology is the Affymetrix GeneChip system [11, 12]. Here, genes are represented by probe sets of short oligonucleotides (typically 11–20 25-mers) that are distributed across the corresponding gene sequences. These oligonucleotides are synthesized in a highly specific manner at defined locations using a photolithographic procedure. After hybridization, the measured intensity for the represented gene is summarized across different probes in the probe set (Figure 5.1). Affymetrix chips have emerged as the pharmaceutical standard and are widely in use because of the highly standardized chip production process. Whole-genome chips are available for a large number of organisms, such as human, mouse, rat, cow, pig, etc. An experiment with Affymetrix technology is typically a single channel experiment, i.e., only one target sample is analyzed in one experiment.

A recently developed technology is the Illumina BeadChip system that utilizes an "array of arrays" format [13, 14]. Each array on the support contains thousands of wells into which up to hundreds of thousands beads self-assemble in a random fashion. Specific 50-mer gene sequences concatenated with an address sequence

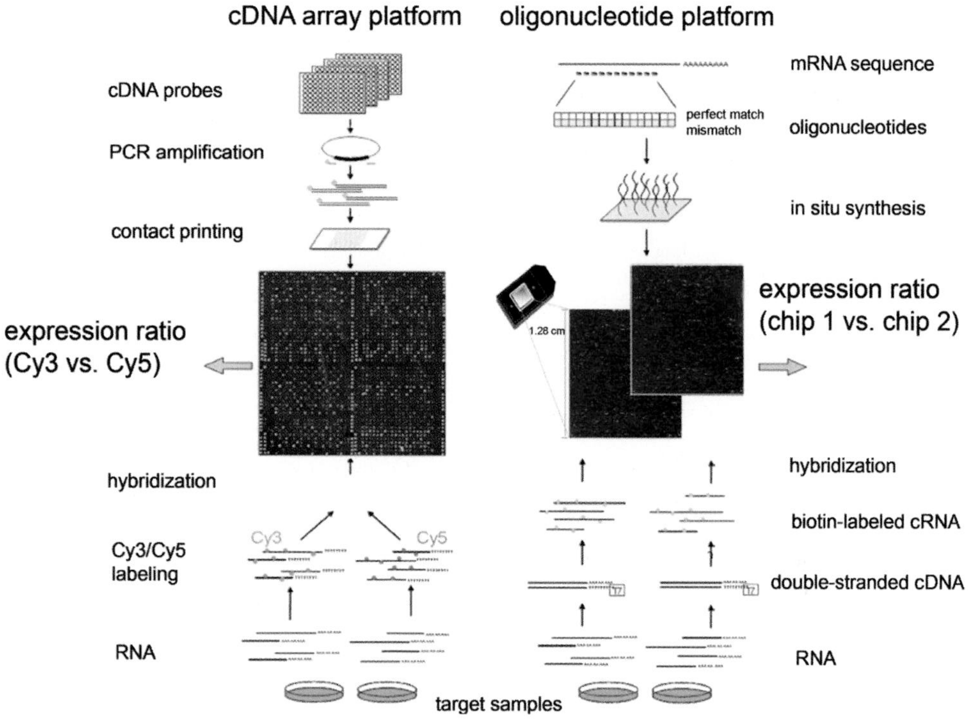

Figure 5.1 Scheme of DNA array analysis using cDNAs (left) and oligonucleotides (right, here Affymetrix technology) as probes. Probe design and construction of the array is shown in the upper part of the figure and the different preparation steps of the target samples are shown in the lower part. In the center of the figure, the strategy for case-control studies is shown using a two-color approach (left panel) and a single-color approach (right panel). Array images were taken from [69] and from http://www.affymetrix.com.

recognize the beads and attach to them. After bead assembly, a hybridization-based procedure is used to map the array in order to determine which bead type resides in each well of the array and to validate the performance of each bead type. An advantage of this technology is that multiple samples can be analyzed on the same chip, thus, preventing experimental artifacts across chips or dye labeling procedures. For example, the recent HumanRef-8 chip offers the possibility to screen eight different samples in parallel.

An alternative technology is the Agilent system [15, 16]. It relies on the immobilization of longer oligonucleotides (60-mers) synthesized *in situ* at or near the surface of the slide by ink jet printing using phosphoramidite chemistry. These probes are highly specific for the represented gene and show, generally, better hybridization properties than systems with shorter oligonculeotides. Experiments are typically double channel experiments, i.e., two target samples are analyzed simultaneously each labeled with a different cyanine dye and quantified with a separate scanning procedure. Agilent offers, similar to Illumina the possibility to perform multiple experiments on a single chip. This platform, as well as other using photolithographic techniques (Nimblegen, Febit), allow synthesis on demand. Chips can be produced from lists of oligonucleotide sequences provided by the customer, simplifying the construction of chips for new experimental systems. But also the construction of chips for many other applications, such as scoring of material from chromatin immune precipitation experiments (ChiP-chip) or the selective enrichment of specific sequences from DNA populations, benefits from this approach.

5.1.2
Platform Comparison

Each platform has pros and cons with respect to hybridization specificity, amounts of necessary material, coverage of the genome, and other factors as pointed out in a recent review [17].

Whole-genome chips contain probes for basically the entire genome. These chips are typically used for screening purposes, when little specific information is available *a priori*. However, if information on markers, specific chromosomal regions, etc, is available, so-called custom arrays are often used. These topic-specific chips are currently available for many diseases (cancer, diabetes), developmental stages or functional classes (kinases).

Several studies have compared chip platforms [18, 19]. Most of these studies discover a rather weak correlation of the global expression patterns resulting from different binding sensitivities caused by different probe lengths and probe-specific characteristics. Other differences result from different loci of the probes in the gene sequence. The most detailed comparison has been performed by the MAQC consortium [20] that compared two very distinct cell types (human brain versus human tissue mixture) with different chip platforms. The study, in contrast, reveals a very good correlation of the oligonucleotide platforms. Correlation between oligonucleotide and cDNA array platforms, however, was found to be much weaker.

Further variation of chip platforms is induced by the different annotation of the probes. Typically probe annotation and design is based on different source databases, for example Unigene, Refseq, LocusLink, ENSEMBL, etc. This probe annotation must be updated regularly which can lead to severe changes in data interpretation [21].

A number of these platforms (Illumina, Agilent, Niimblegen, Febit) allow some flexibility in subdividing chips into smaller "subchip" areas, simplifying the analysis of larger numbers of probes (at a correspondingly lower target number). Chip techniques are, however, increasingly being replaced by next-generation sequencing, providing digital data, with less noise, higher sensitivity, more flexibility, and a wider range of information, which can be collected in parallel.

5.1.3
Next Generation Sequencing

In contrast to the analog detection used in chips, sequencing is digital in providing the number of reads of a specific sequence in the target material. This technology is evolving rapidly. Currently, available commercial systems fall into two groups. One system, the FLX/Titanium system from Roche, uses a miniaturized pyrosequencing protocol to generate reads of up to 500 basepairs (bp) or longer, but still has relatively high costs per base pair. The second group produces relatively short reads at much lower costs and is at the moment mostly represented by the GenomeAnalyser II (GA II) from Illumina/Solexa, as well as by the SOLiD system produced by Applied Biosystems [22]. Both systems are under rapid development, with each new upgrade increasing throughput and decreasing costs. At the moment, these systems produce data in the order of one gigabase raw sequence per day, in short reads of 30 to 50 bp. Both systems are based on different forms of single molecule amplification. In the case of the GAII single molecules are amplified locally with a PCR reaction to give local, ideally well-separated sequence clusters [23]. These sequences are ligated to adaptor sequences that are attached to a solid phase substrate. After complete amplification, multiple chemistry cycles are performed in order to generate the sequence read-out. Four labeled reverse terminators (indicating the four different bases), additional primers and DNA polymerase are added to the flow cell, and after laser excitation the emitted fluorescence from each sequence cluster on the flow cell is recorded by an image in order to capture the first base for each spot on the flow cell image; this step is then repeated to capture the second base, etc., until for each sequence cluster a read of a certain length (typically 35 bp) has been recorded. In the case of the ABI system, this amplification is carried out by an emulsion PCR protocol, generating beads with multiple copies of a single DNA sequence. The sequence is read out based on a stepwise ligation of labeled oligonucleotides to the growing chain [24].

In addition to these systems, a novel "open source" system has been developed by the Harvard University (G007, http://www.polonator.org/). This system, which uses a technology similar to that used in in the SOLiD, promises to further increase specifications and lower sequencing costs compared to the currently available commercial systems.

These new sequencing techniques provide in many cases flexible alternatives to chip techniques in identifying the abundance of specific sequences, providing information on transcript abundance or RNA processing events (RNA-seq). Similarly, sequencing provides a more flexible and, ultimately, more sensitive alternative to chips in, e.g., the analysis of chromatin immunoprecipitation products, providing key information on the binding of regulatory proteins to genomic DNA [25].

In all these applications, sequencing techniques provide a number of advantages over classical, chip-based analysis protocols: The detection of sequences is inherently digital. A sequence is either found or not found. Similar to the superior sound quality of digitally encoded CDs over analog records, noise in the measuremts can be arbitrarily reduced by increasing the number of reads analyzed in an experiment. Conversely, multiple samples can be encoded by adding short sequence tags, mixed, and analyzed together in a single sequencing run, providing small amounts of sequence for multiple samples in parallel. Most importantly, however, sequencing is "hypothesis free." It detects any sequence, which is present in the sample, irrespective, whether the appropriate probe sequence had been considered by the design of the chip or not. In addition, sequencing allows a much easier integration of different types of information than many chip-based protocols. By sequencing, the abundance of trancripts can be measured by counting all reads that map to the transcript sequence, the splice patterns can be identified by detecting reads across splice junctions, the unexpected sequence variants can be identified due to RNA editing or, particularly important, in the case of cancer, solmatic mutation events can be detected [26].

5.1.4
Image Analysis and Data Quality Control

Image analysis is the first bioinformatics module in the data analysis pipeline of either microarrays or sequencing. Here, the digital information stored after the scanning of the arrays is translated into a numerical value for each entity (cDNA, oligonucleotide, sequence cluster) on the array. Commonly, image analysis is a two-step procedure. In the first step, a grid is found whose nodes describe the center positions of the entities and in the second step the digital values for each entity are quantified in a particular pixel neighborhood around its center. Different commercial products for image analysis of microarrays are available, for example, *GenePix* (Axon), *ImaGene* (BioDiscovery), *Genespotter* (MicroDiscovery), *AIDA* (Raytest), or *Visual Grid* (GPC Biotech). Furthermore, academic groups have developed their own software for microarray image analysis, for example, *ScanAlyze* (Stanford University), *FA* (Max-Planck Institute for Molecular Genetics) or *UCSF Spot* (University of California San Francisco). Besides these products, most commercial platforms have already built-in image analysis programs that provide the digital image for each experiment.

5.1.4.1 Grid Finding

Grid finding procedures are mostly geometric operations (rotations, projections, etc.) of the pixel rows and columns. Grid finding is defined differently with different methods, but essential steps are the same. The first step usually identifies the global borders of the originally rectangular grid. In a step-down procedure smaller subgrids are found and finally the individual spot positions are identified (Figure 5.2(a)). Grid finding has to cope with many perturbations of the ideal grid of spot positions, for example, irregular spaces between the blocks in which the spots are grouped, and nonlinear transformations of the original rectangular array to the stored image. Due to spotting problems subgrids can be shifted against each other and spots can distort irregularly in each direction from the virtual ideal position.

Of course, there are many different parameters for finding grids and thus image analysis programs show a lot of variations. However, common basic steps of the grid finding procedure are:

1. preprocessing of the pixel values
2. detection of the spotted area
3. spot finding.

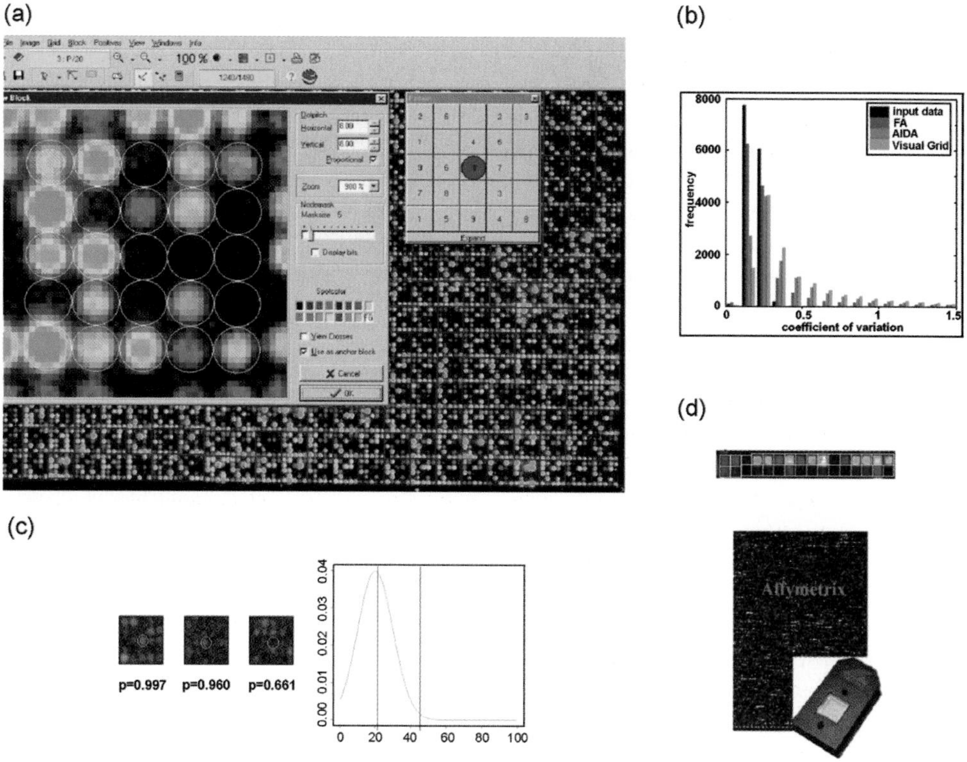

Figure 5.2 Image analysis and data acquisition. (a) Visualization of individual subgrid adjustment with *Visual Grid* (GPC Biotech AG). Spotting patterns show the geometry of the cDNAs organized in subgrids. Local background can be assigned to each spot by defining specific neighborhoods. (b) Image analysis was performed with three image analysis programs classified by manual (green bars), semiautomated (red bars), and automated (blue bars) procedures on simulated data. Purpose of the simulation was to compare the reproducibility of the signals by replicated analysis of perturbed signals (CV value). The histogram shows the frequencies (*Y*-axis) over the range of the CV (*X*-axis). (c) Spot validity can be judged by a negative control sample distributed on the array. After quantification a small, nonzero intensity is assigned to each of these empty spots reflecting the amount of background signal on the array. Since these positions are spread uniformly over the array, the distribution of these signals reflects the distribution of the signal noise for this experiment and is an indicator whether signals are at the background level or reflect reliable expression levels. If the cumulative distribution function for the spot's signal is close to one (blue line), this indicates that the cDNA is expressed in the tissue whereas low values reflect noise (red line). In practice, cDNAs are considered "expressed" when their signal exceeds a proportion of 0.9, a threshold consistent with the limit of visual detection of the spots. (d) Affymetrix geometry employs successive printing of gene representatives (oligonucleotide probes). Approximately 20 different oligonucleotides that are spread across the gene sequence are immobilized (perfect matches) with each PM having a one base-pair mismatch (MM) next to it, which is an estimator for the local background. The pair PM–MM is called an atom. The whole set of PM–MM pairs for the same gene is called a feature. After image analysis the feature values are condensed to a single value reflecting the genes concentration in the target sample.

The purpose of the first step is to amplify the regular structure in the image through robustification of signal-to-noise ratio, for example, by shifting a theoretical spot mask across the image and assigning those pixels to grid center positions that show the highest correlation between the spot mask and the actual pixel neighborhood. In the second step, a quadrilateral is fitted to mark the spotted region of the slide within the image. Several of the above programs require manual user interaction in this step. In the third step, each node of the grid is detected by mapping the quadrilateral to a unit square and to detect local maxima of the projections in x- and y-directions of the pixel intensities (for example in *FA*).

5.1.4.2 Spot Quantification

Once the center of the spot has been determined for each probe a certain pixel area around that spot center is used to compute the signal intensity. Here, the resolution of the image is important as well as the scanner transfer function, i.e., the function that determines how the pixel was calculated from the electronic signals within the scanning device. Quantification is done in two distinct ways. *Segmentation* tries to distinguish foreground from background pixels [27] and to sum up all pixels for the actual signal and the background, respectively. *Spot shape fitting* tries to fit a particular probability distribution (cf. Chapter 13), for example a two-dimensional Gaussian spot shape around the spot center. Then the signal intensity is computed as a weighted sum of the pixel intensities and the fitted density. A reasonable fit can be achieved using the maximum-likelihood estimators of the probability distributional parameters [28]. Not surprisingly, different strategies in spot quantification will lead to different results.

Image analysis methods can be grouped in three different classes, *manual*, *semiautomated*, and *automated* methods. Manual methods rely on the strong supervision of the user by requiring an initial guess on the spot positions. This can be realized by clicking the edges of the grid or by adjusting an ideal grid manually on the screen. Semiautomated methods require less interaction but still need prior information, for example, the definition of the spotted area. Automated methods try to find the spot grid without user interaction. Simulation studies on systematically perturbed artificial images have shown that the data reproducibility increases with the grade of automation of the software [29]. However, for noisy images that show a very irregular structure manual methods might be the best choice (Figure 5.2(b)).

5.1.4.3 Signal Validity

Signal validity testing has two tasks – the detection of *spot artifacts* (for example, overshining of two spots, background artifacts, irregular spot forms, etc.) and the judgement on the *detection limit*, i.e., whether the spot can reasonably be detected and thus if the gene is expressed in the tissue of interest or not.

Spot artifacts are identified by applying morphological feature recognition criteria such as circularity, regularity of spot form, and background artifact detection methods. In the Affymetrix oligo-chip design spot validity is often judged by the comparison of the PM/MM (perfect match/mismatch) pairs using a statistical test. Each gene is represented on the chip by a set of n oligonucleotides (~20-mers) that are distributed across the gene sequence ($PM_1, \ldots, PM_n$). For each perfect match, PM_i, there is an oligonucleotide next to it, MM_i, with a central base pair mismatch in the original PM sequence (Figure 5.2(c)). This value serves as a local background for the probe. For each gene the perfect matches and the mismatches yield two series of values, $PM_1, \ldots, PM_n$ and $MM_1, \ldots, MM_n$ and a Wilcoxon rank test can be calculated for the hypothesis that the two signal series are equal or not (cf. Chapter 13). If the P-value is low then this indicates that the signal series have significantly higher values than the mismatch signal series and thus it is likely that the corresponding gene is expressed in the tissue. Conversely, if the P-value is not significant then there is no great difference in PM- and MM-signals and thus it is likely that the gene is not expressed. In order to calculate a single expression value to the probe it has been assumed that the average of PM–MM differences is a good estimator for the expression of the corresponding gene.

$$y_i - \frac{1}{n}\sum_{j=1}^{n}(PM_{ij} - MM_{ij}). \tag{5.1}$$

Here, y_i corresponds to the ith gene and PM_{ij} and MM_{ij} are the jth perfect match and mismatch probe signals for gene i. This use of the mismatches for analysis has been criticized. It has been reported that the MM probes often interacts with the transcript and thus produces high signal values [30]. This fact is known as cross-hybridization and is a severe practical problem. This has led to alternative computations of the local background, for example, by evaluating local neighborhoods of probes with low expression values (*background zone weighting*) [31].

In cDNA arrays such kinds of significance test for signal validity cannot be performed on the spot level because most commonly each cDNA is spotted only a small number of times such that there are not enough replicates for performing a test. Instead this procedure can be carried out on the pixel level. Here, for each spot a local background area is defined, for example, by separating foreground and background pixels by the segmentation procedure or by defining specific spot neighborhoods (corners, ring, etc.) as the local background. Alternatively, the signals can be compared at the spot level to a negative control sample. For example, several array designs incorporate empty positions on the array (i.e., no material was transferred). The scanning and image analysis will assign each such position a small intensity level that corresponds to the local background. For each regular spot a certain probability can then be calculated that the spot is different from the negative sample (Figure 5.2(d)). This can be done by outlier criteria or by direct comparison to the negative sample [6].

Signal validity indices can be used as an additional qualifier for the expression ratio (Table 5.1). Suppose we compare a gene's expression in two different conditions (A and B), then we distinguish four cases ($1 =$ signal is valid, $0 =$ signal is invalid):

Probes belonging to the fourth case should be removed from further analysis since they represent genes which are either not expressed in both conditions or which cannot be detected using the experimental platform (possibly because the number of molecules is low). This will occur fairly often in practice since only a part of the genes on the array will actually be activated in the tissue under analysis. The other three

Table 5.1 Signal validity in case-control studies.

A	B	Ratio	Interpretation	Possible marker
1	1	Valid	Gene expression is detectable in both conditions	Yes
1	0	Invalid	Gene expression is detectable in condition A but not in B	Yes
0	1	Invalid	Gene expression is detectable in condition B but not in A	Yes
0	0	Invalid	Gene expression is not detectable in both conditions	No

cases may reveal genes with significant changes but the expression ratio is only meaningful in the first case where both conditions generate valid signals.

It should be pointed out that the signal intensities are only crude estimators for the actual concentrations and the interpretation as concentration changes is only valid if the intensity-concentration correspondence is approximately linear. Microarray measurements often show deviations from this assumption. For instance, saturation effects if the spot signals are close to the hardware limit (if a 16-bit scanner is used the highest possible intensity value is 65535) or other nonlinearities if the concentration of the gene is below the detection limit of a microarray.

5.1.5
Preprocessing

The task of data *preprocessing* (or mostly termed *normalization*) is the elimination of influence factors that are not due to the probe–target interaction such as labeling effects (different dyes), background correction, pin effects (spotting characteristics), outlier detection (cross-hybridization of oligonucleotide-probes), etc. Many different algorithms and methods have been proposed to fulfill these tasks. Rather than listing these different methods, we will concentrate here on describing some common fundamental concepts. Data normalization has become a major research component in recent years, resulting in many different methods each claiming specific merits [32].

The purpose of preprocessing methods is to make signal values comparable across different experiments. This involves two steps – the selection of a set of probes (the *normalization sample*) and the calculation of numerical factors that are used to transform the signal values within each experiment (the *normalization parameters*). The selection of a normalization sample is commonly implicitly based on the assumption that the expression for the same probe in the normalization sample will not vary across experiments due to biological reasons. Different methods have been proposed for that purpose:

1. house-keeping genes;
2. selected probes whose mRNA is spiked to the labeled target sample in equal amounts;
3. numerical methods to select a set of nonvarying probes across the batch of experiments.

While the first two cases involve additional biological material, the third is directly based on the probes of interest. Numerical methods try, for example, to calculate a maximal normalization sample by so-called *maximal invariant sets*, i.e., maximal sets of probes whose signals have the same rank order across all experiments under analysis, or by applying an iterative regression approach [31].

5.1.5.1 Global Measures

The weakest transformation of data is given by estimating global factors to eliminate multiplicative noise across arrays. A very robust procedure calculates the median signal of each array and determines a scaling factor that equalizes those medians. In the next step this scaling factor is applied to each individual signal to adjust the raw signals.

Alternatively, an iterative regression method can be applied to normalize the experimental batch. Assume we have two experiments then this algorithm reads as follows:

1. apply a simple linear regression fit of the data from the two experiments;
2. calculate the residual;
3. eliminate those probes that have residuals above a certain threshold;
4. repeat steps 1–3 until the changes in residuals are below a certain threshold.

A batch of more than two experiments can be normalized with this approach by comparing each single experiment with a preselected experiment or with the *in silico* average across the entire batch. Global measures can be used for normalizing for overall influence factors that are approximately linear. Nonlinear and spatial effects (if present) are not addressed by these methods.

5.1.5.2 Linear Models

Linear model approaches have been used for cDNA arrays as well as for oligo chips [33, 34]. A model for a spotted microarray developed by Kerr and Churchill defines several influence factors that contribute to artificial spot signals. The model reads

$$\log(y_{ijkl}) = b + a_i + d_j + v_k + g_l + ag_{il} + vg_{kl} + \varepsilon_{ijkl}. \tag{5.2}$$

This model takes into account a global mean effect, b, the effect a_i of the array i and the effect d_j of the dye j. v_k is the effect of variety k, i.e., the specific cDNA target sample and g_l is the effect of gene l. ε_{ijkl} is the random error assumed to be Gaussian distributed with mean zero. In a simpler model there are no interactions. In practice there might be interactions between gene and array effects, ag_{il}, or between gene and sample effects, vg_{kl}. This can then be solved with ANOVA methods incorporating interaction terms [35].

Li and Wong use a linear model approach for normalizing oligonucleotide chips (d-chip). Here, the model assumes that the intensity signal of a probe j increases linearly with the expression of the corresponding gene in the ith sample. Equations for mismatch oligonucleotides and perfect match oligonucleotides are then given by

$$\begin{aligned} PM_{ij} &= a_j + g_i v_j + g_i w_j + \varepsilon \\ M_{ij} &= a_j + g_i v_j + \varepsilon. \end{aligned} \tag{5.3}$$

Here, a_j is the background response for probe pair j, g_i is the expression of the ith gene, v_j and w_j are the rates of increase for the mismatch and the perfect match probe, respectively. The authors developed a software package for performing analysis and normalization of Affymetrix oligo chips, which is available for academic research (www.dchip.org).

5.1.5.3 Nonlinear and Spatial Effects

Spotted cDNA microarrays commonly incorporate nonlinear and spatial effects due to different characteristics of the pins, the different dyes, and local distortions of the spots.

A very popular normalization method for eliminating the dye effect is *LOWESS* (or LOESS), LOcally WEighted polynomial regreSSion [36]. LOWESS is applied to each experiment with two dyes separately. The data axis is screened with sliding windows and in each window a polynomial is fit

$$y = \beta_0 + \beta_1 x + \beta_2 x^2 + \ldots . \tag{5.4}$$

Parameters of the LOWESS approach are the degree of the polynomial (usually 1 or 2) and the size of the window. The local polynomials fit to each subset of the data are almost always either linear or quadratic. Note that a zero degree polynomial would correspond to a weighted moving average. LOWESS is based on the idea that any function can be well approximated in a small neighborhood by a low-order polynomial. High-degree polynomials would tend to overfit the data in each subset and are numerically unstable, making accurate computations difficult. At each point in the data set the polynomial is fit using weighted least squares, giving more weight to points near the point whose response is being estimated and less weight to points further away. This can be achieved by the standard weight function such as

$$w(x) = \begin{cases} (1-|x-x_i|^3)^3, & |x|<1. \\ 0, |x| \geq 1 \end{cases} \tag{5.5}$$

Here x_i is the current data point. After fitting the polynomial in the current window, the window is moved and a new polynomial is fit. The value of the regression function for the point is then obtained by evaluating the local polynomial using the explanatory variable values for that data point. The LOWESS fit is complete after regression function values have been computed for each of the n data points. The final result is a smooth curve providing a model for the data. An additional user-defined smoothing parameter determines the proportion of data used in each fit. Large values of this parameter produce smooth fits. Typically smoothing parameters lie in the range 0.25 to 0.5 [37].

5.1.5.4 Other Approaches

There are many other approaches to DNA array data normalization. One class of such models employs *variance stabilization* [38, 39]. These methods address the problem that gene expression measurements have an expression-dependent variance and try to overcome this situation by a data transformation that can stabilize the variance across the entire range of expression. The transformation step is usually connected with an error model for the data and a normalization method (such as regression). The most popular of those variance stabilizations is the log transformation. However, the log transformation amplifies errors at small expression values, which has led to the use of alternative transformations.

A lot of the above-discussed normalization methods are included in the R statistical software package (www.r-project.org) and, particularly for microarray data evaluation, in the R software packages distributed by the Bioconductor project – an open source and open development software project to provide tools for microarray data analysis (www.bioconductor.org).

5.2 Analysis of Gene Expression Data

Summary

The analysis of genome-wide gene expression data involves basic concepts from multivariate statistics. Most applications belong to two groups: the first group consists of case-control studies comparing a certain transcriptome state of the biological system (e.g., disease state, perturbed state) to the control situation; the second group of applications consist of multiple case studies involving different states (e.g., drug response time series, groups of patients, etc.). The analysis of case-control studies involves testing of statistical hypotheses. Here, expression changes are observed that deviate from a predefined hypothesis and this deviation is judged for significance. The basic methods for multicase studies are clustering and classification. Here, groups of coexpressed genes serve to identify functionally related groups of genes or experiments. These types of analysis result in the identification of marker genes and their related interactions, which are the basis for further network studies.

5.2.1 Planning and Designing Experiments for Case-Control Studies

The analysis of fold changes is a central part of transcriptome analysis. Questions of interest are whether certain genes can be identified as being differentially expressed when comparing two different conditions (for example, a normal versus a disease condition). Whereas early studies of fold-change analysis were based on the expression ratio of probes derived from the expression in a treatment and a control target sample, it has become a working standard to perform experimental repetitions and to base the identification of differentially expressed genes on statistical testing procedures judging the null hypothesis $H_0: \mu_x = \mu_y$ versus the alternative $H_0: \mu_x \neq \mu_y$, where μ_x, μ_y are the population means of the treatment and the control sample, respectively. Strikingly, it is still very popular to present the expression ratio in published results without any estimate of the error and studies that employ ratio error bounds are hard to find (for an exception see [6]). It should be noted that fold changes without estimates of the error bounds contain only very limited information. For example, probes with low expression values in both conditions can have tremendous ratios but these ratios are meaningless because they reflect only noise. A simple error calculation can be done as follows. Assume that we have replicate series for control and treatment series $x_1, \ldots, x_n$ and $y_1, \ldots, y_m$. A widely used error measure of the sample averages is the *standard error of the mean*

$$S_x = \sqrt{\frac{1}{(n-1)n}\sum_{i=1}^{n}(x_i-\bar{x})^2} \quad \text{and} \quad S_y = \sqrt{\frac{1}{(m-1)m}\sum_{i=1}^{m}(y_i-\bar{y})^2}. \tag{5.6}$$

The *standard error of the ratio* can then be calculated as

$$\frac{\bar{x}}{\bar{y}} \pm \frac{1}{\bar{y}^2}\sqrt{\bar{x}^2 S_y^2 + \bar{y}^2 S_x^2}. \tag{5.7}$$

An important question in the design of such an experiment is how many replicates should be used and what level of fold change can be reliably detected. This is – among other factors – dependent on the experimental noise. Experimental observations indicate that an experimental noise of 15–25% can be assumed in a typical microarray experiment. The experimental noise can be interpreted as the mean CV of replicated series of expression values of the probes. The dependence of the detectable fold change on the number of experimental repetitions and on the experimental error has been discussed in several papers [40, 41].

Figure 5.3 shows a simple simulation that illustrates this fact. Replicate series are sampled from a Gaussian distribution with mean $\mu = 1$ and $\sigma^2 = 0.04$ (i.e., $CV = 0.2$) for the control series. In order to simulate fold changes the mean of the treatment series is changed subsequently holding the CV constant (for example, $\mu = 2$ and $\sigma^2 = 0.16$ (i.e., $CV = 0.2$) if a fold change of factor two is simulated). Then, replicates are sampled from that distribution. A Welsh test is performed and it is marked whether the *P*-value is significant (<0.05) or not. The sampling is repeated 1000 times and the number of positive test results is depicted. The curves show the dependency of the true positive rate on the sample size. For example, a 1.5-fold change is detectable in only 32% of all cases when three repetitions are used. This number increases to 95% when eight replicates are used (black line). The simulation suggests that a fold-change analysis should be performed with at least four independent replicates.

5.2.2
Tests for Differential Expression

5.2.2.1 DNA Arrays

Let, $x_1, \ldots, x_n$ and $y_1, \ldots, y_m$ be two independent samples derived from replicated measurements of the same probe across two conditions (treatment and control). Differential expression of the gene represented by the probe in the two conditions can be judged by location tests (see Chapter 13). It is assumed, as a null hypothesis,

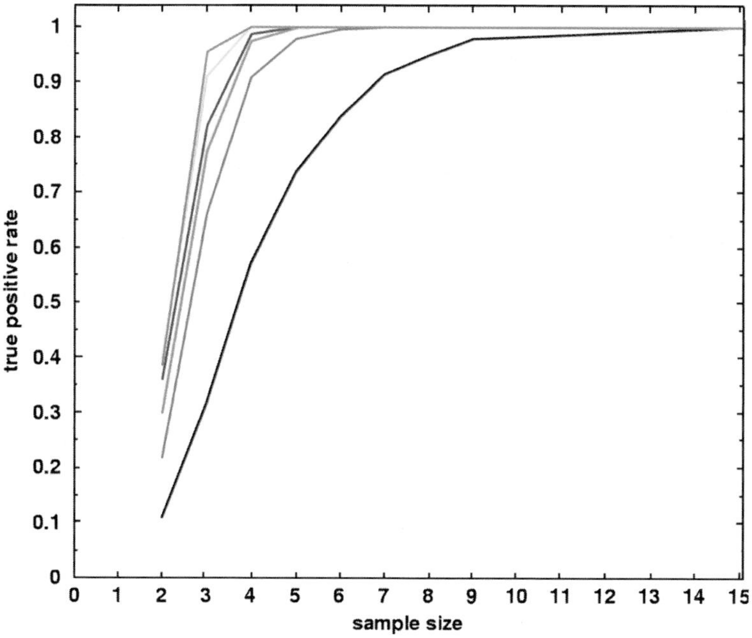

Figure 5.3 Simulation of the dependency of fold change detection on the sample size. Experimental error is assumed to be 20%, i.e., CV of replicated control and treatment series equals 0.2. Samples are drawn from Gaussian distributions with mean equal to 1 for the control series and mean equal to 1.5 (black), 2 (red), 2.5 (green), 3 (blue), 5 (yellow), and 10 (magenta) for the treatment samples, respectively, in order to simulate the fold changes. Sampling is repeated 1000 times and the proportion of true positive test results ($P < 0.05$) is plotted (Y-axis) over the sample size (X-axis).

that the expression values under two conditions have the same expectation value. Deviations from the null hypothesis of equal means are judged by test statistics. These test statistics are real-valued functions on the data samples

$$f(x_1, \ldots, x_n, y_1, \ldots, y_m). \tag{5.8}$$

Test statistics typically follow a certain probability distribution under the null hypothesis, and so, for each given value of the test statistic the probability of an even more extreme observation can be calculated by integrating the respective area under the probability density function. This probability is computed as the P-value that judges the significance of the observation, for example a certain fold change, given the null hypothesis. Thus, observations that have a low P-value indicate that the null hypothesis of equal location of the two samples is very unlikely and should be rejected. These observations are typically called significant results.

It is notable that the P-value is only valid if the assumptions about the underlying probability distributions are valid. For example, if a t-test is applied to a single gene observation resulting in a P-value of 0.01, this value is only true if both series are Gaussian distributed and have equal variances. Furthermore, the test assumes that the replicates are independent of each other. Strikingly, many studies miss this fact entirely, for example, applying a Gaussian-based *t*-test without checking the validity of the distributional assumptions. Thus, replicates on the same array and replicates in different experiments should not be mixed since they have different characteristics and cannot be treated as independent replicates. Important issues are:

- are the distributional assumptions valid?
- are the replicates independent of each other?
- is the number of replicates sufficient to detect the fold change that you are interested in?
- are outliers removed from the samples?

Most commonly, modifications of four different tests are applied in microarray data analysis. These tests are implemented in statistical software packages such as R/Bioconductor or SAS:

1. Student's *t*-test
2. Welch's test
3. Wilcoxon's rank sum test
4. Permutation tests.

While the first two tests assume Gaussian distributed data and the *P*-values are calculated by a probability distribution, the latter two are nonparametric and the *P*-values are calculated based on combinatorial arguments.

Example 5.1

In a microarray study incorporating approximately 15,000 different cDNAs and four independent hybridization experiments the early differentiation event in human blastocysts has been investigated, i.e., the formation of the trophectoderm and the inner cell mass [42]. *HMBG1* is a specific gene of interest because it has been published as a potential stemness gene in human stem cell lines, i.e., a gene that is relevant for remaining pluripotency of cells. *HMBG1* is a member of the high mobility group of transcription factors encoding proteins that act primarily as architectural facilitators in the assembly of nucleoprotein complexes, for example, the initiation of transcription factor target genes.

The four measured expression values are for the trophectoderm (upper row values) and ICM (lower row values), respectively:

32,612	46,741	29,238	32,671
49,966	58,037	94,785	122,044

P-values for differential expression between the two sample groups are 0.037 for Student's *t*-test, 0.068 for the Welch test, and 0.029 for the Wilcoxon test. This example shows how a high variance (ICM sample) can mislead the Gaussian-based tests, whereas the rank-based test is fairly stable. Note that ranking separates the groups perfectly.

Table 5.2 Contingency table for tag-based statistical analysis.

	Tags in condition A	Tags in condition B	Total
Tags for this particular gene	a	b	$a+b$
Tags for all other genes	c	d	$c+d$
Total	$a+c$	$b+d$	$a+b+c+d$

5.2.2.2 Next Generation Sequencing

While the differential analysis of DNA arrays has been well developed through recent years, differential analysis of next generation sequencing data is still being developed. In principle, these analyses can be compared to EST (expressed sequence tag) data analyses and many of the methods proposed there can be extrapolated.

Consider, for a given gene the measurement of a sequence reads in condition A (treatment) and b sequence reads in condition B (control).

We can organize the data in a 2×2 contingency table as shown in Table 5.2.

The question whether or not the difference in read counts for the particular gene in the two conditions is significant can be answered by different statistical approaches [43]:

1. Fisher's exact test
2. Chi-square test
3. Bayesian methods [44].

The latter method has been originally proposed in the analysis of EST libraries. It follows a Poisson assumption of the occurrence of a tag for a particular gene in a large population of tags and uses a Bayesian approach to compute the corresponding conditional probabilities. The probability of observing b reads of the gene in condition B (under the null hypothesis of equal distribution) given that a reads have been observed in condition A is expressed as

$$P(b|a) = \left(\frac{b+d}{a+c}\right)^b \frac{(a+b)!}{a!b!\left(1+\frac{b+d}{a+c}\right)^{a+b+1}}. \tag{5.9}$$

Resulting P-values are computed by

$$P = \min\left\{\sum_{k=0}^{b} P(k|a), \sum_{k=b}^{\infty} P(k|a)\right\}. \tag{5.10}$$

5.2.3 Multiple Testing

The single gene analysis described above has statistically a major drawback. We cannot view each single test separately but have to take into account the fact that we perform thousands of tests in parallel (for example, for each gene on an array).

Thus, a global significance level of $\alpha = 0.05$, for example, performed with $n = 10{,}000$ cDNAs will imply a false positive rate of 5%. This means that we must expect that 500 (!) individual tests yield false positive results and thus that many cDNAs are falsely identified as potential targets. Inclusion of such false positives in the further analysis steps can be extremely costly. To control the trade-off between the numbers of false positives and false negatives, corrections for multiple testing are commonly applied to microarray studies that assure a global significance rate of 5%.

Let α_g be the global significance level and let α_s be the significance level at the single gene level. It is clear that we cannot assure a global significance level α_g without adjusting the single gene levels. For example, the probability of making the correct decision given that we reject the null hypothesis (i.e., the probability that a selected gene is truly differentially expressed) is

$$p_s = (1-\alpha_s). \tag{5.11}$$

The probability of making the correct decision on the global level (i.e., the probability that all selected genes are truly differentially expressed) is the product of the probabilities on the individual levels

$$p_g = (1-\alpha_s)^n. \tag{5.12}$$

The probability of drawing the wrong conclusion in at least one of the n different tests is

$$P(\text{wrong}) = \alpha_g = 1-(1-\alpha_s)^n. \tag{5.13}$$

For example, if we have 100 different genes on the array and we set the gene-wise significance level to 0.05 we will have a probability of 0.994 of making a type-I error. This is the so-called *family-wise error rate* (FWER) of the experiment, i.e., the global type-I error rate. Multiple testing corrections try to adjust the single gene level type-I error rate in a way that the global type-I error rate is below a given threshold. In practice, it means that the calculated P-values have to be corrected.

The most conservative correction is the *Bonferroni correction*. Here, we approximate (5.13) by the first terms of the binomial expansion, i.e.,

$$(1-\alpha_s)^n = \sum_{i=0}^{n} \binom{n}{i} (-1)^{n-i} \alpha_s^i. \tag{5.14}$$

Thus, we rewrite

$$\alpha_g = 1-\sum_{i=0}^{n} \binom{n}{i} (-\alpha_s)^i \approx n\alpha_s \Rightarrow \alpha_s = \frac{\alpha_g}{n}. \tag{5.15}$$

The Bonferroni correction of the single gene level is the global confidence level divided by the number of the tests performed. This, however, is far too conservative for many practical applications. For example, using an array of $n = 10{,}000$ probes and an experiment FWER of 0.01, then only those observations would be judged as *significantly differentially expressed* whose P-value is below $1.0\mathrm{e}-06$. Fairly, few genes would meet this requirement. The result would therefore consist of many false negatives.

The Bonferroni correction is too strict in the sense that we apply the same significance level to all genes. Consider, instead, the following stepwise procedure:

For a given global significance level α_g sort the probes in increasing order after their *P*-values calculated on the single-gene basis. If $p_1 < \frac{\alpha_g}{n}$, then adjust the remaining $n-1$ *P*-values by comparing the next *P*-value $p_2 < \frac{\alpha_g}{n-1}$, etc. If m is the largest integer for which $p_m < \frac{\alpha_g}{n-m+1}$ then we call genes 1, . . ., m significantly differentially expressed. This procedure is called *Holm's stepwise correction* and it assures that the global significance level is valid. Although it is more flexible than the Bonferroni correction it is still too strict for practical purposes.

A widely used method for adjusting *P*-values is the *Westfall and Young step-down correction* [45]. This procedure is essentially based on permutations of the data.

1. Perform $d = 1, \ldots, D$ permutations of the sample labels, and let p_i be the gene-wise *P*-value of the ith probe
2. For each permutation, compute the *P*-value p_{id} from the dth permutation for the ith probe
3. Adjust the *P*-value of probe i by $\tilde{p}_i = \dfrac{\{d; \min_i p_{id} \le p_i\}}{D}$

The advantage of this resampling method is that, unlike the approaches above, it takes into account data dependences.

An alternative to controlling the FWER is the computation of the *false discovery rate* (FDR). The FDR is defined as the expected number of type-I errors among the rejected hypotheses [46].

The procedure follows the scheme

1. As in the case of Holm's procedure sort the probes in increasing order by their *P*-values, calculated on the single-gene basis. Select a level α_g for the FDR.
2. Let $j^* = \max\{j;\ p_j \le j\alpha/n\}$.
3. Reject the hypotheses for $j = 1, \ldots, j^*$.

Recent variations of controlling the FDR with application to microarray data have been published in [47, 48].

The practical use of multiple testing is not entirely clear. Whereas it is useful to select false positive results from true positive results on the one hand, it will on the other hand discard a lot of potentially useful targets and the experimentalist might lose important biological information.

5.2.4
ROC Curve Analysis

In Chapter 13, we introduce the basic types of errors of a statistical test procedure. If, in practice, a training sample is available (for example, a set of gene probes known to be differentially expressed and a set of probes that is known to be unchanged), we can for each test result calculate the true and false positive rates. The performance of a specific test, normalization method, etc., can then be display using a ROC (*receiver*

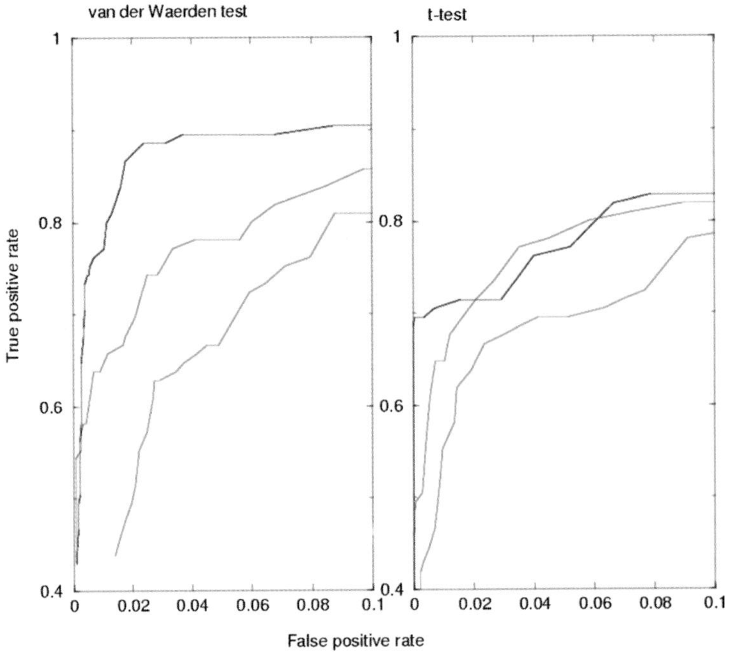

Figure 5.4 ROC curve for visualizing performance of normalization methods and test procedures. Six independent hybridization experiments were performed with wild-type zebrafish embryos (control) and lihtium-treated embryos (treatment). The true positive sample was identified by 105 cDNAs that were verified by an independent experimental technique (*in-situ* hybridization). The false positive sample was estimated by 2304 copies of an *Arabidopsis thaliana* cDNA whose complementary sequence was spiked to the treatment and control target samples, respectively. Left graph: The van der Waerden test is used for judging differential expression on three different normalization methods, global median normalization (black), variance stabilization (red), and linear regression (green). Right graph: Student's *t*-test is used for judging differential expression using the same normalization methods. ROC analysis reveals that the nonparametric test outperforms the Gaussian-based test and furthermore, that the global normalization performs best with both test methods compared to the other methods.

operating characteristic) curve. The purpose and result of a ROC curve analysis is, for example, to evaluate several normalization and test procedures and to choose the best methods.

Figure 5.4 shows a typical example of a ROC curve analysis. Here, we map the false postive rate (*X*-axis) and the true positive rate (*Y*-axis) and compare the performance of three normalization procedures and two statistical tests on an experimental test set with known expression changes. Ideally, the ROC curve has an integral of one and is a straight line (no false positives, maximal sensitivity) and those procedures are preferable that give the highest overall integral. Alternatively, one might select a specific area of interest (for example, a false positive rate below the experimental significance level) and choose that procedure which shows the highest performance in the selected area. Similar ROC curve analysis has been used to compare different normalization strategies [49].

5.2.5
Clustering Algorithms

Clustering algorithms are a general group of tools from multivariate explorative statistics. They are used to group data objects according to their pairwise similarity with respect to a set of characteristics measured on these objects. Clustering algorithms are widely used in order to identify coregulated genes with microarray experiments. There is a simple assumption behind that strategy – the concept of *guilt-by-association*. The rationale behind this concept is that those genes whose probes show a similar profile through a set of experimental conditions will share common regulatory rules. Thus, gene expression clusters are used to identify common functional characteristics of the genes.

Clustering algorithms are explorative statistical methods that group together genes with similar profiles and separate genes with dissimilar profiles, whereby similarity (or dissimilarity) is defined numerically by a real-valued pairwise (dis)similarity function. Consider p experiments have been performed on n different genes on the array, then the profile of gene i is a p-dimensional vector $\boldsymbol{x}_i = (x_{i1}, \ldots, x_{ip})$ and a *pairwise similarity measure* can be any function $d: \Re_p \times \Re_p \rightarrow \Re$. Intuitively, one would prefer functions that reflect some kind of geometric distance such as the *Euclidean distance*, or more general, *Minkowsky*- or l^q*-distances* defined by

$$d_q(\boldsymbol{x}_n, \boldsymbol{x}_m) = \left(\sum_{i=1}^{p} |x_{ni} - x_{mi}|^q \right)^{\frac{1}{q}}. \tag{5.16}$$

Note that for $q = 1$ we have the *Manhattan distance* and for $q = 2$ we have the Euclidean distance. Another class of pairwise similarity measures are correlation measures such as Pearson's- or Spearman's correlation coefficient.

A practical problem occurs with *missing values* since there may be some measurements that yield an unreliable value for a given probe. However, one wants to keep the other reliable measurements of that probe and use its profile in further analysis. The fact that the profile now consists only of $p - 1$ values has to be taken into account. The treatment of missing values is a characteristic of the pairwise similarity measure. For example, one could try to estimate the distance of two vectors with missing values by the valid values. Assume two vectors, $\boldsymbol{x}_n$, $\boldsymbol{x}_m$, then the squared Euclidean distance is given by $d_2^2(\boldsymbol{x}_n, \boldsymbol{x}_m) = \sum_{i=1}^{p} (x_{ni} - x_{mi})^2$ if both vectors have no missing values. If there are missing values, count the number of coordinate pairs that include at least one missing value, k, compute the distance on the remaining coordinate pairs and estimate the distance by a multiplicative factor adapted to the amount of missing pairs, i.e., $d_2^2(\boldsymbol{x}_n, \boldsymbol{x}_m) = \frac{p}{p-k} \sum_i (x_{ni} - x_{mi})^2$. If for example, half of the data is missing the remaining distance is multiplied with 2. Such and other adjustments for missing data can be found in the book of Jain and Dubes [50].

Example 5.2

In practice, it might be useful to transform data prior to computing pairwise distances. Consider the profiles $\boldsymbol{x}_1 = (100, 200, 300)$, $\boldsymbol{x}_2 = (10, 20, 30)$, and $\mathbf{x}_2 = (30, 20, 10)$. Euclidean distance will assign a higher similarity to the pair $\mathbf{x}_2, \mathbf{x}_3$ than to the pair $\mathbf{x}_1, \mathbf{x}_2$ because it only takes into account the geometric distance of the three data vectors. Correlation measures would assign a higher similarity to the pair $\mathbf{x}_1, \mathbf{x}_2$ than to the pair $\mathbf{x}_2, \mathbf{x}_3$ since they take into account whether the components of both vectors change in the same direction. For example, if these data were derived from a time-series measurement one would argue that both vectors $\mathbf{x}_1, \mathbf{x}_2$ increase with time (although on different levels of expression), whereas $\mathbf{x}_3$ decreases with time. In many applications, thus, it makes sense to transform the data vectors before calculating pairwise similarities. A straightforward geometric data transformation would be to divide each component x_j of a p-dimensional data vector $\mathbf{x} = (x_1, \ldots, x_p)^T$ by its Euclidian norm, i.e., perform the transformation $\tilde{x}_j = \frac{x_j}{\|x\|}$. The resulting effect is that after transformation each data vector $\tilde{x}$ has an Euclidean norm of one and is mapped to the unit sphere.

The choice of the similarity measure is important since it influences the output of the clustering algorithm. It should be adapted to the question of interest. Figure 5.5 shows two different clustering results using two different distances.

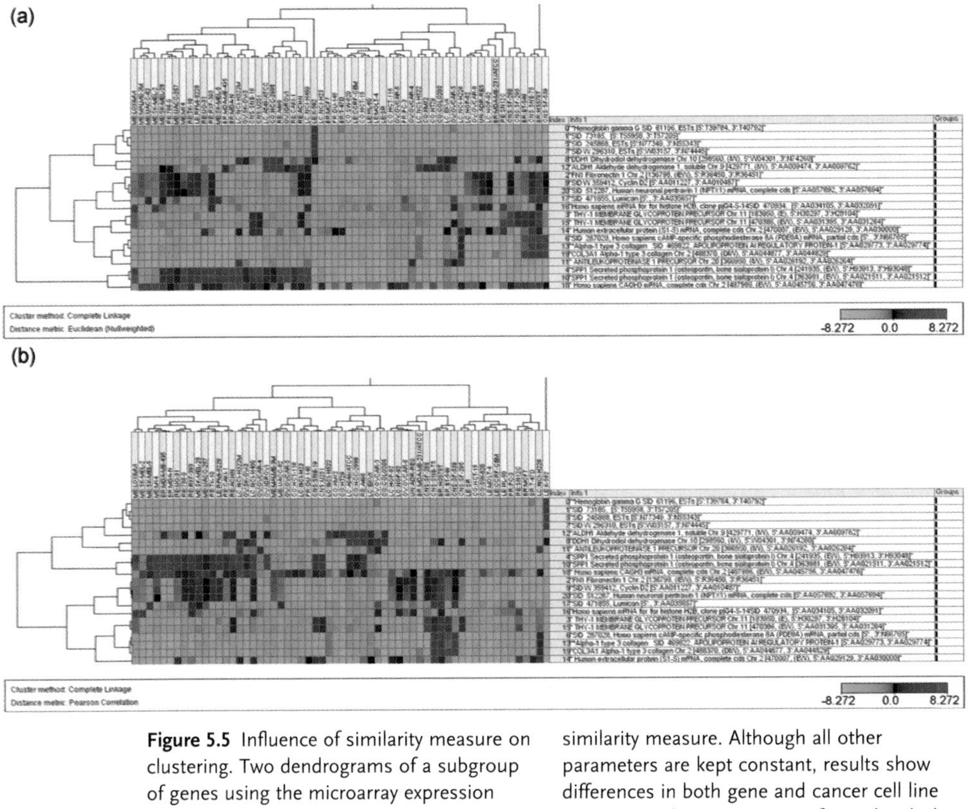

Figure 5.5 Influence of similarity measure on clustering. Two dendrograms of a subgroup of genes using the microarray expression data of Ross *et al.* [70] were generated using hierarchical clustering with Euclidean distance (a) and Pearson correlation (b) as pairwise similarity measure. Although all other parameters are kept constant, results show differences in both gene and cancer cell line groupings. Clustering was performed with the *J-Express Pro* software package (Molmine, Bergen Norway).

Two classes of clustering algorithms are commonly distinguished, *hierarchical* and *partitioning* methods [50]. In contrast to partitioning methods that try to find the "best" partition given a fixed number of clusters, hierarchical methods calculate a full series of partitions starting from n clusters each of which contains one single data point and ending with one cluster that contains all n data points (or vice versa); in each step of the procedure two clusters are merged according to a prespecified rule. In the following, we describe the classical hierarchical algorithm and commonly used partitioning methods (SOM and K-means).

5.2.5.1 Hierarchical Clustering

Let $x_1, \ldots, x_n$ be the p-dimensional data points (expression profiles of n gene representatives across the p experiments). The process of hierarchical clustering algorithms requires a dissimilarity measure, d, between pairs of clusters (related to a dissimilarity measure, $\tilde{d}$, between pairs of data points) and an update procedure for recalculation of the merged clusters. It has then the following scheme:

1. Set the counter variable $\nu = n$ and start with the finest possible partition.
2. Iterate:
   (a) Calculate a new partition by joining two clusters that minimize d.
   (b) Update the distances of the remaining clusters and the joined cluster and decrease the counter variable by 1.
3. Stop, if $\nu = 1$, i.e., all data points are in one cluster otherwise repeat steps 1–3. (5.17)

Several cluster dissimilarity measures are in use:

$$\text{Single linkage} \quad d\left(C_k^{(\nu)}, C_l^{(\nu)}\right) = \min_{x_i \in C_k^{(\nu)}, x_j \in C_l^{(\nu)}} \tilde{d}\,(x_i, x_j). \tag{5.18}$$

$$\text{Complete linkage} \quad d\left(C_k^{(\nu)}, C_l^{(\nu)}\right) = \max_{x_i \in C_k^{(\nu)}, x_j \in C_l^{(\nu)}} \tilde{d}\,(x_i, x_j). \tag{5.19}$$

$$\text{Average linkage} \quad d\left(C_k^{(\nu)}, C_l^{(\nu)}\right) = \frac{1}{\left|C_k^{(\nu)}\right|\left|C_l^{(\nu)}\right|} \sum_{x_i \in C_k^{(\nu)}, x_j \in C_l^{(\nu)}} \tilde{d}\,(x_i, x_j). \tag{5.20}$$

Here, $C_i^{(\upsilon)}$, denotes the ith cluster at the νth iteration step ($i = k, l$). In the single-linkage procedure the distance of two clusters is given by the minimal pairwise distance of the members of the first and second cluster, in the complete linkage the distance of two clusters is given by the maximal pairwise distance of the members of the first and second cluster and in the average-linkage procedure the distance of two clusters is given by the pairwise distance of the arithmetic means of the clusters. In all three procedures those two clusters that minimize the cluster distance over all possible pairs of clusters are merged.

Once two clusters have been merged to a new cluster the distances to all other clusters must be recomputed. This is usually implemented using the following

Table 5.3 Parameters in hierarchical clustering.

Method	α_i ($i=k, l$)	β	γ
Single linkage	0.5	0	−0.5
Complete linkage	0.5	0	0.5
Average linkage	$\dfrac{\lvert C_i^{(v)}\rvert}{\lvert C_k^{(v)}\rvert+\lvert C_l^{(v)}\rvert}$	0	0

recursive formula:

$$d(C_m^{(v-1)}, C_k^{(v)} \cup C_l^{(v)}) = \alpha_k d(C_m^{(v)}, C_k^{(v)}) + \alpha_l d(C_m^{(v)}, C_l^{(v)}) + \beta d(C_k^{(v)}, C_l^{(v)}) + \gamma \left| d(C_m^{(v)}, C_l^{(v)}) - d(C_m^{(v)}, C_k^{(v)}) \right|, \tag{5.21}$$

where the parameters depend on the cluster distance measure. The parameters for the update procedure are summarized in Table 5.3.

The parameter β is zero in these examples, but there exist other update methods (for example, the centroid and the Ward method) that incorporate a positive β.

Hierarchical methods have been applied in the context of clustering gene-expression profiles [51]. They are memory intensive with increasing data size because all pairwise distances must be calculated and stored. Hierarchical methods suffer from the fact that they do not "repair" false joining of data points from previous steps, indeed they follow a determined path for a given rule. Figure 5.6 displays this problem. In a recent study [6], the gene-expression profiles of chromosome 21 mouse orthologues were studied in nine different mouse tissues from a mouse model for trisomy 21 (TS65Dn mouse). Among genes predominantly active in the brain they found *DSCAM*, a cell surface protein acting as an axon guidance receptor. A hierarchical clustering using average linkage as an update rule was performed and the resulting dendrogram is displayed. This cluster is significantly nonrandom, however, several of the profiles numerically close to *DSCAM* are missing (black bars) due to false joining in previous steps.

Another problem with hierarchical clustering methods is that it may be difficult to decide on a representative member for each cluster, especially when using the

Figure 5.6 Practical example of a dendrogram from nine different mouse tissues. For each cDNA the logarithm (base 2) of the ratio between the normalized intensity in the specific tissue and the average of intensities of this cDNA across the nine control tissues was calculated. Ratios are represented with a color gradient spanning from green (under-expressed) to red (overexpressed). Hierarchical clustering was performed with the average-linkage update rule and Pearson correlation as similarity measure (*J*-Express, Molmine, Bergen Norway). Additionally, clones with the most similar expression profiles to *Dscam* (with respect to the Pearson correlation) are displayed: 10%-closest (13 clones, left column), 15%-closest (20 clones, middle column), and 20%-closest (26 clones, right column). Note that in hierarchical clustering procedures, clones with similar expression profiles can be split to different parts of the dendrogram (e.g., *Olig2*), and vice versa (e.g., *Abcg1*).

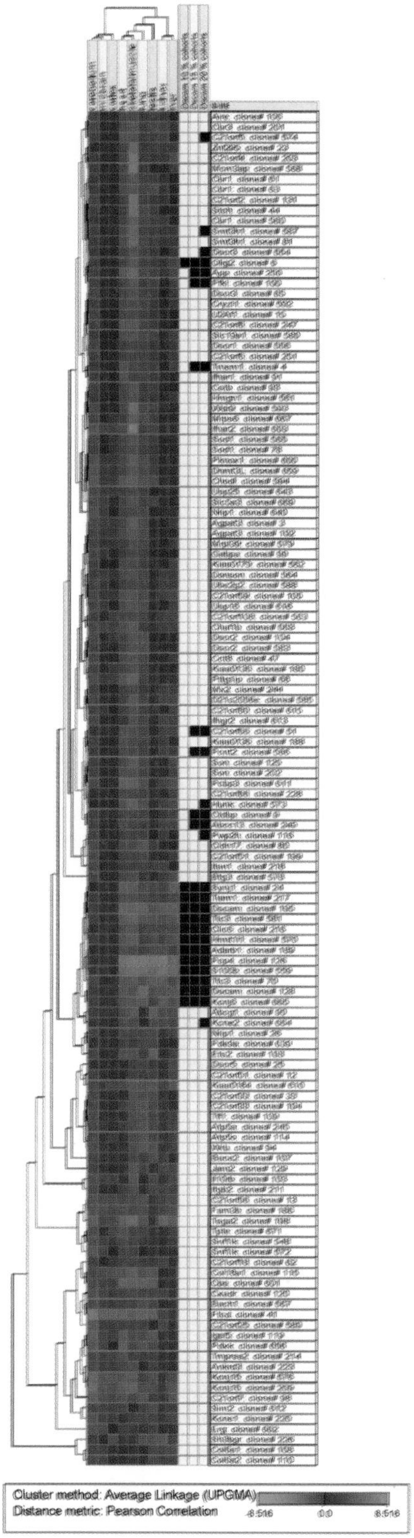
Cluster method: Average Linkage (UPGMA)
Distance metric: Pearson Correlation
-8.516
0.0
8.516

single-linkage algorithm. In contrast when a partitioning algorithm is used, the center of each cluster is a natural representation of the cluster's feature.

5.2.5.2 Self-Organizing Maps (SOMs)

Clustering methods are implicitly used in the construction of self-organizing maps (SOMs), a method in the neural network framework introduced by Kohonen [52]. Kohonen's algorithm tries to find an illustrative display of n-dimensional data points in a given lattice, L, of points, usually in two or three dimensions such that the high dimensional data structure (neighborhoods, topological ordering, and clusters) are preserved and can be detected in this low dimensional structure. The points $r_j \in L$ are called nodes (neurons). Each node r_j has a representation in the n-dimensional space of the data points; this representation is called reference vector, $\boldsymbol{c}_j$, (or weight vector of the neuron). Basically there are two main steps which are repeated for each data vector for a number of iterations, in the order of tens of thousands iterations.

1. Randomly initialize the reference vector $\boldsymbol{c}_j^{(1)}$ for each node
2. For each iteration step $\nu + 1$ do:
   (a) Randomly pick an input data vector $\boldsymbol{x}_{\nu+1}$. Denote by $\boldsymbol{c}_j^{(\nu)}$ the weight vector of the jth node at iteration ν. The matching node is defined by $\boldsymbol{c}_{j_0}^{(\nu)} \in \operatorname{argmin}\{d_2(\boldsymbol{x}_{\nu+1}, \boldsymbol{c}_j^{(\nu)}); j\}$, where d_2 is defined in (5.16)
   (b) Update the reference vector of the matching node and its neighbors by the update formula $\boldsymbol{c}_j^{(\nu+1)} = \boldsymbol{c}_j^{(\nu)} + \eta^{(\nu)} h_{j_0 j}^{(\nu)} (\boldsymbol{x}_{\nu+1} - \boldsymbol{c}_j^{(\nu)})$.
3. Assign each data vector to the cluster with the most similar reference vector.

$0 < \eta^{(\upsilon)} < 1$, the so-called learning function, monotonically decreases with the number of iterations; $0 < h_{j_0 j}^{(\upsilon)} < 1$ is called the neighborhood function, which decreases monotonically with the distance between two nodes.

The main task of the neighborhood function is to provide learning, i.e., updating of the weights, not only for the best matching node, but also for its neighbors. The task of the learning function is to shrink in time as iterations increase.

The result of Kohonen's algorithm is that nodes that are spatially close tend to develop similar weight vectors. Of course, the rate at which the neighborhood shrinks is critical. If the neighborhood is large and it shrinks slowly, the cluster centers will tend to stick close to the overall mean of all of the samples.

Commonly used neighborhood functions are $h_{j_0 j}^{(\upsilon)} = e^{-\frac{d_2(r_{j0}, r_j)^2}{2\sigma^2(\upsilon)}}$ and $h_{j_0 j}^{(\upsilon)} = \begin{cases} 1, d_2(r_{j_0}, r_j) < \sigma(\upsilon) \\ 1, d_2(r_{j_0}, r_j) \geq \sigma(\upsilon) \end{cases}$, where r_{j_0} is the matching node, r_j is the adapted node whose reference vector is updated and $\sigma^2(\upsilon)$ is the neighborhood radius, which is decreasing with the number of iterations. Self-organizing maps have been used in the context of clustering gene-expression profiles in [53, 54].

5.2.5.3 K-Means

K-means algorithms are a fast and large-scale applicable clustering method. The main idea behind these techniques is the optimization of an objective function, which is usually a function of the deviations between all patterns of the data points from their respective cluster centers. The most commonly used optimization is the minimization of the within-cluster sum of squared Euclidean distances utilizing an iterative scheme, which starts with a random initialization of the cluster centers, then alters the clustering of the data to obtain a better value of the objective function.

K-means algorithms alternate between two steps until a stopping criterion is satisfied. These steps are a pairwise distance measure of the data vectors and the cluster centers related to the optimization criterion and an update procedure for the cluster centers.

Euclidean distance has been used in most cases as the pairwise similarity measure because of its computational simplicity. The cluster center at each iteration can be calculated in a straightforward manner by the arithmetic mean of the data vectors currently assigned to the cluster, which is known to minimize the within-cluster sum of squared Euclidean distances.

The original *K*-means algorithm reads:

1. Start with an initial partition of the data points in K clusters with cluster centers $c_1^{(1)}, \ldots, c_K^{(1)}$ and let $W^{(1)}$ be the value of the initial objective function.
2. At the νth step of the iteration, assign each data point to the cluster with the lowest pairwise distance.
3. Recompute the cluster centers $c_1^{(\nu+1)}, \ldots, c_K^{(\nu+1)}$ by minimizing $W^{(\nu+1)}$.
4. If for all K, $|c_k^{(\nu)} - c_k^{(\nu+1)}| < \varepsilon$ stop; else go to step 2.
5. Assign each data vector to the nearest cluster center. (5.22)

If the Euclidean distance is used as the distance measure, the algorithm minimizes the within-cluster sum of squares of the K clusters. In this case, the cluster centers are recomputed in every iteration as the arithmetic means of the respective data points. Other pairwise distance measures are the l_1-metric (*K*-median clustering) and the l_∞-metric (*K*-midranges clustering). A common criticism on *K*-means algorithms concerns the fact that the number of centers has to be fixed from beginning of the procedure. Furthermore, the results are highly dependent on the initialized set of centers. Alternative algorithms have been published that do not require to determine the number of clusters in advance and thus overcome this criticism [55].

A simple approach of refining the *K*-means algorithm employs two thresholding parameters (*sequential K-means*). The original idea dates back to MacQueen [56]. A parameter ρ controlling the distance within the clusters is used to define new cluster centers and a parameter σ controlling the distance between cluster centers is used to merge cluster centers. The algorithm reads as follows:

1. Initialize K cluster centers $c_1^{(1)}, \ldots, c_K^{(1)}$.
2. Select a new data point x_i at the $\nu + 1$th step.
3. Compute the distances to all cluster centers from the previous step $c_1^{(\nu)}, \ldots, c_K^{(\nu)}$. Let $w_1^{(\nu)}, \ldots, w_K^{(\nu)}$ be the weights of the clusters in that step, i.e., the number of data points already assigned to the cluster centers.

   If $\min\{d(c_j^{(\nu)}, x_i); j = 1, \ldots, K\} < \rho$ then

(a) Assign $\boldsymbol{x}_i$ to the cluster center with the minimal distance, $\boldsymbol{c}_{j_0}^{(\nu)}$ and update the centroid and its weight by $w_{j_0}^{(\nu+1)} = w_{j_0}^{(\nu)} + 1$ and $\boldsymbol{c}_{j_0}^{(\nu+1)} = \frac{w_{j_0}^{(\nu)} \boldsymbol{c}_{j_0}^{(\nu)} + \boldsymbol{x}_i}{w_{j_0}^{(\nu+1)}}$.

(b) Compute the distance of the updated center to each of the other cluster centers. If $\min\{d(\boldsymbol{c}_j^{(\nu)}, \boldsymbol{c}_{j_0}^{(\nu+1)}); j = 1, \ldots, K\} < \sigma$, merge the center with the minimal distance and update the centroid and the weight again according to a. Repeat this step until for all centers, the condition $d(\boldsymbol{c}_j^{(\nu)}, \boldsymbol{c}_{j_0}^{(\nu+1)}) \geq \sigma$ is satisfied.

If $\min\{d(\boldsymbol{c}_j^{(\nu)}, \boldsymbol{x}_i); j = 1, \ldots, K\} \geq \rho$, initialize a new cluster center by $\boldsymbol{c}_{K+1}^{(\nu+1)} = \boldsymbol{x}_i$ and $w_{K+1}^{(\nu+1)} = 1$.

4. Reclassify the data points.

The above algorithm iteratively allows to join clusters that are similar to each other and to introduce new cluster centers in each step of the iteration and is thus a very flexible alternative. It should be pointed out that *K*-means algorithms are not very stable in their solutions, i.e., running the same algorithm with different parameters will lead to different results. Thus, this algorithm should be applied not just one time on the data set but rather several times with several initializations of cluster centers. In a postprocessing step the stable clusters can then be retrieved.

5.2.6 Cluster Validation

Many clustering algorithms are currently available each of which claims special merits and has some interpretation that makes it suitable for a class of applications. However, it is important to compare the output of cluster algorithms in order to decide which one gives best results for the current problem. For that purpose *cluster validation measures* are used. In principle, two groups of measures can be separated, external and internal measures. *External validation measures* incorporate *a priori* knowledge on the clustering structure of the data, for example in simulation experiments when the true partition of the data is known, or in real experiments when specific gene clusters are known. Typically, an external cluster validation measure is a numerical function that evaluates two different groupings of the same data set. This is done by the following scheme:

Assume that we have n p-dimensional data vectors $\boldsymbol{x}_1, \ldots, \boldsymbol{x}_n$ and that a clustering result generates a partition of this data set in disjoint subsets. This is implicitly done with partitioning algorithms, whereas with hierarchical algorithms the dendrogram has to be cut in a suitable postprocessing step. Each partition can be represented by a binary $n \times n$-partitioning matrix, $\boldsymbol{C} = (c_{ij})$, with

$$c_{ij} = \begin{cases} 0, & \text{if data vectors } \boldsymbol{i} \text{ and } \boldsymbol{j} \text{ are not in the same cluster} \\ 1, & \text{if data vectors } \boldsymbol{i} \text{ and } \boldsymbol{j} \text{ are not in the same cluster} \end{cases}$$

Let $\boldsymbol{C}$ and $\boldsymbol{T}$ be two partitioning matrices computed from two different clustering algorithms, then most external indices are defined as numerical functions on the 2×2 contingency table (Table 5.4).

Table 5.4 Contingency table for judging clustering quality.

C/T	0	1	Total
0	n_{00}	n_{01}	$n_{0.}$
1	n_{10}	n_{11}	$n_{1.}$
Total	$n_{.0}$	$n_{.1}$	n^2

Here, n_{11} denotes the number of pairs that are in a common cluster in both partitions, $n_{1.}$ and $n_{.1}$ are the marginals of the partition matrices $T$and C, respectively. Likewise, the other cell entries are defined. A commonly used index is, for example, the *Jaccard coefficient*

$$J(T, C) = \frac{n_{11}}{n_{11} + n_{01} + n_{10}} \tag{5.23}$$

that measures the data pairs clustered together proportionally to the marginals. Other examples are Hubert's Γ statistic, the goodness-of-fit statistic or measures based on information theory [50].

Internal validation measures compare the quality of the calculated clusters solely by the data itself. Indices of quality are topological concepts, for example compactness or isolation, that are computed by numerical functions, information theoretic concepts that quantify, for example, highly informative clusters and variance concepts that quantify the overall variance explained by the cluster. A widely used topological measure is the *Silhouette index* [57]. Consider a clustering of n data vectors that results in Kclusters, $S_1, \ldots, S_K$. For each data vector, $\boldsymbol{x}_i$, we can calculate two topological values. Let S_l be the cluster that is assigned to $\boldsymbol{x}_i$, then the *compactness* value describes the average distance of $\boldsymbol{x}_i$ to all other data points in the same cluster, i.e.,

$$a_i = \frac{1}{|S_l|-1} \sum_{\boldsymbol{x}_k \in S_l, k \neq i} d(\boldsymbol{x}_i, \boldsymbol{x}_k), \tag{5.24}$$

where d is a suitable distance measure. The *isolation* value describes the minimal average distance to all other clusters, i.e.,

$$b_i = \min\left\{ \frac{1}{|S_j|} \sum_{\boldsymbol{x}_k \in S_l} d(\boldsymbol{x}_i, \boldsymbol{x}_k); j = 1, \ldots, K, j \neq l \right\}. \tag{5.25}$$

The compactness (isolation) of a cluster is defined as the average compactness- (isolation-) values of its cluster members. Apparently, clusters of high quality are compact and isolated. The Silhouette index for a data point combines compactness and isolation by

$$SI(\boldsymbol{x}_i) = \frac{b_i - a_i}{\max\{a_i, b_i\}}. \tag{5.26}$$

The value of the Silhouette Index is bound to the interval $[-1, 1]$. Negative values indicate that this data vector should belong to a different cluster rather than the computed one. Figure 5.7 shows a visualization of the above measures.

Cluster validation is an important topic that has drawn insufficient attention in gene-expression analysis. Currently, the situation is somewhat troublesome for the user of clustering software packages. On the one hand there is the choice between a multitude of sophisticated algorithms, multiple algorithmic parameters, and visualization tools. However, each of these methods will generate a different result contributing to the confusion and frustration of the user and there are too few tools that validate and compare results and select the best one. Thus, future research will focus on the comparison and integration of different methods in order to reduce the bias of the individual methods.

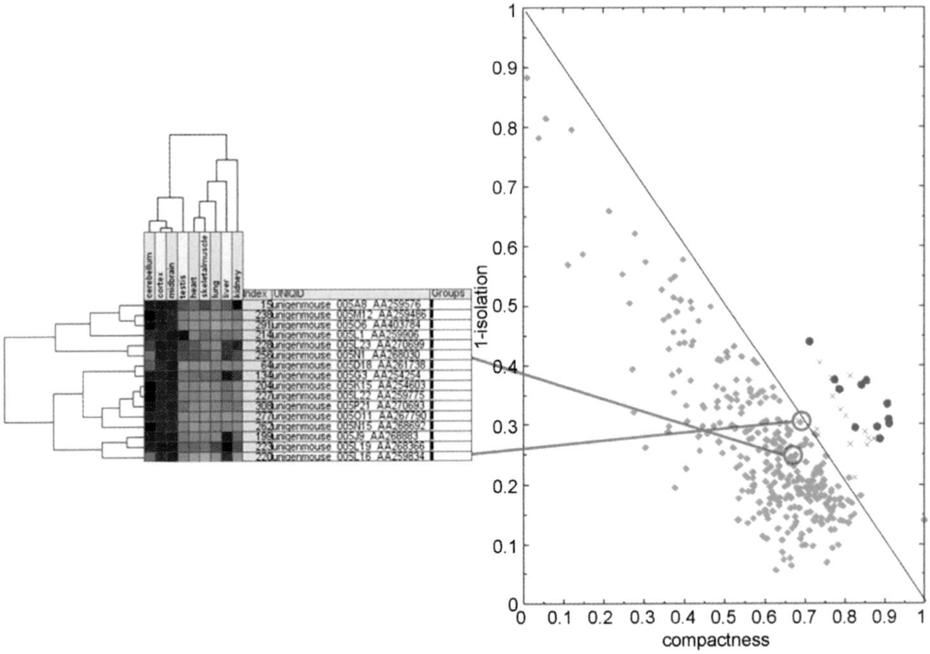

Figure 5.7 Visualization of cluster quality. Left: cluster of cDNA sequences that have a tissue-specific expression in brain tissue. In this study nine different tissues have been compared in the mouse using a whole-genome approach. Genes in that specific cluster show a high expression in three brain regions (cortex, cerebellum, and midbrain). Right: Compactness (*X*-axis) and isolation (*Y*-axis) can be used to visualize the cluster quality in a two-dimensional plot. Crosses represent the brain-specific cDNAs and circles represent another cluster of liver-specific sequences. Green diamonds represent random assignments of compactness and isolation. The visualization allows the identification of false positives in each cluster which can enhance following analyses, for example with respect of promoter searches.

5.2.7
Overrepresentation and Enrichment Analyses

Essentially, case-control studies (Section 5.2.2) and multicase studies (Section 5.2.6) result in lists of genes that are significant for the study under analysis and functional categorization of these lists of genes is a fundamental issue. Adding functional attributes to the selected genes gives a first impression of the molecular interactions that are involved in the problem. Since more and more functional annotations are available for genes, for example through the GeneOntology Consortium [58] or through many different pathway databases, these annotations are used to validate clustering results.

Measuring the statistical significance of functional categorization is essentially based on a simple statistical method. Consider a cluster of n genes out of which k genes belong to a certain functional class and $n-k$ belong to other classes. Let N be the total number of genes under analysis and K be the total number of genes annotated for that class. Is the observed number untypical or does it rather express a random distribution of the specific functional class? This problem can be translated into an urn model. If the n genes were randomly drawn from the total of N genes then the probability of having exactly k out of K genes from the functional class would be given by the *hypergeometric distribution*

$$P(k) = \frac{\binom{K}{k}\binom{n-K}{m-K}}{\binom{n}{m}}. \tag{5.27}$$

The P-value for the cluster can then be calculated as the probability of having more than the observed number of hits of that functional group using (5.27), i.e.,

$$p = \sum_{j \geq k} P(j). \tag{5.28}$$

Example 5.3

In a recent work a core set of 213 marker genes with respect to type-2 diabetes mellitus has been identified with a meta-analysis across different microarray resources [59]. Enrichment analyses based on the hypergeometric distribution were carried out in order to assess whether certain biochemical pathways were overrepresented in the functional annotations of the candidate list (Table 5.5).

The results show that the fundamental pathways associated with type-2 diabetes mellitus (annotated in the KEGG database) are significantly enriched by the selected marker sets such as PPAR signaling and Insulin signaling. These kinds of overrepresentation analyses are often used to judge a specific selection of marker genes or – vice versa – to identify new pathways potentially relevant for the disease under study.

Table 5.5 Overrepresentation analysis.[a]

Pathway ID	SigSet	Set	Sig	All	*P*-value	*Q*-value	Pathway description
path:mmu03320	13	69	213	15274	1.02E − 11	1.37E − 09	PPAR signaling pathway
path:mmu04920	12	73	213	15274	3.46E − 10	1.66E − 08	Adipocytokine signaling pathway
path:mmu04930	10	44	213	15274	3.69E − 10	1.66E − 08	Type-2 diabetes mellitus
path:mmu04910	13	128	213	15274	2.70E − 08	9.09E − 07	Insulin signaling pathway
path:mmu04612	6	38	213	15274	1.30E − 05	0.000351	Antigen processing and presentation
path:mmu00280	6	44	213	15274	3.11E − 05	0.000697	Valine, leucine and isoleucine deg.
path:mmu04610	7	67	213	15274	3.98E − 05	0.000764	Complement and coagulation casc.

[a]All are the genes under consideration, Sig the number of candidate genes, Set is the number of genes in the pathway under study, and SigSet the overlap of genes in the pathway and the candidate genes. *P*-values were computed with the upper tail of the hypergeometric distribution indicating the probability of observing this overlap by chance. *Q*-values are the *P*-values corrected for multiple testing.

Overrepresentation analysis described in Eq. (5.27) does not take into account the specific fold-changes of a gene in the experiments so that each gene in the list is weighted equally. In contrast, gene-enrichment analysis weights the genes according to the experimental observations (fold-change, expression differences, etc.). A simple approach is, for example, a weighting of the gene according to its fold-change and significance *P*-value (cf. Section 5.2.2). Let p_i be the *P*-value and r_i be the ratio of the gene in a case-control study, then the quantity

$$|\log_{10}(p_i)||\log_2(r_i)| \tag{5.29}$$

is an indicator for the influence of the gene in the study. These scores can be used for gene-enrichment analysis in order to assess the importance of entire pathways for the study. An example is shown in Figure 5.8.

Gene-enrichment scores have been proposed in order to extrapolate differential analysis of genes to the differential analysis of entire pathways. A statistical argument based on a nonparametric, robust hypothesis test has been proposed in [42]. Here, array data were used to test whether specific pathways showed differential expression in human blastocyst differentiation. Pathways were taken from the KEGG database. Consider for each pathway i, the set of related genes $(x_{i1}, y_{i1}), \ldots, (x_{in_i}, y_{in_i})$. Here, x_{ij}, y_{ij} denote the expression level of the jth gene in two different samples (case control). Wilcoxon's matched pairs signed rank test was used to calculate a Z-score for the differences $d_{ij} = x_{ij} - y_{ij}$ for each pathway i. These differences were ranked, and the ranks of differences with negative signs, R_{neg}, and those with positive signs, R_{pos}, were summed. The test statistic is the smaller of the two numbers,

$$R = \min\{R_{\text{pos}}, R_{\text{neg}}\}. \tag{5.30}$$

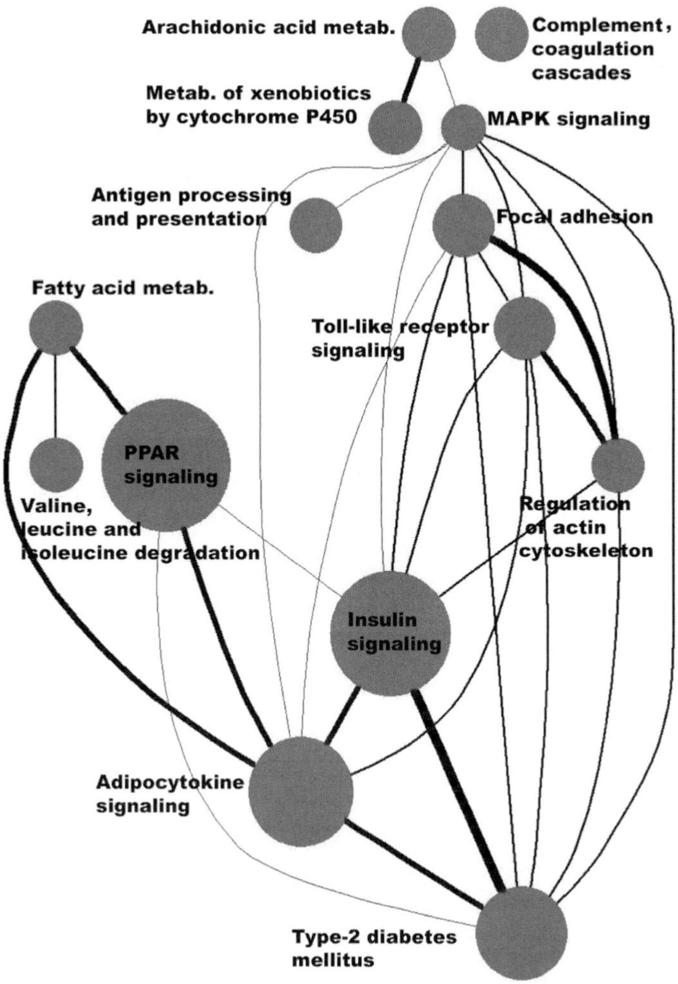

Figure 5.8 Pathway crosstalk with respect to the type-2 diabetes mellitus candidate gene set (identified by -[59]). Pathways were derived from the KEGG database. Each pathway has been weighted according to the total disease score reflected by the size of the nodes. Only pathways with a total score > 20 were selected for display. The thickness of the edges between different pathway nodes reflects the overlap score derived from the sum of the scores of the overlapping genes. The graph was generated with the graphviz package (www.graphviz.org).

If the pathway is not affected by the treatments R_{neg} and R_{pos} will be fairly equal, but, if there is a trend of under- or overexpression, the test statistic will be small. The Z-score is defined as

$$z = \frac{|R - E(R)|}{\sqrt{\mathrm{Var}(R)}}, \tag{5.31}$$

where E is the expectation and Var is the variance of R. These were calculated as

$$E(R) = \frac{n_i(n_i+1)}{4} \tag{5.32}$$

and

$$\mathrm{Var}(R) = \frac{n_i(n_i+1)(2n_i+1)}{24}, \tag{5.33}$$

respectively.

5.2.8 Classification Methods

An important medical application of microarray analysis is the diagnosis of diseases and subtypes of a disease, for example cancer. Normal cells can evolve into malignant cancer cells by mutations of genes that control cell cycle, apoptosis, and other processes [60]. To determine the exact cancer type and stage is essential for the correct medical treatment of the patient. The task of sample diagnostics cannot be treated by the methods discussed so far. This task requires a complementary set of mathematical algorithms for gene expression, namely classification procedures. Recall that the purpose of clustering is to partition genes (and possibly conditions) into coexpression groups by a suitable optimization method based on the expression matrix. The purpose of classification is to assign a given condition (for example, a patient's expression profile across a set of genes) to preexisting classes of conditions (for example, groups of patient samples from known disease stages). The clustering methods discussed so far do not utilize any supporting tissue annotation (e.g., tumor vs. normal). This information is only used to assess the performance of the method. Such methods are often referred to as *unsupervised*. In contrast, *supervised* methods, attempt to predict the classification of new tissues based on their gene expression profiles after training on examples that have been classified by an external "supervisor."

The practical problems underlying the classification of patients to disease subtypes are:

1. new/unknown disease classes have to be identified;
2. marker genes have to be found that separate the disease classes;
3. patients have to be classified by assigning them to one of the classes.

The general classification problem can be stated as follows: Let T be a set of n training samples consisting of pairs $(\boldsymbol{x}_i, z_i)$, $T = \{(\boldsymbol{x}_1, z_1), \ldots, (\boldsymbol{x}_n, z_n)\}$, where $\boldsymbol{x}_i$ is a p-dimensional vector and $z_i \in \{-1, 1\}$ is a binary label (class label). Each vector consists of the expression profile of the patient sample across the p marker genes and each label assigns this vector to one the classes. Given a new query vector, $\boldsymbol{x} \in \Re_p$, the classification method (*classifier*) has to predict the group label, z, of $\boldsymbol{x}$ given the training set. Thus, each classification method can be interpreted as a function $F : \Re_p \times T \rightarrow \{-1, 1\}$.

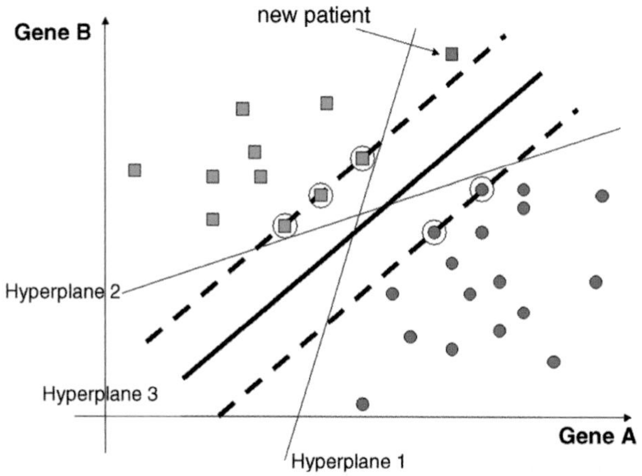

Figure 5.9 Support vector machines. Two classes of patient data with are separated by the plane that is spanned by the expression levels according to two genes. Hyperplanes 1 and 2 yield two perfect linear separations of the groups; however, when classifying a new patient they disagree in the classification. Hyperplane 1 assigns the patinet to group 1 (circles) whereas hyperplane 2 assigns the patient to group 2 (squares) due to the fact that both hyperplanes are geometrically too close to each of the subsets. The support vector machine classifier tries to maximize the margin between the two groups by defining support vectors (circled data points) and a hyperplane that maximizes the minimum distances to these support vectors (hyperplane 3).

5.2.8.1 Support Vector Machines

Support vector machines (SVMs) are the most widely used group of methods for classification [61]. Different studies have been published using SVMs in recent years, in particular for cancer diagnostics [62, 63].

The basic underlying principle of support vector machines is a linear decision rule. Consider two different groups of vectors in $\Re_p$. We want to find a hyperplane that separates these two samples by making the least possible error. Even if perfect separation is possible, the usual problem is that there are many such separating hyperplanes so that we have to define some kind of optimization criterion. Figure 5.9 illustrates the problem with the simple case of a two-dimensional space spanned by the expression levels of the patients according to two marker genes (A and B). Hyperplanes 1 and 2 are both separating the two samples perfectly. However, given a new patient profile (red square) both methods would lead to different classification results. The problem here is that both hyperplanes are geometrically too close to one of the samples and thus risk misassignment of a future datum.

The idea behind SVMs is to select a hyperplane that is more likely to generalize on future data. This is achieved by finding a hyperplane that maximizes the minimum distances of the closest points and thus to maximize the width of the margin between the two classes. The hyperplane is specified by the boundary training vectors (*support vectors*).

Recall the classification problem from the previous section. A hyperplane can be described by $H(\boldsymbol{w}, b) = \{\boldsymbol{x}; \boldsymbol{wx} + b = 0\}$, with a vector $\boldsymbol{w} \in \Re_p$ that determines the orientation of the hyperplane and a scalar b that determines the offset of the hyperplane from the origin. Here, $\boldsymbol{wx}$ denotes the inner- or dot-product of the two vectors. A hyperplane in two dimensions is given by a straight line (Figure 9.9) and in three dimensions by a plane. We say that a hyperplane supports a class if all points in that class fall on one side. Thus, we would like to find a pair $\boldsymbol{w}$, b so that $\boldsymbol{wx}_i + b \geq 1$ for the points with class label $z_i = 1$ and $\boldsymbol{wx}_i + b \leq 1$ for the points with class label $z_i = -1$. To compute the hyperplane with the largest margin, we search two supporting hyperplanes for the two classes. The support planes are pushed apart until they hit into a specified proportion of the data vectors from each class (the support vectors marked with a circle in Figure 5.9). Thus, the solution depends only on these support vectors. The distance between the supporting hyperplanes $\boldsymbol{wx} + b = 1$ and $\boldsymbol{wx} + b = -1$ is equal to $\frac{2}{||\boldsymbol{w}||}$, where $||\cdot||$ denotes the Euclidean norm. Thus, maximizing the margin is equivalent of the following problem:

$$\begin{aligned}&\text{Minimize } ||\boldsymbol{w}||^2 \text{ and } b\\&\text{subject to } z_i(\boldsymbol{x}_i\boldsymbol{w} + b) \geq 1 \text{ for } i = 1, \ldots, n.\end{aligned} \tag{5.34}$$

This problem can be represented by the Langrangian dual problem

$$\begin{aligned}&\text{Minimize } \alpha \text{ values } \frac{1}{2}\sum_{i,j} z_i z_j \alpha_i \alpha_j \boldsymbol{x}_i \boldsymbol{x}_j - \sum_i \alpha_i\\&\text{subject to } \sum_i z_i \alpha_i = 0 \text{ and } \alpha_i \geq 0.\end{aligned} \tag{5.35}$$

Both problems lead to the same solution, i.e., a hyperplane with the property that $\boldsymbol{w} = \sum_i z_i \alpha_i \boldsymbol{x}_i$. The classification rule found by the algorithm then reads for any new datum

$$F_T(\boldsymbol{x}) = \text{sign}\left(\sum_i z_i \alpha_i \boldsymbol{x}_i \boldsymbol{x} + b\right). \tag{5.36}$$

It should be noted that this classification rule depends only on the support vectors since the dual problem assigns values $\alpha_i = 0$ to all other data vectors.

In practice, it may occur that in the original dimension, p, no linear separation can be performed on the training data. SVMs then map the data to a higher dimensional space where a linear separation is possible, using a map $\Phi: \Re_p \to \Re_m$, $m > p$. Since the optimization problem involves only inner products of the vectors an optimal separating hyperplane in the projected space can be found by solving the problem for the inner products $\Phi(\boldsymbol{x}_i)\Phi(\boldsymbol{x}_j)$. Fortunately, (due to Mercer's theorem which is beyond the scope of this book) it is known that for certain mappings and any two vectors the inner product in the projected dimension can be calculated using a *kernel function* $K: \Re_p \times \Re_p \to \Re$ such that

$$K(\boldsymbol{x}_i, \boldsymbol{x}) = \Phi(\boldsymbol{x}_i)\Phi(\boldsymbol{x}_j). \tag{5.37}$$

Two kernels are widely used

- Linear kernel: $K(\boldsymbol{x}_i, \boldsymbol{x}_j) = \boldsymbol{x}_i \boldsymbol{x}_j$
- Polynomial kernel: $K(\boldsymbol{x}_i, \boldsymbol{x}_j) = (\gamma \boldsymbol{x}_i \boldsymbol{x}_j + \varepsilon)^d$.

In practice, misclassifications will occur. To avoid this, one may modify the algorithm and introduce an error parameter, C, in the optimization problem (5.35) and the dual problem (5.35). This error parameter represents the trade-off between the training set misclassification error and the size of the margin. The optimization problem involving the kernel and this parameter reads

$$\begin{aligned} &\text{Minimize } \alpha \text{ values} \quad \frac{1}{2}\sum_{i,j} z_i z_j \alpha_i \alpha_j K(x_i, x_j) - \sum_i \alpha_i \\ &\text{subject to} \quad \sum_i z_i \alpha_i = 0 \text{ and } C \geq \alpha_i \geq 0 \end{aligned} \tag{5.38}$$

and the classification is based on

$$F_T(x) = \text{sign}\left(\sum_i z_i \alpha_i K(x_i, x) + b\right) \tag{5.39}$$

Further information on SVMs can be found in [64]. SVMs seem to be the method of choice for classifying samples according to gene-expression profiles. They have proven to outperform other procedures, in particular, in cancer diagnosis in several independent studies [62, 63].

5.2.8.2 Other Approaches

A very simple classification approach is the *k-nearest neighbor* classification method [65]. Consider a training data set of n pairs (x_i, z_i), $i = 1, \ldots, n$, of p-dimensional expression profiles and group labels. If a query, x, is to be classified, then it is likely that the group label of x equals the group label of the most similar training datum. Thus, the classification rule is given by

$$\begin{aligned} &F_T(x) = z_{i_0}, \text{ where} \\ &i_0 \in \arg\max\{S(x, x_i); x_i \in T\}. \end{aligned} \tag{5.40}$$

S is a suitable similarity function between the expression profiles, for example the Pearson correlation coefficient. Taking into account the high error rates in microarray experiments it is not reasonable to base the classification on just the nearest neighbor of the query in the training set but rather on the k-nearest neighbors. Thus, the result of the classification of the query is defined as the majority vote of these k data vectors. Further refinements are performed by weighting the group labels of the data vectors according to their similarity to the query vector x. K-nearest neighbor methods yield good results in many classification procedures and can be used as a benchmark for more sophisticated algorithms.

Classification can also be combined with clustering methods using *clustering-based classification* [66]. If we consider the n training samples (tumor subtypes, cell lines, etc.) as expression vectors whose coordinates are the expression levels of some genes, i.e., essentially transposing the expression matrix discussed in Section 5.2.5, then we can perform a clustering of the training sample in two or more clusters. This yields groups of samples that are similar to each other based on the selected set of genes. Clustering-based classification method simply cluster the query sample together with the training samples and assign the label of the highest confidence calculated from all training labels in the same cluster to the query.

A third group of algorithms is based on *boosting* [67]. The idea of boosting is to construct a good classifier by repeated calls of weak classifiers. An example for a Boosting algorithm is the AdaBoost algorithm by Freund and Shapire.

Exercises and Problems

1. Robust statistical testing:

   Let, $x_1, \ldots, x_n$ and $y_1, \ldots, y_m$ be two independent samples of observations. Wilcoxon's rank test is a robust alternative to Gaussian-based tests. The test statistic T is based on the ranks of the first sample across the combined samples, i.e., $T(x_1, \ldots, x_n, y_1, \ldots, y_m) = \sum_{i=1}^{n} R(x_i)$, where $R(x_i)$ is the rank of x_i in the combined sample of observations.

   Write a computer program that computes the exact P-values for this test. *Hint:* Implement a recursive algorithm. Let $w(z, n, m)$ be the number of possible rank orderings that result in a value of T equal to z. This number is a sum of the number of possible rank orderings of T containing the highest rank, $m + n$, and those that do not, which can be described as

   $$w(z, n, m) = w(z-(m+n), n-1, m) + w(z, n, m-1).$$

   The P-value can be derived by counting all combinations of rank orderings that yield a more extreme value of T divided by the total number of possible rank orderings.

2. Comparison of tests:

   Expression of a specific gene was measured in two different patient groups yielding the following series of observations:

Group 1:	2434	2289	5599	2518	1123	1768	2304	2509	14820	2489	1349	1494
Group 2:	3107	3365	4704	3667	2414	4268	3600	3084	3997	3673	2281	3166

   Compute the significance of the group differences with the Student's t-test and Wilcoxon's rank sum test. Why is the gene significantly changed (at the 0.05 level) according to the rank test but not according to the t-test? What result is more reliable? What can be done in order to robustify Student's t-test?

3. Distance metrics:

   In Section 5.2.5, we discuss the *Minkowsky-* or *l^q-distances* defined by

   $$d_q(\mathbf{x}_n, \mathbf{x}_m) = \left(\sum_{i=1}^{p} |x_{ni} - x_{mi}|^q \right)^{\frac{1}{q}},$$

   where $\mathbf{x}_n$, $\mathbf{x}_m$ are two p-dimensional data vectors. Show that the inequality holds

   $$\frac{1}{\sqrt{p}} d_1(\mathbf{x}_n, \mathbf{x}_m) \le d_2(\mathbf{x}_n, \mathbf{x}_m) \le \sqrt{p} \cdot d_1(\mathbf{x}_n, \mathbf{x}_m).$$

Hint: Show that for each finite series $z_1, \ldots, z_p$ of real values the inequality holds

$$\frac{1}{\sqrt{p}}\sum_{i=1}^{p}|a_i| \leq \left(\sum_{i=1}^{p} a_i^2\right)^{\frac{1}{2}} \leq \sqrt{p}\cdot\max(|a_1|,\ldots,|a_p|).$$

This can be deduced from the *Cauchy–Schwartz-inequality*:

$$\sum_{i=1}^{p}|a_i b_i| \leq \left(\sum_{i=1}^{p} a_i^2\right)^{\frac{1}{2}}\left(\sum_{i=1}^{p} b_i^2\right)^{\frac{1}{2}} \tag{5.41}$$

for any two series of real values.

4. Clustering (practical exercise):

   The Gene Expression Omnibus (http://www.ncbi.nlm.nih.gov/geo/) contains a large collection of publicly available expression data. Search for expression data generated on the NCI-60 panel of cancer cell lines [68]. Download the preprocessed and normalized data and perform hierarchical clustering. Use different metrics and observe changes in cluster composition. Identify groups of genes that are specific for certain cancer types. Identify the most variable and the most constant expression patterns in the data set.

5. Urn models:

   In Section 5.2.7, we have introduced the hypergeometric distribution in the context of overrepresentation analyses. This, and many other practical problems, can be described with so-called *urn models*. Consider an urn containing N balls out of which K are red and N–K are black. The experiment consists of n draws from that urn. If the ball is replaced in the urn after each draw we call the experiment *drawing with replacement* otherwise *drawing without replacement*. Of practical interest is the calculation of the probability of having exactly k red balls among the n balls drawn. This is given by $p(k) = \binom{n}{k} p^k (1-p)^{n-k}$ (Binomial distribution), $p = \frac{K}{N}$, if we draw with replacement, i.e., each ball is placed back in the urn after drawing, and $p(k) = \frac{\binom{K}{k}\binom{N-K}{n-k}}{\binom{N}{n}}$ (Hypergeometric distribution), if we draw without replacement.

(a) Compute the expectations and variances of both distributions. What differences do you observe between drawing with replacement and drawing without replacement?

(b) Limit theorem for the hypergeometric distribution: Let $q_k = \frac{\binom{K}{k}\binom{N-K}{n-k}}{\binom{N}{n}}$ and show that, for large N, the hypergeometric distribution can be approximated by the binomial distribution by proving

$$\binom{n}{k}\left(p-\frac{k}{N}\right)^k\left((1-p)-\frac{n-k}{N}\right)^{n-k} \leq q_k \leq \binom{n}{k}p^k(1-p)^{n-k}\left(1-\frac{n}{N}\right)^{-n}.$$

What can you deduce from this calculation?

References

1 Poustka, A. *et al.* (1986) Molecular approaches to mammalian genetics, *Cold Spring Harbor Symposia on Quantum Biology*, Cold Spring Harbor, New York, pp. 131–139.

2 Lehrach, H. *et al.* (1990) Hybridization fingerprinting in genome mapping and sequencing, in *Genome Analysis*, (ed. K.E.Da.S. Tilghman), Cold Spring Harbor, New York, pp. 39–81.

3 Lennon, G. and Lehrach, H. (1991) Hybridization analyses of arrayed cDNA libraries. *Trends in Genetics*, **7**, 314–317.

4 Gress, T. *et al.* (1992) Hybridization fingerprinting of high-density cDNA library arrays with cDNA pools derived from whole tissues. *Mammalian Genome*, **3**, 609–619.

5 Granjeaud, S. *et al.* (1996) From hybridisation image to numerical values: a practical high-throughput quantification system for high density filter hybridisations. *Genetic Analysis: Biomolecular Engineering*, **12**, 151–162.

6 Kahlem, P. *et al.* (2004) Transcript level alterations reflect gene dosage effects across multiple tissues in a mouse model of down syndrome. *Genome Research*, **14**, 1258–1267.

7 Schena, M. *et al.* (1995) Quantitative monitoring of gene expression patterns with a complementary DNA microarray. *Science*, **270**, 467–470.

8 DeRisi, J. *et al.* (1996) Use of cDNA microarray to analyse gene expression patterns in human cancer. *Nature Genetics*, **14**, 457–460.

9 Spellman, P. *et al.* (1998) Comprehensive identification of cell cycle-regulated genes of the yeast *Saccharomyces cerevisiae* by microarray hybridisation. *Molecular Biology of the Cell*, **9**, 3273–3297.

10 Whitfield, M.L. *et al.* (2002) Identification of genes periodically expressed in the human cell cycle and their expression in tumors. *Molecular Biology of the Cell*, **13**, 1977–2000.

11 Lockhart, D.J. *et al.* (1996) Expression monitoring by hybridizaion to high-density oligonucleotide arrays. *Nature Biotechnology*, **14**, 1675–1680.

12 Wodicka, L. *et al.* (1997) Genome-wide expression monitoring in Saccharomyces cerevisiae. *Nature Biotechnology*, **15**, 1359–1367.

13 Gunderson, K.L. *et al.* (2004) Decoding randomly ordered DNA arrays. *Genome Research*, **14**, 870–877.

14 Kuhn, K. *et al.* (2004) A novel, high-performance random array platform for quantitative gene expression profiling. *Genome Research*, **14**, 2347–2356.

15 Hughes, T. *et al.* (2000) Functional discovery via a compendium of expression profiles. *Cell*, **102**, 109–126.

16 Hughes, T. *et al.* (2001) Expression profiling using microarrays fabricated by an ink-jet oligonucleotide synthesizer. *Nature Biotechnology*, **19**, 342–347.

17 Hardiman, G. (2004) Microarray platforms – comparisons and contrasts. *Pharmacogenomics*, **5**, 487–502.

18 Kuo, W.P. *et al.* (2002) Analysis of matched mRNA measurements from two different microarray technologies. *Bioinformatics (Oxford, England)*, **18**, 405–412.

19 Tan, P.K. *et al.* (2003) Evaluation of gene expression measurements from commercial microarray platforms. *Nucleic Acids Research*, **31**, 5676–5684.

20 Shi, L. *et al.* (2006) The MicroArray Quality Control (MAQC) project shows inter- and intraplatform reproducibility of gene

expression measurements. *Nature Biotechnology*, **24**, 1151–1161.

21 Dai, M. *et al.* (2005) Evolving gene/transcript definitions significantly alter the interpretation of GeneChip data. *Nucleic Acids Research*, **33**, e175.

22 Shendure, J. *et al.* (2004) Advanced sequencing technologies: methods and goals. *Nature Reviews. Genetics*, **5**, 335–344.

23 Bennett, S. (2004) Solexa Ltd. *Pharmacogenomics*, **5**, 433–438.

24 Cloonan, N. *et al.* (2008) Stem cell transcriptome profiling via massive-scale mRNA sequencing. *Nature Methods*, **5**, 613–619.

25 Wold, B. and Myers, R.M. (2008) Sequence census methods for functional genomics. *Nature Methods*, **5**, 19–21.

26 Sultan, M. *et al.* (2008) A global view of gene activity and alternative splicing by deep sequencing of the human transcriptome. *Science*, **321**, 956–960.

27 Jain, A.N. *et al.* (2002) Fully automated quantification of microarray image data. *Genome Research*, **12**, 325–332.

28 Steinfath, M. *et al.* (2001) Automated image analysis for array hybridization experiments. *Bioinformatics (Oxford, England)*, **17**, 634–641.

29 Wierling, C.K. *et al.* (2002) Simulation of DNA array hybridization experiments and evaluation of critical parameters during subsequent image and data analysis. *BMC Bioinformatics*, **3**, 29.

30 Chudin, E. *et al.* (2001) Assessment of the relationship between signal intensities and transcript concentration for Affymetrix GeneChip arrays. *Genome Biology*, **3**, RESEARCH0005.

31 Draghici, S. (2003) *Data Analysis Tools for DNA Microarrays*, Chapman & Hall/CRC Press, Boca Raton, FL.

32 Quakenbush, J. (2002) Microarray data normalization and transformation. *Nature Genetics*, **32** Suppl, 496–501.

33 Kerr, M.K. *et al.* (2000) Analysis of variance for gene expression microarray data. *Journal of Computational Biology: A Journal of Computational Molecular Cell Biology*, **7**, 819–837.

34 Li, C. and Wong, W.H. (2001) Model-based analysis of oligonucleotide arrays: expression index computation and outlier detection. *Proceedings of the National Academy of Sciences of the United States of America*, **98**, 31–36.

35 Christensen, R. (1996) *Plane answers to complex questions*, 2nd Edition, Springer, New York.

36 Cleveland, W.S. and Devlin, S.J. (1983) Locally weighted regression: an approach to regression analysis by local fitting. *Journal of the American Statistical Association*, **83**, 596–610.

37 Yang, H. *et al.* (2002) Normalization for cDNA microarray data: a robust composite method addressing single and multiple slide systematic variations. *Nucleic Acids Research*, **30**, e15.

38 Durbin, B.P. *et al.* (2002) A variance-stabilizing transformation for gene-expression microarray data. *Bioinformatics (Oxford, England)*, **18** (1), S105–S110.

39 Huber, W. *et al.* (2002) Variance stabilisation applied to microarray data calibration and to the quantification of differential expression. *Bioinformatics (Oxford, England)*, **18** (1), S96–S104.

40 Herwig, R. *et al.* (2001) Statistical evaluation of differential expression on cDNA nylon arrays with replicated experiments. *Nucleic Acids Research*, **29**, E117.

41 Zien, A. *et al.* (2003) Microarrays: How many do you need? *Journal of Computational Biology: A Journal of Computational Molecular Cell Biology*, **10**, 653–667.

42 Adjaye, J. *et al.* (2005) Primary differentiation in the human blastocyst: comparative molecular portraits of inner cell mass and trophectoderm cells. *Stem Cells (Dayton, Ohio)*, **23**, 1514–1525.

43 Man, M.Z. *et al.* (2000) POWER_SAGE: comparing statistical tests for SAGE experiments. *Bioinformatics (Oxford, England)*, **16**, 953–959.

44 Audic, S. and Claverie, J.M. (1997) Significance of digital gene expression profiles. *Genome Research*, **7**, 986–995.

45 Westfall, P.H. and Young, S.S. (1993) *Resampling-Based Multiple Testing:*

Examples and Methods for p-Value Adjustment, Wiley, New York.

46 Benjamini, Y. and Hochberg, Y. (1995) Controlling the false discovery rate: a practical and powerful approach to multiple testing. *The Journal of the Royal Statistical Society. Series B*, **57**, 289–300.

47 Tusher, V.G. *et al.* (2001) Significance analysis of microarrays applied to the ionizing radiation response. *PNAS*, **98**, 5116–5121.

48 Storey, J.D. and Tibshirani, R. (2003) Statistical significance for genome-wide studies. *PNAS*, **100**, 9440–9445.

49 Irizarry, R.A. *et al.* (2003) Summaries of Affymetrix GeneChip probe level data. *Nucleic Acids Research*, **31**, e15.

50 Jain, A.K. and Dubes, R.C. (1988) *Algorithms for Clustering Data*, Prentice-Hall, Englewood Cliffs, NJ.

51 Eisen, M.B. *et al.* (1998) Cluster analysis and display of genome-wide expression patterns. *Proceedings of the National Academy of Science USA*, **95**, 14863–14868.

52 Kohonen, T. (1997) *Self-Organizing Maps*, Springer, Berlin.

53 Tamayo, P. *et al.* (1999) Interpreting patterns of gene expression with self-organizing maps: Methods and application to hematopoietic differentiation. *Proceedings of the National Academy of Science USA*, **96**, 2907–2912.

54 Törönen, P. *et al.* (1999) Analysis of gene expression data using self-organizing maps. *FEBS Letters*, **451**, 142–146.

55 Herwig, R. *et al.* (1999) Large-scale clustering of cDNA-fingerprinting data. *Genome Research*, **9**, 1093–1105.

56 MacQueen, J.B. (1967) Some methods for classification and analysis of multivariate observations, in *Proceedings of the 5th Berkeley Symposium on Mathematical Statistics and Probability* (eds L.M. LeCam and J. Neymann), UCLA Press, Los Angeles.

57 Rousseeuw, P.J. (1984) Least median of squares regression. *Journal of the American Statistical Association*, **79**, 871–880.

58 Consortium, G.O. (2003) The gene ontology (GO) database and information resource. *Nucleic Acids Research*, **32**, D258–D261.

59 Rasche, A. *et al.* (2008) Meta-analysis approach identifies candidate genes and associated molecular networks for type-2 diabetes mellitus. *BMC Genomics*, **9**, 310.

60 Hanahan, D. and Weinberg, R.A. (2000) The hallmarks of cancer. *Cell*, **100**, 57–70.

61 Vapnik, V.N. (1995) *The Nature of Statistical Learning Theory*, Springer, New York.

62 Furey, T.S. *et al.* (2000) Support vector machine classification and validation of cancer tissue samples usng microarray expression data. *Bioinformatics (Oxford, England)*, **16**, 906–914.

63 Statnikov, A. *et al.* (2004) A comprehensive evaluation of multicategory classification methods for microarray gene expression cancer diagnosis. *Bioinformatics*, **21**, 631–643.

64 Cristianini, N. and Shawe-Taylor, J. (2000) *An Introduction to Support Vector Machines*, Cambridge University Press, Cambridge.

65 Duda, R.O. and Hart, P.E. (1973) *Pattern Classification and Scene Analysis*, John Wiley & Sons, New York.

66 Alon, U. *et al.* (1999) Broad patterns of gene expression revealed by clustering analysis of tumor and normal colon tissues probed by oligonucleotide arrays. *Proceedings of the National Academy of Science USA*, **96**, 6745–6750.

67 Freund, J. and Shapire, R. (1996) Experiments with a new boosting algorithm. Machine Learning. Proceedings to the 13th International Conference, Morgan Kaufmann, San Francisco.

68 Ross, D.T. *et al.* (2000) Systematic variation in gene expression patterns in human cancer cell lines. *Nature Genetics*, **24**, 227–235.

69 Adjaye, J. *et al.* (2004) Cross-species hybridisation of human and bovine orthologous genes on high density cDNA microarrays. *BMC Genomics*, **5**, 83.

70 Ross, D.T. *et al.* (2000) Systematic variation in gene expression patterns in human cancer cell lines. *Nature Genetics*, **24**, 227–235.

6
Gene Expression Models

6.1
Mechanisms of Gene Expression Regulation

Summary

The expression of genes is a highly regulated process in eukaryotic as well as in prokaryotic cells and has a profound impact on the ability of the cells to maintain vitality, perform cell division and respond to environmental changes or stimuli. In this section we describe two basic mechanisms of gene expression regulation: the transcriptional regulation through transcription factors that bind to DNA motifs upstream of the transcription start site and, thus, initiate transcription of the DNA sequence to mRNA, and the posttranscriptional regulation through microRNAs that bind to the mRNA sequences and act as translational repressors. These two mechanisms of gene expression regulation have been intensively studied in recent years giving rise to many different computational methods, data resources and databases for the analysis of specific gene regulatory pathways.

6.1.1
Transcription-Factor Initiated Gene Regulation

Gene expression is a fundamental process that involves many different molecular processes from the activation of transcriptional regulators to the synthesis of a functional protein [1, 2]. Hundreds of different cell types exist and fulfill specific roles in the organism. Each cell type contains the entire genomic information, but only a proportion of the genes is expressed determining the specific role of the cells of this type. Gene expression in eukaryotes is controlled at six different steps (cf. Section 10.4). These steps determine the diversity and specification of the organism [3]:

1. transcriptional control: when and how often is a gene transcribed,
2. RNA processing control: how is the RNA transcript spliced,

Systems Biology: A Textbook. Edda Klipp, Wolfram Liebermeister, Christoph Wierling, Axel Kowald, Hans Lehrach, and Ralf Herwig

ISBN: 978-3-527-31874-2

3. RNA transport and localization control: which mRNAs in the nucleus are exported to cytosol and where in the cytosol are they localized,
4. translational control: which mRNAs in the cytosol are translated by ribosomes,
5. mRNA degradation control: which mRNAs in the cytosol are destabilized,
6. protein activity control: decide upon activation, inactivation, compartmentalization, degradation of the translated protein.

Each single step is complex and has been studied extensively in isolation. In computational analyses the entire gene regulation process is typically approximated with a linear structure of more or less independent modules where the output of the previous module is the input for the current module.

The expression level of the majority of genes is controlled by transcription factors. Transcription factors are proteins that bind to DNA regulatory sequences upstream of the site at which transcription is initiated. Various regulatory pathways control their activities. More than 5% of human genes encode transcription factors [4]. Once activated, transcription factors bind to gene regulatory elements and, through interactions with other components of the transcription machinery, promote access to DNA and facilitate the recruitment of the RNA polymerase enzymes to the transcriptional start site.

In eukaryotes, there are three RNA polymerases, namely RNAP I, II, and III. RNAP II catalyzes the transcription of protein-coding genes and is responsible for the synthesis of mRNAs and certain small nuclear RNAs while the others are responsible for generating tRNAs (RNAP III) and ribosomal RNAs (RNAP I) [5].

The RNAP II enzyme itself is unable to initiate promoter dependent transcription in the absence of complementing factors. It needs to be supplemented by so-called *general transcription factors* (GTFs) [1]. RNAP II together with these GTFs and the DNA template form the preinitiation complex and the assembly of this complex is nucleated by binding of TBP (a component of TFIID) to the *TATA-box* [6]. The TATA-box is a core promoter (or minimal promoter) that directs transcriptional initiation at a short distance (about 30 bp downstream). Soon after RNAP II initiates transcription, the nascent RNA is modified by the addition of a *cap* structure at its 5′ end. This cap serves initially to protect the new transcript from attack by nucleases and later serves as a binding site for proteins involved in export of the mature mRNA into the cytoplasm and its translation into protein.

The start of RNA synthesis catalyzed by RNAP II is the *transcription initiation*. During *transcription elongation* the polymerase moves along the gene sequence from the 5′ to the 3′ end and extends the transcript. The transition between these early transcriptional events, initiation and elongation, seems to be coordinated by the capping process. A family of elongation factors then regulates the elongation phase. Upon reaching the end of a gene, RNAP II stops transcription (*termination*), the newly RNA is cleaved (*cleavage*) and a polyadenosine (*poly(A)*) tail is added to the 3′ end of the transcript (*polyadenylation*).

The resulting pre-mRNA contains coding sequences in the gene (*exons*) that are divided by long noncoding sequences (*introns*). These introns are removed by pre-mRNA splicing.

Transcription, i.e., the transfer of information from DNA to RNA, and translation, i.e., the transfer of information from RNA to protein, are spatially separated in eukaryotes by the nuclear membrane; transcription occurs in the nucleus, whereas translation is a cytoplasmic event. For that reason, processed mRNAs must be transported from the nucleus to the cytoplasm before translation can occur. The bidirectional transport of macromolecules between nucleus and cytoplasm occurs through protein-covered pores in the nuclear membrane. The export of mRNA is mediated by factors that interact with proteins of the nuclear pores and bind to mRNA molecules in the nucleus and direct them into the cytoplasm. Translation of mRNA into protein takes place on *ribosomes*, i.e., large ribonucleoprotein complexes, and follows the similar principles as transcription. Important for the translation process is the presence of transfer RNA molecules (tRNAs) that deliver the correct amino acid to the currently considered nucleotide triplet. tRNAs have a common characteristic secondary structure and are bound to the mRNA by means of anticodons complementary to the triplet for which they carry the appropriate amino acid. Subsequently, tRNAs are recruited and the polypeptide is synthesized until the first stop codon is present. The first step is the location of the start codon in conjunction with subunits of the ribosome triggered by translational initiation factors. Subsequent phases are elongation and termination. The nascent polypeptide chain then undergoes folding and often posttranslational chemical modification to generate the final active protein (cf. Section 10.4).

The transcriptional control is the most important in gene expression what makes biological sense since the cell invests energy to synthesize products and this energy should not be wasted through subsequent termination of the activity of these products. Gene transcription is controlled by RNAP II and it depends on the presence of several additional proteins in order to transcribe the gene in the proper cellular context. In eukaryotes, gene expression requires a complex regulatory region that defines the transcription starting point and controls the initiation of transcription, the *promoter*. Several algorithms are available that try to identify promoters for specific genes. Some of these algorithms are discussed in this section.

6.1.2 General Promoter Structure

Promoter prediction algorithms implicitly assume a specific model for a typical promoter. The general structure of a RNAP II promoter is described in Figure 6.1(a). The typical promoter is composed of three levels of regulatory sequence signals: The first level contains sequence motifs that enable the binding of specific transcription factors. The next level is the combination of binding sites to promoter modules that jointly act as functional units. The third level consists of the complete promoter that modulates gene transcription depending on cell type, tissue type, developmental stage, or activation by signaling pathways.

The promoter must contain binding sites for the GTFs such as the TATA-box. These proximate regulatory motifs constitute the *core promoter* that is able to bind the preinitiation complex and to determine the exact transcription start site. The core

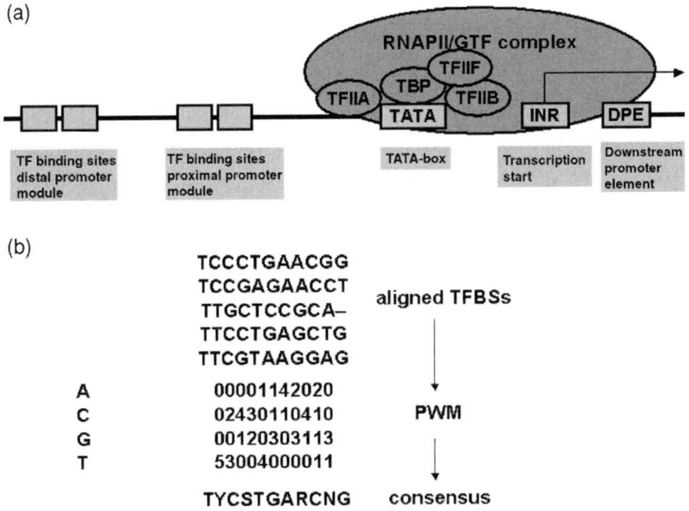

Figure 6.1 (a) General structure of a eukaryotic gene promoter. (b) Example of a positional weight matrix and a consensus sequence derived from different transcription factor binding sites.

promoter needs additional regulatory motifs at varying distances from the transcriptional start point, the regulatory binding sites (transcription factor binding sites, TFBSs). These sites can be situated nearby or kilobases away from the core promoter.

Transcription initiation can be viewed as a process involving successive forming of protein complexes. In the first step transcription factors bind to upstream promoter and enhancer sequence motifs and form a multiprotein complex. In the next step this complex recruits the RNAPII/GTF complex to the core promoter and the transcription start site. This is done through protein–protein interactions either directly or by adaptor proteins [7]. The full complex then starts the transcription process.

The *core promoter* is located in the direct neighborhood of the transcription start site (approximately 30 bp). The core promoter is the best characterized part of the promoter and is defined as a set of binding sites sufficient for the assembly of the RNAPII/GTF complex and for specifying transcriptional initiation. Several core classes of promoters are known [8, 9].

1. TATA-box: If TBP is present in the RNAPII/GTF complex then this protein binds to the sequence motif and the transcription starts approximately 30 bp downstream.
2. TATA-less: No TATA-box is present. The start site is determined by a sequence motif INR (initiator region) surrounding the start site [10].
3. A combination of both INR and TATA-box.
4. Null promoter: None of the two sequence motifs are present. Transcription initiation is solely based on upstream (or downstream) promoter elements [11].
5. Additionally, to INR in some cases there exist a downstream promoter element (DPE) and both elements are able to specify the transcription start site [12].

Whereas the core promoter determines the transcription start site this function cannot explain how genes whose protein products are needed in parallel are coregulated, for example from genes that are located on different chromosomes. Thus additional regulatory elements are necessary that meet the requirement of higher flexibility and coordinated gene expression.

Typically a few hundred bp upstream of the core promoter is the proximate promoter module that contains transcription factor binding sites for proteins responsible for the modulation of the transcription [13]. The corresponding factors can either influence the binding of the core promoter components or the chromatin structure (or both). Furthermore, a promoter can contain a distal promoter module (in the order of kb apart from the transcription start site). Although these modules cannot act as promoters on their own they are able to enhance or suppress the activity of transcription up to orders of magnitude (enhancer or silencer). Enhancer and silencer often exhibit a tissue-specific activity. Likewise to the transcription factors binding to the proximate module of the promoter the factors binding to the distal module influence gene expression by interactions with the factors in the RNAPII/GTF complex or by changing the chromatin structure. There is no clear boundary for the promoter in the 5′-direction and the common explanation of interactions with distal factors to the transcription apparatus is given by the formation of large loops in the DNA. The function of a promoter is to increase or repress the transcription from the core promoter (basal transcription). Thus, any given gene will have a specific regulatory region determined by the binding sites of the transcription factors that ensure that the gene is transcribed in the appropriate cell type and at the proper point in development. The transcriptional activation is not simply determined by the presence of the binding sites but also through the availability of the corresponding transcription factors. These transcription factors are themselves subjected to regulation and activation, for example through signaling pathways and the whole process can entail complex procedures such as transcriptional cascades and feedback control loops [14].

6.1.3 Prediction and Analysis of Promoter Elements

As described in the previous section, promoters are complex and diverse what makes promoter prediction a difficult task. Several reviews have been published that compare the performances of promoter recognition programs [15–18].

6.1.3.1 Sequence-Based Analysis

The modeling of gene transcription regulation follows its combinatorial nature starting from the detection of individual binding sites (5–25 bp in length), to the detection of specific combinations of binding sites, so-called composite regulatory elements [19], to the detection of the promoter.

The detection of *individual binding sites* is the first level in that process. TFBSs have high sequence variability what distinguishes them for example from restriction sites, i.e., the recognition sequences of a restriction enzyme. Whereas restriction sites are almost exact in the sense that sites which vary by only a single mismatch will be cut less well by orders of magnitude, transcription factor binding can tolerate high sequence variability of the TFBSs. This variation makes biologically sense in that it allows a higher flexibility of the regulatory system and assigns the promoters different activity levels [20].

In order to meet this flexibility known TFBSs for the same transcription factor that may vary slightly are often represented by a *consensus sequence* that is close to each single motif according to some criterion. There is a trade-off in the consensus sequences between the number of mismatches that are allowed and the precision of the representation and thus a trade-off between the specificity and the sensitivity of the algorithms. A consensus sequence is typically denoted in the *IUPAC* code to describe ambiguities in nucleotide composition (Figure 6.1(b)).

Alternatively to consensus sequences is the use of *positional weight matrices* (PWM). A PWM is a matrix representation of a TFBS, with rows representing one of the bases, "A," "C," "G", and "T," and columns representing the position within the motif (Figure 6.1(b)). Each entry in the matrix corresponds to a numerical value indicating the confidence for the specific base at that position. The PWM approach is somewhat more general than the consensus sequence approach in the sense that each consensus can be represented by a PWM (for example, through frequency counts across the aligned motifs) such that the same set of sites can be matched but not vice versa. The calculation of the matrix elements can be performed in different ways. Stormo *et al.* [16] applied a neural network learning algorithm to determine the weights of a PWM to distinguish known sites from nonsites in a training sample of *E. coli* sequences. Afterward they predicted new sequences using the calculated weights. Other approaches used thermodynamical considerations to compute the weights of a PWM [8]. The authors showed that the logarithms of the base frequencies should be proportional to the binding energy contribution of the bases assuming an equal distribution of base pairs through the genome.

Recognition of composite regulatory elements has been proposed in order to meet the combinatorial nature of gene regulation, for example of two transcription factors that interact with each other in gene regulation. Statistical approaches have been made to reveal common pairs of TFBSs from DNA sequences by weighing matrices for two corresponding transcription factors. Methods take into account, for example, the matching distances of the matrices on the DNA sequence and the mutual orientation and combines this with binding energy considerations. A number of examples of composite regulatory elements have been collected in the TRANSCompel database [21].

The general principle of *promoter recognition* methods is based on the strategy to determine a promoter model by features that are trained on a set of known promoter sequences and nonpromoter sequences. These features are subsequently used to search for an unknown number of promoters in a contiguous DNA sequence. The methods differ by the way the features are determined. Typically, they fall into two groups. The first group uses the pure sequence composition and is based on scoring moving sequence windows, whereas the second group employs prediction based on the detection of motifs from the core promoter element such as TATA-box or INR.

The first group of algorithms can be exemplified by the PromFind method described in Hutchinson [22]. This method is based on the idea of discriminative counts of sequence groups. PromFind uses the frequency of heptamers (sequences of length 7) in coding and noncoding sequences trained on sequences of 300 bp in length. Discrimination is based on the following measure

$$d_i(s) = \frac{f(s)}{f(s) + f_i(s)}, \quad i = 1, 2. \tag{6.1}$$

Here, $f(s)$ denotes the frequency of heptamer s in the promoter sequences and $f_i(s)$ corresponds to the frequency of the heptamer in the training sample ($i = 1$: noncoding, $i = 2$: coding). For each sequence in a window of size 300 bp the two measures are calculated and the window with the highest value is returned. Another way of computing discriminative counts is employed in PromoterInspector [23].

The second group of algorithms uses biological sequence features from the core promoter [24]. The hit ratio of known TFBSs within promoters and nonpromoters is used as an indicator for the identification of a promoter. The combined ratio scores of all TFBSs in a certain sequence window are used to build a scoring profile. This profile combined with a weight matrix for TATA-boxes is used for predicting the transcription start site. Further methods model the core promoter with artificial neural networks [25], ensembles of multilayer perceptrons for binding sites or hidden Markov models.

There are worldwide initiatives that – among other goals – try to interpret and annotate genome-wide promoter structure such as the ENCODE project (Encyclopedia of DNA Elements). The ENCODE consortium aims in its pilot phase at the in-depth analysis of 30 Mb of genomic DNA corresponding to 1% of the human genome. Functional experiments along with intensive computational analyses have led to a comprehensive characterization of the human genome function [26]. A recent study within the ENCODE region of the human genome has predicted more than 900 putative human promoters and analyzed its function in different human cell lines. Promoter activity analyses showed that, on average, regions up to 300 bp upstream of the transcription start site contributed positively to promoter activity whereas regions from 500 to 1000 bp contributed rather negatively [27].

6.1.3.2 Approaches that Incorporate Additional Information

Since it has been shown that the error rates of the promoter prediction programs are fairly unsatisfactory [15], new developments try to incorporate additional information, in particular gene expression data, as a back up when predicting TFBSs.

A first class of approaches *combines binding site prediction with gene expression data* derived from DNA arrays. The widespread use of DNA arrays (cf. Chapter 5) has given rise to the following general program [28]:

1. Identify coexpression groups by clustering or other statistical methods.
2. Search in the upstream regions of the grouped genes for common regulatory motifs.

This approach has been utilized for the first time for identifying novel regulatory networks in *Saccharomyces cerevisiae*. The authors used a *K*-means clustering algorithm to identify groups of coregulated genes. They identified common sequence motifs in the upstream sequences of the genes and identified 18 motifs in 12 clusters that were highly overrepresented within their own cluster and absent in the others, thus indicating the existence of different regulation patterns.

This and other studies demonstrated that genes that are coexpressed across multiple experimental conditions underlie often common regulatory mechanisms, and, thus, share common TFBSs in their promoters. Although these results are promising, methods that work well in yeast are difficult to extend to higher eukaryotes. This is mainly due to the fact that in yeast regulatory sequences are fairly proximal to the transcription start site, whereas in higher eukaryotes these sequences can be located many kilobases on either side of the coding region. A recent approach to human data has been published [29]. Here, the authors used DNA array data and human genome sequence data to identify putative regulatory elements that control the transcriptional program of the human cell cycle. They identified several transcription factors (such as E2F, NF-Y, and CREB) whose target sequences appear, with increased probability, in the promoters of cell-cycle regulated genes and assigned these factors to certain phases of the cell cycle.

There are several other computational methods described that incorporate gene coexpression signature among a range of expression experiments, for example derived from microarrays. Clusters of genes are evaluated for overrepresented sequence motifs [30]. Several software packages offer multifunctional series of algorithms that can be applied including higher level data analysis such as the comparison of the motifs, the assignment of motifs to known positional weight matrices, and the clustering of motifs [31]. TF specific motifs are collected in dedicated databases such as TRANSFAC [20] or JASPAR [32].

Another class of approaches uses *comparative sequence analysis* from upstream sequences of orthologous genes through different organisms [33]. These authors investigated skeletal-muscle specific transcription factors and found that their binding sites are highly conserved in human and mouse DNA sequences. The general observation of conserved noncoding regions throughout different organisms has given rise to a number of recent developments that incorporate cross-species analysis of promoter elements [34].

A combination of the two approaches has been applied to the detection and experimental verification of a novel *cis*-regulatory element involved in the heat shock response in *C. elegans* [35]. The authors identified coregulated genes with DNA arrays and investigated the upstream regions of these genes for putative binding sites by pattern recognition algorithms. Either in the case of significant overrepresentation or in the case of cross-species conservation they built biological assays of the regulatory motifs using GFP reporter transgenes.

Additional sequence information is also sometimes incorporated in promoter identification, in particular the identification of CpG islands. It has been reported that these CpG islands correlate with promoters in vertebrates so that their features are used in the computational process [36, 37]. By definition CpG islands are genomic regions with

1. longer than 200 bp
2. nucleotide frequencies of C and G in that region greater than 50%

3. CpG dinucleotide frequency in that region is higher than 0.6 of that expected from mononucleotide frequencies.

Despite all these developments the recognition and identification of promoter elements remains an error-prone task implied by the highly complex nature of eukaryotic gene regulation. Future approaches will thus have to incorporate additional information to a much larger extent than it is currently done.

6.1.4
Posttranscriptional Regulation Through microRNAs

MicroRNAs (miRNAs) are small RNA molecules that regulate gene expression at the posttranscriptional level. MicroRNAs are about 20–25 nucleotides (nt) long and have been identified in plants, animals, and viruses [38]. A microRNA binds specifically at an mRNA and controls gene expression through the regulation of mRNA stability and translation. The general mechanism of microRNA gene regulation is shown in Figure 6.2(a). Most miRNAs are transcribed from their DNA sequences as primary miRNAs (pri-miRNAs) by RNA polymerase II. In animals, pri-miRNAs are converted to mature miRNAs by two successive endonucleolytic cleavages. The pri-miRNA is first cut in the nucleus the ribonuclease III (RNase III) enzyme Drosha into an approximately 70 nt long stem loop, the precursor miRNA (pre-miRNA). This precursor miRNA is exported to cytoplasm by Exportin-5 and cut into mature miRNA by another RNase III enzyme called Dicer. The mature miRNA is then loaded into an effector complex, the RNA-induced silencing complex (RISC), whose core component is a member of the Argonaute (Ago) family of RNA regulatory proteins [39]. MiRNAs match with their mRNA targets by sequence complementarity. In plants this match is very well positioned in either the coding or the 3′UTR regions of the targets. This nearly perfect binding initiates mRNA degradation. In animals miRNAs typically regulate gene expression by imperfect binding to the 3′UTRs of the target mRNAs effecting inihibition of protein synthesis or causing mRNA degradation (Figure 6.2(a)). The 5′-region (seed region) of the miRNA (approximately nucleotides 2–8) is the primary determinant of binding specificity. The effect of the rather imperfect binding of the rest of the miRNA sequence enables regulation of hundreds of different mRNAs per miRNA; thus, providing each miRNA with a powerful regulatory potential. A common consequence of such seed-mediated miRNA binding is a decrease in the amount of the protein encoded by the target mRNA. However, the precise molecular mechanisms of miRNA-mediated translational repression are still under discussion. In fact, distinct mechanisms of repression have been proposed by different laboratories for different miRNA-target pairs and even for the same miRNAs.

For most of the detected miRNAs their functional roles are still unknown. MiRNA target discovery is a major issue in that respect. However, for a few cases it has already been shown that deregulation of miRNA expression has multiple implications for developmental processes and human diseases. For example, it had been shown that de-regulation of miRNAs can affect cancer pathways through an interaction with genes that are involved in proliferation and apoptosis [40]. The authors showed that

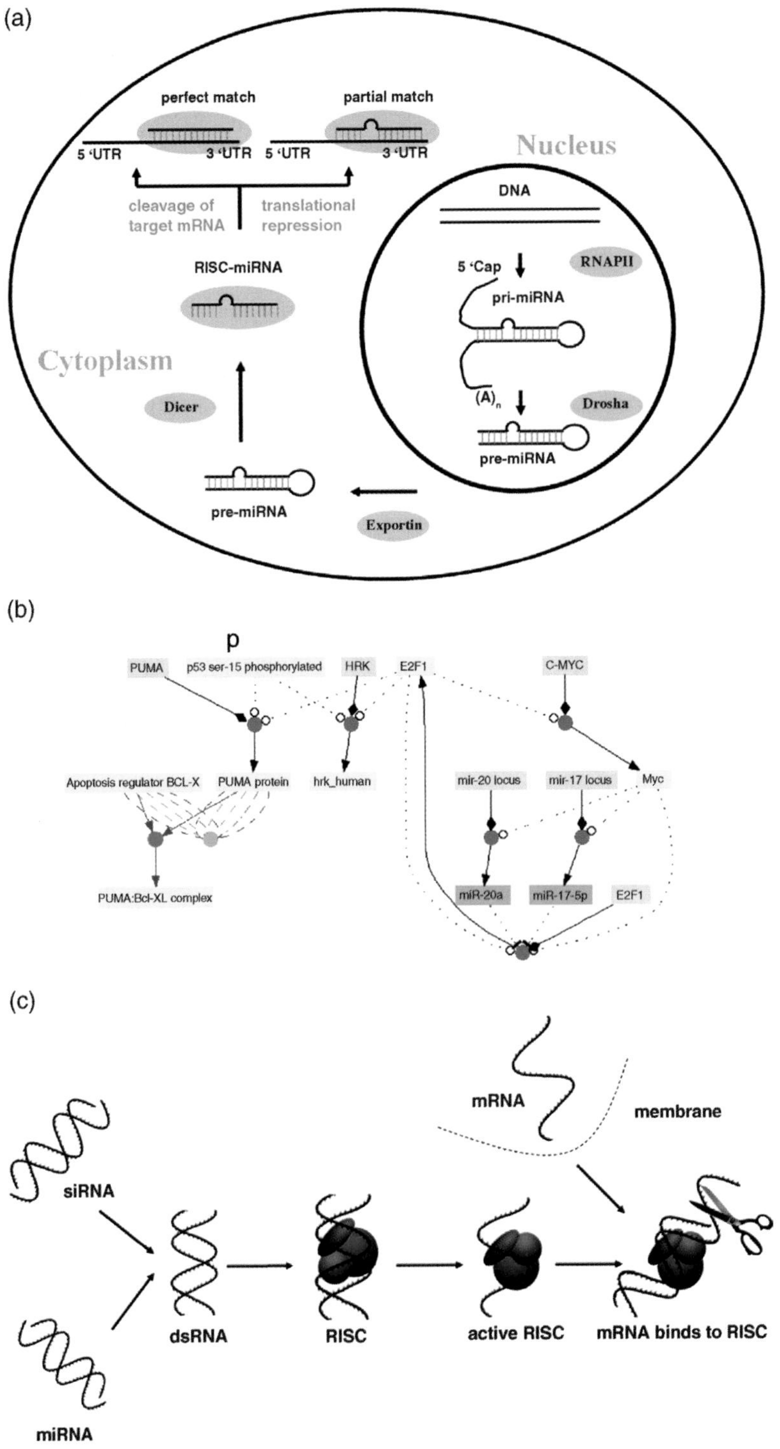
(a)
perfect match
partial match
5 'UTR
3 'UTR
5 'UTR
3 'UTR
Nucleus
cleavage of target mRNA
translational repression
DNA
5 'Cap
RNAPII
RISC-miRNA
pri-miRNA
Cytoplasm
Dicer
(A)n
Drosha
pre-miRNA
pre-miRNA
Exportin
(b)
p
PUMA
p53 ser-15 phosphorylated
HRK
E2F1
C-MYC
Apoptosis regulator BCL-X
PUMA protein
hrk_human
mir-20 locus
mir-17 locus
Myc
PUMA:Bcl-XL complex
miR-20a
miR-17-5p
E2F1
(c)
mRNA
membrane
siRNA
dsRNA
RISC
active RISC
mRNA binds to RISC
miRNA

two miRNAs, miR-17-5p and miR-20a, negatively regulate the E2F1 transcription factor expression. These miRNAs are among six miRNAs that are activated by the transcription factor c-MYC, which is also an activator of E2F1. The work gives an example of the complex interaction between transcriptional and translational control of gene expression: c-MYC simultaneously activates E2F1 transcription and downgrades its translation through the activation of additional miRNAs giving rise to a tightly controlled proliferative signal. Additional implications and potential downstream effects of this regulatory process are shown in Figure 6.2(b).

6.1.4.1 Identification of microRNAs in the Genome Sequence

Identification of miRNAs in the genome sequences incorporates a set of characteristic criteria that define miRNAs and that are usually involving the identification of pre-miRNA [41]:

1. The presence of a characteristic secondary structure involving hairpin modules;
2. Phylogenetic conservation;
3. Thermodynamic stability of hairpins and sequence comparison to known miRNA.

These characteristics can be encoded into sequence alignment algorithms. Mostly, computational prediction of miRNAs is based on machine learning techniques (cf. Section 5.2.8) that use known miRNAs as a training set for the algorithm and then try to identify novel miRNAs. These miRNAs are then validated experimentally, for example by PCR. Computer programs commonly utilize the hairpin shape of the precursor sequence of the mature miRNA. Multiple of these structures can be found in the genome and the majority of them are assumed not to be miRNA precursors. The programs thus search for predictive properties that distinguish the known miRNAs from this control group. Most algorithms depend on evolutionary conservation of miRNAs in different species. Common programs are MirScan, RNAFold, or PalGrade [42].

There are several public databases and resources for the analysis of miRNAs, the most common of which is MiRBase (http://microrna.sanger.ac.uk), the central online repository for miRNA nomenclature, sequences, annotation and target prediction of the Sanger centre. Currently, miRBase contains 5071 miRNA loci from 58 species. The number of known miRNAs in the genome is increasing rapidly and is under constant discussion. Whereas early studies estimated the number of mature miRNAs in the human genome with 255 [43]; recently this number has been increased to 555 [44]. Numbers for other species are: *M. musculus* (455), *Danio rerio* (183), *C. elegans* (135), *D. melanogaster* (85), and the plant *A. thaliana* (199).

Figure 6.2 (a) Biogenesis of miRNA. (b) Network diagram that shows the tight interaction of two miRNAs with E2F1 and c-MYC regulatory networks. Different colors refer to different interaction types (blue: gene regulatory interaction, orange: protein-protein interactions, green: biochemical interaction). Different edge colors refer to different databases where these interactions had been retrieved from. The edge style refers to the interaction type. The network has been constructed with ConsensusPathDB, a database for pathway intergration (http://cpdb.molgen.mpg.de <http://cpdb.molgen.mpg.de/>. [80]). (c) Basic mechanism of RNAi.

6.1.4.2 MicroRNA Target Prediction

The identification of miRNA targets uses the fact that miRNAs recognize their targets by partial sequence complementarity and, thus, that these targets can be identified by using the miRNA sequence itself. There are several programs available for miRNA target predictions (for example, DIANAmicro, TargetScans, MiRanda, PicTar, and MicroInspector). These programs essentially perform two steps. In the first step they identify potential miRNA binding sites according to specific base-pairing rules using different algorithmic approaches such as maximum-likelihood and dynamic programming. Different programs distinguish between 5′ and 3′ base pairing of the miRNA and also on the proportion of identity of these base pairings. A typical observation of miRNA–mRNA interactions in animals is a contiguous pairing in the miRNA 5′-region (proximal seed at positions 2–8) and less complementarity in the central part of miRNA (positions 10 and 11) that precludes the cleavage of the target mRNA in the middle of the duplex. In the second step, the programs implement cross-species conservation requirements taking advantage of the fact that miRNA regulation is highly conserved. Different programs have been compared with experimentally verified benchmark data sets [45]. Benchmarking data was taken from public data repositories and consisted of 84 experimentally verified miRNA–target interactions involving 23 different miRNAs. As a result of this, relatively small, benchmarking study authors observed a rather bad performance of all programs. The sensitivity (defined as the number of true positive interactions divided by the number of all known interactions) was <50% in all cases. More severely, the three programs that came close to this figure (MiRanda, TargetScan, PicTar) predicted more than 10,000 different interactions, and, thus, generated high false positive rates.

6.1.4.3 Experimental Implications – RNA Interference

RNA interference uses the above-mentioned mechanism of posttranscriptional translation repression (*gene silencing, knock-down*) by reducing the concentration of the mRNA sequence and, thus, the quantity of the protein [46, 47]. Using RNAi it is possible to specifically degrade mRNA and reduce the activity of the corresponding protein (cf. Section 11.11). This has multiple implications for modeling gene regulatory pathways since it allows deducing, for example, target genes of certain transcription factors and enables the experimental measurement of functional gene interdependences. The degradation of mRNA is initiated by short double-stranded RNA molecules (dsRNA). Originally, these molecules were observed in the model organisms *Caenorhabditis elegans, Drosophila melanogaster,* and *Arabidopsis thaliana* [48–50]; later also in vertebrates [51].

Different classes of regulatory dsRNAs are known, such as miRNAs and siRNAs. Gene silencing is induced as shown in Figure 6.2(c). The dsRNA fragments are loaded into the silencing complex RISC and hybridize to the protein coding RNA. The catalytic component of the RISC, the argonaut proteins, are endonucleases and degrade the mRNA molecule [47].

RNAi has been developed as a routine and powerful experimental procedure, in particular, if it is combined with high-throughput experiments to screen the inhibition effects on a genome-wide scale. Through transfection of a cell culture with transcription factor specific siRNAs it is possible to reduce the activity of the

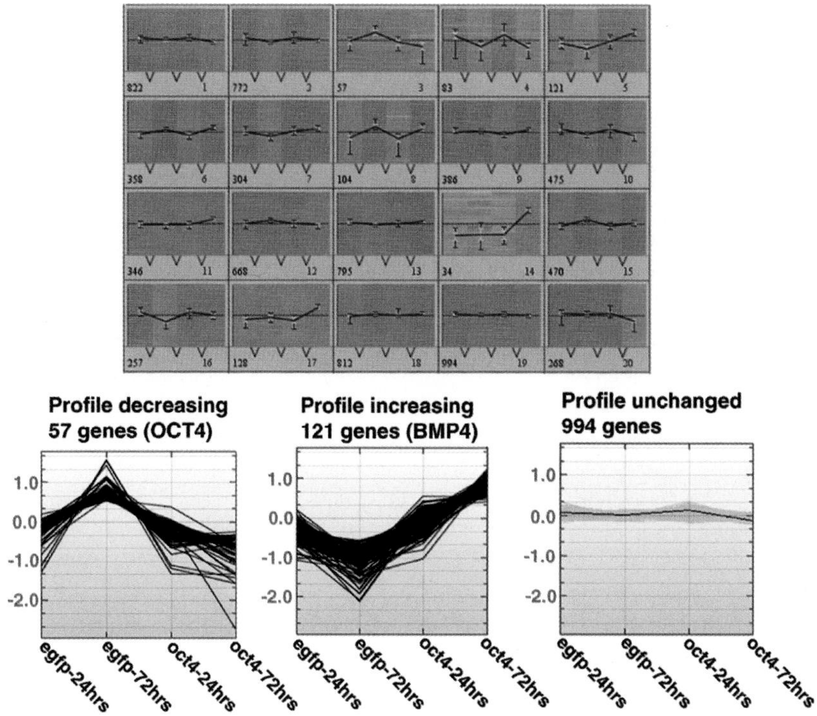

Figure 6.3 Resulting expression patterns from an RNAi experiment. Microarray experiments have been carried out using an OCT-4 knock-down at 24 hrs and 72 hrs and an unspecific EGFR knock-down as a control at the same time points after transfection. The resulting expression values were clustered using a K-means algorithm what resulted in twenty clusters, each of which contained genes with a typical expression profile (upper part). The lower panel shows three examples of clusters with decreasing expression pattern (OCT-4 like genes), increasing expression patterns (BMP4-like genes) and constant expression patterns.

transcription factor to a large amount, thus, allowing to measure the transcriptional consequences for its potential target genes. Figure 6.3 shows an example of an RNAi experiment with the transcription factor OCT-4, a crucial factor in early embryonic development [52]. Recent studies on reprogramming human somatic cells to induced pluripotent stem cells emphasize the function of the transcription factor OCT-4 as key regulator of pluripotency. It is supposed that pluripotency and self-renewal is controlled by a transcription regulatory network governed by OCT-4 regulation and the down-regulation of OCT-4 is crucial in initiating for early embryonic differentiation. Clustering (cf. Section 5.2.5) has been applied to identify genes that change their expression patterns according to the knock-down measured at 24 and 72 h in comparison to an unspecific knock-down at the same time points. Expression profiles and expression fold-changes can then be interpreted as effects of the knock-down on the underlying molecular network structure.

Figure 6.3 shows specific clusters of coexpressed genes across different experiments. One cluster, for example, shows genes with a continuous down-regulation through time including the transcription factor OCT-4 itself and many of its known target genes. Another cluster shows a continuous upregulation of genes that are downstream effects of the loss of stemness characteristic and indicative of cell differentiation such as BMP4. Most genes show no expression differences indicating the specificity of the knock-down.

It should be noted that RNAi analysis cannot distinguish between direct and indirect targets of a transcription factor since no information on DNA–protein binding is given. The experiment gives an impression on all potential downstream effects of the knock-down and, thus, the number of predicted targets is typically large. In order to reveal the exact transcriptional dependencies these measurements must be complemented by other techniques, for example chromatin immunoprecipitation (ChIP) followed by microarray analysis or sequencing and by computational analysis of the promoter sequences.

6.2 Gene Regulation Functions

Summary

The expression of genes is controlled individually by regulatory proteins. *Gene regulation functions*, which describe the kinetics of transcription in mathematical terms, result from microscopic binding states of the promoter. They have been determined accurately for individual promoters – for instance, for the Lac operon in *E. coli* – by fitting plausible mathematical functions to measured transcription data. Based on high-throughput expression data, simple gene regulation functions and regulator activities can be estimated even for larger transcription networks.

Regulation of gene expression is one of the main control mechanisms in cells [53]. Biochemically, mRNA transcription is controlled by regulatory proteins (e.g., σ factors and transcription factors), which bind to regulatory sites on the DNA and modulate the promoter activities of genes or operons. A small genetic network comprising the dual regulator MetR in *E. coli* together with its target genes and other regulators controlling them is shown in Figure 6.4.

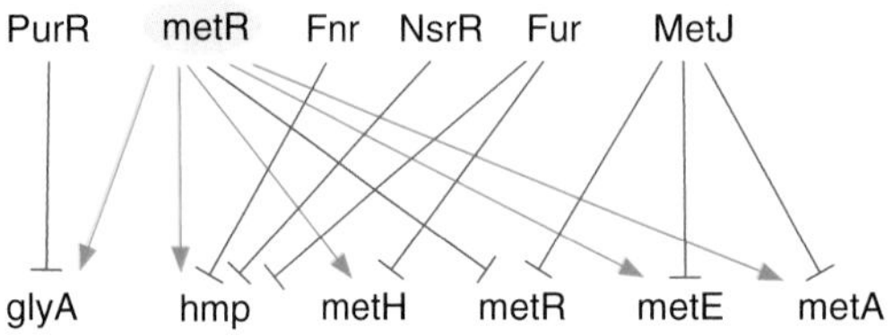

Figure 6.4 Genetic network in *E. coli* comprising the transcriptional regulator MetR and its known target genes. MetR (gray ellipse) regulates a number of target genes (bottom), which therefore form the MetR regulon. Other regulators controlling these genes are shown on top. Arrows denote transcriptional regulation (blue: repression, red: activation). Data taken from the EcoCyc database [54].

The quantitative impact of regulators on genes may be either positive or negative, weak or strong. In addition, the influences of several regulators can be processed in complicated ways. To obtain dynamic models of gene networks (see Sections 6.3 and 8.2), the simple qualitative arrows need to be replaced by quantitative *gene regulation functions*, the rate laws of transcription. We shall discuss in this section how such functions arise from the promoter sequence and how they can be determined from data.

6.2.1
The Lac Operon in *Escherichia coli*

Metabolites can control the enzymes that catalyze their own production or consumption. The resulting feedback loops can constantly adapt the protein levels to the current needs of the cell. A classic example of such regulation, the diauxic growth of bacteria, was discovered by J. Monod in 1941. *Escherichia coli* bacteria prefer glucose as their energy source and maintain enzymes for glucose metabolism under all conditions. Besides glucose, the bacteria can utilize other sugars such as lactose. Three enzymes are necessary for consumption of lactose: β-galactosidase, permease, and thiogalactoside transacetylase. They are coded and regulated together in a transcription unit called the *Lac operon*.

However, when cells are shifted from a glucose-rich medium to a glucose-free, but lactose-rich medium, they need a certain time before they can assimilate lactose at a high rate. The expression level of the Lac operon is usually low; it is only increased on demand, i.e., if glucose is missing and lactose is present in the medium. In a rough approximation, strong Lac expression follows the logical rule "low glucose AND high lactose." Biochemically, the transcription rate is controlled by a combination of two signals (see Figure 6.5(a)). On the one hand, a high glucose level decreases the concentration of cyclic AMP (cAMP), an intracellular messenger that activates the transcriptional activator CRP. Thus, at high glucose levels, CRP remains inactive, and Lac transcription is low. Lactose, on the other hand, is sensed via allolactose, an

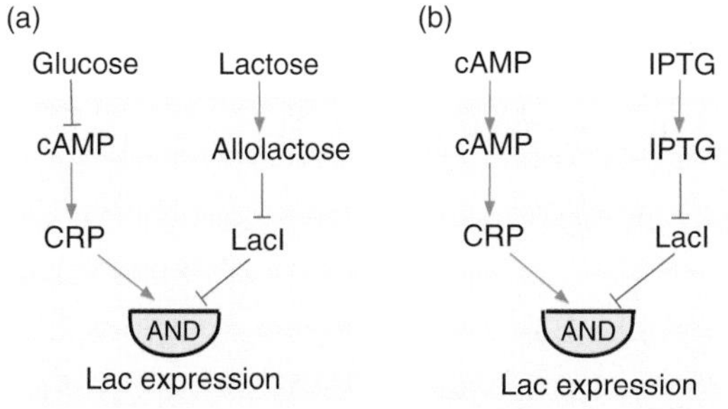

Figure 6.5 Regulation of the Lac operon. (a) The Lac operon is controlled by the transcriptional regulators CRP and LacI, which respond to extracellular levels of lactose and glucose. High expression of the Lac operon requires that lactose is present and glucose is absent. (b) In an experiment [55], the activities of CRP and LacI are regulated by extracellular levels of the ligands cAMP and IPTG. Effectively, both substances activate Lac expression.

isomer formed by converting the 1–4 bond of lactose into a 1–6 bond. Allolactose activates the transcriptional repressor LacI, which shuts down Lac expression by blocking the binding of polymerase and by promoting a DNA loop. Therefore, if no lactose is present, Lac expression will also be low.

For strong expression of the Lac operon (Fig. 6.5, bottom), the repression must be released and the activator CRP has to be bound. In nature, this requires that glucose is absent and lactose is present, just as stated in the logical function. In experiments, however, the regulators CRP and LacI can also be controlled by extracellular levels of cAMP and IPTG, a substitute for allolactose (Figure 6.5(b)). Dynamical models of the Lac operon and the lactose utilization pathway are described in the web supplement.

6.2.2
Gene Regulation Functions Derived from Equilibrium Binding

To describe gene expression by a kinetic model, we need kinetic laws for the transcription rates. For simplicity, we may assume that the transcription rate y of a gene depends on regulator activities x_l while any other influences on transcription are neglected. The rate y is then given by a *gene regulation function*

$$y(t) = f(\boldsymbol{x}(t), \boldsymbol{p}). \tag{6.2}$$

The parameter vector $\boldsymbol{p}$ and the mathematical function f are specific for each gene; however, different genes may also be modeled with the same form of f. The vector $\boldsymbol{x}$ contains the activities of all regulators for the gene in question. Promoters in eukaryotes can process a large number of inputs, which implies complicated input functions [56]. For simple prokaryotic genes, however, fairly plausible gene regulation functions can be derived from theoretical models [57, 58] and fitted to experimental data [55, 59, 60].

A gene regulation function f_i effectively describes microscopic processes like binding of regulators and is determined to a large extent by the nucleotide sequence of the promoter region. As an example, Figure 6.6 shows different binding states of the Lac promoter in a simplified scheme with five states.

The relationship between promoter sequence and gene regulation function is schematically shown in Figure 6.7: a gene promoter can assume various microscopic

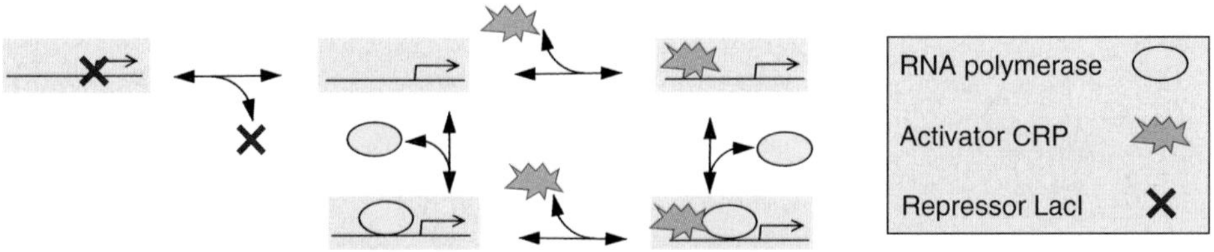

Figure 6.6 Microscopic states of the Lac promoter (schematic model). The promoter can be bound by RNA polymerase, the activator CRP, and the repressor LacI. Bound activator increases the probability of polymerase binding (right). Transcription only occurs in states with bound polymerase (bottom). Bound repressor LacI inhibits binding of other molecules (left). In reality, the promoter sequence is much more complex: LacI can bind to several binding sites and cause DNA looping. A detailed model with 50 states is described in [61].

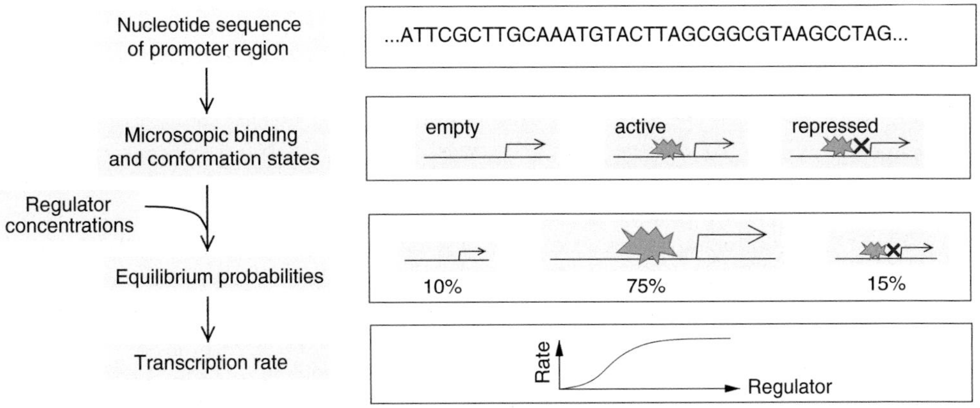

Figure 6.7 Schematic relation between nucleotide sequence and transcription rates.

states, characterized by different regulators bound to their binding sites and by different conformations of the DNA. For a quantitative model, we make two basic assumptions: (i) on the time scale of interest, there is a thermodynamic equilibrium between different states; the probability for each state depends on its binding energy and on the concentration of the regulator molecules present. (ii) In each of the states, transcription initiation occurs randomly at a certain rate.

With these assumptions, the mathematical form of the gene regulation function f_i follows from an analysis of the conformation states. Each state is characterized by a free energy $F = E - TS$, where E and S denote the energy and the entropy of the state, respectively, and T is the temperature. The free energy captures energies related to regulator binding or bending in DNA loops; these energies depend on the promoter sequence, in particular, on presence and sequences of regulator binding sites. The entropy term depends, among other things, on the number of free regulator molecules. The free energy F of a promoter state determines its statistical weight $w_i = \exp(-F_i/(K_B T))$ in the Boltzmann distribution, and the total transcription rate

$$y = \frac{\sum_i w_i\, v_i}{\sum_i w_i} \tag{6.3}$$

is computed as the weighted average over the synthesis rates in all different states.

If we write this transcription rate as a function of regulator concentrations, we obtain an expression for the gene regulation function. Its mathematical form and the parameters are determined by the microscopic states and their energies. In practice, however, the parameters have to be estimated from measured transcription rates because it is hard to directly measure or compute the microscopic energies.

6.2.3
Occupation Probability Derived from Statistical Thermodynamics

To illustrate the link between the microscopic binding states and a macroscopic gene regulation function, we now reconsider protein–DNA binding in a statistical model by Bintu *et al.* [57]. Proteins can bind either specifically or unspecifically to DNA: at a specific binding site, a protein is bound tightly with a large negative binding energy E_1; unspecific binding sites have a smaller binding energy E_0. In the simple model, we assume that all regulator proteins are bound to DNA, either to a single specific site or to one of the many unspecific sites.

In equilibrium, the occupation probability of the specific site depends on the number of protein molecules present. For the calculation, we first assume that n protein molecules are distributed over N unspecific sites: there are $\binom{N}{n} = N!/(n!(N-n)!)$ possible microstates, each representing a pattern of proteins bound to the DNA. Each microstate has a Boltzmann weight $\exp(-\beta n E_0)$, with $\beta = (k_B T)^{-1}$, Boltzmann's constant k_B, and temperature T. To compute the probability for specific binding, we compare two macrostates, X_0 and X_1: in X_0, the specific site is empty, all n proteins are bound nonspecifically, and the total free energy is nE_0. In state X_1, the specific site is occupied and only $n-1$ proteins are bound non-specifically, so the total free energy is $(n-1)E_0 + E_1$. The probability weights for the two states read

$$Z_0 = \binom{N}{n} e^{-n\beta E_0}, \quad Z_1 = \binom{N}{n-1} e^{-(n-1)\beta E_0} e^{-\beta E_1} \tag{6.4}$$

and the corresponding free energies are given by the formula $F_i = -k_B T \ln Z_i$. The occupation probability for the specific site reads $p_1 = Z_1/(Z_1 + Z_0)$ and for $n \ll N$, we obtain the approximation

$$p_1 \approx \frac{n/N}{n/N + e^{\beta \Delta E}}, \tag{6.5}$$

where $\Delta E = E_1 - E_0 < 0$ denotes the energy gain in case of specific binding.

To rewrite this result in terms of concentrations, we introduce the total regulator concentration $x_{tot} = n/(VN_A)$, where V is the cell volume and N_A is Avogadro's constant. Furthermore, we assume that only a small fraction of the regulator molecules is specifically bound, so we approximate x_{tot} by x, the concentration of nonspecifically bound regulators. By defining the effective dissociation constant $K_D = Ne^{\beta \Delta E}/(VN_A)$, we obtain the formula

$$p_1 = \frac{x}{x + K_D}, \tag{6.6}$$

which could also be obtained from a simple binding kinetics (see Section 2.1.4).

Bintu *et al.* have used the above statistical approach to calculate gene regulation functions for promoters with several binding sites and regulators [57, 58]. The resulting gene regulation functions are rational functions, for instance,

$$f(x_1, x_2) = \frac{1 + a_1 x_1 + a_2 x_2}{1 + b_1 x_1 + b_2 x_2} y^* \tag{6.7}$$

for two activators X_1 and X_2, where x_1 and x_2 denote the respective fractions of active regulators. The positive parameters a_1, a_2, b_1, b_2, and y^* in such gene regulation functions depend on the binding energies in the microscopic model.

6.2.4
Gene Regulation Function of the Lac Operon

What remains to be shown now is whether actual gene regulation functions in reality follow the above prediction. Setty *et al.* [55, 62] have experimentally determined the regulation function of the Lac operon in living *E. coli* cells [57, 60, 62]. In the experiment, transcription rates were measured by a fluorescent reporter protein (GFP) under the control of the Lac promoter (see Section 4.1.2). The regulator activities were regulated via extracellular levels of cAMP and IPTG, a substitute for allolactose (see Figure 6.5, right). The transcription rate, plotted against logarithmic concentrations of extracellular cAMP and IPTG, shows four plateaus corresponding to the possible combinations of low and high concentrations (Figure 6.8(a)). As expected, the transcription rate is high at high cAMP and IPTG levels, mimicking a physiological situation with low glucose and high lactose concentrations. In contrast to the Boolean regulation function, the expression rates for low cAMP and low IPTG are not exactly zero. This baseline activity has an important biological function: in order to switch the Lac system to a high expression level, some lactose has to be imported into the cell to produce the messenger allolactose. That requires that the lactose transporter LacY is already present before, at least at a low level.

If the levels of cAMP and IPTG are regarded as proxies for transcriptional activators (inhibition of the repressor LacI effectively counts as activation), the simplified microscopic model in Figure 6.6 leads to a gene regulation function of the form (6.7) shown in Figure 6.8(a). The measured transcription rates can be fitted well by this function, and parameters can be obtained from the data fit.

Mutations in regulator binding sites will change the energies of the binding states and therefore the shape of the regulation function. This has been shown experimentally for the promoter sequence of the Lac operon [62] (see Figure 6.8). In the same way, evolution can adapt and optimize the performance of genetic networks by modifying the promoters' nucleotide sequences; the plasticity of gene regulation functions allows for evolutionary fine-tuning of the gene regulatory system. In the case of the Lac operon, a

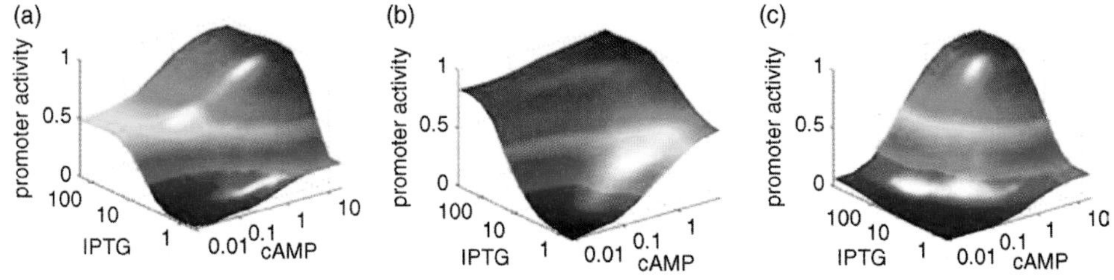

Figure 6.8 Gene regulation functions of the wild type Lac operon and two variants obtained by altered promoter sequences. (a) Measured gene regulation function in an *E. coli* wild-type strain. (b) The strain U340 (obtained from a screen of *E. coli* strains with point mutations in the Lac promoter) shows an OR-like regulation function. (c) Another strain, U339, shows an AND-like regulation function. From [62].

pure AND-like regulation function (Figure 6.8) could have evolved rather easily. Kaplan *et al.* [60] have extended this analysis to a number of *E. coli* operons involved in sugar utilization. Each of them responds effectively to extracellular cAMP and its cognate sugar. Although the regulation functions differ quite remarkably, most of them share a common feature: the two-dimensional regulation functions can be approximately obtained by multiplying two regulation functions for the individual inputs.

6.2.5
Transcriptional Regulation in Larger Networks

If the regulator activities $\boldsymbol{x}(t)$ and the transcription rate $y(t)$ for a gene regulation function (6.2) have been measured, the parameters $\boldsymbol{p}$ can be obtained from nonlinear regression. However, it is difficult to measure or control the active form of transcription factors. In the Lac operon study [55], for instance, external levels of IPTG and cAMP had to be used as controllable proxies. Alternatively, in case that the regulator activities are completely unknown, one can compare the levels of different target genes and estimate the regulator activities along with the gene regulation functions. This has, for instance, been used to determine gene regulation functions for the SOS system [63] and the flagella system [59] in *E. coli* and for target genes of the mammalian cell cycle regulator p53 [64].

Microarrays allow to measure the mRNA levels of thousands of genes at the same time. The expression levels of a single gene, measured in different cell samples, form an expression profile. Such data contain, in principle, valuable information about the regulators of a gene, their activities, and the corresponding gene regulation functions. Data-driven methods like clustering or biclustering compute similarity measures between the expression profiles of different genes and assess their statistical significance. One may hypothesize that genes with similar expression profiles may be coregulated (i.e., regulated by common transcription factors), but the two findings not necessarily coincide. Even if genes respond to the same regulators, their expression profiles may differ due to (i) different gene regulation functions [60]; (ii) additional transcription factors that control only some of the genes; (iii) different rates of mRNA degradation. Dynamical models of gene expression can account for these effects and help to infer coregulation more reliably than by using simple similarity scores.

Most genes respond to several transcription factors, and transcription factors can regulate large numbers of target genes. Thus to determine the gene regulation functions from expression data, the effects of different transcription factors have to be disentangled. One such method is network component analysis, which is based on simple linear gene regulation functions and applicable to fairly large networks.

6.2.6
Network Component Analysis

Network component analysis (NCA) [65, 66] is a method to translate a known genetic network structure into a quantitative model of gene regulation. It employs gene expression data to estimate all gene regulation functions and regulator activities in parallel. In the NCA model, we assume linear gene regulation functions, so the temporal activity $y_{it} = y_i(t)$ of a promoter is a weighted sum of the regulator activities $x_{lt} = x_l(t)$

$$y_i(t) = \sum_l a_{il}\, x_l(t). \tag{6.8}$$

The index t refers to different samples and can, for instance, represent time points in an experiment. The input weights a_{il} indicate whether a regulator acts as an activator ($a_{il} > 0$), as a repressor ($a_{il} < 0$), or has no effect ($a_{il} = 0$) on the promoter activity. Network structures can be obtained from databases [54, 67] or from experiments (e.g., [68]). By the network structure, many of the coefficients a_{il} are already restricted to zero values, and known modes of regulation (activation/repression) may further restrict the signs of the remaining elements a_{il}. The linear NCA model (6.8) resembles statistical models used in principal component analysis [69] or independent component analysis [70], but in contrast to these methods, it includes biological knowledge about the structure of the genetic network.

To estimate the model parameters, we rewrite Eq. (6.8) as a matrix product

$$\boldsymbol{Y} = \boldsymbol{A}\boldsymbol{X}. \tag{6.9}$$

The aim of NCA is to estimate the regulator activities $x_l(t)$ and the input weights a_{il} from measured expression values $y_i^{\exp}(t)$. We require that

$$\boldsymbol{Y}^{\exp} \approx \boldsymbol{A}\boldsymbol{X}. \tag{6.10}$$

with least-squares errors. Given a data matrix $\boldsymbol{Y}^{\exp}$ and the above-mentioned constraints on $\boldsymbol{A}$, the matrices $\boldsymbol{A}$ and $\boldsymbol{X}$ can be determined by an iterative optimization: first, $\boldsymbol{A}$ is initialized with random values and $\boldsymbol{X}$ is chosen by least-squares estimation, then $\boldsymbol{X}$ is kept fixed and $\boldsymbol{A}$ is updated. This mutual updating is iterated until convergence. For ideal data (artificial data obtained from an NCA model without noise), this biquadratic optimization converges to a global optimum for both matrices $\boldsymbol{A}$ and $\boldsymbol{X}$. However, this optimum may be nonunique: depending on the network topology, different parameter choices will lead to equally good results, so the NCA model may be non-identifiable. Consider, for example, two regulators that soley control a single gene. From its expression profile, we can determine a linear combination of the regulator activities, but their individual profiles and the corresponding input weights cannot be reconstructed. Identifiability of the NCA model depends on the network structure and can be checked by analyzing the wiring between regulators and their target genes [65].

The linear NCA model can also be interpreted in terms of nonlinear gene regulation functions: if the inputs x_l and outputs y_l represent logarithmic regulator activities $x_l = \ln c_l$ and logarithmic promoter activities $y_l = \ln v_l$, Eq. (6.8) is equivalent to a nonlinear gene regulation function of the form

$$v_i(t) = \prod_l (c_l(t))^{a_{il}} \tag{6.11}$$

This function describes multiplicative effects between regulators, but it does not account for saturation.

6.3
Dynamic Models of Gene Regulation

Summary

In order to comprehend the functioning of organisms at the molecular level, we wish to know which genes are expressed, to what level, where, and when. A network of interactions between DNA, mRNA, proteins, and other molecules realizes the regulation of gene expression. This network comprises many components. According to the central dogma of molecular biology formulated by Francis Crick [71], there is a forward flow of information from gene to mRNA to protein. Moreover, positive and negative feedback loops and information exchange with signaling pathways and energy metabolism ensure the appropriate regulation of expression according to the current state of the cell and the environment.

Modeling of gene expression is used here as an example to apply different modeling techniques. The dynamics and the regulatory patterns of gene expression will be mathematically described with various graphs, Boolean networks, Bayesian networks, ordinary and partial differential equation systems, stochastic processes, and with rule-based formalisms.

6.3.1
One Gene Regulatory Network: Different Approaches

In the following, we present an overview of modeling approaches for gene regulation and the scientific questions that can be tackled with different techniques. For the sake of clarity, we use only examples with a small number of components (genes and proteins), although the presented approaches can also be applied to larger systems.

The example genetic network shown in Figure 6.9 contains four genes, **a** through **d**, which code for transcription to mRNA, which in turn serves *via* translation as a template for the proteins, **A** through **D**. The proteins **A** and **B** may form a heterodimer that activates the expression of gene **c**. Protein **C** inhibits the expression of genes **b** and **d**, which are thereby coregulated. Protein **D** activates the translation of protein **B**.

6.3.2
Representation of a Gene Regulatory Network as Graph

A directed graph G is a tuple (i.e., an ordered set) $G = (V, E)$, where V denotes a set of vertices and E a set of edges. In a gene network model, the vertices $i \in V$ correspond to the genes and the edges correspond to their regulatory interactions. An edge is a pair (i, j) of vertices. It is directed if i regulates the expression of j or, in other words, i and j

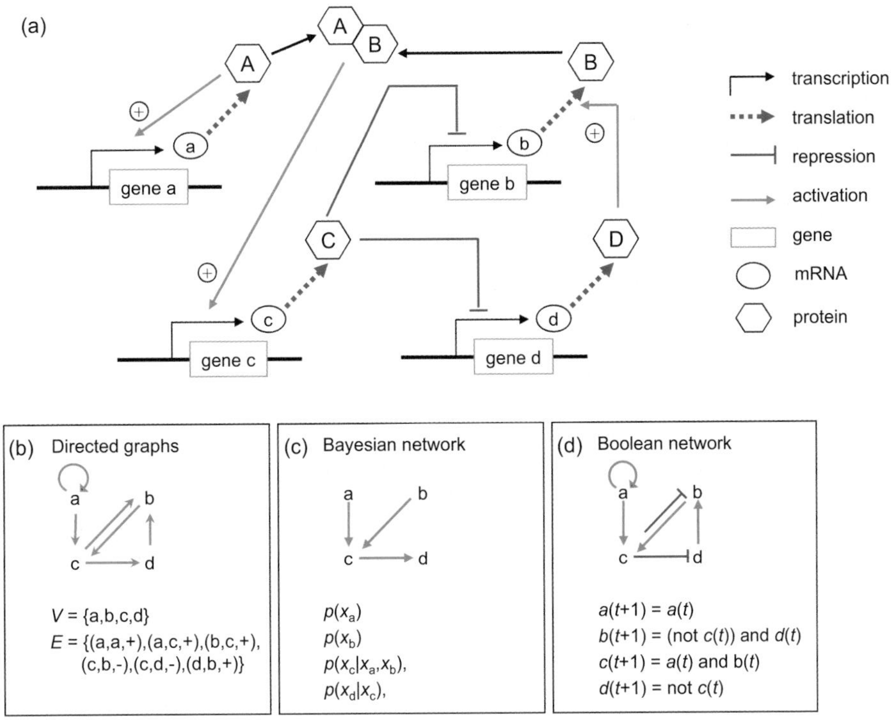

Figure 6.9 Gene regulatory network with four genes and mutual regulation.

can be assigned to tail and head of the edge, respectively. The labels of edges or vertices may be expanded to contain information about the genes and their interactions. In general, one may express an edge as a tuple (*i*, *j*, *properties*). The entry *properties* can simply indicate whether gene *i* activates (+) or inhibits (−) expression of gene *j*, as shown in Figure 6.9(c). But it can also be a list of regulators and their influence on that specific edge, such as (*i*, *j*,(*k*, activation), (*l*, inhibition as homodimeric protein)).

In principle, many databases that provide information about genetic regulation are organized as richly annotated directed graphs (e.g., Transfac, KEGG, see Chapter 16).

Directed graphs do not suffice to describe the dynamics of a network. But they may contain information that allows certain predictions about network properties, for example:

- Tracing paths between genes yields sequences of regulatory events, shows redundancy in the regulation or indicates missing regulatory interactions (that are, for example, known from experiment).
- A cycle in the graph may indicate feedback regulation.

- Comparison of gene regulatory networks of different organisms may reveal evolutionary relations and reveal targets for bioengineering and for pharmaceutical applications [72].
- The network complexity can be measured by the connectivity, i.e., the distribution and the average value of the numbers of regulators per gene or the target genes per regulator.

6.3.3 Bayesian Networks

For modeling gene expression, a Bayesian conditioning can be applied in different ways: given expression data one may attempt (i) to learn the network structure (see Section 5.2), (ii) to learn parameters of the network, or (iii) to predict its dynamics. We consider here the latter case and represent the regulatory connections in the gene network as a directed acyclic graph $\boldsymbol{G}=(V, \boldsymbol{E})$. Again, the vertices $i \in V$ represent genes and edges $\boldsymbol{E}$ denote regulatory interactions. Variables x_i belonging to the vertices i denote a property relevant to the regulation, e.g., the expression level of a gene or the amount of active protein. A conditional probability distribution $p(x_i|\boldsymbol{L}(x_i))$ is defined for each x_i, where $\boldsymbol{L}(x_i)$ is the (possibly empty) vector of *parent* variables belonging to the direct regulators of i. The directed graph $\boldsymbol{G}$ and the conditional distributions together specify a joint probability distribution $p(\boldsymbol{x})$ that characterizes the Bayesian network. The joint probability distribution can be decomposed into

$$p(\boldsymbol{x}) = \prod_i p(x_i|\boldsymbol{L}(x_i)). \qquad (6.12)$$

The directed graph expresses dependences of probabilities: The expression level of a gene represented by a child vertex depends on the expression levels of genes belonging to the parent vertices in a statistical sense. Hence, the graph structure also describes conditional independences $i(x_i;y|z)$, meaning that x_i is independent of the set of variables $\boldsymbol{y}$ given the set of variables $\boldsymbol{z}$. Two graphs or Bayesian network topologies are equivalent, if they imply the same set of independences. In this case they can be considered as the same undirected graph, but with varying direction of edges. Equivalent graphs cannot be distinguished by observation of the variables $\boldsymbol{x}$ [73].

Example 6.1

For the network given in Figure 6.9(c) the conditional independence relations are $i(x_a;x_b)$ and $i(x_d;x_a,x_b|x_c)$. The joint probability distribution of the network is

$$p(x_a, x_b, x_c, x_d) = p(x_a) \cdot p(x_b) \cdot p(x_c|x_a, x_b) \cdot p(x_d|x_c)$$

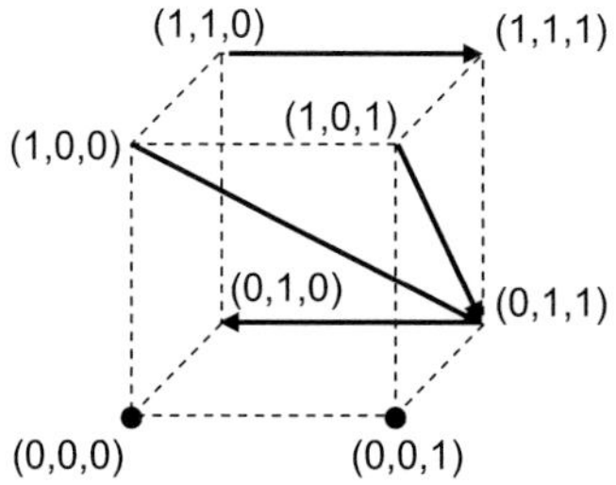

Figure 6.10 The eight possible states for a Boolean network of $N = 3$ elements (see Figure 6.15) are represented as corners of a cube. The possible transitions are symbolized by arrows. The isolated attractors are marked by black dots.

Bayesian networks have been used to deduce gene regulatory networks from gene expression data. The aim is to find the network or equivalence class of networks that best explains the measured data. A problem is the determination of initial probability distributions.

6.3.4
Boolean Networks

Boolean models are based on proposition logic formalized by George Boole, 1815–1864. This type of logic entails the principle of bivalence: any statement is either true or false. A third possibility or contradictions are excluded. Statements can be combined using the operators "and," "or," or "not" and combinations thereof. The truth value of combined statements depends only on the truth value of the individual statements and on the operation between them.

Boolean logic has been applied to biological processes such as regulation of gene expression in the framework of Kauffman's *NK* Boolean networks [74–77]. Genes are the elements of the network. Levels of gene expression are approximated by only two states: each gene is either expressed (is assigned the value "1") or not expressed ("0"). The network has N elements or *nodes*. Each element has K inputs (regulatory interactions) and one output. Inputs and output have binary values (1 or 0). Since every node can be in one of two different states, a network of N genes can assume 2^N different states. An N-dimensional vector of elements can describe the state at time t. The values are updated in discrete time steps, i.e., the value of each element at time $t + 1$ depends on the values of its inputs at time t. Boolean networks have always a finite (although possibly large) number of possible states and hence only a finite number of possible state changes. The state changes of an individual element are specified by the Boolean rules that relate the output to the inputs. There are 2^{2^K} possible Boolean rules for a node with K inputs. The rules can be labeled by numbers representing the respective binary numbers of output or rules can be associated to their meaning in normal life (*and*, *or*) (see Tables 6.1 and 6.2).

Table 6.1 Boolean rules for a node with $K = 1$ input.

Input	**Output**			
A	**0**	**A**	**not A**	**1**
0	0	0	1	1
1	0	1	0	1
Rule	0	1	2	3

Table 6.2 Boolean rules for a node with $K = 2$ inputs.

Input		**Output**															
A	**B**	**0**	**AND**		**A**		**B**	**XOR**	**OR**	**NOR**		**NOT B**		**NOT A**		**NAND**	**1**
0	0	0	0	0	0	0	0	0	0	1	1	1	1	1	1	1	1
0	1	0	0	0	0	1	1	1	1	0	0	0	0	1	1	1	1
1	0	0	0	1	1	0	0	1	1	0	0	1	1	0	0	1	1
1	1	0	1	0	1	0	1	0	1	0	1	0	1	0	1	0	1
Rule		0	1	2	3	4	5	6	7	8	9	10	11	12	13	14	15

Example 6.2

The network

$$A \rightarrow B \rightarrow C \rightarrow D \tag{6.13}$$

has the maximal connectivity $K = 1$. Let be $A = \text{const.}$, $B = f_B(A) = \text{not } A$, $C = f_C(B) = \text{not } B$, and $D = f_D(C) = C$ with the initial state $(A,B,C,D)(t_0) = (1,0,0,0)$. The following states are

$$(A, B, C, D)(t_1) = (1, 0, 1, 0)$$
$$(A, B, C, D)(t_2) = (1, 0, 1, 1)$$
$$\ldots$$
$$(A, B, C, D)(t_i) = (1, 0, 1, 1) \text{ for } i = 2, \ldots, \infty.$$

After two steps the system has attained a fixed point.

Example 6.3

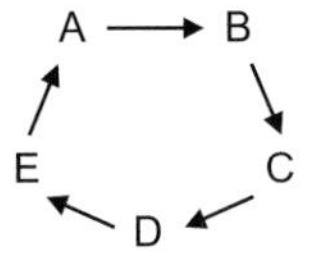

(6.14)

Another possible structure of a Boolean network with $K = 1$ is the closed loop, in which the input of the first element is the output of the last element.

Periodic behavior can occur if all elements obey rules 1 or 2 (see Table 6.1). Assume, for example, that all elements follow rule 1 and the initial state is $(ABCDE) = (10000)$. The states for the following time steps will be (01000), (00100), (00010), (00001), and again (10000), which closes the cycle. Rules 0 or 3 break the periodic behavior, since the output of the respective element is no longer dependent on the input, so they and lead to constant behavior.

Example 6.4

The network

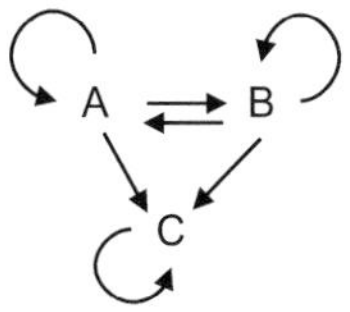

(6.15)

has $N = 3$ elements and may assume $2^N = 8$ different states. Let the rules be

$$A(t+1) = A(t) \text{ and } B(t)$$
$$B(t+1) = A(t) \text{ or } B(t)$$
$$C(t+1) = A(t) \text{ or } (\text{not } B(t) \text{ and } C(t))$$

Table 6.3 lists the possible actual states and the respective following states for (ABC). It can be seen that the states (000), (001), (010), and (111) are fixed points, since they will not be left. The states (000), (001), (100), (101), and (110) cannot be reached from other states. See also Figure 6.10.

Table 6.3 Successive states for the Boolean network depicted in (6.15).

Current state	000	001	010	011	100	101	110	111
Next state	000	001	010	010	011	011	111	111

For the network presented in Figure 6.9(d), the following Boolean rules apply:

$$\begin{aligned}
a(t+1) &= f_a(a(t)) = a(t) && \text{rule 1 for } K = 1 \\
b(t+1) &= f_b(c(t), d(t)) = (\text{not } c(t)) \text{ and } d(t) && \text{rule 2 for } K = 2 \\
c(t+1) &= f_c(a(t), b(t)) = a(t) \text{ and } b(t) && \text{rule 2 for } K = 2 \\
d(t+1) &= f_d(c(t)) = (\text{not } c(t)) && \text{rule 0 for } K = 1.
\end{aligned} \tag{6.16}$$

The temporal behavior is determined by the sequence of states (a,b,c,d) given in an initial state.

From Table 6.4 it is easy to see that this network has two different types of stationary behavior. If the initial state of **a** is 0, then the system evolves toward the steady state 0101, meaning that genes **a** and **c** are switched off, while genes **b** and **d** are switched on. If the initial state of **a** is 1, then the system evolves toward a cyclic behavior consisting of the following sequence of states: 1000 → 1001 → 1101 → 1111 → 1010 → 1000.

The sequence of states given by the Boolean transitions represents the trajectory of the system. Since the number of states in the state space is finite, the number of possible transitions is also finite. Therefore, each trajectory will lead either to a steady state or to a state cycle. These state sequences are called *attractors*. *Transient states* are those states that do not belong to an attractor. All states that lead to the same attractor constitute its *basin of attraction*.

Boolean networks have been used to explore general and global properties of large gene expression networks. Studying random networks (i.e., each gene has K inputs, and each gene is controlled by a randomly assigned Boolean function), Kauffman [75, 78] has shown that the systems exhibit highly ordered dynamics for small K and certain choices of rules. Both the median number of attractors and the cycle length of attractors are on the order of $\sqrt{N}$. Kauffman suggested to interpret the number of possible attractors as the number of possible cell types arising from the same genome.

6.3.5 Description with Ordinary Differential Equations

Gene expression can be mathematically described with systems of ordinary differential equations in the same way as dynamical systems (Section 2.1) in metabolism,

Table 6.4 Successive states for the Boolean network depicted in Figure 6.9(d).

0000 → 0001	1000 → 1001
0001 → 0101	1001 → 1101
0010 → 0000	1010 → 1000
0011 → 0000	1011 → 1000
0100 → 0001	1100 → 1011
0101 → 0101	1101 → 1111
0110 → 0000	1110 → 1010
0111 → 0000	1111 → 1010

signaling, and other cellular processes. We consider the equation system

$$\frac{dx_i}{dt} = f_i(x_1, \ldots, x_n), \quad i = 1, \ldots, n. \tag{6.17}$$

The variables x_i denote the concentrations of mRNAs, proteins, or other molecules. The functions f_i comprise the rate laws that express the changes of x_i due to transcription, translation, or other individual processes. Production terms for transcription are discussed in more detail in Section 7.2. More information about how to specify the rate equations and how to analyze the resulting ODE systems is given in Section 2.3.

Example 6.5

The dynamics of the system depicted in Figure 6.9 can be described in several ways depending on the desired level of detail. If we consider only the mRNA abundances a, b, c, d, we obtain

$$\begin{aligned}
\frac{da}{dt} &= f_a(a) \\
\frac{db}{dt} &= f_b(b, c, d) \\
\frac{dc}{dt} &= f_c(a, b, c) \\
\frac{dd}{dt} &= f_d(c, d).
\end{aligned} \tag{6.18}$$

Specific expressions for the functions f under the depicted regulatory interactions can use gene regulation functions and a linear function (i.e., mass action) for mRNA degradation, such as in the following equations:

$$\begin{aligned}
f_a(a) &= v_a - k_a \cdot a \\
f_b(b, c, d) &= \frac{V_b \cdot (d/K_b)^{n_d}}{(1 + (d/K_b)^{n_d})(1 + (c/K_{Ic})^{n_c})} - k_b \cdot b \\
f_c(a, b, c) &= \frac{V_c \cdot (a \cdot b/K_c)^{n_{ab}}}{1 + (a \cdot b/K_c)^{n_{ab}}} - k_c \cdot c \\
f_d(c, d) &= \frac{V_d}{1 + (c/K_{Ic})^{n_c}} - k_d \cdot d.
\end{aligned} \tag{6.19}$$

Here, k_a, k_b, k_c, and k_d are the first order rate constants of the degradation of mRNAs a, b, c, and d, respectively. v_a denotes the constant rate of expression of gene **a**, the Hill term $\frac{V_b \cdot (d/K_b)^{n_d}}{1 + (d/K_b)^{n_d}}$ describes the formation of **b** activated by **d** with maximal rate V_b, dissociation constant K_b, and Hill coefficient n_b. The inhibition by **c** is expressed by the term $(1 + (c/K_{Ic})^{n_c})$ in the denominator. The formation of **c** is modeled with a Hill expression that indicates a threshold (K_{Ic}) of the formation of c depending on the concentrations of **a** and **b** (Section 1.1). V_c and K_c are maximal rate and dissociation constant, respectively, and n_{ab} is the Hill coefficient. The production of **d** depends on the maximal rate V_d and on the inhibition by **c**. The dynamics for a specific choice of parameters is shown in Figure 6.11.

The ODE formalism allows for involving more details, for example the explicit consideration of the protein concentrations. Considering specifically the mRNA of gene **b** and protein **B** and assuming for the individual reaction steps either Hill, Michealis–Menten, or mass action kinetics, respectively, we get

$$\begin{aligned} \frac{d}{dt}b &= \frac{V_b}{(1+(C/K_{Ic})^{n_c})} - k_b \cdot b \\ \frac{d}{dt}B &= D \cdot \frac{V_B \cdot b}{K_B + b} - k_B \cdot B - k_{AB} \cdot A \cdot B. \end{aligned} \tag{6.20}$$

Here, we have distinguished between the processes determining the velocity of translation (basic rate V_b and inhibition by protein **C**) and of transcription (dependence on mRNA concentration **b** and on the activator concentration **D**) and on the degradation or consumption on both levels (degradation of **b** and **B** with mass action rate constants k_b and k_B, respectively, and formation of complex **AB** with rate constant k_{AB}).

Using the description with ODE systems one may take into account detailed knowledge about gene regulatory mechanisms, such as known regulation functions, individual interactions of proteins with proteins or proteins with mRNA and so on. An obstacle is the current lack of exactly this type of knowledge, the lack of kinetic constants, or time-resolved concentration data due to measurement difficulties and uncertainties in the function of many proteins and their interactions.

6.3.6
Gene Expression Modeling with Stochastic Processes

For gene expression, it can be argued that the assumptions of continuous and deterministic concentration changes employed in the description with ODEs are not valid. Each gene is present in only one, two, or a few copies. The number of transcription factor molecules is usually small (on the order of tens or hundreds).

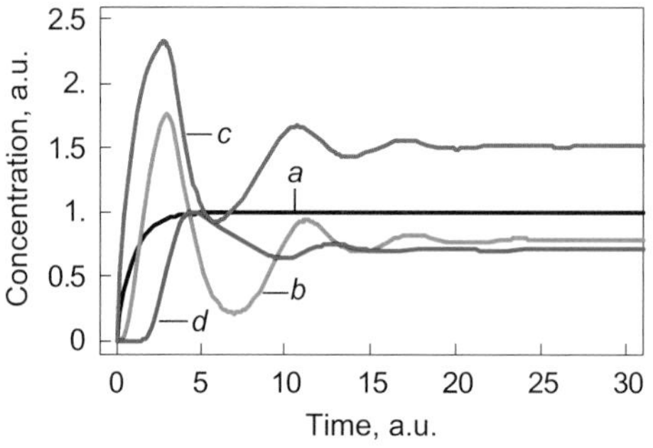

Figure 6.11 Dynamics of the mRNA concentrations of the system presented in Figure 6.9 according to Eq. (6.19). Parameters: $v_a = 1$, $k_a = 1$, $v_b = 1$, $K_b = 5$, $k_{Ic} = 0.4$, $K_b = 0.1$, $V_c = 1$, $K_c = 5$, $K_c = 0.1$, $V_d = 1$, $k_d = 1$, $n_{ab} = 4$, $n_c = 4$, $n_d = 4$. Initial conditions: $a(0) = b(0) = c(0) = d(0) = 0$.

Even the abundance of mRNA molecules is often below the detection limit. Therefore, it is not sure whether the objects of the considered processes are actually present, and the character of the events becomes probabilistic. Furthermore, the involved processes can hardly be regarded as continuous. In transcription, for instance, it takes certain time from the initiation until termination. The discrete and probabilistic character of processes is taken into account in stochastic modeling of gene regulation, which will be discussed in more detail in the next chapter. In the most common approach, the state variables are discrete molecules numbers x. The number of molecules of each species can change only by simple reaction steps (formation of a molecule, complex formation, degradation). A convenient way to simulate the dynamics of such a stochastic system is the Gillespie algorithm [74], see Section 7.2. This algorithm provides an individual realization, i.e., trace of the system through the states space as time evolves. It computes molecule numbers for each chemical species along the time axis. Repeated execution of the algorithm with the same initial conditions yields several realizations that can be used to compute means and percentile or the probability $p(x,t)$ that there are x molecules of type x present at time t.

Example 6.6

Stochastic simulation of the network presented in Figure 6.9 is shown in Figure 6.12 using the following set of reactions and parameters:

Expression of protein A from gene a,	$a \to a + A$,	$k_A = 1.0$
Expression of protein B from gene b,	$b \to b + B$,	$k_B = 1.0$
Expression of protein C from gene c,	$c \to c + C$,	$k_C = 0.2$
Expression of protein D from gene d,	$d \to d + D$,	$k_D = 1.0$
Formation of protein complex AB,	$A + B \to AB$,	$k_{AB} = 1.0$
Inhibition of gene b	$b + C \to b_I + C$,	$k_{bI} = 1.0$
Activation of gene b,	$b_I \to b$,	$k_{bA} = 0.1$
Inhibition of gene c,	$c \to c_I$,	$k_{cI} = 0.1$
Activation of gene c,	$c_I + AB \to c + AB$,	$k_{cA} = 1.0$
Inhibition of gene d,	$d + C \to d_I + C$,	$k_{dI} = 1.0$
Activation of gene d,	$d_I \to d$,	$k_{dA} = 0.1$
Degradation of protein A,	$A \to$,	$k_{Ad} = 1.0$
Degradation of protein B,	$B \to$,	$k_{Bd} = 0.1$
Degradation of protein C,	$C \to$,	$k_{Cd} = 1.0$
Degradation of protein D,	$D \to$,	$k_{Dd} = 1.0$
Degradation of protein complex AB,	$AB \to$,	$k_{ABd} = 1.0$

(6.21)

The parameters $k\ldots$ times the current numbers of substrate molecules provide the probability that the respective reaction occurs in the next time step. Figure 6.12 shows protein abundances for an individual simulation run (a), the average over 100 simulation runs (b), both done with Gillespie's direct method, and the deterministic simulation (c).

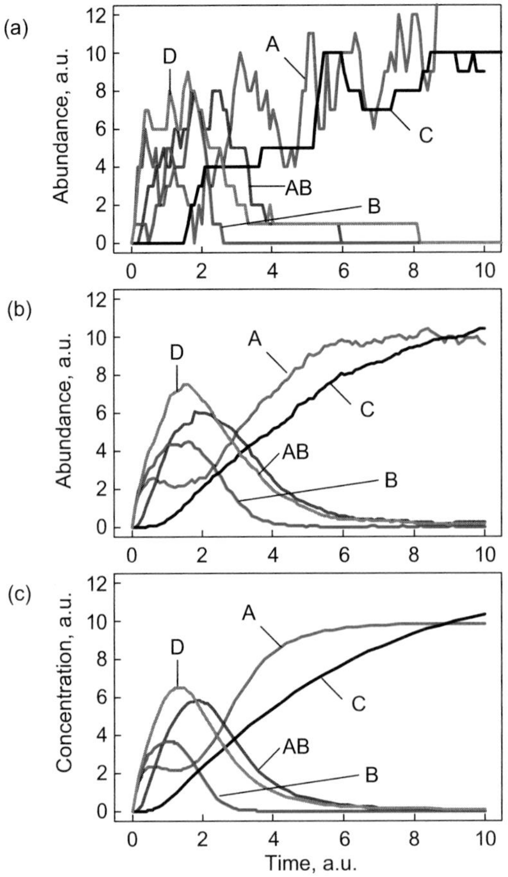

Figure 6.12 Stochastic simulations of the reaction network shown in Figure 6.9 using the system (6.21). (a) Individual simulation run, (b) average over 100 simulation runs, both simulated with Gillespie's direct method, and (c) deterministic simulation. Parameters: see text, initial abundances: gene a = 10; protein A = 0; gene b = 10; gene bi = 0; protein B = 0; gene c = 0; gene ci = 10; protein C = 0; gene d = 10; gene di = 0; protein D = 0; complex AB = 0.

Exercises and Problems

1. Show that the occupation probability $\frac{Z_1}{Z_1+Z_0}$ in Section 6.2.3, with $n \ll N$, yields approximately Eq. (6.5).

2. Assume that the concentration of mRNA follows a kinetic model

$$\frac{dc(t)}{dt} = \nu(t) - \mu\, c(t)$$

with a constant degradation rate μ. How can the transcription rate $\nu(t)$ be computed from experimental measurements of $c(t)$? Assume that $c(t)$ is given as a continuous curve and that the measurements are exact. Describe the limiting cases $\mu \to 0$ and $\mu \to \infty$. Which difficulties will arise with real-world data?

3. In a genetic network, gene C is regulated by genes A and B with an AND function, D by A and C with an OR function, A by D and C with XOR function (rule 6, Table 6.2), and B by B and D with NAND function (rule 14). Sketch the network. Find out all possible states and all attractors (steady states).

4. Two genes A and B regulate each other negatively. Describe their interaction with ODEs with increasing detail: (i) A directly inhibits B and vice versa. (ii) Both code for mRNA, which acts as an inhibitor. (iii) Both code for mRNA, which is translated to protein, which in turn act as transcription factors downregulating their targets. Formulate the ODE systems in the most simple way. What are the effects of including increasing number of levels in the analysis?

References

1 Orphanides, G. and Reinberg, D. (2002) A unified theory of gene expression. *Cell*, **108**, 439–451.

2 Proudfoot, N.J. *et al.* (2002) Integrating mRNA processing with transcription. *Cell*, **108**, 501–512.

3 Alberts, B. *et al.* (2002) *Molecular Biology of the Cell*, 4th Edition, Garland Science, New York.

4 Tupler, R. *et al.* (2001) Expressing the human genome. *Nature*, **409**, 832–833.

5 Allison, L.A. *et al.* (1985) Extensive homology among the largest subunits of eukaryotic and prokaryotic RNA polymerases. *Cell*, **42**, 599–610.

6 Woychik, N.A. and Hampsey, M. (2002) The RNA polymerase II machinery: structure illuminates function. *Cell*, **108**, 453–463.

7 Ptashne, M. and Gann, A. (1997) Transcriptional activation by recruitment. *Nature*, **386**, 569–577.

8 Berg, O.G. and von Hippel, P.H. (1987) Selection of DNA binding sites by regulatory proteins. Statistical mechanical theory and application to operators and promoters. *J Mol Biol*, **193**, 723–750.

9 Juven-Gershon, T. *et al.* (2008) The RNA polymerase II core promoter – the gateway to transcription. *Curr Opin Cell Biol*, **20**, 253–259.

10 Smale, S.T. (1994) Core promoter architecture for eukaryotic protein-coding genes, in *Transcription: Mechanisms and Regulation* (eds R.C. Conaway and J.W. Conaway), Raven Press, New York, pp. 63–81.

11 Novina, C.D. and Roy, A.L. (1997) Core promoters and transcriptional control. *Trends Genet*, **12**, 351–355.

12 Burke, T.W. and Kadonga, J.T. (1997) The downstream promoter element, DPE, is conserved from *Drosophila* to humans and is recognized by TAF-II60 of *Drosophila*. *Genes Dev*, **11**, 3020–3031.

13 Kadonaga, J.T. (2004) Regulation of RNA polymerase II transcription by sequence-specific DNA binding factors. *Cell*, **116**, 247–257.

14 Pedersen, A.G. *et al.* (1999) The biology of eukaryotic promoter prediction – a review. *Comput Chem 1999*, 191–207.

15 Fickett, J.W. and Hatzigeorgiou, A.C. (1997) *Eukaryotic promoter recognition, Genome Res,* **7**, 861–878.

16 Stormo, G.D. (2000) DNA binding sites: representation and discovery. *Bioinformatics,* **16**, 16–23.

17 Werner, T. (2003) The state-of-the-art of mammalian promoter recognition. *Briefings Bioinf,* **4**, 22–30.

18 Bajic, V.B. *et al.* (2006) Performance assessment of promoter predictions on ENCODE regions in the EGASP experiment. *Genome Biol,* **7** (1), S3 1–13.

19 Kel, A. *et al.* (1995) Computer tool FUNSITE for analysis of eukaryotic regulatory genomic sequences. *ISMB,* **3**, 197–205.

20 Matys, V. *et al.* (2006) TRANSFAC and its module TRANSCompel: transcriptional gene regulation in eukaryotes. *Nucleic Acids Res,* **34**, D108–D110.

21 Kel-Margoulis, O.V. *et al.* (2002) TRANSCompel: a database on composite regulatory elements in eukaryotic genes. *Nucleic Acids Res,* **30**, 332–334.

22 Hutchinson, G.B. (1996) The prediction of vertebrate promoter regions using differential hexamer frequency analysis. *CABIOS,* **12**, 391–398.

23 Scherf, M. *et al.* (2000) Highly specific localization of promoter regions in large genomic sequences by PromoterInspector: a novel context analysis approach. *J Mol Biol,* **297**, 599–606.

24 Prestridge, D.S. (1995) Prediction of pol II promoter sequences using transcription factor binding sites. *J Mol Biol,* **249**, 923–932.

25 Reese, M.G. (2001) Application of a time-delay neural network to promoter annotation in the Drosophila melanogaster genome. *Comput Chem,* **26**, 51–56.

26 Birney, E. *et al.* (2007) Identification and analysis of functional elements in 1% of the human genome by the ENCODE pilot project. *Nature,* **447**, 799–816.

27 Cooper, S.J. *et al.* (2006) Comprehensive analysis of transcriptional promoter structure and function in 1% of the human genome. *Genome Res,* **16**, 1–10.

28 Tavazoie, S. *et al.* (1999) Systematic determination of genetic network architecture. *Nat Genet,* **22**, 281–285.

29 Elkon, R. *et al.* (2003) Genome-wide in silico identification of transcriptional regulatiors controlling the cell cycle in human cells. *Genome Res,* **13**, 773–780.

30 Macisaac, K.D. *et al.* (2006) A hypothesis-based approach for identifying the binding specificity of regulatory proteins from chromatin immunoprecipitation data. *Bioinformatics,* **22**, 423–429.

31 Gordon, D.B. *et al.* (2005) TAMO: a flexible, object-oriented framework for analyzing transcriptional regulation using DNA-sequence motifs. *Bioinformatics,* **21**, 3164–3165.

32 Sandelin, A. *et al.* (2004) JASPAR: an open-access database for eukaryotic transcription factor binding profiles. *Nucleic Acids Res,* **32**, D91–D94.

33 Wasserman, W.W. *et al.* (2000) Human-mouse genome comparisons to locate regulatory sites. *Nat Genet,* **26**, 225–228.

34 Dieterich, C. *et al.* (2003) CORG: a database for COmparative Regulatory Genomics. *Nucleic Acids Res,* **31**, 55–57.

35 Thakurta, D.G. *et al.* (2002) Identification of a novel cis-regulatory element involved in the heat shock response in *C. elegans* using microarray gene expression and computational methods. *Genome Res,* **12**, 701–712.

36 Fatemi, M. *et al.* (2005) Footprinting of mammalian promoters: use of a CpG DNA methyltransferase revealing nucleosome positions at a single molecule level. *Nucleic Acids Res,* **33**, e176.

37 Saxonov, S. *et al.* (2006) A genome-wide analysis of CpG dinucleotides in the human genome distinguishes two distinct classes of promoters. *Proc Natl Acad Sci USA,* **103**, 1412–1417.

38 Ambros, V. (2004) The functions of animal microRNAs, *Nature*, **431**, 350–355.

39 Bartel, D.P. (2004) MicroRNAs: genomics, biogenesis, mechanism, and function. *Cell*, **116**, 281–297.

40 O'Donnell, K.A. *et al.* (2005) c-Myc-regulated microRNAs modulate E2F1 expression, *Nature*, **435**, 839–843.

41 Berezikov, E. *et al.* (2006) Approaches to microRNA discovery. *Nat Genet*, **38**, S2–S7.

42 Bentwich, I. (2005) Prediction and validation of microRNAs and their targets. *FEBS Lett*, **579**, 5904–5910.

43 Lim, L.P. *et al.* (2003a) Vertebrate microRNA genes. *Science*, **299**, 1540.

44 Griffiths-Jones, S. *et al.* (2008) miRBase: tools for microRNA genomics. *Nucleic Acids Res*, **36**, D154–D158.

45 Sethupathy, P. *et al.* (2006) A guide through present computational approaches for the identification of mammalian microRNA targets. *Nat Methods*, **3**, 881–886.

46 Paddison, P.J. and Hannon, G.J. (2002) RNA interference: the new somatic cell genetics? *Cancer Cell*, **2**, 17–23.

47 Carrington, J.C. and Ambros, V. (2003) Role of microRNAs in plant and animal development. *Science*, **301**, 336–338.

48 Fire, A. *et al.* (1998) Potent and specific genetic interference by double-stranded RNA *in Caenorhabditis elegans*. *Nature*, **391**, 806–811.

49 Reinhart, B.J. *et al.* (2002) MicroRNAs in plants. *Genes Dev*, **16**, 1616–1626.

50 Lim, L.P. *et al.* (2003b) The microRNAs of Caenorhabditis elegans, *Genes Dev*, **17**, 991–1008.

51 Lagos-Quintana, M. *et al.* (2002) Identification of tissue-specific microRNAs from mouse. *Curr Biol*, **12**, 735–739.

52 Babaie, Y. *et al.* (2007) Analysis of Oct4-dependent transcriptional networks regulating self-renewal and pluripotency in human embryonic stem cells. *Stem Cells*, **25**, 500–510.

53 Ptashne, M. and Gann, A. (2002) *Genes and Signals*, Cold Spring Harbor Laboratory Press, Cold Spring Harbor, NY.

54 Keseler, I.M., Collado-Vides, J., Gama-Castro, S., Ingraham, J., Paley, S., Paulsen, I.T., Peralta-Gil, M. and Karp, P.D. (2005) EcoCyc: A comprehensive database resource for *Escherichia coli*. *Nucleic Acids Research*, **33** (Database issue): D334–D337.

55 Setty, Y., Mayo, A.E., Surette, M.G. and Alon, U. (2003) Detailed map of a *cis*-regulatory input function. *Proc Natl Acad Sci USA*, **100** (13), 7702–7707.

56 Yuh, C.H., Bolouri, H. and Davidson, E.H. (1998) Genomic cis-regulatory logic: experimental and computational analysis of a sea urchin gene. *Science*, **279**, 1896–1902.

57 Bintu, L., Buchler, N.E., Garcia, H.G., Gerland, U., Hwa, T., Kondev, J. and Phillips, R. (2005) Transcriptional regulation by numbers: models. *Curr Opin Genet Dev*, **15**, 116–124.

58 Bintu, L., Buchler, N.E., Garcia, H.G., Gerland, U., Hwa, T., Kondev, J., Kuhlman, T. and Phillips, R. (2005) Transcriptional regulation by numbers: applications. *Curr Opin Genet Dev*, **15**, 125–135.

59 Kalir, S. and Alon, U. (2004) Using a quantitative blueprint to reprogram the dynamics of the flagella gene network. *Cell*, **117**, 713–720.

60 Kaplan, S., Bren, A., Zaslaver, A., Dekel, E. and Alon, U. (2008) Diverse two-dimensional input functions control bacterial sugar genes. *Molecular Cell*, **29**, 786–792.

61 Santillán, M. and Mackey, M.C. (2004) Influence of catabolite repression and inducer exclusion on the bistable behavior of the Lac operon. *Biophys J*, **86**, 1282–1292.

62 Mayo, A.E., Setty, Y., Shavit, S., Zaslaver, A. and Alon, U. (2006) Plasticity of the *cis*-regulatory input function of a gene. *PLoS Biol*, **4** (4), e45.

63 Ronen, M., Rosenberg, R., Shraiman, B.I. and Alon, U. (2002) Assigning numbers to the arrows: parametrizing a gene regulation network by using accurate expression kinetics. *Proc Natl Acad Sci USA*, **99** (16), 10555–10560.

64 Barenco, M., Tomescu, D., Brewer, D., Callard, R., Stark, J. and Hubank, M. (2006) Ranked prediction of p53 targets using hidden variable dynamic modelling. *Genome Biology*, **7** (3), R25.

65 Liao, J.C., Boscolo, R., Yang, Y., Tran, L.M., Sabatti, C. and Roychowdhury, V.P. (2003) Network component analysis: Reconstruction of regulatory signals in biological systems. *Proc Natl Acad Sci USA*, **100** (26), 15522–15527.

66 Kao, K.C. *et al.* (2004) Transcriptome-based determination of multiple transcription regulator activities in *Escherichia coli* by using network component analysis. *Proc Natl Acad Sci USA*, **101** (2), 641–646.

67 Salgado, H., Gama-Castro, S., Martínez-Antonio, A., Díaz-Peredo, E., Sánchez-Solano, F., Peralta-Gil, M., Garcia-Alonso, D., Jiménez-Jacinto, V., Santos-Zavaleta, A., Bonavides-Martínez, C. and Collado-Vides, J. (2004) RegulonDB (version 4.0): Transcriptional regulation, operon organization and growth conditions in *Escherichia coli* K-12. *Nucleic Acids Res*, 303–306.

68 Lee, T.I., Rinaldi, N.J., Robert, F., Odom, D.T., Bar-Joseph, Z., Gerber, G.K., Hannett, N.M., Harbison, C.T., Thompson, C.M., Simon, I., Zeitlinger, J., Jennings, E.G., Murray, H.L., Gordon, D.B., Ren, B., Wyrick, J.J., Tagne, J.B., Volkert, T.L., Fraenkel, E., Gifford, D.K. and Young, R.A. 2002 Transcriptional regulatory networks in *Saccharomyces cerevisiae*. *Science*, **298**, 799–804.

69 Alter, O., Brown, P.O. and Botstein, D. (2000) Singular value decomposition for genome-wide expression data processing and modelling. *Proc Natl Acad Sci USA*, **97** (18), 10101–10106.

70 Liebermeister, W. (2002) Linear modes of gene expression determined by independent component analysis. *Bioinformatics*, **18**, 51–60.

71 Crick, F. (1970) Central dogma of molecular biology. *Nature*, **227**, 561–563.

72 Dandekar, T. *et al.* (1999) Pathway alignment: application to the comparative analysis of glycolytic enzymes. *Biochem J*, **343**, (Pt 1) 115–124.

73 Friedman, N. *et al.* (2000) Using Bayesian networks to analyze expression data. *J Comput Biol*, **7**, 601–620.

74 Kauffman, S.A. and Weinberger, E.D. (1989) The NK model of rugged fitness landscapes and its application to maturation of the immune response. *J Theor Biol*, **141**, 211–245.

75 Kauffman, S.A. and Johnsen, S. (1991) Coevolution to the edge of chaos: coupled fitness landscapes, poised states, and coevolutionary avalanches. *J Theor Biol*, **149**, 467–505.

76 Kauffman, S.A. (1993) *The Origins of Order: Self-Organization and Selection in Evolution*, Oxford University Press, New York.

77 Kauffman, S.A. and Macready, W.G. (1995) Search strategies for applied molecular evolution. *J Theor Biol*, **173**, 427–440.

78 Kauffman, S.A. (1991) Antichaos and adaptation. *Sci Am*, **265**, 78–84.

79 Gillespie, D.T. (1977) Exact stochastic simulation of coupled chemical chemical reactions. *J Phys Chem*, **81**, 2340–2361.

80 Kamburov, A., Wierling, C., Lehrach, H., Herwig, R. (2009) ConsensusPathDB – A database for integrating human functional interaction networks. *Nucleic Acids Res.*, **37** (Database issue): D623–D628.

7
Stochastic Systems and Variability

7.1
Stochastic Modeling of Biochemical Reactions

Summary

On a microscopic level, chemical reactions are random events that lead to fluctuating amounts of substance molecules. The dynamics of chemical systems can be modeled by different types of mathematical random processes, based on individual reaction events (calculation by the chemical Master equation or direct simulation), their frequencies in given time intervals (calculation by the τ-leaping method), or randomly drifting substance concentrations (chemical Langevin equation). These random processes entail deterministic kinetic models as a limiting case. Temporal fluctuations of substance amounts can be characterized by autocorrelations and spectral densities.

The cellular machinery differs a lot from the machines we see in our everyday life: on a microscopic level, individual molecules are constantly formed and destroyed by chemical reactions. Proteins and other molecules tumble back and forth, diffuse, change their conformations, assemble and disassemble in permanent thermal movement. Thermal movement and chemical reactions can be described mathematically by random processes (see Chapter 14): reactions happen unpredictably, and each sequence of random events leads to a different history of the system. Stochastic models allow us to compute mean values, fluctuations, and temporal correlations of system states [1]. Furthermore, individual realizations of random processes can be obtained by stochastic simulation.

On larger space and time scales, the microscopic processes translate into an effective macroscopic behavior, for instance, the dynamics of metabolic pathways governed by kinetic laws. Random models provide a more detailed description than the deterministic kinetic models presented in the chapters before. Whenever the random fluctuations remain small, deterministic models provide a good and numerically cheap approximation. However, random fluctuations can become important if

Systems Biology: A Textbook. Edda Klipp, Wolfram Liebermeister, Christoph Wierling, Axel Kowald, Hans Lehrach, and Ralf Herwig

ISBN: 978-3-527-31874-2

molecule numbers are low – which typically happens in gene expression – or in models with nonlinear and unstable dynamics.

In this chapter, we shall discuss stochastic models of biochemical systems. They are based on (i) individual stochastic reaction events; (ii) randomly varying count numbers of reactions within discrete time intervals; (iii) randomly fluctuating reaction velocities in continuous time. For large particle numbers in well-mixed systems, the random dynamics lead to (iv) deterministic laws as a limiting case [2]. Stochastic biochemical models apply to all kinds of biochemical systems including metabolic and gene expression networks. A given biochemical system can be described in all four frameworks, each being an approximation of the previous one.

7.1.1 Chemical Random Process for Molecule Numbers

Molecule numbers in cells fluctuate in time due to random production and degradation events. As a simple case, let us consider a single type of molecules described by an integer number $x(t)$. In a chemical random process, we assume that production occurs with a constant propensity (probability per time unit), while the degradation propensity is proportional to the number of molecules present. Such a process may serve as a simple model for mRNA turnover (constitutive transcription, linear degradation), but it can also describe how molecules enter or leave a spatial volume by diffusion. Mathematically, it is defined as a Markov process (see Chapter 14) with continuous time and the transitions:

Event	Transition	Propensity
Production	$x \rightarrow x+1$	$a_+(x) = w_+$
Degradation	$x \rightarrow x-1$	$a_-(x) = w_- x$

(7.1)

At time point t, the system is in a state $x(t)$ and the next reaction event can occur at any moment in time. To quantify the probabilities for different events, we consider a short time interval $[t, t + \Delta t]$. In the limit $[\Delta t \rightarrow 0]$ (infinitely short interval), each possible event $l = +$ (production) or $l = -$ (degradation) would occur with a probability $p_l \approx a_l \Delta t$, and we can neglect the possibility that more than one event occurs.

In Eq. (7.1), we thus distinguish between two kinds of rate: the *propensities* $a_\pm(t)$ refer to the absolute rate of reaction events (for all molecules together), while the degradation rate w_- refers to single molecules. The degradation rate $a_-(x)$, for example, is proportional to x because each of the existing x molecules can be degraded with rate w_-; it is zero if no molecule is present. Production events, on the other hand, occur with a constant rate $a_+ = w_+$ (in units of 1/s). We assume that both rates w_l are constant, but the propensity a_- will change in time because it depends on the system state $x(t)$.

The random process (7.1) gives rise to a time-dependent probability distribution $p_x(t)$ on the state space, which assigns a probability to each possible molecule number x.

For a large ensemble of cells, this probability corresponds to the percentage of cells that show a particular state at time t. The distribution $p_x(t)$ changes in time according to the chemical Master equation (see Chapter 14)

$$\begin{aligned}\frac{dp_x}{dt} &= a_+(x-1)p_{x-1}+a_-(x+1)p_{x+1} \\ &\quad -a_+(x)p_x-a_-(x)p_x.\end{aligned} \tag{7.2}$$

The terms on the right-hand side correspond to the four possible events that may change the probability of state x: the system can move to the state x from the states $x-1$ (by production) or $x+1$ (by degradation), and it can leave the state x by the production or degradation of a molecule. To solve Eq. (7.2), we need to specify an initial condition: for instance, if the system starts with exactly one molecule at $t=0$ for all realizations of the ensemble, we choose $p_1(0)=1$ and $p_j(0)=0$ for all $j\neq 1$. The stationary distribution of Eq. (7.2) is a Poisson distribution $p(x,\lambda)=(\lambda^x e^{-\lambda})/x!$ with average value and variance

$$\lambda=\langle x\rangle=\mathrm{var}(x)=w_+/w_-. \tag{7.3}$$

The random process (7.1) corresponds to a macroscopic kinetic model

$$\frac{ds}{dt}=v_+-v_-=\alpha-\beta s \tag{7.4}$$

for the production and degradation of a substance (concentration s) in a volume V. The stoichiometric matrix $\mathbf{N}=(1,-1)$ and the velocity vector $v=(\alpha,\ \beta s)^T$ correspond to the events and rates in model (7.1), and the parameters of the two models are related by $V\alpha=w_+$ and $\beta=w_-$. The kinetic model (7.4) yields a steady-state concentration $s^{st}=\alpha/\beta$ corresponding to a molecule number $x^{st}=V\alpha/\beta$, which equals – in this linear model – the mean value (7.3) of the stochastic process. If we consider large volume sizes $V\to\infty$ while keeping this mean concentration fixed (the so-called *thermodynamic limit*), the relative fluctuation width $\sqrt{\mathrm{var}(x)}/\langle x\rangle$ of the stochastic model tends to zero. We can thus regard the kinetic model as a limiting case of the stochastic model (7.1) for infinite volumes V.

7.1.2
The Chemical Master Equation

The above approach can be generalized to arbitrary biochemical systems with irreversible kinetics [3]. If a model contains reversible reactions, they have to be split first into irreversible forward and backward reactions. To translate a kinetic model into a stochastic process, we define the states x and state transitions, specify the propensities $a_l(\mathbf{x})$, and determine the chemical Master equation. For a well-mixed system, substrate molecules hit each other with a rate proportional to the substrate concentrations, which leads to a mass-action law for the propensities. Complex reactions can be described by breaking them down into elementary steps following a mass-action law or, approximately, by computing the propensities by effective (e.g., Michaelis–Menten) kinetic laws [4].

In general, we consider a biochemical reaction system with m substance species S_i, irreversible reactions R_l, and the stoichiometric matrix $\boldsymbol{N}$. The system state, a vector $x \in \mathbb{N}^m$, contains the molecule numbers of all substances, and a reaction R_l changes the molecule numbers by

$$x_i \rightarrow x_i + n_{il} \quad \text{or} \quad \boldsymbol{x} \rightarrow \boldsymbol{x} + \boldsymbol{n}_l, \tag{7.5}$$

where $\boldsymbol{n}_l$ is the lth column of $\boldsymbol{N}$. As above, we assume that reactions occur randomly with propensities a_l: to compute them, we consider a well-stirred mixture of molecules in a volume V. Formulae for the propensities follow from kinetic theory: each reaction rate depends on how many substrate molecules are available, how often the substrates of a reaction come into close vicinity, and how often such a contact leads to a successful reaction. A unimolecular reaction R_l with a single substrate S_i occurs with a constant rate w_l per substrate molecule, leading to a propensity $a_l(\boldsymbol{x}) = w_l\, x_i$. The rate w_l (measured in units 1/s) is identical to the mass-action rate constant k_l in the corresponding kinetic model, irrespective of the system volume. For other reaction stoichiometries, however, k_l has to be rescaled with the system volume in order to obtain w_l. Propensities for different types of reaction and their relation to rate constants are listed in Table 7.1. If a reaction R_l is catalyzed by a substance S_i, the formula for the propensity $a_l(\boldsymbol{x})$ has to be modified: the molecule number x_i appears as another prefactor in a_l, and the scaling with V changes accordingly.

Like in the process (7.1), the time-dependent distribution $p(x_1, \ldots, x_m, t)$ of system states is governed by the *chemical Master equation*, a differential equation system for the probabilities in state space:

$$\frac{\mathrm{d}p(\boldsymbol{x}, t)}{\mathrm{d}t} = \sum_l a_l(\boldsymbol{x} - \boldsymbol{n}_l)p(\boldsymbol{x} - \boldsymbol{n}_l, t) - \sum_l a_l(\boldsymbol{x})p(\boldsymbol{x}, t). \tag{7.6}$$

Each state $\boldsymbol{x}$ gives rise to one differential equation (7.6), and all these equations together are called the chemical Master equation. If we consider the process (7.1) as a simple biochemical reaction system, we can easily recognize Eq. (7.2) as a special case of Eq. (7.6). In Eq. (7.6), the states $\boldsymbol{x}$ are written symbolically as function arguments;

Table 7.1 Rates for different types of biochemical reaction (no substrate, one substrate, two substrates, two substrate molecules of the same type).

Reaction	Formula	Propensity	Scaling
No substrate	$0 \rightarrow \cdots$	$a_l = w_l$	$w_l = k_l V$
Unimolecular	$A \rightarrow \cdots$	$a_l = w_l\, x_A$	$w_l = k_l$
Bimolecular	$A + B \rightarrow \cdots$	$a_l = w_l\, x_A x_B$	$w_l = k_l / V$
Bimolecular	$A + A \rightarrow \cdots$	$a_l = \frac{1}{2} w_l\, x_A(x_A - 1)$	$w_l = k_l / V$

alternatively, they also could be written as discrete subscripts (e.g., $P\boldsymbol{x}(t)$). The first positive term in Eq. (7.6) enumerates all realizations that start in a state $\boldsymbol{x} - \boldsymbol{n}_l$ and lead to state $\boldsymbol{x}$ via a reaction R_l; the second, negative term collects all realizations that exit state $\boldsymbol{x}$. The propensities for impossible states $\boldsymbol{x} - \boldsymbol{n}_l$ with negative molecule numbers are defined as zero. For analytical solutions of the chemical Master equation, see [5].

7.1.3 Stochastic Simulation

Individual realizations of a random process can be obtained from stochastic (or "Monte Carlo") simulation: just like random numbers are realizations of a random variable, stochastic simulation draws random histories from the process according to their probability density. Gillespie has introduced various simulation methods for chemical random models with continuous time and discrete particle numbers [6, 7], which also apply to other Markov jump processes (see Chapter 14). The methods yield individual realizations of the process or, in other words, possible histories of the system. Stochastic simulation methods for biochemical systems are implemented, e.g., in the software tools Dizzy and Copasi (see Chapter 17).

7.1.3.1 Direct Method

The *direct method* [6] simulates a series of individual transitions (e.g., chemical reaction events in continuous time). First, we choose an initial state $x(t=0)$. Then, we iteratively simulate individual transitions; each of them is simulated as follows:

1. Determine all possible transitions R_l from the current state and compute their rates $w_l(x)$.
2. To simulate the next transition, decide *when* it will happen and *which* reaction will happen: the waiting time Δt is drawn from an exponential random distribution with characteristic time $\tau = 1/\sum_l a_l(x)$. Then, one of the possible transitions is chosen randomly; the propensities $a_l(x)$ are used as probability weights, i.e., probabilities for the transitions are calculated as $p_l = a_l(x)/\left(\sum_j a_j(x)\right)$, where the sum runs over all possible transitions starting in x.
3. Update the system state x and the time t and then choose the next transition (step 2).

The simulation of single transitions continues until a history of duration T has been completed. By repeating the simulations, we obtain a large collection of realizations; statistical properties of the process itself – like mean behavior, time correlations, and probabilities for specific qualitative behavior – can then be estimated from a statistics over the realizations.

The direct method becomes numerically expensive if certain reactions (e.g., a fast conversion between two substances) occur very frequently while others are much slower. In this case, it will take many steps until all possible reactions have occurred in considerable numbers. This problem can be avoided by using either the explicit τ-leaping method or hybrid methods in which fast reactions are effectively described by ordinary differential equations [8].

7.1.3.2 Explicit τ-Leaping Method

In the *explicit τ-leaping method* [9, 10], we do not simulate individual events; instead, we consider time intervals of fixed length τ and compute how often each reaction occurs in the current time interval. As an approximation, we assume that the propensities remain constant within each time interval: in this case, the numbers of reaction events follow independent Poisson distributions, so we can simulate them by Poisson-distributed random variables. To compute an entire realization of the process, an initial state is picked at random; then one iteratively computes the reaction propensities, chooses the numbers of events for the next interval (by drawing them from a Poisson distribution), and updates the system state. A series of such time intervals yields a complete simulation of the process.

The efficiency and the approximation error of the explicit τ-leaping method depend on the size of τ: if the time intervals are large, many reaction events will occur within each interval, and the τ-leaping method becomes much faster than the direct method. At the same time, however, the assumption of constant propensities within each interval may lose its justification and the approximation error increases. The method is justified best for large particle numbers because in this case, many reaction events can occur without considerably changing the propensities.

7.1.3.3 Stochastic Simulation and Spatial Models

To justify the above random models for chemical reactions, we assumed a well-stirred mixture in which molecules move freely and diffusion is much faster than the chemical reactions. In reality, however, heterogeneous distribution of substances, special geometries, and compartment structure can affect the overall reaction rates. To model spatially heterogeneous systems, we can employ the same stochastic methods as for well-mixed systems; we just have to split the cell into many spatial subvolumes and describe the cell state by molecule numbers for the individual volumes. Mixing within the cell is modeled explicitly by diffusion events between subvolumes, but we still assume fast mixing within the subvolumes.

Spatial modeling enlarges the state space considerably: to describe m molecular species by their numbers in n volume elements, we need a state vector of length $m{\cdot}n$. Instead of describing molecules by count numbers, we may also track the fate of individual molecules. If the number of molecules is small and their detailed positions and conformations play a role, each of them can be characterized by an individual state, and Gillespie's algorithms can be used.

7.1.4 The Chemical Langevin Equation

The stochastic model given by Eq. (7.5) describes the molecules by discrete numbers that are changed by individual reaction events. Gillespie has proposed another approximation in which molecule numbers are represented by real-valued variables

x_i following a Brownian-motion-like dynamics in state space [3]. The resulting model is described by a Langevin equation (see Chapter 14)

$$\frac{dx_i(t)}{dt} = \sum_l n_{il}\, a_l(\boldsymbol{x}(t)) + \sum_l n_{il} \sqrt{a_l(\boldsymbol{x}(t))}\, \xi_l(t) \tag{7.7}$$

called the *chemical Langevin equation*. The term $\xi_l(t)$ denotes Gaussian white noise with mean $\langle \xi_l \rangle = 0$ and covariance function $\left\langle \xi_j(t_1)\, \xi_l(t_2) \right\rangle = \delta_{jl}\, \delta(t_1 - t_2)$ with Kronecker's δ_{jl} and Dirac's $\delta(t)$ distribution.

By introducing the substance concentrations $s_i = x_i/V$ (measured here in molecules per volume, not moles per volume) and reaction velocities $v_l(\boldsymbol{s}(\boldsymbol{x})) = a_l(\boldsymbol{x})/V$ and dividing Eq. (7.7) by the available volume V, we obtain a Langevin equation for concentrations:

$$\frac{ds_i(t)}{dt} = \sum_l n_{il}\, v_l(\boldsymbol{s}(t)) + \sum_l n_{il} \sqrt{v_l(\boldsymbol{s}(t))/V}\, \xi_l(t). \tag{7.8}$$

In contrast to the corresponding kinetic model – which would contain only the first term (see Section 2.3.1) – each reaction velocity contains an additive noise term. The noise amplitude scales with the square root of the mean reaction velocity and inversely with the square root of the volume. If the volume is increased at fixed mean concentrations, the relative contribution of the second term will decrease, and for very large systems (thermodynamic limit), the noise term becomes arbitrarily small.

The noise term in the chemical Langevin equation leads to deviations from the deterministic trajectory in state space. If the Jacobian along the trajectory is stable (negative real parts of the eigenvalues) and if particle numbers are very high, the system will show small fluctuations around the mean trajectory. Fluctuations around a (macroscopic) stable steady state can be computed using a linear approximation: with reaction velocities $v_l = a_l/V$, we can linearize Eqs. (7.7) for particle numbers and (7.8) for concentrations, which yields

$$\frac{d\boldsymbol{x}}{dt} \approx \boldsymbol{A}\boldsymbol{x} + V\boldsymbol{B}\,\xi \tag{7.9}$$

$$\frac{d\boldsymbol{s}}{dt} \approx \boldsymbol{A}\boldsymbol{s} + \boldsymbol{B}\,\xi, \tag{7.10}$$

with the Jacobian $\boldsymbol{A} = \boldsymbol{N}\,\tilde{\boldsymbol{\varepsilon}}$ (see Section 2.3.1) and the matrix $\boldsymbol{B} = V^{-1/2}\boldsymbol{N}\,\mathrm{Dg}(\boldsymbol{v})^{1/2}$. We obtain the same elasticity matrix for concentrations and reaction rates ($\tilde{\boldsymbol{\varepsilon}} = \partial \boldsymbol{v}/\partial \boldsymbol{c}$) and for molecule numbers and propensities ($\tilde{\boldsymbol{\varepsilon}} = \partial \boldsymbol{a}/\partial \boldsymbol{x}$). Given the matrices $\boldsymbol{A}$ and $\boldsymbol{B}$, we can compute the covariance matrix of $\boldsymbol{x}$, $\boldsymbol{Q} = \mathrm{cov}(\boldsymbol{x})$ from the Lyapunov equation (see Chapter 15)

$$\boldsymbol{A}\boldsymbol{Q} + \boldsymbol{Q}\boldsymbol{A}^{\mathrm{T}} + \boldsymbol{B}\boldsymbol{B}^{\mathrm{T}} = 0. \tag{7.11}$$

From the covariance matrix, we obtain individual noise levels for all substances in the system (diagonal elements of $\boldsymbol{Q}$) and the linear correlations between pairs of substances. Another way to derive the mean values and covariances is the *linear noise approximation* (see [11–14]).

Equation (7.11) also shows that upon rescaling the $\boldsymbol{A} \rightarrow \lambda \boldsymbol{A}$, the covariance matrix will scale as $\boldsymbol{Q} \rightarrow 1/\lambda \boldsymbol{Q}$; hence, for very stable systems (large negative eigenvalues of the Jacobian), the covariance of fluctuations will remain small. For large volumes V, on the other hand, the noise matrix $\boldsymbol{B}$ becomes small, and the error of the linear approximation diminishes. For smaller volumes, however, low particle numbers may lead to larger fluctuations which can even enable the system to escape from the steady state. In this case, the above approximations break down [14, 15]. For instance, fluctuations may enable a bistable system to switch randomly between its stable states (see Section 4.3.5).

7.1.5
Deterministic and Stochastic Modeling Frameworks

Biochemical reaction systems can be described by stochastic or deterministic models. Usually, stochastic simulations are computationally more expensive, so they should only be used when random fluctuations play a role. For well-mixed systems of infinite volume (i.e., infinite particle numbers), the fluctuations tend to zero and the random process is well approximated by a macroscopic deterministic model. For finite particle numbers and linear kinetics, the macroscopic model still represents the expected value of the random process. For nonlinear systems, however, random fluctuations can be important, for instance, enabling a bistable system to jump randomly between its stable steady states.

As an example, Figure 7.1 shows simulation results from both types of modeling framework for a simple gene expression model (treated in more detail in Section 7.2.1). In the macroscopic deterministic model, mRNA concentration x and

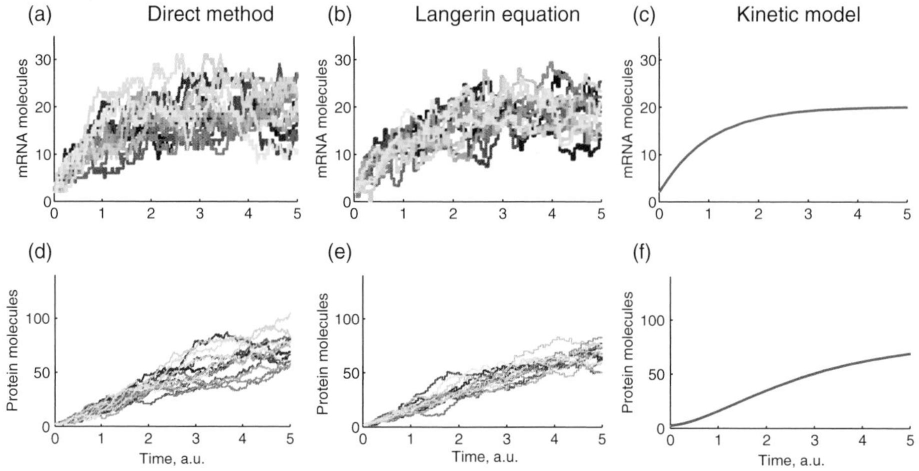

Figure 7.1 Simulations of molecule numbers for an mRNA species (top: (a), (b), (c)) and the corresponding protein (bottom: (d), (e), (f)). Time series were computed with Gillespie's direct method (left: (a), (d)), chemical Langevin equation (center: (b), (e)), and a deterministic kinetic model (right: (c), (f)). For the two stochastic models, 10 realizations are shown in different colors. Parameters: $k_x^+ = 20$, $k_x^- = 1$, $k_y^+ = 2$, and $k_y^- = 5$. Initial molecule numbers $x = 2$, $y = 2$, volume $V = 1$.

protein concentration y follow the rate equations

$$\begin{aligned}\frac{dx}{dt} &= k_{+x} - k_{-x}\,x \\ \frac{dy}{dt} &= k_{+y}\,x - k_{-y}\,y.\end{aligned} \tag{7.12}$$

For simplicity, we assume a volume $V = 1$, so the concentrations in the deterministic model (measured as molecules per volume) correspond directly to molecule numbers. This model will be studied in more detail in the Section 7.2.

7.1.6 Temporal Fluctuations

The chemical Langevin equation (7.7) describes intrinsic noise due to stochastic reaction events. Besides this, Langevin equations can also be used to describe extrinsic noise, i.e., random influences from outside the system. If the parameter vector $\boldsymbol{k}(t)$ in a kinetic model

$$\frac{d\boldsymbol{s}(t)}{dt} = \boldsymbol{N}\boldsymbol{v}(\boldsymbol{s}(t), \boldsymbol{k}(t)) \tag{7.13}$$

follows a random process, the substance levels $\boldsymbol{s}(t)$ will also behave randomly. To compute their statistical properties, we assume that for constant parameters $\boldsymbol{k}_0$, the equation system (7.13) has a stable steady state with concentrations $\boldsymbol{s}^{st}(\boldsymbol{k}_0)$. We linearize Eq. (7.13) around this reference state and for the fluctuations $\boldsymbol{u}(t) = \boldsymbol{k}(t) - \boldsymbol{k}_0$ and $\boldsymbol{x}(t) = \boldsymbol{s}(t) - \boldsymbol{s}^{st}(\boldsymbol{k}_0)$, we obtain the approximation

$$\frac{d\boldsymbol{x}(t)}{dt} = \boldsymbol{N}\,\tilde{\varepsilon}\boldsymbol{x}(t) + \boldsymbol{N}\,\tilde{\pi}\boldsymbol{u}(t), \tag{7.14}$$

with the substrate elasticity matrix $\tilde{\varepsilon} = \partial\boldsymbol{v}/\partial\boldsymbol{s}$ and the parameter elasticity matrix $\tilde{\pi} = \partial\boldsymbol{v}/\partial\boldsymbol{k}$. By collecting all concentrations and fluxes in an output vector

$$\boldsymbol{y} = \begin{pmatrix} \boldsymbol{s}(t) - \boldsymbol{s}^{st} \\ \boldsymbol{v}(t) - \boldsymbol{v}^{st} \end{pmatrix} = \begin{pmatrix} \boldsymbol{I} \\ \tilde{\varepsilon} \end{pmatrix} \boldsymbol{x} + \begin{pmatrix} 0 \\ \tilde{\pi} \end{pmatrix} \boldsymbol{u}, \tag{7.15}$$

and abbreviating the matrices in Eqs. (7.14) and (7.15) by $\boldsymbol{A}, \boldsymbol{B}, \boldsymbol{C}$, and $\boldsymbol{D}$, we obtain the standard form of a linear model (see Chapter 15)

$$\begin{aligned}\frac{d\boldsymbol{x}(t)}{dt} &= \boldsymbol{A}\boldsymbol{x}(t) + \boldsymbol{B}\,\boldsymbol{u}(t) \\ \boldsymbol{y} &= \boldsymbol{C}\,\boldsymbol{x}(t) + \boldsymbol{D}\,\boldsymbol{u}(t).\end{aligned} \tag{7.16}$$

The propagation of noise in a linear, time-invariant system of the form (7.16) can be described by the frequency response function (see Chapter 15)

$$\boldsymbol{H}(i\omega) = -\boldsymbol{C}(\boldsymbol{A} - i\omega\boldsymbol{I})^{-1}\boldsymbol{B}. \tag{7.17}$$

If the output $\boldsymbol{y}$ represents metabolic concentrations or fluxes, the frequency responses are given, respectively, by the spectral response matrices [16, 17]

$$\begin{aligned}\tilde{\boldsymbol{R}}^{S}(\omega) &= -(\boldsymbol{N}\,\tilde{\varepsilon} - i\omega\boldsymbol{I})^{-1}\boldsymbol{N}\tilde{\pi} \\ \tilde{\boldsymbol{R}}^{J}(\omega) &= (\boldsymbol{I} - \tilde{\varepsilon}(\boldsymbol{N}\,\tilde{\varepsilon} - i\omega\boldsymbol{I})^{-1}\boldsymbol{N})\tilde{\pi}.\end{aligned} \tag{7.18}$$

Like the usual metabolic response matrices for steady states, the matrices (7.18) characterize the response to small perturbations, but at finite frequencies ω. Their elements are complex numbers describing the amplitudes and phases of output variables relative to the parameter perturbation (compare Chapter 15).

If the parameters follow a stationary Gauss–Markov process with mean values $\boldsymbol{k}_0$ and a small fluctuation amplitude, the spectral density Φ_y of $\boldsymbol{y}$ can be computed from the spectral density of the parameter fluctuations $\boldsymbol{u}$ and the frequency response as (see Chapter 15)

$$\Phi_y(\omega) = \tilde{\boldsymbol{R}}(\omega)\Phi_u(\omega)\tilde{\boldsymbol{R}}(\omega)^{\dagger}, \tag{7.19}$$

where the symbol † denotes the adjoint (conjugate transpose) matrix. If we assume that the parameter fluctuations follow a white noise process with spectral density $\Phi_u(\omega) = \boldsymbol{I}$, the spectral density of the substance concentrations reads $\Phi_y(\omega) = \boldsymbol{R}(\omega)\boldsymbol{R}(\omega)^{\dagger}$.

Example 7.1 Minimal biochemical system with Hopf bifurcation

Figure 7.2 shows the minimal biochemical reaction system with a Hopf bifurcation [18]. The rate equations for metabolite concentrations a, b, and c in this system read

$$\begin{aligned} \frac{da}{dt} &= (k_1 x - k_4)a - k_2 ac \\ \frac{db}{dt} &= k_4 a - k_5 b \\ \frac{dc}{dt} &= k_5 b - k_3 c. \end{aligned} \tag{7.20}$$

The external substrate concentration x acts as a bifurcation parameter: if x is small, the system has a stable steady state, but if it reaches the critical value x_{crit}, this state will become unstable and the metabolite levels will start oscillating at a frequency ω_0. This type of change from a stable to an unstable focus is known as a *supercritical Hopf bifurcation* (see Section 2.3.1).

However, the system reveals its tendency to oscillate already below the bifurcation point: as it approaches the bifurcation, it becomes more and more susceptible to periodic perturbations, amplifying parameter oscillations and noise at frequencies around ω_0 [17]. Hence, the spectral densities of metabolite levels caused by intrinsic chemical noise show a resonance peak near the frequency ω_0 (see Figure 7.3(a)).

Both bifurcation and resonance are related to an eigenvalue of the Jacobian. Figure 7.3(b) shows the eigenvalues as points in the complex plane: in a stable steady state, all eigenvalues have negative real parts, so they are located in the left half-plane. Close to the Hopf bifurcation – with x just below its critical value – a pair of complex eigenvalues comes close to the imaginary axis. These eigenvalues are responsible for the resonance behavior: according to Eq. (7.18), the spectral response coefficients contain the term $\boldsymbol{A} - i\omega\boldsymbol{I}$ in which the eigenvalues of $\boldsymbol{A}$ are shifted down by $i\omega$. At a frequency $\omega \approx \omega_0$, the upper eigenvalue becomes almost zero, giving rise to a very large eigenvalue in the inverse matrix $(\boldsymbol{A} - i\omega\boldsymbol{I})^{-1}$ (see Figure 7.3(c)). This amplification leads to a resonance peak in the spectral response matrix and, as a consequence, in the spectral densities.

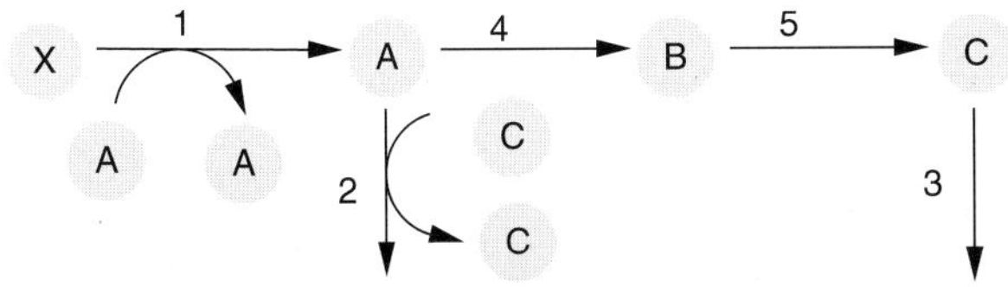

Figure 7.2 Minimal biochemical system with Hopf bifurcation [18]. If the level of the external substrate X exceeds a critical value, the levels of A, B, and C show sustained oscillations.

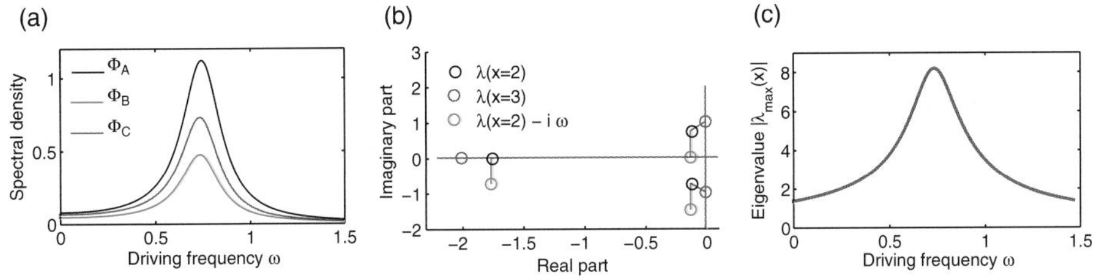

Figure 7.3 Resonance in the minimal biochemical system with Hopf bifurcation (see Figure 7.2). (a) Spectral densities of metabolite concentrations due to chemical noise. (b) Eigenvalues of the Jacobian in the complex plane. Eigenvalues for a bifurcation parameter below and at the critical value are shown in black and blue, respectively. The term $-i\omega$ in the spectral response coefficient shifts the upper-right eigenvalue λ^* (black) toward the origin (red). (c) Resonance in the curve $|(\lambda^* - i\omega)^{-1}|$. All quantities in arbitrary units. From Liebermeister [17].

Figure 7.3(b) illustrates another general feature of biochemical systems. If a system is driven by periodic perturbations above its own highest resonance frequency, all eigenvalues of $(A - i\omega I)^{-1}$ will finally decrease with the frequency ω. Therefore, linearized biochemical models act as low-pass filters in the range of high-frequency perturbations or noise.

7.2 Fluctuations in Gene Expression

Summary

Experiments show that protein levels fluctuate in time and can differ strongly between similar cells. Random fluctuations in transcription and translation can lead to temporal bursts in protein levels, associated with a non-Poisson distribution of molecule numbers and characteristic temporal correlations. In general, random fluctuations in living systems consist of two contributions: extrinsic variation due to influences by other systems and intrinsic variation arising from random dynamics in the system itself. Random behavior enables cells to create diversity, e.g., to maintain a subpopulation of persistor cells in bacterial cultures. The contribution of intrinsic and extrinsic variability can be measured in living cells by single-cell measurements with fluorescent reporter proteins.

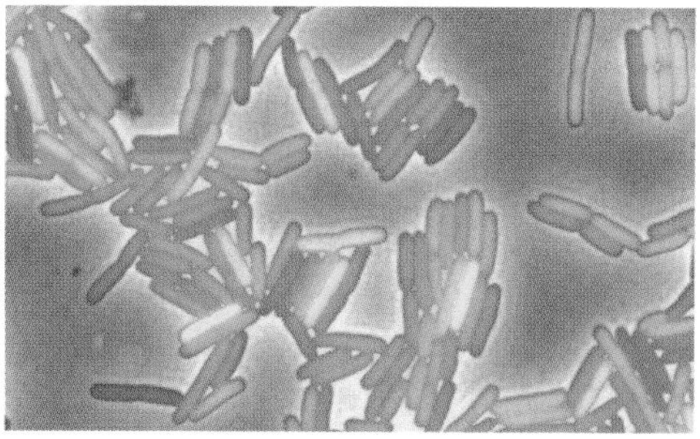

Figure 7.4 *Escherichia coli* bacteria expressing different fluorescent proteins (see Section 4.1.2). With two proteins shown in red and green, the total brightness depends on the sum of both proteins. Depending on the expression ratio, cells appear in red, yellow, or green. Different expression levels are partly caused by random events in the cell (Courtesy of M. Elowitz).

Different cells behave differently, even if they are genetically identical and have been grown under the same conditions (see Figure 7.4). The variability of protein levels, metabolic state, and cell morphology is caused by internal factors like cell cycle phase and by changes in the environment (e.g., nutrients, temperature, cell density). But cells also generate random behavior by themselves. Random fluctuations in gene expression and in other microscopic processes enable cells to switch spontaneously between different states, which allows them to create diversity in their populations.

Random dynamics can be created in microscopic processes, such as gene transcription, which involve small molecule numbers. If molecules act as catalysts (as mRNA does in translation), fluctuations in their numbers will influence downstream processes; chemical noise propagates through the biochemical networks, adds up, and contributes to the total variability. We can generally distinguish between *intrinsic noise*, which is generated in a system itself, and *extrinsic noise*, which is imported from other random processes that influence the system. Transcription, for instance, is intrinsically stochastic, but it also depends on transcription factor levels and other cell variables that fluctuate and contribute additional extrinsic noise.

In this chapter, we shall study the random nature of gene expression and see how it can be observed by single-cell measurements (see Section 11.14). Flow cytometry allows us to measure protein levels for different cells, while the temporal behavior within single cells can be measured by fluorescence microscopy (see Figure 7.4).

Random dynamics in gene expression can be modeled by stochastic processes as described in Section 7.1. In such models, we implicitly assume that cells represent individual realizations of the same stochastic process. Models for stochastic gene expression have been validated in experiments with artificial genetic circuits [19–22].

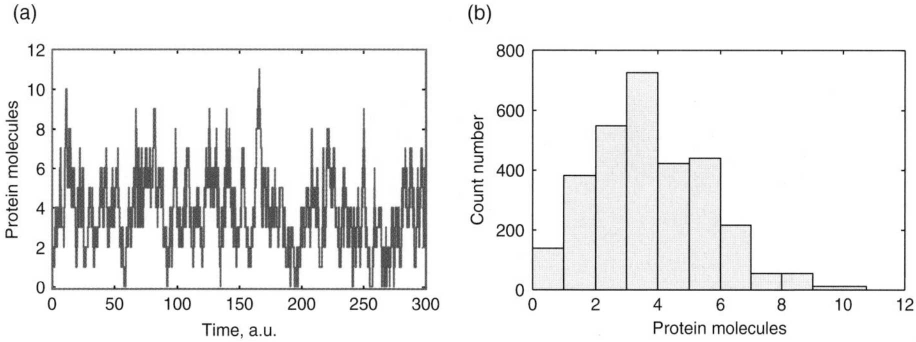

Figure 7.5 Simple stochastic model of protein production. (a) Temporal changes of molecule numbers, simulated by a simple chemical random process with constant translation rate (see Section 7.1.1, parameters $w_+ = 2, w_- = 0.5$). (b) Histogram of molecule numbers, sampled over time. Asymptotically – i.e. for infinite time intervals – the numbers follow a Poisson distribution.

7.2.1 Stochastic Model of Transcription and Translation

If proteins were produced and degraded according to a simple chemical random process (see Section 7.1.1), their numbers would follow a Poisson distribution as shown in Figure 7.5. In reality, protein levels are regulated by various processes including transcription, transcription factor activation, chromatin remodeling, mRNA splicing, translation, and degradation of mRNA and proteins. All such processes produce noise, which can propagate along the entire chain of protein synthesis and contribute to the variability of protein levels. The noise, however, does not only accumulate, but also changes its statistical properties: we shall study this phenomenon in a simple model describing transcription and translation (see Section 7.1.6).

7.2.1.1 Macroscopic Kinetic Model

We consider a gene that is transcribed constitutively at a fixed rate k_{+x}, while translation occurs with a fixed rate k_{+y} per mRNA molecule. A kinetic model of this process (with mRNA concentration s_x, protein concentration s_y, and respective degradation rates k_{-x} and k_{-y}) reads

$$\begin{aligned} \frac{ds_x}{dt} &= k_{+x} - k_{-x}\, s_x \\ \frac{ds_y}{dt} &= k_{+y} s_x - k_{-y}\, s_y. \end{aligned} \tag{7.21}$$

The transcription rate k_{+x} may vary in time depending on the presence of transcriptional activators. For constant rate k_{+x} (constitutive expression), the

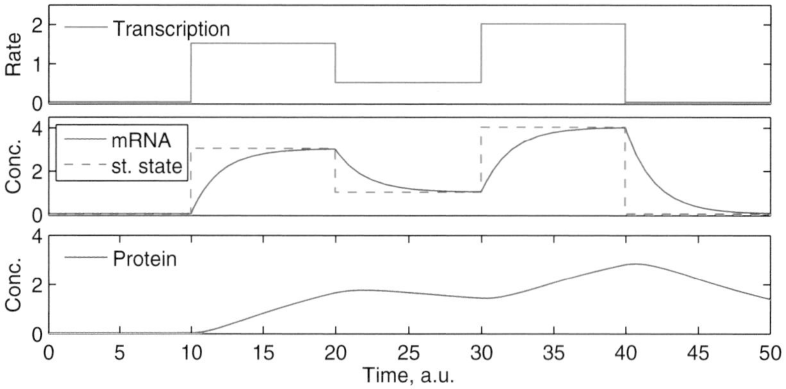

Figure 7.6 Deterministic model of transcription and translation (compare Figure 7.7, parameters $k_x^+ = k_{-x} = 0.5$, $k_{+y} = k_{-y} = 0.1$). The curves show time simulations with a predefined step-like profile for the transcription rate k_{+x} (arbitrary units). After each change, the mRNA level approaches its steady-state value (dashed). The protein level changes more slowly.

concentrations converge to their stationary values

$$s_x^{st} = \frac{k_{+x}}{k_{-x}}, \quad s_y^{st} = \frac{s_x^{st} k_{+y}}{k_{-y}}. \tag{7.22}$$

Figure 7.6 shows the temporal concentration profiles that would result from a predefined, piecewise constant transcription rate k_{+x} (top). After each jump, the mRNA level (center) relaxes exponentially to the respective steady state, and the protein level follows more slowly (bottom).

7.2.1.2 Microscopic Stochastic Model

On the microscopic level, transcription and translation are random processes that produce single molecules. In our model, we can thus describe the molecule numbers by coupled chemical random processes for mRNA and protein amounts (Figure 7.7). A realization of this process can be interpreted as a walk on a two-dimensional

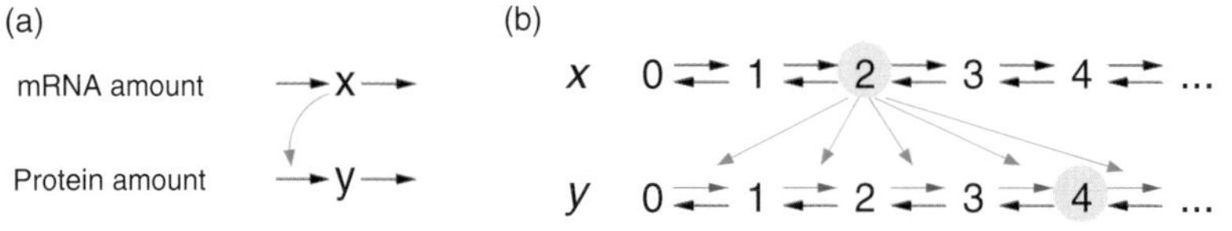

Figure 7.7 Stochastic model of transcription and translation. (a) Transcription and translation are modeled as coupled random processes for molecule numbers of mRNA and protein. Present mRNA molecules (molecule number x) activate translation of protein (molecule number y). (b) The processes for x and y are coupled. Current numbers of mRNA and protein molecules are marked by circles. The rate a_y^+ for protein synthesis (blue arrows) depends on the number of mRNA molecules present (red arrows).

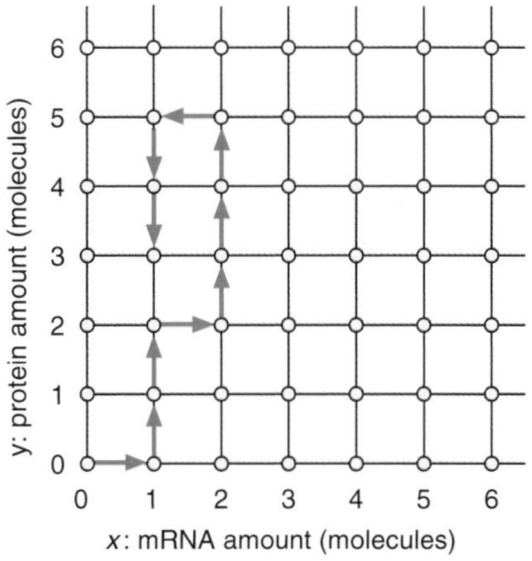

Figure 7.8 State space for the model of transcription and translation (see Figure 7.7). The state space consists of pairs (x,y) of mRNA numbers x and protein numbers y. A single realization of the process can be seen as a path through state space (example path shown in red, time not shown).

grid (Figure 7.8) with transition rates given by

Process	Transition	Rate
Transcription	$x \to x+1$	$a_x^+ = w_{+x}$
mRNA degradation	$x \to x-1$	$a_x^- = w_{-x}\, x$
Translation	$y \to y+1$	$a_y^+ = w_{+y}\, x$
Protein degradation	$y \to y-1$	$a_y^- = w_{-y}\, y$

(7.23)

The number of mRNA molecules x follows a simple chemical random process, and its stationary ensemble is described by a Poisson distribution. The protein production rate is not constant, but depends on the varying amount of mRNA molecules present (Figure 7.9). Therefore, the protein level y shows a more complicated dynamics. Models of the same type can be used to describe other two-level processes [23] and regulatory circuits consisting of several genes [24] (see the web supplement).

7.2.1.3 Fluctuations and Protein Bursts

The stationary distribution of this process can be computed using the generating function [24] (see the web supplement) or by solving the chemical Langevin equation (see exercise 3). We obtain the mean values

$$\langle x \rangle = \frac{w_{+x}}{w_{-x}}, \qquad \langle y \rangle = \langle x \rangle \frac{w_{+y}}{w_{-y}} \tag{7.24}$$

similar to Eq. (7.22), while the variances are determined by

$$\frac{\mathrm{var}(x)}{\langle x \rangle} = 1, \qquad \frac{\mathrm{var}(y)}{\langle y \rangle} = 1 + \frac{w_{+y}}{w_{-x} + w_{-y}}. \tag{7.25}$$

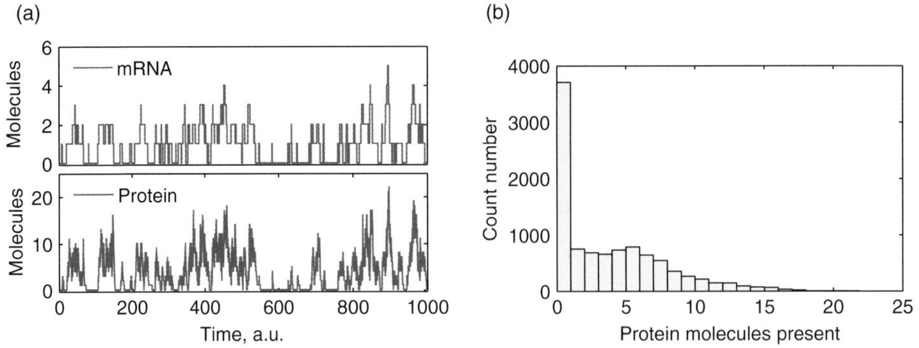

Figure 7.9 Stochastic dynamics of transcription and translation (model shown in Figure 7.7, with parameters $w_{+x} = w_{-x} = 0.1$, $w_{+y} = 2$, $w_{-y} = 0.5$). (a) Simulated time series for numbers of mRNA and protein molecules. Bursts of protein expression occur when several mRNA molecules are present. (b) Histogram of protein numbers. Because of the bursts, the protein numbers do not follow a Poisson distribution.

The ratio between variance and average value, called the *Fano factor*, has a value of 1 for the mRNA molecules, as expected for a Poisson distribution. For the proteins, however, it is larger than 1, indicating that the distribution is broader than a Poisson distribution of the same mean value. According to Eqs. (7.24) and (7.25), the average value and the variance of y can be adjusted separately by tuning the four rates w_{+x}, w_{-x}, w_y, and w_{+y} [24].

In simulations of the process (7.23), the protein number y shows temporal bursts (see Figure 7.9). Such bursts, which have also been observed in experiments [25], arise in periods of high mRNA abundance and lead to a broader, non-Poisson distribution of protein levels. This can be understood as follows. Assume that the number of mRNA molecules remains constant for long periods of time; in each such period, the protein number y follows a random process with constant translation rate $w_{+y}\,x$, so the values in a time series will asymptotically follow a Poisson distribution. After many such periods with different mRNA numbers, the distribution of protein numbers will resemble a mixture of Poisson distributions with different mean values, which is broader than a single Poisson distribution.

7.2.2
Measuring the Intrinsic and Extrinsic Variability

Is the behavior of cells completely predetermined by their internal state and their environment, or is there something fundamentally stochastic in it? And if there are random events, how much do they contribute to the differences between cells? To answer this question, one might try to create two cells in exactly the same initial state and expose them to exactly the same environment, but this is not possible in practice. However, Elowitz *et al.* [21] were able to answer this question at least partially, for individual genes within a cell. To quantify the random effects in gene expression, they integrated two fluorescent reporter proteins, CFP and YFP, into the genome of *E. coli*

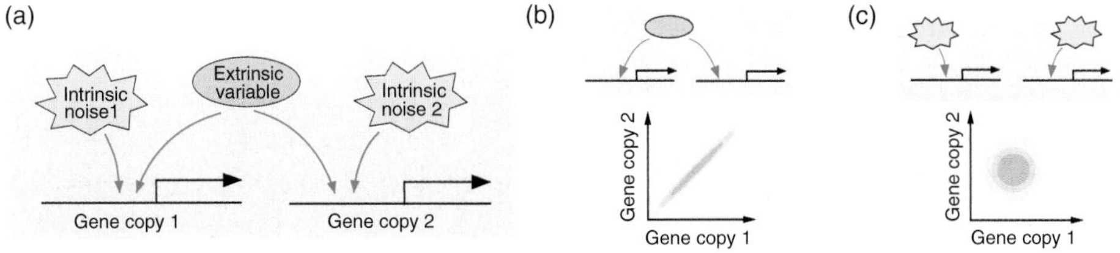

Figure 7.10 Expression of reporter genes reveals the contributions of intrinsic and extrinsic noise. (a) Two gene copies with the same promoter sequence are regulated by extrinsic variables (e.g., transcription factors). In addition, both transcription rates show intrinsic fluctuations, represented by uncorrelated noise variables. (b) With extrinsic noise alone, expression levels will be completely correlated, so the scatter plot will yield a line. (c) Intrinsic noise alone leads to uncorrelated expression levels.

bacteria. The genes were controlled by two copies of the same promoter, located in the same cell, and thus exposed to the same cell state.

In this experiment, any difference between the expression levels will indicate essential random behavior, as illustrated in Figure 7.10. If expression was completely determined by factors extrinsic to transcription, the gene product levels should be correlated. On the other hand, if expression is dominated by intrinsic processes, the two copies should show uncorrelated expression. A general definition of intrinsic and extrinsic noise [26] is described in the web supplement.

The levels of both protein copies were recorded in single cells by fluorescence microscopy. Scatter plots between CFP and YFP intensities (Figure 7.11) allow us

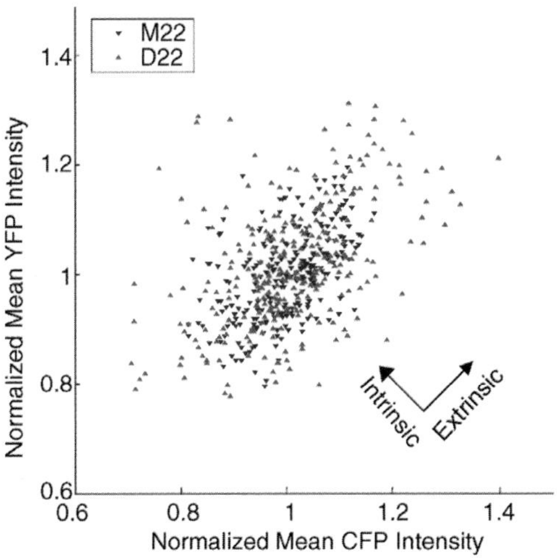

Figure 7.11 Expression levels arising from two copies of the same gene promoter (see Figure 7.10). The scatter plot shows levels of the two reporter proteins CFP (*x*-axis) and YFP (*y*-axis). The shape of the cloud indicates the amounts of intrinsic and extrinsic noise in protein production. Data from a quiet strain (M22, with constitutive Lac expression, $\eta_{int} = 5.5 \pm 0.5\%$, $\eta_{ext} = 5.1 \pm 0.5\%$) and a noisy strain (D22, $\eta_{int} = 10.5 \pm 1\%$, $\eta_{ext} = 4.6 \pm 1.2\%$) are shown. From Elowitz *et al.* [21].

to estimate the contribution of intrinsic (uncorrelated) and extrinsic (correlated) influences on gene expression. It was found that both contributions depend on the mean expression level; at high expression levels (derepressed Lac promoter), the cell-to-cell variation is about $\eta_{tot} = 8\%$, including about $\eta_{int} = 5\%$ caused by intrinsic noise. At normal expression levels (from a wild-type Lac promoter), which are about 20 times lower, the relative variation reaches about $\eta_{tot} = 40\%$ in total and $\eta_{int} = 20\%$ from intrinsic noise alone. As predicted, the intrinsic noise decreases with the expression level as $\eta^2_{int} \approx c_1/\langle x \rangle + c_2$ with constants c_1 and c_2 [26]. The first term would be expected from a Poisson distribution (Fano factor 1), while the constant term may reflect fluctuations of extrinsic noise. The same methodology can also be applied to entire cellular subsystems [27] (see the web supplement).

7.2.3
Temporal Fluctuations in a Gene Cascade

Protein levels do not only differ between cells, but they also fluctuate in time. We can compare the protein level in a single cell to the average value in the cell population: if a level is above average in a certain moment, it will stay above average for some time. This fact is expressed by the temporal autocorrelations (see Chapter 15), which define a time scale for fluctuations. The statistic properties of fluctuations reflect the dynamics of the regulation network. If a genetic circuit is driven by extrinsic fluctuations, then also protein levels will fluctuate, and we can compute their frequency spectrum and time correlations from a Langevin equation (see Section 7.1.6).

7.2.3.1 Linear Model of Two Genes

As an example, we consider a gene X_1 that activates a second gene X_2; synthesis of gene X_1 is subject to extrinsic, time-dependent noise. If transcription and translation are modeled as a single step, we can describe the gene expression levels s_1 and s_2 by a kinetic model similar to Eq. (7.21),

$$\begin{aligned} \frac{ds_1}{dt} &= \alpha_1(1+\xi)-\beta s_1 \\ \frac{ds_2}{dt} &= \alpha_2 s_1-\beta s_2 \end{aligned} \tag{7.26}$$

The production rate of X_1 fluctuates with a noise term ξ, and for simplicity, we assume equal degradation constants β for both genes. Without the noise ($\xi = 0$), the system would have a steady state with concentrations $s_1^{st} = \alpha_1/\beta$ and $s_2^{st} = s_1^{st}\alpha_2/\beta$. The fluctuation ξ, however, leads to deviations $x_1(t) = s_1(t)-s_1^{st}$ and $x_2(t) = s_2(t)-s_2^{st}$ from the steady state, which obey the rate equation (in the vectorial form)

$$\frac{d}{dt}\begin{pmatrix} x_1 \\ x_2 \end{pmatrix} = \begin{pmatrix} -\beta & 0 \\ \alpha_2 & -\beta \end{pmatrix}\begin{pmatrix} x_1 \\ x_2 \end{pmatrix} + \begin{pmatrix} \alpha_1 \\ 0 \end{pmatrix}\xi. \tag{7.27}$$

We can rewrite this equation as a standard linear system (7.16) with the nomenclature $\boldsymbol{u}=\xi$, $\boldsymbol{y}=\boldsymbol{x}$, and the matrices

$$A=\begin{pmatrix}-\beta & 0\\ \alpha_2 & -\beta\end{pmatrix},\ B=\begin{pmatrix}\alpha_1\\ 0\end{pmatrix},\ C=I,\ D=0 \tag{7.28}$$

Given these matrices, we can compute the frequency response function $\boldsymbol{H}(i\omega)$ as well as the spectral densities $\Phi(\omega)$ and the autocorrelation function $R(\tau)=\Phi(\tau)/\Phi(0)$ for both genes (see Chapter 15). If the input is modeled by white noise ξ, we obtain the spectral density functions (compare Section 7.1.6)

$$\Phi_{x_1}(\omega)=\frac{\alpha_1^2}{\beta^2+\omega^2},\quad \Phi_{x_2}(\omega)=\frac{\alpha_1^2a_2^2}{(\beta^2+\omega^2)^2}. \tag{7.29}$$

Inverse Fourier transformation of these spectral densities yields the autocorrelation functions [28]

$$R_{x_1}(\tau)=e^{-\beta|\tau|},\quad R_{x_2}(\tau)=e^{-\beta|\tau|}(1+\beta|\tau|). \tag{7.30}$$

The spectral densities (7.29) and the autocorrelation functions (7.30) are shown in Figure 7.12 with parameter values $\alpha_1=\alpha_2=\beta=1$. The white noise process ξ has a constant spectral density $\Phi_u(\omega)=1$ for all frequencies ω. In gene X_1, fluctuations at higher frequencies become damped, so the spectral density decreases. In gene X_2, this effect is even more pronounced. The restriction to lower frequencies leads to longer fluctuations in time, as can be seen in the autocorrelation function. The autocorrelation curves of the two genes show qualitatively different shapes, corresponding to the direct and indirect perturbation by the white noise.

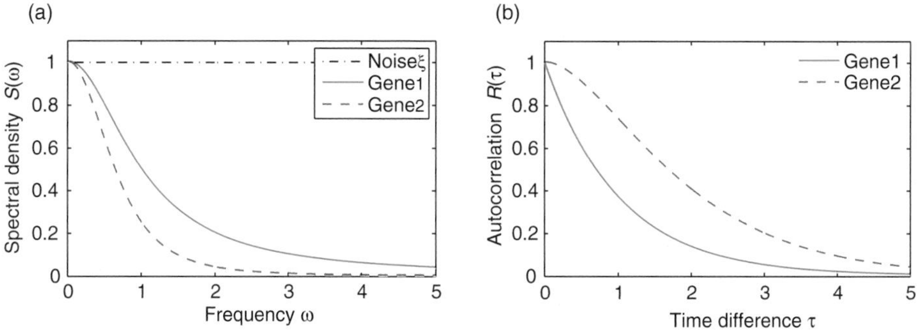

Figure 7.12 Expression fluctuations in a cascade of two genes. (a) Spectral densities for noise ξ and both genes. (b) Autocorrelation functions of both genes. As the effects of noise propagate down the cascade, high-frequency noise is filtered out and the autocorrelation functions – which are related to the spectral densities *via* Fourier transformation – become broader. All quantities are shown in arbitrary units.

7.2.3.2 Measuring the Time Correlations in Protein Levels

According to the above model, the time scale of fluctuations is mainly determined by protein degradation. The degradation term, however, can be a proxy for different biological processes: the effective degradation constant β can be changed by different types of protein degradation, dilution in growing cells (with cell cycle time $T_{1/2}$) effectively resembles degradation with $\beta = \ln 2/T_{1/2}$, and feedback control on production can lead to additional linear production terms $\alpha_X^{act}x$ or $-\alpha_X^{inh}x$. All these processes will influence the time scale of fluctuations.

Measurements in single cells allow us to estimate the time scale of protein fluctuations *in vivo* [28]. Figure 7.13(c) shows rank autocorrelations for the protein USP7, which can be compared to the autocorrelations predicted from Eq. (7.30). The correlation curve qualitatively resembles protein X_1 in the model, with white noise fluctuations in the production rate. Another protein, HMGA2 (Figure 7.13(d)), shows different time correlations and rather resembles protein X_2 with pink (low frequency) noise in the production rate.

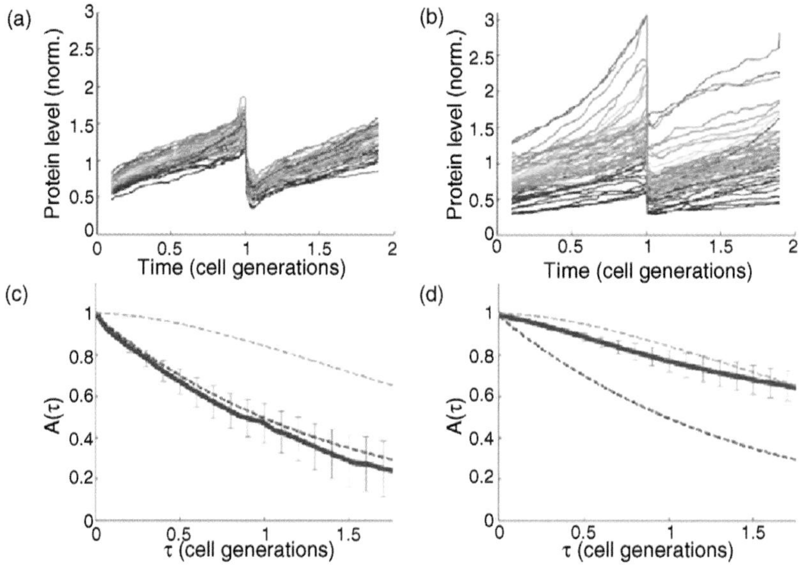

Figure 7.13 Time correlation of protein levels in human cells. Sigal *et al.* [28] have measured time-dependent protein levels by tracking single cells in time-lapse microscopy images. (a) Level of the protein USP7 in different cells (colors) over two cell cycles. The protein content (measured by fluorescence of YFP-labeled proteins) increases during the cell cycle and is approximately split into halves in each cell division. (b) To compare data from different cells, time was rescaled to cell cycle periods; then, for each moment in time, a rank order of protein levels was computed for a set of cells. (c) Experimental rank autocorrelation between time points (blue line) for the protein USP7. The curve resembles the predicted correlation for proteins with white noise input (lower dashed line, compare Figure 7.12(b)). (d) Result for the protein HMGA2. The form of the autocorrelation function suggests time-correlated input noise (upper dashed line). From Sigal *et al.* [28].

7.2.4 Biological Functions of Noise

Cells are built from noisy parts and exposed to fluctuating environments. However, noise need not always be a disadvantage for them – in contrast, it can be used by cells to create necessary diversity in cell populations.

7.2.4.1 Random Switching

If two genes inhibit each other, they can form a bistable switch (see Section 4.3.5 and 8.2.7). By their action on downstream processes, genetic switches are able to trigger "decisions" between different types of behavior, like the lysogenic and the lytic state in the λ phage [29]. Gene expression noise can induce spontaneous transitions in a bistable switch: in state space, random fluctuations move the system from one stable state over the separatrix into the basin of attraction of the other stable state. Such spontaneous switching can help to generate diversity. For example, some bacteria populations contain small fractions of *persistor* cells, which are less susceptible to antibiotics, at the expense of a smaller growth rate [30]. In contrast to genetic resistance, this behavior is based on reversible switching between wild-type and persistor state [31]. It allows bacterial colonies to maintain a percentage of such persistors even if the colony is not challenged with drugs for a long time [32].

7.2.4.2 Exploration Strategies

Control of noise levels can be seen as part of an exploration strategy [33]: by behaving more randomly in hard situations, a system can increase its probability of evading them. This strategy is the basis of *bacterial chemotaxis*, a mechanism to move toward the source of a chemical attractant. In chemotaxis, bacteria move in a sequence of straight runs, but in between they randomly change their direction (they "tumble"). On their way, bacteria monitor the local attractant level to adjust their tumbling probability: as long as the concentration increases, the tumbling frequency is kept low, and the bacterium is likely to stay on track. However, if it moves down a gradient, it will increase its tumbling frequency and thereby the probability of changing its direction. On average, this biased random walk leads to a movement toward regions of high attractant concentration.

A similar principle prevails at the evolutionary level in stress-induced mutagenesis [34]: under stress, bacteria can switch to an increased error rate of DNA replication and thereby increase their mutation own rate – which may be the limiting factor for genetic adaptation. If we regard a cell population as a cloud of points in genotype space, a higher mutation rate corresponds to faster diffusion. By adapting the mutation rate to its current fitness level, a cell population can explore possible genetic changes more rapidly in order to evade the stress situation.

7.3
Variability and Uncertainty

Summary

The behavior of individual cells depends on internal, e.g., enzymatic, parameters and on the environmental conditions. In uncertainty analysis, parameter values are drawn from a probability distribution to study the variability of the resulting model predictions. The probability distributions of metabolite levels and other cell variables can be characterized by their average values, variances, and correlations. Uncertainty analysis helps to study variability in cell populations, to obtain probabilistic model predictions, and to assess to what extent the dynamics of a system is predetermined by its network structure.

Diversity in cell populations can have various reasons, including genetic differences, fluctuating gene expression, varying supply of nutrients, changes during the cell cycle, or temperature changes. All these factors will influence the state of the metabolic network, and their variation will lead to varying, correlated metabolite levels – which are in fact observed in metabolome data [35]. In models, we can try to simulate how random variation of parameters – kinetic constants, enzyme levels, or external metabolite levels – perturbs the metabolic state, how these perturbations spread in the network, and which variability of metabolic fluxes and concentrations will result from them. Let us consider a kinetic model (see Section 2.3.1)

$$\frac{\mathrm{d}s(t)}{\mathrm{d}t} = \boldsymbol{N}\boldsymbol{v}(s(t), \boldsymbol{k}), \tag{7.31}$$

with stoichiometric matrix $\boldsymbol{N}$, reaction rate vector $\boldsymbol{v}$, and a vector $\boldsymbol{k}$ containing the varying kinetic parameters. If the model has a stable steady state and $\boldsymbol{k}$ is randomly distributed, the steady-state concentrations $s^{\mathrm{st}}(\boldsymbol{k})$ will also follow a probability distribution, which determines the variances and correlations of metabolite levels. Alternatively, we may assume that the parameters in Eq. (7.31) fluctuate in time according to a random process $\boldsymbol{k}(t)$. In this case, the concentrations are driven by the temporal perturbations and will also follow a random process.

A probability distribution for $\boldsymbol{k}$ can describe (i) parameter variability within a cell for different time points, (ii) variability within cell populations, or (iii) subjective uncertainty about parameter values. The aim of uncertainty analysis is to study the resulting uncertainty of the system behavior. It can be used to simulate cell populations, to assess the relation between network structures and dynamic behavior, to detect robustness properties, and to obtain probabilistic predictions when parameters are uncertain or unknown.

7.3.1
Models with Uncertain Constant Parameters

To model diversity in a cell population, we may assume that all cells follow the same model, but with different – yet constant – parameters. We can assume that the model

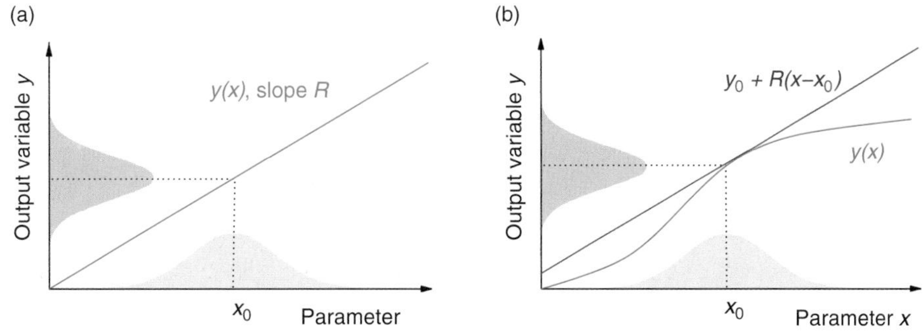

Figure 7.14 Model with parameter distribution. (a) An output variable y depends linearly on the parameter x. In this case, the distributions of x and y have the same shape except for scaling by the slope R of $y(x)$. (b) In most systems biology models, observables y (e.g., steady-state fluxes) depend nonlinearly on parameters x (e.g., enzyme levels). The response curve $y(x)$ can be approximated by its tangent at the reference point (mean parameter value); in this approximation, the width of y depends on the slope R, i.e., the metabolic response coefficient.

behavior is summarized in a response function $\mathbf{y}(\mathbf{x})$. The output vector $\mathbf{y}$ may comprise different kinds of variables such as steady-state concentrations, entire time series, or quantities like maximal values or response times, while the parameter vector $\mathbf{x}$ contains kinetic parameters and initial values, possibly in logarithmic form.

For a population model, the parameter vector $\mathbf{x}$ is described by a joint probability distribution, with probabilities corresponding to percentages in a large cell population. For positive parameters (e.g., concentrations and most kinetic constants), it is convenient and fairly plausible to work with the logarithmic values. Multiplicative relationships between parameters, like the constraint $k_+/k_- = K^{\mathrm{eq}}$ for mass-action rate constants $k_\pm$ and the equilibrium constant K^{eq}, translate to simple additive relationships for the logarithms ($\ln k_+ - \ln k_- = \ln K^{\mathrm{eq}}$) [36, 37].

If we assume a Gaussian distribution for these logarithmic parameters, we imply that the original parameters follow log-normal distributions. A multivariate Gaussian distribution for logarithmic parameters $x_m = \ln k_m$ can be specified by its mean value $\langle \mathbf{x} \rangle$ and the covariance matrix $\mathrm{cov}(\mathbf{x})$. Any linear combination of Gaussian random variables will be Gaussian-distributed again, so various kinds of model parameter (e.g., $\ln k_+$, $\ln k_-$, and $\ln K^{\mathrm{eq}}$ in the above example) can be specified by a joint Gaussian distribution [38]. The probability density $p(\mathbf{x})$ together with the shape of the function $y(\mathbf{x})$ determine the distribution of the output variables (see Figure 7.14).

7.3.2 Computing the Distribution of Output Variables

7.3.2.1 Monte Carlo Simulation

If the parameters of a model are uncertain, the resulting distribution of model outputs can be computed by Monte Carlo simulation [39]. Let y be a quantitative or qualitative system property that depends on the parameter set $\mathbf{x}$ (e.g., as shown in Figure 7.14). By drawing Monte Carlo samples $\mathbf{x}_\alpha, \alpha = 1, \ldots, n$, and computing the respective outcomes $y(\mathbf{x}_\alpha)$, one obtains a histogram of y. As the number of samples goes to infinity, this empirical distribution will approximate the true distribution $p(y)$. Monte Carlo simulation works for systems with discrete or continuous parameters and output variables; however, the repeated calculation of $y(\boldsymbol{x})$ may become costly – for instance, if it involves computation of steady states. Moreover, for finite sample sizes n, the statistical error has to be taken into account (see exercise 6).

7.3.2.2 Approximation for Narrow Parameter Distributions

For sharp parameter distributions, we can alternatively employ the approximation shown in Figure 7.14(b). In the case of a linear response function $y(x) = R\,x$ (as in Figure 7.14(a)), the distribution of y will resemble the distribution of x, but stretched in width by a factor $R = \mathrm{d}y/\mathrm{d}x$, the slope of $y(x)$. To keep the probability density $p(y)$ normalized (its the integral must have a value of 1), it has to be divided by the same factor, so we obtain as probability density $p(y(x)) = p(x)/R$. If the response curve $y(x)$, however, is nonlinear, we can approximate it by its tangent at the value x_0,

$$y(x) \approx y(x_0) + R(x - x_0), \tag{7.32}$$

with the sensitivity $R = \mathrm{d}y/\mathrm{d}x|_{x=x_0}$. If the parameter x is Gaussian distributed with the mean value x_0 and a small width σ_x and if the approximation (7.32) is valid in this parameter region, the values of y will approximately follow a Gaussian distribution with mean $y(x_0)$ and standard deviation $\sigma_y = R\,\sigma_x$. The same approximation can be applied to larger systems with several observables y_i and parameters x_m following a multivariate Gaussian distribution. If $\boldsymbol{y}(\boldsymbol{x})$ is smooth enough and the parameter distribution is narrow, the response function can be approximated by a first-order expansion

$$y_l(\boldsymbol{x}^0 + \Delta\boldsymbol{x}) \approx y_l(\boldsymbol{x}^0) + \sum_m R_{lm}\Delta x_m, \tag{7.33}$$

with the sensitivities R_{lm}. In this approximation, the observables y_i follow a Gaussian distribution [36] determined by

$$\langle \boldsymbol{y} \rangle \approx \boldsymbol{y}(\boldsymbol{x}^0) \tag{7.34}$$

$$\mathrm{cov}(\boldsymbol{y}) = \langle \boldsymbol{y}\,\boldsymbol{y}^{\mathrm{T}} \rangle \approx \boldsymbol{R}\langle \boldsymbol{x}\,\boldsymbol{x}^{\mathrm{T}} \rangle \boldsymbol{R}^{\mathrm{T}} = \boldsymbol{R}\,\mathrm{cov}(\boldsymbol{x})\boldsymbol{R}^{\mathrm{T}}. \tag{7.35}$$

According to Eq. (7.35), the variability of the outputs $\boldsymbol{y}$ depends on two factors, the parameter variability (covariance matrix $\mathrm{cov}(\boldsymbol{x})$) and the sensitivity matrix $\boldsymbol{R}$. If a variable responds weakly to parameter changes, it will also show little overall variability and thus be robust. Formulae (7.34) and (7.35) are not restricted to steady-state quantities. For computing the variability of time-dependent concentrations, for instance, we can use the time-dependent response coefficients [40]

$$\tilde{R}^{s_l}_{k_m}(t) = \frac{\partial s_l(t;k)}{\partial k_m}, \tag{7.36}$$

where $s_l\,(t;k)$ denotes a time-dependent solution of Eq. (7.31).

If the parameters x_m in Eq. (7.33) represent logarithmic kinetic constants $x_m = \ln k_m$ of a biochemical system and the outputs denote logarithmic steady-state concentrations $y_l = \ln s_l^{\mathrm{st}}$, the sensitivities in (7.33) will be the scaled response coefficients $R^{s_l}_{k_m}$. With Gaussian-distributed parameters x_m and the linear approximation (7.33), the original kinetic parameters k_m and the concentrations s_l follow log-normal distributions. A second-order approximation of the response function [36] shows that nonlinearities can shift the average output value $\langle y_l \rangle$ (corresponding to an average over the biological sample) away from the output $y(\langle \boldsymbol{x} \rangle)$ expected from the average parameters (see the web supplement). This exemplifies the difficulties that arise when single-cell models are fitted to cell population data.

7.3.2.3 Temporal Parameter Fluctuations

If parameters fluctuate in time, they can be described by random processes (see Chapter 14 and Section 7.1.6) and their impact on the output variables will depend on the frequency of the fluctuations. If enzyme levels change slowly, the metabolic system will follow the perturbations in a quasi-steady state, so we can approximate this situation with static (yet uncertain) parameters. On the other hand, if parameters fluctuate fast, the system cannot adapt itself to their changes and will effectively respond to their mean values. In between, on the timescale of the system's own dynamics, parameter fluctuations can propagate through the network, be damped or amplified, and may possibly lead to resonance.

For linearized biochemical models, these effects can be computed as shown in Sections 7.1.6 and 7.2.3. If the parameters are modeled by a stationary Gauss–Markov process, all information about their variances and correlations is summarized in the spectral density matrices, which are related by Eq. (7.19),

$$\Phi_y(\omega) = \tilde{R}^y_x(\omega)\Phi_x(\omega)\tilde{R}^y_x(\omega)^\dagger$$

for non-logarithmic perturbation parameters $\boldsymbol{x}$ and output variables $\boldsymbol{y}$. This equation resembles Eq. (7.35) for the static parameter variability, but the covariance matrix and response coefficients are replaced, respectively, by spectral density matrices and spectral response coefficients. Noise, represented by $\Phi_x(\omega)$, is translated into fluctuations of the observables, represented by $\Phi_y(\omega)$. The linearized system acts as a frequency filter: small spectral response coefficients $\tilde{R}_{im}$ lead to dampening of the noise effects, whereas large response coefficients lead to amplification.

7.3.3 Uncertainty Analysis of Biochemical Models

The dynamics of a biochemical system depends on its network structure, the kinetic laws, and the kinetic parameters. Some system properties, like the set of stationary fluxes (see Section 2.2.2), follow directly from the stoichiometric structure. Also the summation theorems of metabolic control theory rely on the stoichiometric structure alone, while the connectivity theorems also depend on the specific kinetics (see Section 2.3.2). But many quantitative properties like steady-state concentrations or control coefficients can be tuned by the choice of parameters, and parameter changes can also alter the system's qualitative behavior. If a quantity depends on the kinetics, is this dependence weak or strong? Are there quantities with very weak dependences? Such questions can be answered by uncertainty analysis.

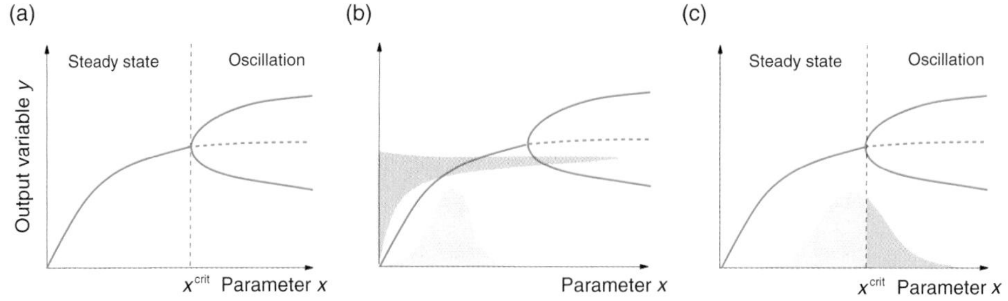

Figure 7.15 Parameter dependence in a system with Hopf bifurcation. (a) Bifurcation analysis. Depending on the parameter x, the system shows a stable steady-state (left region) or sustained oscillations (right region). A bifurcation (change of qualitative behavior) happens at a critical value x^{crit} (dashed line). (b) In uncertainty analysis, a distribution of the parameter x (probability density shown in light gray) leads to a distribution of the steady-state value $y(x)$ (density in dark gray, attached to the y-axis). Oscillations are improbable in this case. (c) Uncertainty analysis for a qualitative property: the probability for oscillations is given by the area of the parameter density above the critical value x_{crit} (dark grey).

Depending on its parameter values, a dynamical system can show different types of qualitative behavior; the transitions, called bifurcations, are studied in *bifurcation analysis* (Figure 7.15(a)). *Local sensitivity analysis,* in contrast, concerns the quantitative effect of small parameter changes: if the system response is a differentiable function $y(\mathbf{x})$, the relationship between parameters and output variables can be described by the sensitivities $\partial y/\partial x_m$, for example, the metabolic response coefficients of biochemical systems. *Global sensitivity analysis* deals with the effects of larger parameter variability. In *uncertainty analysis,* in particular, we assume a given statistical distribution for the parameters and compute probabilities for the resulting quantitative and qualitative behavior. If an output variable or a model property – for instance, robustness – shows little or no variability, we can conclude that it is mainly determined by the model structure.

Even if the actual distribution of parameters is unknown, uncertainty analysis can be of practical use. If a biochemical model predicts a certain behavior – for instance, inhibition of an enzyme A decreases a flux B – it may be arguable if this result is generic or if it only holds for a specific choice of parameters. An uncertainty analysis with uniformly distributed parameters may suffice as a simple test.

Example 7.2 Sampling of stationary flux distributions

As an example, let us consider a variant of flux balance analysis (see Section 9.1.3). In the model shown in Figure 7.16(a), a metabolite X (with concentration s_x) participates in three reactions. To balance it, the stationary fluxes have to satisfy

$$\frac{ds_x}{dt} = \nu_1 + \nu_2 + \nu_3 = 0. \tag{7.37}$$

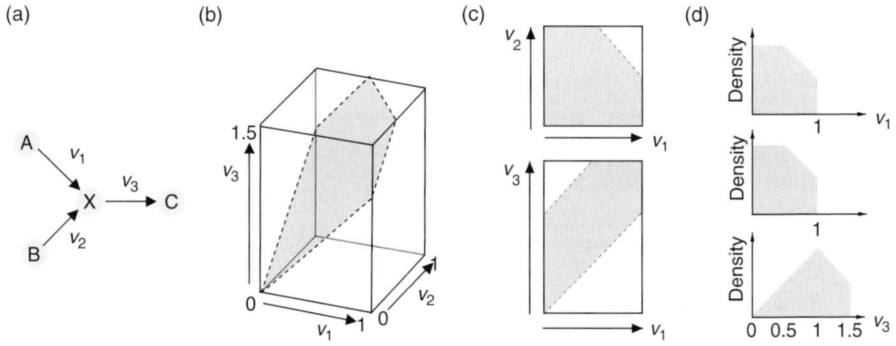

Figure 7.16 Polyhedron of stationary fluxes. (a) Metabolic branch point with three reactions and one balanced metabolite X. (b) Feasible fluxes are defined by the stationarity conditions and inequality constraints (see the main text). They form a polyhedron in flux space. (c) The same polyhedron, projected to the plane spanned by the basis vectors for ν_1 and ν_2 (top) or ν_1 and ν_3 (bottom). (d) The individual fluxes ν_1, ν_2, ν_3 show nonuniform probability distributions. As the flux vectors are uniformly distributed in the polyhedron, these distributions arise from the projections of the polyhedron to the three coordinate axes.

We now impose the additional constraints $0 \leq \nu_1 \leq 1, 0 \leq \nu_2 \leq 1, 0 \leq \nu_3 \leq 1.5$, restricting the fluxes to be nonnegative and bounded by maximal values. The resulting allowed flux combinations form a convex polyhedron in flux space (Figure 7.16(b)).

In usual flux balance analysis, we would pick one of these flux distributions by an optimality criterion. As an alternative, flux distributions can be sampled uniformly from the polyhedron [41]. If we assume equal probabilities for all allowed flux vectors $\boldsymbol{\nu}$, the distributions of the individual fluxes ν_1, ν_2, and ν_3 follow from the projections of the polyhedron to the respective directions in flux space (Figures 7.16(c) and (d)). These distributions will be nonuniform: for instance, the maximality constraint on ν_3 leads to a drop in probability for high values of ν_1 and ν_2. Moreover, different fluxes are correlated, e.g., high values of ν_1 and ν_3 are likely to appear together (Figure 7.16(c), bottom). This kind of analysis also applies to high-dimensional problems: in large metabolic networks, the probability distributions and correlations of individual fluxes can be computed by Monte Carlo sampling [41].

7.3.3.1 Sampling of Reaction Elasticities

The dynamics of a metabolic system depends both on its structure (reaction stoichiometries and wiring pattern of allosteric regulation) and on the kinetic laws and constants. But how strongly does the structure alone determine the dynamic behavior? For a given network, this question can be studied by an uncertainty analysis with kinetic parameters drawn from a random distribution: to determine the qualitative behavior around a steady state (stable or instable, node or focus?), one may draw random parameter values, solve the model for its steady state, and compute the reaction elasticities. Once the stoichiometric matrix **N** and the elasticity matrix $\tilde{\varepsilon}$

are known, the qualitative behavior follows from a fairly simple analysis of the Jacobian $\mathbf{A} = \mathbf{N}\,\tilde{\varepsilon}$ (see Section 2.3.1).

The calculation of steady states, however, is numerically quite expensive. Steuer *et al.* [42] have therefore proposed an alternative method of uncertainty analysis based on a sampling of scaled elasticities. The unscaled elasticity coefficients $\tilde{\varepsilon}_{li}$ can be written in terms of scaled elasticities ε_{li} as

$$\tilde{\varepsilon}_{li} = \frac{\partial v_l}{\partial s_i} = v_l \frac{\partial \ln|v_l|}{\partial \ln s_i} s_i^{-1} = v_l\, \varepsilon_{li}\, s_i^{-1}. \tag{7.38}$$

A scaled elasticity ε_{li} represents an apparent reaction order: in a linear or bilinear reaction, it has a value of 1 for substrates and -1 for products. For Michaelis–Menten kinetics and common modes of activation and inhibition, the absolute values vary between 1 (resembling mass-action kinetics) and 0 (saturation).

For uncertainty analysis using Eq. (7.38), the scaled elasticities ε_{li} are drawn randomly and independently from a uniform distribution. Stationary fluxes and concentrations can also be sampled, with the fluxes satisfying stationarity and constraints imposed by thermodynamics (see Section 9.1.4). If fluxes or concentrations are known from experiments, they can be inserted directly into the model. The unscaled elasticities are computed by (7.38), and with the stoichiometric matrix, the Jacobian can be computed. It is instructive to study a scaled version of the Jacobian, $\mathrm{Dg}(\mathbf{s})^{-1}\mathbf{A}\,\mathrm{Dg}(\mathbf{s})$, as this matrix allows us to compare kinetic models directly for their qualitative behavior – e.g., the occurrence of bifurcations – irrespective of their particular steady-state concentrations.

7.3.4
Distributions for Kinetic Parameters

Parameter distributions can describe actual variability in cell populations as seen in single-cell measurements (see Section 11.14). Flow cytometry or fluorescence microscopy reveal distributions and correlations of enzyme levels, which can then be used for uncertainty analysis. On the other hand, a distribution can also describe our limited knowledge about parameter values: if upper and lower bounds for an enzyme level are known, we may assume a uniform distribution in this range. By exploring the consequences of different values, uncertainty analysis will tell us which of the model results are well determined and which would require more accurate parameter values.

In both cases, the results of uncertainty analysis depend crucially on the shape and size of the assumptive parameter distribution. A narrow distribution will induce little variability, and correlations between parameters can also make a big difference. Therefore, the parameter distribution should be chosen carefully and with a meaningful interpretation.

7.3.4.1 Principle of Minimal Information

If a parameter distribution is supposed to describe our subjective knowledge, it should express all implied information and nothing more. According to the *principle of minimal information* [43], this can be achieved by choosing a distribution with maximal Shannon entropy, given all constraints that arise from our present knowledge (for details on entropies, see web supplement). If reliable upper and lower bounds for a parameter are available, the entropy is maximized by a uniform distribution, so the parameter should be drawn uniformly from the interval in question. On the other hand, if the mean value and variance are known, application of the same information principle leads to a Gaussian distribution. In either case, we need to decide in advance how to parametrize the model: use of logarithmic or nonlogarithmic parameters, for instance, will lead to different results.

7.3.4.2 Thermodynamic Constraints on Parameters

Whenever kinetic parameter values are fitted, optimized, or drawn from a random distribution, one needs to make sure that only valid parameter combinations are considered. In metabolic networks with mass-action kinetics, for instance, the rate constants $k_{\pm l}$ and the equilibrium constant K_l^{eq} for each reaction l have to satisfy the relation $k_{+l}/k_{-l} = K_l^{eq}$. The equilibrium constants, in turn, depend on the standard chemical potentials $\mu_i^{(0)}$ via $\ln K_l^{eq} = -\beta \sum_i n_{il}\, \mu_i^{(0)}$ with $\beta = 1/(RT)$, which yields the condition

$$k_{+l}/k_{-l} = e^{-\beta \sum_i n_{il}\, \mu_i^{(0)}}. \tag{7.39}$$

A set of rate constants will only be feasible if there exists a set of chemical potentials $\mu_l^{(0)}$ that fulfills condition (7.39). For a densely connected network, it is unlikely that randomly chosen rate constants will pass this test. Instead of testing condition (7.39), we can directly employ it for a different parametrization of the model [36, 44]: values of the chemical potentials $\mu_i^{(0)}$ are directly sampled from a Gaussian distribution; these values determine the equilibrium constants. Next, prefactors r_l are sampled from a log-normal distribution and the kinetic constants are computed by $k_{\pm l} = r_l (K_l^{eq})^{\pm 1/2}$. This sampling procedure yields rate constants $k_{\pm l}$ with dependent log-normal distributions, which are thermodynamically feasible by construction. The convenience kinetics [37] and the thermodynamic-kinetic modeling approach [44] parametrize kinetic models in such a way, which ensures thermodynamic feasibility.

7.3.4.3 Obtaining Parameter Distributions from Experimental Data

Distributions of kinetic parameters are needed for uncertainty analysis, but they are also useful for parameter estimation. In maximum likelihood estimation, upper and lower bounds on parameters can restrict the parameters to biologically plausible values and decrease the numerical effort; in Bayesian estimation, uncertain prior knowledge can be directly traded against a good data fit.

So how can we specify meaningful parameter distributions for unknown or uncertain parameters? A simple possibility is to choose a plausible value for each parameter and to allow for some variation around it, e.g., by using a Gaussian distribution for the logarithmic parameter values. One question here is how to determine realistic values and variances; another question is how to choose correlations between the parameters and to ensure that the parameter sets satisfy all relevant constraints.

Data on thermodynamic and enzyme kinetic parameters can be found in publications or databases like NIST [45] or Brenda [46]. Simple distributions for positive parameters can be obtained from them as follows [38]. Parameters that have been measured are described by a log-normal distribution representing the measured value and error bar; if experimental conditions are not exactly comparable, the error bar may be artificially increased. If a parameter has not been measured, one may describe it by a broader distribution: for instance, the empirical distribution of Michaelis constants in the Brenda database, which is roughly log-normal, could be used to describe a specific, but unknown Michaelis constant. Multivariate Gaussian distributions accounting for constraints between kinetic parameters can be obtained by Bayesian estimation [38] (see Section 4.4.7).

7.4 Robustness

Summary

Robustness – the ability to maintain biological function despite external variation, internal fluctuations, or failure of system parts – is an essential feature of biological systems. During evolution, networks have developed structures that contribute to robustness, such as feedback loops or redundant elements. Robustness and control properties, as described by the summation theorems of metabolic control theory, can also result from the scaling behavior of the system. If robustness properties of biological systems are known or have been hypothesized, they can be a helpful guideline for model building.

Living organisms must be able to tolerate noise, unpredictable changes in their environment, and imperfections of their own components. In addition, individual pathways within cells need to work properly under varying external conditions (temperature, nutrients, stress conditions) and cope with various internal changes (e.g., metabolic status, different cell cycle phases). The cellular machinery itself can be perturbed by fluctuating gene expression and by mutations, which may change the parameters and even the structure of the cellular network.

Robustness, the ability to work reliably under varying conditions, is an important and characteristic property of living systems [47, 48, 49]. Although robustness is a mechanistic concept, it also plays an important evolutionary role: if a certain behavior maximizes the biological fitness, then any deviation from it will lead to a fitness loss. Hence, evolution will not only select for systems that work optimally under standard conditions (typical states of cell and environment, complete system), but in addition, for systems that can deal with deviations from the ideal situation. Probably, systems will be adapted to typical and frequent perturbations rather than to extremely unusual conditions.

Besides being robust, cells also need to be *sensitive* to certain signals, e.g., to respond precisely and adequately to external stimuli. There is a subtle interplay between robustness and sensitivity: in order to be sensitive to its input signals, a sensory system must be robust against other influences. On the other hand, sensitive signaling systems can trigger adaptation and thereby enhance the overall robustness of the cell. Robustness and sensitivity are two sides of a coin, and their proper balance is vital for the functioning of cells.

Robustness in cells can be achieved by robust parts and by network structures that promote robustness, such as backup elements or feedback loops. If a robustness mechanism is added to an existing network, it can destroy the robustness of other quantities: for instance, a feedback system that suppresses low-frequency noise may increase the noise at higher frequencies [47].

7.4.1 Robustness Properties in Biochemical Systems

7.4.1.1 Biological Robustness Properties

The notion of robustness always refers to two quantities: an influencing quantity x that is perturbed and an output quantity $y(x)$ to be stabilized. Depending on the nature of x, we can distinguish between different kinds of robustness [48]: *parameter insensitivity* implies that qualitative behavior depends little on details of the reaction kinetics and the kinetic constants; *homeostasis* stabilizes a quantity against external dynamic perturbations; *canalization* ensures that the system reaches a specific outcome from arbitrary initial conditions; *failure tolerance* means that a network remains functional if some of its parts are deleted. Mathematically, an output y is robust to an influence x if deviations of x from its reference value have little (or no) effect on y. This implies that a random variation of x_m leads to little (or no) variability in y and that many possible values of x will yield similar (or identical) values of y.

7.4.1.2 Mathematical Robustness Criteria

Various mathematical methods have been devised to quantify robustness in different cases. Robustness to small parameter changes in kinetic models can be estimated by the (scaled or unscaled) metabolic response coefficients. According to Eq. (7.35), the response matrix $\boldsymbol{R}_{\mathrm{x}}^{\mathrm{y}}$ determines how much variability is caused by narrow parameter distributions. To estimate how strongly a specific output behavior is affected by large perturbations, we can quantify the range of parameter sets that lead to this behavior. Robustness of a dynamical property (e.g., oscillations), for instance, can be quantified by the area in parameter space in which this behavior occurs [48]. Likewise, robustness of a steady-state (or another dynamical attractor) against the initial conditions can be measured by the size of its basin of attraction, and robustness against gene deletions can be quantified by the number of single-gene deletions that leave a certain network property intact. In all three cases, the areas or numbers can be estimated by random sampling.

7.4.1.3 Precise Robustness in a Bacterial Two-Component System

A quantity y in a model is *precisely robust* to a parameter x if this parameter does not influence y at all. Certain model structures can ensure precise robustness: examples

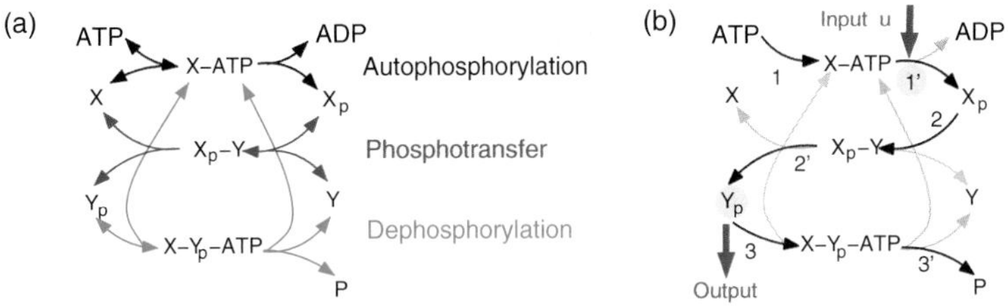

Figure 7.17 Model of the EnvZ/OmpR two-component system in *E. coli*. [53] (a) The model describes three subsequent reactions: autophos-phorylation (black), phosphotransfer (gray), and dephos-phorylation (red). (b) The same model, with the flow of phosphate groups highlighted in black. Numbers denote reaction steps in the model; input and output variables are marked by blue arrows.

occur in a model of the bacterial chemotaxis pathway [50–52] and in a model of the two-component signaling system [53], which we shall discuss now.

Two-component systems are an important form of signaling systems in bacteria: in the EnvZ/OmpR system in *E. coli*, the membrane-bound sensor EnvZ senses osmolarity and activates the diffusible transcription factor OmpR, which then triggers the osmotic stress response. Experiments [54] have shown that a system output (in this case, expression of target genes of OmpR) is remarkably robust against overexpression of both signaling proteins: it changes by roughly 20% even if the EnvZ and OmpR levels are increased by a factor of 10.

Shinar *et al.* [53] have proposed a robust kinetic model of the EnvZ/OmpR system (see Figure 7.17): (i) first, the sensor EnvZ (called X) is phosphorylated by consumption of ATP; (ii) its phosphate group is transferred to the regulator OmpR (called Y); (iii) finally, the phosphorylated regulator (called Y_P) is dephosphorylated again.

In the model equations, each reaction consists of two elementary steps, a reversible binding step and an irreversible dissociation step, both with mass-action kinetics: the three reactions correspond to pairs of elementary reactions (1, 1′), (2, 2′) and (3, 3′) (numbers shown in Figure 7.17(b)) with reaction velocities

$$\begin{array}{llcl} \text{Autophosphorylation :} & v_1 & = & k_1[\mathrm{X}][\mathrm{ATP}]-k_{-1}[\mathrm{X}\cdot\mathrm{ATP}] \\ & v_{1'} & = & k_{1'}(u)[\mathrm{X}\cdot\mathrm{ATP}] \\ \text{Phosphotransfer :} & v_2 & = & k_2[\mathrm{X_P}][\mathrm{Y}]-k_{-2}[\mathrm{X_P}\cdot\mathrm{Y}] \\ & v_{2'} & = & k_{2'}[\mathrm{X_P}\cdot\mathrm{Y}] \\ \text{Dephosphorylation :} & v_3 & = & k_3[\mathrm{Y_P}][\mathrm{X}\cdot\mathrm{ATP}]-k_{-3}[\mathrm{X}\cdot\mathrm{Y_P}\cdot\mathrm{ATP}] \\ & v_{3'} & = & k_{3'}[\mathrm{X}\cdot\mathrm{Y_P}\cdot\mathrm{ATP}]. \end{array} \tag{7.40}$$

The binding steps are described by forward and backward rate constants $k_{\pm 1}, k_{\pm 2}, k_{\pm 3}$, while the covalent modification steps have only forward rate constants $k_{1'}$, $k_{2'}$, and $k_{3'}$.

In some two-component systems, the dephosphorylation requires the presence of ATP, although ATP is not needed in this step as an energy source. This requirement for ATP has been shown experimentally for the EnvZ/OmpR system itself, for the envelope stress system CpxA/CpxR in *E. coli*, and for the oxygen limitation system PrrB/PrrA in *R. sphaeroides* (see [53]). The need for ATP in dephosphorylation is modeled in a very particular way: it is assumed that the first intermediate complex, X·ATP, is needed as a catalyst in the dephosphorylation step. The external osmolarity signal u regulates the autophosphorylation rate *via* the parameter $k_{1'}(u)$. A given value of $k_{1'}$ will lead to a certain steady-state level of Y_P, which is regarded as the system output (blue arrows in Figure 7.17(b)).

The model shows a single steady-state flux, in which phosphate groups from ATP are converted into inorganic phosphate (see Figure 7.17(b)). The presence of an external stress signal changes the phosphorylation rate of X, which shifts the steady state and changes the output concentration $[Y_P]$. The system output reads

$$s^{ss}_{Y_P}(u) = \frac{(k_{-3}+k_{3'})}{k_{+3}}\frac{k_{1'}(u)}{k_{3'}}. \tag{7.41}$$

The output signal depends on the kinetic parameters, but not on the total concentrations of X, Y, and ATP, and is therefore completely robust against changes of these three quantities. Robustness in this system only breaks down if the total concentration of Y is below the value given by Eq. (7.41): in this case, the flux stops and Y is completely phosphorylated (reaching a lower concentration than in Eq. (7.41)). The remarkable thing about this model is that its robustness properties do not rely on fine-tuned parameters. On the contrary, they are "hard-coded" by the system structure and it will not be affected by parameter variation between cells.

7.4.2 Structural Robustness in Large Networks

About 300 out of 4000 genes in *E. coli* have been classified as *essential* [47] – the cell needs them to survive – so most loss-of-function mutations have relatively little effect on cell viability. On the one hand, many cell systems are only needed in special situations – e.g., a synthesis pathway may be necessary in growth on minimal medium, but not in growth on a full medium. On the other hand, different proteins (e.g., isoenzymes) and metabolic pathways can also compensate for each other.

7.4.2.1 Backup Genes

Biological and technical systems can be made more robust by backup strategies: if a system component exists twice (e.g., an enzyme is coded by two alleles in a diploid cell), the two copies are redundant, and one of them may fail without compromising the system's performance. Multiple enzyme copies can evolve by gene duplication, and many genes (about 60% of the genes in yeast [55]) have duplicates. If one copy is lost, we may expect the enzyme amount to decrease and the physiological effect of the gene to be weaker. This effect can be avoided by quantitative robustness – as manifested, for instance, by the phenomenon of recessive genes. Quantitative robustness of enzyme levels can be ensured by gene silencing (e.g., in one copy of the X chromosomes in women) or by feedback control of expression levels. Furthermore, the biochemical effect of enzymes can be partially robust against the enzyme level, as we saw in Section 7.4.1.3.

After a gene duplication, genes can be expressed to higher amounts and backup genes are available for the case of loss-of-function mutations. However, gene duplication comes at a cost, especially in cells that replicate fast and therefore need to keep their genome small. Under strong selection pressure on genome size, even antibackup strategies may evolve: obligate intracellular parasites have lost many genes that are dispensable under the constant conditions in host cells. Also virus strains can lose some of their own genes and profit from gene products produced by wild-type viruses residing in the same host cell [56]. By reducing their genome, these "selfish" mutants gain a fitness advantage, but at the same time, they completely depend on other viruses and thus become extremely vulnerable. Similarly, as soon as cells lose the ability to produce certain substances (e.g., amino acids), these substances become essential, i.e., they have to be taken up from food.

7.4.2.2 Backup Pathways

There is not only redundancy between individual genes, but also on the level of pathways. For example, many cells can use two pathways – glycolysis and the TCA cycle – for producing ATP. If one of the pathways cannot be used (e.g., because either glucose or oxygen is missing), there is still a chance to use the second pathway. Many pathways are dispensable in appropriate environments: peripheral anabolic pathways are only needed if their product is not provided by the environment, so their action can often be replaced by transporters [48]. If a pathway is blocked by the loss of a gene, it may be bypassed by redirecting of metabolic fluxes. The importance of both kinds of backup mechanisms, redundancy between gene copies and by higher level mechanisms, has been estimated for the yeast *S. cerevisiae*. It turned out that in this case, redundancy of individual genes plays a minor role [55].

Certain network structures are particularly robust against failure of elements. In metabolic networks, for instance, the mean distance between metabolites – that is, the number of reactions between them – is remarkably small, and it increases little even if a considerable fraction of nodes is removed at random. However, if a few highly connected metabolites (such as ATP) are removed, the network diameter rises rapidly.

7.4.3 Quantitative Robustness by Feedback

7.4.3.1 Negative Feedback

A basic task in control engineering is to keep a certain quantity constant despite external perturbations and noise or variation in the system components. This problem of homeostasis also arose in evolution of biological networks. A simple and powerful way to buffer a quantity against perturbations is *negative feedback*. Let us consider a linear model

$$\frac{dx}{dt} = \boldsymbol{A}\boldsymbol{x} + \boldsymbol{B}\,\boldsymbol{u}, \tag{7.42}$$

with Jacobian matrix $\boldsymbol{A}$ and an input vector $\boldsymbol{u}(t)$, obtained from a metabolic network (see Section 4.3.4). The output $\boldsymbol{x}$ will be affected by fluctuations of $\boldsymbol{u}$, and the robustness of the system depends on the eigenvalues of $\boldsymbol{A}$.

In a technical system, this eigenvalue spectrum could be modified by adding a feedback controller that measures the current state $\boldsymbol{x}$, computes a linear function $z = \boldsymbol{F}\boldsymbol{x}$, and adds it to the system input. The resulting *closed-loop system* reads

$$\frac{\mathrm{d}x}{\mathrm{d}t} = \boldsymbol{A}\boldsymbol{x} + \boldsymbol{B}(\boldsymbol{u} + \boldsymbol{z}) = (\boldsymbol{A} + \boldsymbol{B}\boldsymbol{F})\boldsymbol{x} + \boldsymbol{B}\boldsymbol{u}, \tag{7.43}$$

with the Jacobian matrix $\boldsymbol{A} + \boldsymbol{B}\boldsymbol{F}$. With an appropriate choice of the feedback matrix $\boldsymbol{F}$, eigenvalues can be shifted to have large negative real parts and the system will become more stable. However, a single negative feedback loop will not move an individual eigenvalue, but change all of them in different ways: depending on the system, it may also destabilize a stable system, e.g., by moving a pair of complex eigenvalues to the right-hand side of the complex plane, enabling the system to show sustained oscillations (see Section 8.2).

If the Jacobian $\boldsymbol{A}$ stems from a metabolic system, its diagonal elements describe the effect that substance concentrations exert on themselves. For the enzymatic chain shown in Figure 7.18 with fixed reaction rate $v_0 > 0$, the Jacobian $\boldsymbol{A} = \boldsymbol{N}\tilde{\varepsilon}$ reads

$$\boldsymbol{A} = \begin{pmatrix} 1 & -1 & 0 \\ 0 & 1 & -1 \end{pmatrix} \begin{pmatrix} 0 & 0 \\ \tilde{\varepsilon}_{11} & \tilde{\varepsilon}_{12} \\ 0 & \tilde{\varepsilon}_{22} \end{pmatrix} = \begin{pmatrix} -\tilde{\varepsilon}_{11} & -\tilde{\varepsilon}_{12} \\ \tilde{\varepsilon}_{11} & \tilde{\varepsilon}_{12} - \tilde{\varepsilon}_{22} \end{pmatrix}, \tag{7.44}$$

where typically $\tilde{\varepsilon}_{11}$ and $\tilde{\varepsilon}_{22}$ are positive while $\tilde{\varepsilon}_{12}$ is negative. Negative diagonal elements arise from the reaction kinetics: if a reaction consumes a substrate (stoichiometric coefficient -1) and the reaction rate increases with the substrate concentration (positive reaction elasticity), it will contribute negatively to the substance's diagonal element in the Jacobian. This also holds for a reaction product (which has a positive stoichiometric coefficient and a negative elasticity). This effect can be further enhanced by allosteric control (substrate activation or product inhibition), which in this case enlarges the magnitude of the elasticity coefficients. In genetic network models, protein levels can be stabilized in a similar way by a negative feedback to their own transcription.

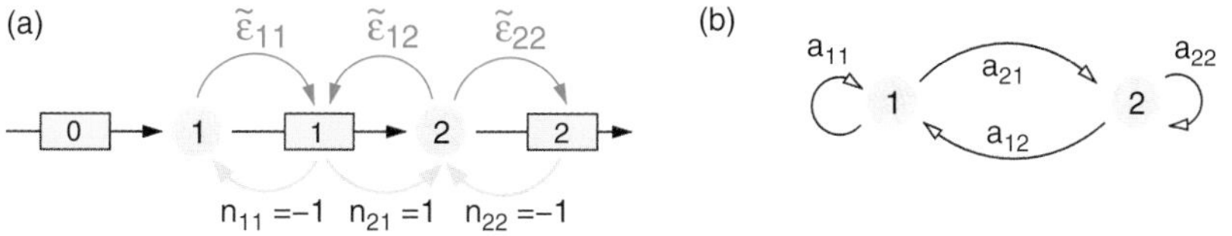

Figure 7.18 Interpretation of the Jacobian matrix. (a) A chain of metabolic reactions (boxes 0, 1, 2) and metabolites (circles). Around a steady state, concentration fluctuations affect the reaction rates *via* the elasticity coefficients (red). In the balance equation, reaction rates act back on the concentrations *via* stoichiometric coefficients (gray). (b) The Jacobian matrix reads $\boldsymbol{A} = \boldsymbol{N}\tilde{\varepsilon}$. Individual elements arise from paths of length 2 in scheme (a): the element $a_{11} = -\tilde{\varepsilon}_{11}$, for instance, is the product of $\tilde{\varepsilon}_{11}$ and n_{11} on the way from metabolite 1 to reaction 2 and back. If there are several paths with the same start and end point, the resulting values are added.

7.4.3.2 Integral Feedback

Integral feedback, a special type of negative feedback, is a popular stabilization method in control engineering. By adding a feedback controller to an existing linear system, the steady-state output of this system can be kept at a prescribed value. Whenever the output deviates from the desired value, the feedback controller senses the deviation and steers the system in the desired direction. To be more specific, let us consider a simple linear system with an output variable $y(t) = ku(t)$ that depends on the input variable $u(t)$. Our goal is to stabilize the steady-state output y^{st} at a predefined value y_0. In integral feedback, a sensor continuously measures the current difference $\Delta y(t) = y(t) - y_0$ and computes its negative time integral $z(t)$. This integral is then fed back into the system by adding it to the input. The resulting differential equations read

$$\begin{aligned} z(t) &= -\int_{t_0}^{t} y(t) - y_0 t \\ y(t) &= ku(t) + k'z(t). \end{aligned} \tag{7.45}$$

If k and u assume arbitrary stationary values, this specific feedback will stabilize the steady-state value at $y^{st} = y_0$ (exercise 9). It has been shown that the mechanism for precise adaptation in the chemotaxis model [50], for instance, implements an integral feedback [57].

7.4.4 Scaling Laws, Invariance, and Dimensional Analysis

The notion of robustness concerns the quantitative relationship between output variables y and inputs or parameters x. In some cases, a dependence between them can be inferred from symmetries or from scaling laws of the system. Some important properties of biological systems can be inferred from their scaling behavior under a change of physical units, in particular, rescaling of time.

Symmetries describe the behavior of physical systems under transformations. If a rotation or mirror reflection leaves a geometric shape unchanged, the shape is *symmetric* or *invariant* with respect to the transformation. Physical laws can also show symmetries, for instance, with respect to translation or rotation in space. Shapes like the fractal Sierpinski triangle (Figure 7.19) which resemble their own rescaled parts are called *self-similar*.

Many quantities in nature are related to each other by power laws of the form

$$y(x) = y_0 (x/x_0)^{\gamma}, \tag{7.46}$$

with reference values x_0 and y_0 and a scaling exponent γ. In a double-logarithmic plot log y against log x, this translates into a linear relationship $\log y = \gamma \log x +$ const. Simple scaling laws hold for geometric shapes under rescaling of space co-ordinates. If x represents a length, then geometric scaling of shapes implies integer exponents (see Figure 7.19): the area of a square (side length L) scales as L^2, a cube volume scales as L^3. Physically, the scaling transformation can have two

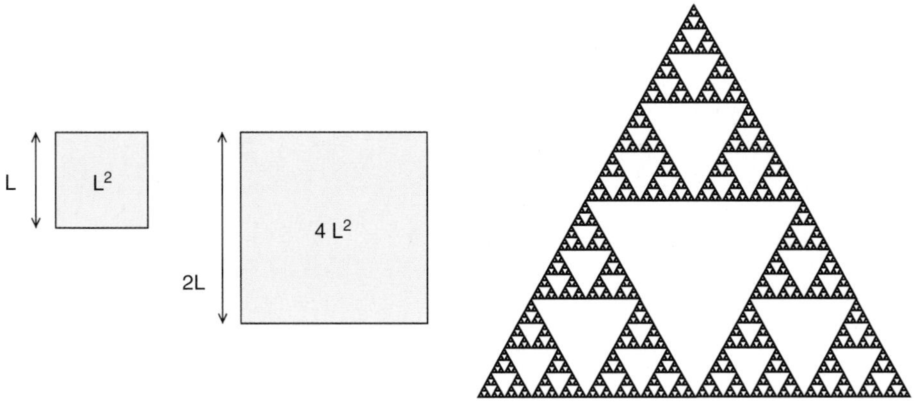

Figure 7.19 (a) The area of a square scales quadratically with the side length. (b) The Sierpinski triangle, a self-similar fractal, is built from smaller copies of itself. Being a fractal, it shows an unusual scaling behavior: if its side length is doubled, its area increases by a factor of 3.

interpretations: we can either think of a shape that is actually enlarged, or we consider the same size, but under a change of length units (e.g., from meters to centimeters) – importantly, the numerical result is the same in both cases.

If the scaling exponent has a value of 0, y remains constant and is called *scale-invariant*. Such quantities can be constructed mathematically from quantities with known scaling behavior: e.g., if the surface area A and the volume V of a body show geometric scaling, $A \sim L^2$ and $V \sim L^3$, then $y = A^{1/2}/V^{1/3}$ is a scale-invariant quantity. We could also infer this from the physical units: while the area and volume are measured in m^2 and m^3, respectively, y is dimensionless. As pointed out above, this means two things: (i) if y is a numerical quantity in a model, it will not be affected by a change of length units. (ii) In the real system, it will not change by actually enlarging or shrinking the system. The use of such dimensionless quantities (e.g., the Mach number in fluid dynamics) can allow us to treat various similar systems by a single unifying law.

Many physiological quantities – such as metabolic rate or lifespan of animals – are related to the body mass by allometric scaling laws of the form (7.46), where x denotes the body mass and the scaling exponents are typically multiples of $1/4$. This is rather surprising because geometric scaling (with body mass proportional to body volume) would imply multiples of $1/3$. This nongeometric scaling in physiology has been explained by a self-similar, fractal geometry of the blood circulation system and related supply systems [58]. Fractals are geometric shapes with non-integer scaling exponents: if the side length of the Sierpinski triangle (in Figure 7.19, right) doubles, for instance, its its size is increased by a factor of 3 (in between 2 for the length of a line, and 4 for the area of a square). Its scaling exponent is $\log 3/\log 2$, a non-integer measure of its dimensionality.

7.4.5
Summation Laws and Homogeneous Functions

A *homogeneous* mathematical function $f(x_1,\ldots,x_n)$ with degree k satisfies the equation

$$f(\lambda x_1,\ldots,\lambda x_n)=\lambda^k f(x_1,\ldots,x_n). \tag{7.47}$$

If we differentiate this equation by λ and then set $\lambda=1$, we obtain a sum rule for the normalized derivatives

$$k=\sum_l \frac{x_l}{f}\frac{\partial f}{\partial x_l}=\sum_l \frac{\partial \ln f}{\partial \ln x_l}. \tag{7.48}$$

For a scale-invariant quantity f (with $k=0$), the normalized derivatives sum to 0, while for linear scaling ($k=1$), the normalized derivatives sum to 1.

7.4.5.1 Summation Theorems

The summation theorems of metabolic control theory can be obtained as special cases of the sum rule (7.48). If all reaction rates v_l in a metabolic model contain an enzyme concentration E_l as a prefactor, $v_l=E_l\, w_l(\mathbf{s},t)$ (with concentration vector $\mathbf{s}$ and time t), then rescaling all enzyme concentrations by a factor λ will linearly rescale all reaction velocities: by replacing $E_i\rightarrow\lambda E_i$, we obtain the system equation $d\mathbf{s}/dt=\lambda \mathbf{N}\mathbf{v}(\mathbf{s})$ or equivalently, $d\mathbf{s}/d(\lambda t)=\mathbf{N}\mathbf{v}(\mathbf{s})$, so effectively, time is rescaled by the factor λ.

As the steady-state concentrations remain unchanged under time rescaling they satisfy summation theorems of the form (7.48) with $k=0$, $f=s_i^{st}$, and $x_l=E_l$. A scaling law with exponent $k=0$ indicates a quantity that is precisely robust against a simultaneous overexpression of all enzymes. The steady-state fluxes, on the other hand, scale linearly with time, so they satisfy Eq. (7.48) with $k=1, f=J_i$, and $x_l=E_l$. Thus the normalized response coefficients, which are identical to the normalized control coefficients, obey the summation theorems

$$\sum_l \frac{\partial J_i}{\partial E_l}\frac{E_l}{J_i}=\sum_l C_{v_l}^{J_i}=1,\quad \sum_l \frac{\partial s_i}{\partial E_l}\frac{E_l}{s_i}=\sum_l C_{v_l}^{S_i}=0. \tag{7.49}$$

7.4.5.2 Conservation Laws for Sensitivity

The sum rules arising from scaling laws represent a limit for overall robustness. The summation theorems (7.49), for instance, state that there is a fixed total amount of non-robustness appear in a system. In particular, a steady-state flux is always sensitive to some of the enzymes abundances – no matter which specific kinetic laws are chosen in the model or a real-world system. Therefore, a change of kinetics, e.g., by allosteric feedback, can redistribute the sensitivities, but it can never remove them completely. Likewise, feedback loops can make a system robust against parameter variation. However, the same feedback loops make the system more susceptible to high-frequency perturbations [47]. Thus if some properties of a system are very robust due to parameter optimization or feedback, this may reduce robustness of other system properties. Under these circumstances, robust design will not necessarily *generate* robustness, but *redistribute* it to those pairs of parameters and outputs that need to be most robust. Redistribution of nonrobustness can also take place on higher levels of organization: for example, by maintaining a constant metabolic state (robustness), cells provide a favorable environment to intracellular parasites and therefore become more susceptible to infection (fragility).

7.4.5.3 **Compensation of Correlated Fluctuations**

Enzyme amounts in cells can vary dramatically, both temporally and between different cells. However, this variability is not completely at random: in particular, enzymes that are encoded by the same bacterial operon are produced from a common mRNA transcript, so their fluctuations are strongly correlated. These correlations allow for a powerful robustness mechanism: the system coded by the operon can be robust against a common over- or underexpression of *all* enzymes if the effects of different enzymes compensate each other; in this case, the effects of a common over- or underexpression may just cancel out. In this mechanism, the overall expression level of the operon may not exert any control on the output, i.e., the scaling exponent between operon expression and system output has a value $k = 0$. This behavior can be achieved by a combination of feedback loops (as it has been proposed for the bacterial chemotaxis system [52]) and it can also arise automatically in metabolic systems (see Section 7.4.5.1).

7.4.6
Robustness and Evolvability

Cellular networks are highly complex, and some of this complexity has been attributed to their need for robustness [47]. The presence of robustness mechanisms depends on which perturbations occur in the typical life of the cell type in question. Some metabolic pathways and regulation mechanisms are only needed under rare circumstances. Robustness mechanisms like gene redundancy or regulatory proteins come at a cost (genome size, protein production), so they will only be preserved if there there are enough situations in which they are needed and selected for. Intracellular parasites, for instance, live under relatively constant conditions and can survive with much simpler networks and smaller genomes.

Besides its direct fitness effects, robustness can also contribute to evolvability [33]. If cell functions are robust against changes in a specific pathway A, then mutations in A will not compromise the function of the rest of the cell; this allows cell populations to explore a variety of versions for A, which makes this pathway better evolvable. In general, if phenotypes are relatively robust against genotypic changes, then genotypic variability can be increased until, possibly, a combination of silent mutations suddenly turns out to provide a fitness advantage. Higher evolvability may provide a second-order selection advantage for robust systems. In periods of fast evolution, on the other hand – after drastic changes in external conditions or within unfavorable environments – robustness may become an obstacle. In this case, evolution requires strong selection, which is impossible without clear phenotypic changes.

7.4.7
Robustness and Modeling

In modeling, the analysis of sensitivity and robustness links three important aspects of biological systems: the environment (which parameters show strong variation?); the biological mechanism (how does parameter variation affect the system outputs?); and the biological function (how do different kinds of variation affect the cell fitness?). This can lead to relevant predictions: for instance, sensitivities computed from a model can indicate the most efficient ways to manipulate a system, predicting, for instance, oncogenes [59] or drug targets.

But robustness can also be helpful for the modeling process itself: if details of a biological mechanism are not known, then by postulating certain robustness properties, the model structure can be restricted (for examples, see [50, 52, 53]). For example, Eldar *et al.* [60] generated many variants of a morphogen model by random parameter sampling and then screened them for models that met a certain robustness criterion. This allowed them to determine model properties that are required for, or at least are strongly correlated with, robustness.

Moreover, robustness and sensitivity play a role in parameter estimation: if a quantity y is insensitive to a parameter x, then data on y will not be useful to determine the parameter. On the other hand, for prediction of y, no accurate estimate of x is needed. As a consequence, it may be easier to study robust systems: think of x as a quantity outside the system of interest. If the system itself is robust, then also the mathematical model describing it will depend little on wrong model assumptions about parameter values, genotypic variation in the surrounding network, initial conditions, or boundary conditions. This can be helpful for modeling because then the simplifying assumption of an isolated system will be justified.

Exercises and Problems

1. Typical concentrations in metabolic pathways are of the order of mM, while mRNA concentrations in gene regulatory are rather of the order of nM. Compute the corresponding orders of magnitude for the particle numbers: compare a prokaryotic cell (diameter 1 μm) to a eukaryotic cell (5 μm). Estimate roughly the range of fluctuations. Which of the modeling frameworks (deterministic or stochastic) should be used in these cases?

2. The ith substance in a biochemical system participates in a number of chemical reactions, with stoichiometric coefficients n_{il} for lth reaction. Consider a macroscopic steady state with average molecule number $\bar{x}_i$ and corresponding reaction velocities ν_l and elasticities $\tilde{\varepsilon}_{li}$. Compute the variance of the fluctuating molecule

number x_i due to chemical reaction noise, assuming that all other substance levels in the system are fixed at predefined values (no fluctuations). Hint: Linearize the chemical Langevin equation around the steady-state value and use the Lyapunov equation to compute the variance.

3. Derive the mean values and Fano factors $\langle x\rangle = w_x^+/w_x^-$, $\langle y\rangle = \langle x\rangle\, w_y^+/w_y^-$, $\mathrm{var}(x)/\langle x\rangle = 1$, $\mathrm{var}(y)/\langle y\rangle = 1 + \frac{w_y^+}{w_x^- + w_y^-}$ for the model of transcription and translation in the Langevin equation framework. Hint: Introduce the constant DNA concentration $g = 1$ as an auxiliary variable in the variable vector $z = (g, x, y)^{\mathrm{T}}$, express the propensities by a linear function $a = Wz$, and use the Lyapunov equation.

4. (a) Derive the spectral densities (Eq. (7.29)) for the two-gene model. (b) Use the result to compute the correlation functions (7.30).

5. (a) An unknown parameter value is assumed to be in the interval $[a, b]$. Apply the principle of minimal information and show that it leads to a uniform distribution in this interval. (b) For another parameter, only its expected value and variance are known. Show that the information principle leads to a Gaussian distribution for the parameter. (c) Show that applying the information principle to a parameter itself or to its logarithm will lead to different results.

6. (a) Implement the following Monte Carlo sampling procedure. A circle (diameter L) is surrounded by a square (side length L); to estimate the circle area relative to the square area (true value $\pi/4$), sample N points $\mathbf{x}_i$ uniformly and randomly from the square and count how many of them (number n) are inside the circle (i.e., $|\mathbf{x}_i - \mathbf{x}_{\text{center}}| \leq L/2$). Use n/N as an estimate of $\pi/4$ and plot its empirical value for increasing sample numbers N. Repeat the numerical experiment several times. (b) Which probability distribution of n/N arises from the random sampling? Compute its average value and standard deviation. (c) Describe how you would use Monte Carlo sampling to compute the probability of oscillations in a kinetic model. (c) Does the error estimate for Monte Carlo sampling also hold for nonuniform parameter distributions?

7. Derive the steady-state output (Eq. (7.41)) of the two-component system.

8. Consider a substance concentration x following the rate equation $dx/dt = E_a\, a - E_b\, b\, x$ with the enzyme concentrations E_a and E_b. Use dimensionality analysis (not an explicit calculation) to show that the steady-state value of x remains unchanged if both enzyme levels change by the same percentage.

9. Consider the system (7.45) and prove that for time-constant u and k, integral feedback stabilizes the output y at the prescribed steady-state value y_0.

10. Consider a signaling pathway that responds to a step-like input stimulus. The transient response $y_i(t)$ of the ith component is characterized by its maximal amplitude y_i^* and the time point t_i^* at which this maximum is reached. Derive the summation theorems for both quantities from time-scaling considerations.

References

1 Turner, T.E., Schnell, S. and Burrage, K. (2004) Stochastic approaches for modelling *in vivo* reactions. *Computational Biology and Chemistry*, **28** (3), 165–178.

2 Kurtz, T.G. (1971) Limit theorems for sequences of jump Markov processes approximating ordinary differential processes. *Journal of Applied Probability*, **8**, 344–356.

3 Gillespie, D.T. (2000) The chemical Langevin equation. *Journal of Chemical Physics*, **113** (1), 297–306.

4 Rao, C.V. and Arkin, A.P. (2003) Stochastic chemical kinetics and the quasi-steady-state assumption: application to the Gillespie algorithm. *Journal of Chemical Physics*, **118** (11), 4999.

5 Jahnke, T. and Huisinga, W. (2007) Solving the chemical master equation for monomolecular reaction systems analytically. *Journal of Mathematical Biology*, **54**, 1–26.

6 Gillespie, D.T. (1976) A general method for numerically simulating the stochastic time evolution of coupled chemical reactions. *Journal of Computational Physics*, **22**, 403–434.

7 Gillespie, D.T. (1977) Exact stochastic simulation of coupled chemical reactions. *The Journal of Physical Chemistry*, **81**, 2340–2361.

8 Alfonsi, A., Cances, E., Turinici, G., Di Ventura, B. and Huisinga, W. (2005) Adaptive simulation of hybrid stochastic and deterministic models for biochemical systems. *ESAIM: Proceedings*, **14**, 1–13.

9 Gillespie, D.T. (2001) Approximate accelerated stochastic simulation of chemically reacting systems. *Journal of Chemical Physics*, **115** (4), 1716–1733.

10 Cao, Y., Gillespie, D.T. and Petzold, L.R. (2006) Efficient step size selection for the tau-leaping simulation method. *Journal of Chemical Physics*, **124**, 044109.

11 van Kampen, N.G. (1997) *Stochastic Processes in Physics and Chemistry*, 2nd edition, North-Holland, Amsterdam.

12 Thattai, M. and van Oudenaarden, A. (2001) Intrinsic noise in gene regulatory networks. *Proceedings of the National Academy of Sciences of the United States of America*, **98** (15), 8614–8619.

13 Elf, J. and Ehrenberg, M. (2003) Fast evaluation of fluctuations in biochemical networks with the linear noise approximation. *Genome Research*, **13**, 2475- 2484.

14 Hayot, F. and Jayaprakash, C. (2004) The linear noise approximation for molecular fluctuations within cells. *Physical Biology*, **1**, 205–210.

15 Samoilov, M.S. and Arkin, A.P. (2006) Deviant effects in molecular reaction pathways. *Nature Biotechnology*, **24** (10), 1235–1240.

16 Ingalls, B.P. (2004) A frequency domain approach to sensitivity analysis of biochemical systems. *The Journal of Physical Chemistry. B*, **108**, 1143–1152.

17 Liebermeister, W. (2005) Metabolic response to temporal parameter fluctuations in biochemical networks. *Journal of Theoretical Biology*, **234** (3), 423–438.

18 Wilhelm, T. and Heinrich, R. (1995) The smallest chemical reaction systems with Hopfbifurcation. *Journal of Mathematical Chemistry*, **17**, 1–14.

19 Elowitz, M.B. and Leibler, S. (2000) A synthetic oscillatory network of transcriptional regulators. *Nature*, **403**, 335–338.

20 Becskei, A. and Serrano, L. (2000) Engineering stability in gene networks by autoregulation. *Nature*, **405**, 590–592.

21 Elowitz, M. *et al.* (2002) Stochastic gene expression in a single cell. *Science*, **297**, 1183.

22 Pedraza, J.M. and van Oudenaarden, A. (2005) Noise propagation in gene networks. *Science*, **307**, 1965–1969.

23 Paulsson, J. (2004) Summing up the noise in gene networks. *Nature*, **427**, 415.

24 Thattai, M. and van Oudenaarden, A. (2001) Intrinsic noise in gene regulatory networks. *Proceedings of the National Academy of Sciences of the United States of America*, **98** (15), 8614–8619.

25 Ozbudak, E.M., Thattai, M., Kurtser, I., Grossman, A.D. and van Oudenaarden, A. (2002) Regulation of noise in the expression of a single gene. *Nature Genetics*, **31**, 69–73.

26 Swain, P.S., Elowitz, M.B. and Siggia, E.D., (2002) Intrinsic and extrinsic contributions to stochasticity in gene expression. *Proceedings of the National Academy of Sciences of the United States of America*, **99** (20), 12795.

27 Colman-Lerner, A. *et al.* (2005) Regulated cell-to-cell variation in a cell-fate decision system. *Nature*, **437**, 699–706.

28 Sigal, A., Milo, R., Cohen, A., Geva-Zatorsky, N., Klein, Y., Liron, Y., Rosenfeld, N., Danon, T., Perzov N. and Alon U. (2006) Variability and memory of protein levels in human cells. *Nature*, **444**, 643–646.

29 Arkin, A., Ross, J. and McAdams H.H. (1998) Stochastic kinetic analysis of developmental pathway bifurcation in phage lambda-infected Escherichia coli cells. *Genetics*, **149** (4).

30 Bigger, W.B. (1944) Treatment of staphylococcal infections with penicillin. *Lancet*, **244** (6320), 497–500.

31 Balaban, N.Q., Merrin, J., Chait, R., Kowalik, L. and Leibler, S. (2004) Bacterial persistence as a phenotypic switch. *Science*, **305**, 1622–1625.

32 Kussell, E., Kishony, R., Balaban, N.Q. and Leibler, S. (2005) Bacterial persistence: a model of survival in changing environments. *Genetics*, **169** (4), 1807–1814.

33 Kirschner, M. and Gerhart, J. (1998) Evolvability. *Proceedings of the National Academy of Sciences of the United States of America*, **95** (15), 8420–8427.

34 Bjedov, I., Tenaillon, O., Géerard, B., Souza, V., Denamur, E., Radman, M. Taddei, F. and Matic, I. (2003) Stress-induced mutagenesis in bacteria. *Science*, **300**, 1404–1409.

35 Steuer, R., Kurths, J., Fiehn, O. and Weckwerth, W. (2003) Observing and interpreting correlations in metabolomics networks. *Bioinformatics (Oxford, England)*, **19** (8), 1019–1026.

36 Liebermeister, W. and Klipp, E. (2005) Biochemical networks with uncertain parameters. *IEE Proceedings - Systems Biology*, **152** (3), 97–107.

37 Liebermeister, W. and Klipp, E. (2006) Bringing metabolic networks to life: convenience rate law and thermodynamic constraints. *Theoretical Biology Medical Modelling*, **3**, 41.

38 Liebermeister, W. and Klipp, E. (2006) Bringing metabolic networks to life: integration of kinetic, metabolic, and proteomic data. *Theoretical Biology Medical Modelling*, **3**, 42.

39 Trigg G.L. (ed) (2005) *Mathematical Tools for Physicists*, Wiley-VCH, Weinheim.

40 Ingalls, B.P. and Sauro, H.M. (2003) Sensitivity analysis of stoichiometric networks: an extension of metabolic control analysis to non-steady state trajectories. *Journal of Theoretical Biology*, **222** (1), 23–36.

41 Price, N.D., Schellenberger, J. and Palsson, B.Ø. (2004) Uniform sampling of steady-state flux spaces: means to design experiments and to interpret enzymopathies. *Biophysical Journal*, **87**, 2172–2186.

42 Steuer, R., Gross, T., Selbig, J. and Blasius, B. (2006) Structural kinetic modeling of metabolic networks. *Proceedings of the National Academy of Sciences of the United States of America*, **103** (32), 11868–11873.

43 Jaynes, E.T. (1957) Information theory and statistical mechanics. *Physical Review*, **106**, 620–630.

44 Ederer, M. and Gilles, E.D. (2007) Thermodynamically feasible kinetic models of reaction networks. *Biophysical Journal*, **92**, 1846–1857.

45 Goldberg, R.N. (1999) Thermodynamics of enzyme-catalyzed reactions: Part 6 – 1999 update. *Journal of Physical and Chemical Reference Data*, **28**, 931.

46 Schomburg, I., Chang, A., Ebeling, C., Gremse, M., Heldt, C., Huhn, G. and Schomburg, D. (2004) BRENDA, the enzyme database: updates and major new developments. *Nucleic Acids Research*, **32**, (Database issue), D431–D433.

47 Csete, M.E. and Doyle, J.C. (2002) Reverse engineering of biological complexity. *Science*, **295** (5560), 1664–1669.

48 Stelling, J., Sauer, U., Szallasi, Z., Doyle, F.J. and Doyle, J. (2004) Robustness of cellular functions. *Cell*, **118**, 675–685.

49 Rao, C., Wolf, D. and Arkin, A. (2002) Control, exploitation and tolerance of intracellular noise, *Nature*, **420**, 231–237.

50 Barkai, N. and Leibler, S. (1997) Robustness in simple biochemical networks. *Nature*, **387**, 913–917.

51 Alon, U., Surette, M.G., Barkai, N. and Leibler, S. (1999) Robustness in bacterial chemotaxis. *Nature*, **397**, 168–171.

52 Kollmann, M., Lovdok, L., Bartholome, K., Timmer, J. and Sourjik, V. (2005) Design principles of a bacterial chemotaxis network. *Nature*, **438**, 504–507.

53 Shinar, G., Milo, R., Martinez, M.R. and Alon, U. (2007) Input–output robustness in simple bacterial signaling systems. *Proceedings of the National Academy of Sciences of the United States of America*, **104** (50), 19931–19935.

54 Batchelor, E., Silhavy, T.J. and Goulian, M. (2004) Continuous control in bacterial regulatory circuits. *Journal of Bacteriology*, **186** (22), 7618–7625.

55 Wagner, A. (2000) Robustness against mutations in genetic networks of yeast. *Nature Genetics*, **24**, 355–361.

56 Turner, P.E. (2005) Cheating viruses and game theory. *American Scientist*, **93**, 428–435.

57 Yi, T., Huang, Y., Simon, M.I. and Doyle, J. (2000) Robust perfect adaptation in bacterial chemotaxis through integral feedback control. *Proceedings of the National Academy of Sciences of the United States of America*, **97** (9), 4649–4653.

58 West, G.B., Brown, J.H. and Enquist, B.J. (1997) A general model for the origin of allometric scaling laws in biology. *Science*, **276**, 122–126.

59 Lee, E., Salic, A., Krüger, R., Heinrich, R. and Kirschner, M.W. (2003) The roles of APC and axin derived from experimental and theoretical analysis of the Wnt pathway. *PLoS Biology*, **1** (1), 116–132.

60 Eldar, A., Rosin, D., Shilo, B.Z. and Barkai, N. (2003) Self-enhanced ligand degradation underlies robustness of morphogen gradients. *Developmental Cell*, **5**, 635–646.

8
Network Structures, Dynamics, and Function

8.1
Structure of Biochemical Networks

Summary

The structure of complex biochemical systems – e.g., metabolism or transcriptional regulation – can be represented by networks. Nodes typically correspond to molecule types or genes, while edges represent, for instance, molecular interactions, causal influences, or correlations in high-throughput data. To detect significant structures that deserve further explanation, networks can be compared to random graphs with defined statistical properties. Various characteristic structures have been found in biological networks, including scale-free degree distributions, small average path lengths, modules and clustering, as well as network motifs.

Living cells employ thousands of biochemical processes to produce and transform substances, to sense environmental stimuli and the internal cell state, and to transmit and process this information. *E. coli* bacteria contain about 4000 genes in total, so the actual number of enzyme-catalyzed reactions (including transcription and translation for all genes) and of compounds involved is at least on the order of 10^5. All these processes are regulated in an orchestrated and adaptive manner. To gain an overview over such highly complex systems, we can visualize them in the form of networks. As an example, a network representing the physical interactions among proteins in yeast is shown in Figure 8.1(a).

An analysis of network topologies emphasizes the structure of interactions rather than the detailed quantitative values. This chapter introduces some basic notions for the statistical analysis of network structures; a comprehensive treatment can be found in [1–3]. Cellular networks are based on different biochemical processes, serve different functions and evolve in different ways..

1. Metabolic networks are characterized by the set of metabolites and by the set of chemical reactions connecting these metabolites. To some extent, their structure can be predicted from the enzymes coded in the genome. Besides that, it is also

Systems Biology: A Textbook. Edda Klipp, Wolfram Liebermeister, Christoph Wierling, Axel Kowald, Hans Lehrach, and Ralf Herwig

ISBN: 978-3-527-31874-2

(a) (b)

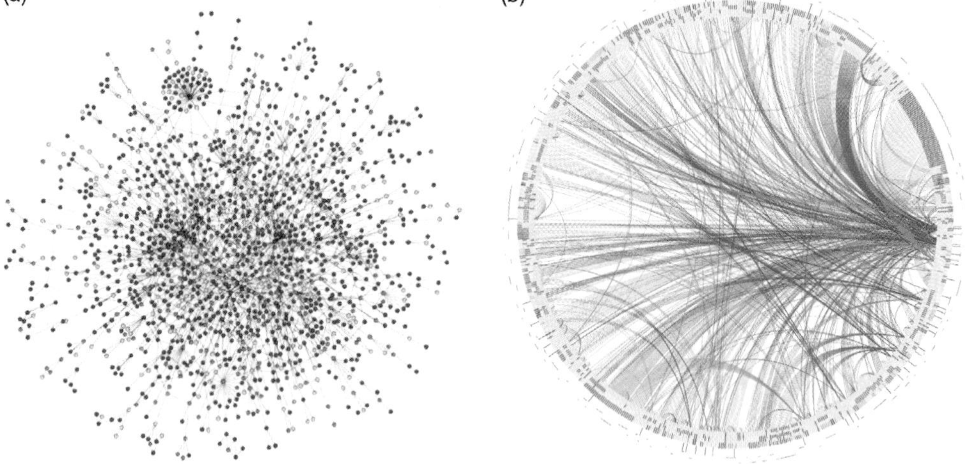

Figure 8.1 Biological networks. (a) Network of protein–protein interactions in yeast. From Jeong et al. [4]. (b) Regulatory interactions between *E. coli* genes. Genes shown as colored segments associated with the structural description of the gene's main function. Curve colors express the nature of relation (red: inhibition, blue: activation, green: dual regulation), and the traces around the circle indicate autoregulation. Courtesy of S. Ortiz, L. Rico, and A. Valencia.

restricted by the laws of chemistry, in particular, the conservation of atom numbers. Depending on their lifestyles, different species have very different metabolic networks, but some central metabolic pathways – e.g., glycolysis – are conserved across many species and all known metabolic networks use a core set of important cofactors. The most comprehensive metabolic model of *E. coli* to date [5] contains 1260 genes, 1148 unique functional proteins with 346 reactions catalyzed by isoenzymes, 167 multigene complexes (involving 415 genes), 2077 reactions, including 1387 chemical and 690 transport reactions, and 1039 unique metabolites. The model distinguishes between three compartments, namely cytoplasm, periplasm, and the extracellular space.

2. Transcription networks (Figure 8.1(b) and Section 8.2.1) summarize the transcriptional regulation of genes by transcription factors. Biochemically, the network structure is determined by transcription factor binding sites. In bacteria, their nucleotide sequences can evolve quite rapidly, which leads to rewiring of the network.

3. Protein–protein interaction networks (see Figure 8.1) represent the physical interactions like binding and complex formation derived, for instance, from yeast-two-hybrid screens (see Section 11.8).

In all three types of network, connections (enzymes or binding sites) may get lost by mutation, so network structures have to be actively preserved by selection.

Therefore, it is plausible to assume that existing connections in a network serve a biological function.

In practice, biological networks are often inferred from high-throughput data or text-mining screens. The results are similarity measures (e.g., statistical correlations, evolutionary relatedness, or co-occurrence in scientific articles). A correlation network, for instance, can be constructed from quantitative data by thresholding: an edge is drawn whenever a correlation exceeds a certain threshold value (e.g., related to statistical significance).

8.1.1 Mathematical Graphs

The structure of a network can be described by a mathematical *graph*. A graph consists of a discrete set of *nodes* and a set of *edges*, which are defined as pairs of nodes. In a directed graph, edges are ordered pairs and usually represented by arrows. In an undirected graph, edges are unordered pairs and displayed as lines. Three small graphs are shown in Figure 8.2.

A graph can be specified by its adjacency matrix $A = (a_{ij})$: edges from node i to node j are represented by elements $a_{ij} = 1$, all other elements have a value of 0; for undirected graphs, the adjacency matrix is symmetric. A directed graph with n nodes can have a maximum of n^2 edges (corresponding to the elements of the adjacency matrix A), n of which are self-edges (diagonal elements of A).

The arrangement of nodes and edges in drawings is a matter of convenience and not defined by the graph itself. If a graph can be drawn in a plane without intersecting edges, it is called *planar*. Complex biological networks are usually nonplanar, and finding a well-drawn layout for them can be a challenge (see Sections 2.4.2 and 2.4.3; for an overview over drawing tools for biological networks, see [6]). In drawings of metabolic networks, cofactors are often omitted or shown multiple times (at each reaction in which they participate), which greatly simplifies the graphical layout.

A graph can be characterized by its statistical properties (see Table 8.1). The nodes that share an edge with node i are called its *neighbors* and the number of neighbors is called the *degree* or *node size* k_i. In directed graphs, we distinguish between in-degrees k_i^{in} and out-degrees k_i^{out} referring, respectively, to incoming

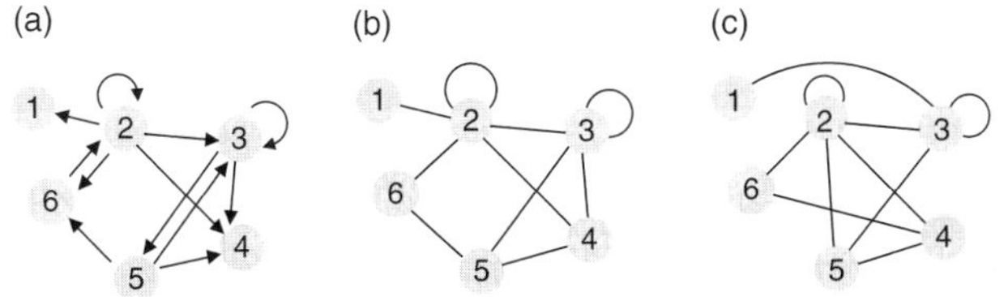

Figure 8.2 Small graphs. (a) Directed graph with 6 nodes and 9 edges. (b) An undirected graph with similar topology. (c) By rewiring, we can obtain a new graph without changing the degrees k_i.

Table 8.1 Statistical properties of graphs.

Graph	n	$\langle k \rangle$	ℓ	$\langle c \rangle$
Example Figure 8.2(b)	6	3	23/15	1/5
E. coli metabolite graph [7]	282	7.35	2.9	0.32
Movie actors [8]	225, 226	61	3.65	0.79
Power grid [8]	4941	2.67	18.7	0.08

The structure of an n-node graph can be characterized by the mean degree $\langle k \rangle$, the diameter ℓ, and the mean clustering coefficient $\langle c \rangle$ (definitions see Section 8.1.4). Self-edges are disregarded in the calculation of the clustering coefficient. The table shows statistics of three real-world graphs. In the movie actors network, two actors share a link if they ever played together in a movie. Data from Albert and Barabási [2].

and outgoing edges. In a finite graph – a graph with a finite number of nodes – the count numbers of nodes with degree k form the *degree sequence* $n_K(k)$. A directed graph with n nodes and m edges has an average degree of $\langle k_{\mathrm{in}} \rangle = \langle k_{\mathrm{out}} \rangle = m/n$, and the probability of finding an edge from node i to node j (both chosen at random) is $m/n^2 = \langle k \rangle / n$. In an infinite or random graph (see below), the *degree distribution* $p(k)$ describes the probability that a randomly picked node has the degree k. A cycle in a directed graph is a sequence of arrows that starts from a node i, follows the arrows in their proper direction, and returns to node i; a graph without cycles is called *acyclic*.

8.1.2 Random Graphs

A random graph represents a distribution over a set of graphs, just like random numbers represent probability distributions over numbers. The probabilities of the individual graphs – the possible realizations of the random graph – can be specified directly: for instance, for a random graph with n nodes, we may assume equal probabilities for all possible graphs with m edges and zero probability for all other graphs. Probabilities can also be defined *via* a random process that generates realizations, typically by starting with a set of nodes and adding edges according to a random law. Random graphs are an important tool for testing the significance of network structures. For brevity, we will use the term "random graph" also for the realizations, and we will sometimes call the random graph itself an "ensemble."

8.1.2.1 Erdős–Rényi Random Graphs

In an *Erdős–Rényi* random graph $\mathcal{G}(n, q)$ with n nodes, each possible edge is realized independently with probability q, so the elements of the adjacency matrix are independent binary variables with probability $p(a_{ij} = 1) = q$. The number of edges in an Erdős–Rényi graph follows a binomial distribution $p(m) = \binom{n^2}{m} q^m (1-q)^{n^2-m}$ with a maximum edge number n^2; similarly, the out-degrees follow a binomial distribution

$p(k) = \binom{n}{k} q^k (1-q)^{n-k}$. This distribution has a peak at the mean degree $\langle k \rangle = qn$ and a standard deviation $\sigma_k = \sqrt{nq(1-q)}$. For large graphs ($n \to \infty$) and fixed mean degree, the degree distribution converges to a Poisson distribution, which decreases exponentially for large degrees. A related random graph, called here $\mathcal{G}_E(n, m)$, contains exactly m edges, which are distributed randomly over the possible positions. In the following, we will consider large directed graphs ($n \to \infty$) with predefined mean degree $\langle k \rangle$. In this case, both types of random graph yield similar results if the parameters are chosen such that $\langle k \rangle = qn = m/n^2$.

8.1.2.2 Geometric Random Graphs

Some network topologies implicitly reflect, an underlying spatial structure: for instance, the connections between nerve cells (which can be represented as a graph) depend on their distances in space. Geometric random graphs [9] are defined based on spatial relationships: (i) The nodes correspond to points in a space (e.g., the plane $\mathbb{R}^2$), with geometric distances d_{ik} between them. (ii) Two nodes are connected with a probability $p(d_{ik})$, which depends on their geometric distance. With a Gaussian probability density $p(d_{ik}) \sim \exp(-d_{ik}^2/(2\sigma^2))$, for instance, typical realizations of the random graph will contain many local connections, but only few connections between distant points.

8.1.2.3 Random Graphs with Predefined Degree Sequence

For statistical tests, we need to construct random graphs that resemble a given network in its basic statistical properties. One possibility is to fix the in- and out-degrees for every node, but no additional structure. Such random graphs can be constructed from a given network by random flipping of edge pairs [10]: in each step, two edges are chosen at random and replaced by two edges with the same origin nodes, but with their target nodes flipped. This flipping changes the graph, but leaves the degree of each node unchanged (see Figures 8.2(b) and (c)). After many such randomization steps, we obtain a randomized graph with the initial in- and out-degrees, but all higher order structure is destroyed by the randomization. More complex random graphs, in which other properties are preserved, can be obtained by simulated annealing [10].

8.1.3 Scale-Free Networks

Many real-world networks, including metabolic networks, social networks, and the world wide web, show a characteristic power-law degree distribution [11]

$$p(k) \sim k^{-\gamma} \tag{8.1}$$

for $k \geq 1$ with scaling exponents $2 < \gamma < 3$ (see Section 7.4.4). By taking the logarithm on both sides of Eq. (8.1), we obtain

$$\log p(k_i = k) = -\gamma \log k + \text{const.}, \tag{8.2}$$

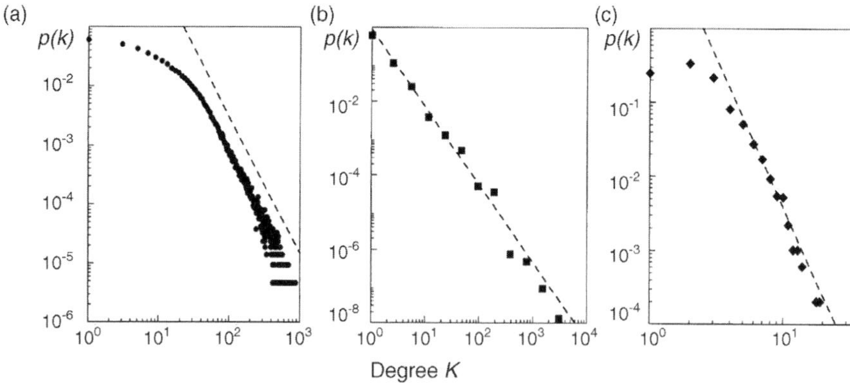

Figure 8.3 Scale-free degree distribution in different networks (see Table 8.1). (a) Movie actors ($n = 212250$, $\langle k \rangle = 28.78$, $\gamma = 2.3$). (b) World wide web ($n = 325729$, $\langle k \rangle = 5.46$, $\gamma = 2.1$). (c) Power grid ($n = 4941$, $\langle k \rangle = 2.67$, $\gamma = 4$). From Barabási and Albert (1999) [11].

so in a double-logarithmic histogram plot, a power-law distribution will show a linear decrease (see Figure 8.3). Thus, a power-law distribution may be hypothesized if linearity holds over several orders of magnitude, in particular for large degrees k. The power-law property can also be tested vigorously by statistical model selection [12].

Power-law distributions appear in various contexts, for instance, in word frequencies in natural language (Zipf's law: the frequency of a word is inversely proportional to its count number rank) or economy (Pareto's law: the number of people with income larger than x scales with x according to a power law). The power-law distribution (8.1) is *self-similar* under rescaling of k ($p(\lambda k) = \lambda^{-\gamma} p(k)$, see Section 7.4.5), so the distribution does not define a typical range for the degrees: for finite network the mean value $\langle k \rangle$ increases with the network size, and for infinite networks, it diverges. Power-law distributions do not show a typical scale for k and are therefore called *scale-free*. Scale-free networks contain a few very large nodes called *hubs*, many nodes with very small degrees, and in between, a hierarchy of nodes of different size. Such a hierarchy can be obtained, for instance, by a iterative, hierarchical construction of networks [13]. Erdös–Rényi networks, in contrast, show a peaked degree distribution characterized by a mean degree $\langle k \rangle$: most nodes have relatively similar degree, and there are virtually no nodes with very large degrees.

Many real-world networks show scale-free degree distributions, which clearly distinguishes them from Erdös–Rényi random graphs. A possible explanation comes from the growth process of networks. In the *preferential attachment* model [11], an existing network grows by successive addition of nodes: a new node connects itself randomly to one of the existing nodes, but with a preference for nodes that already have many connections. Therefore, nodes of large degree have higher chances to increase their degree even further ("The rich get richer"). In simulations, preferential attachment with linear relation between preference and node size leads to graphs with scale-free degree distributions.

Is preferential attachment a possible explanation for scale-freeness in biochemical networks? For metabolic networks, this would mean that new enzymes tend to metabolize reactants that already participate in many reactions – which might be the case, but has not been shown yet. However, it seems that the present hub metabolites arose early in evolution [7], as predicted by the preferential attachment model. In protein–protein interaction networks, preferential attachment can be realized by *gene duplication* [14, 15]. If a protein A is copied by a gene duplication, then all its interaction partners B will obtain a new edge. Now assume that genes are duplicated at random: if a protein B has many interaction partners, it is likely that one of them will be duplicated next; if B has few interaction partners, this is less probable. In total, the probability of obtaining a new interaction partner is proportional to the current number of interaction partners – just as required in the preferential attachment model.

The evolution of real-world networks is of course much more complex than preferential attachment, involving specific preferences between nodes, dynamic rewiring, and removal of nodes and edges. However, the preferential attachment model demonstrates that scale-free networks can emerge already from a simple evolutionary mechanism – and without selection for a specific biological function.

8.1.4
Clustering and Local Structure

8.1.4.1 Clustering Coefficient

In a geometric random graph, common neighbors of a node are more likely to share an edge than arbitrary pairs of nodes. This phenomenon, called *clustering*, also appears in many real-world graphs and can be quantified by the *mean clustering coefficient*. For a node i, the number r_i counts all connections between the neighboring nodes or, in other words, the number of triangles (3-loops) involving node i. In an undirected graph, a node with degree k_i can have a maximal value of $r_i^{\max} = k(k-1)/2$. Watts and Strogatz [8] defined the clustering coefficient of a node as $c_i = r_i/r_i^{\max}$, stating which fraction of possible edges between neighbors are actually realized.

Clustering in graphs may indicate an underlying similarity relation between nodes. In social networks, people who live close to each other or have similar interests (small distance in an abstract "interest space") are also more likely to share other relationships. Clustering can also arise from collapsing a bipartite graph (compare Figure 8.4): in a *bipartite graph*, there are two types of nodes (e.g., A and B, black or white), and each edge connects nodes of different types. In the collapsed graph, all nodes of type B are removed, and all neighbors of a removed node become mutually connected. A co-authorship graph, for instance, implicitly results from a bipartite graph of authors and publications. In such graphs, each collapsed node gives rise to a fully connected subgraph, which leads to high clustering coefficients.

8.1.4.2 Small-World Networks

If there is a shortest path between two nodes, its length is called the *topological distance* The *diameter* ℓ of a graph is the average distance between nodes. In an

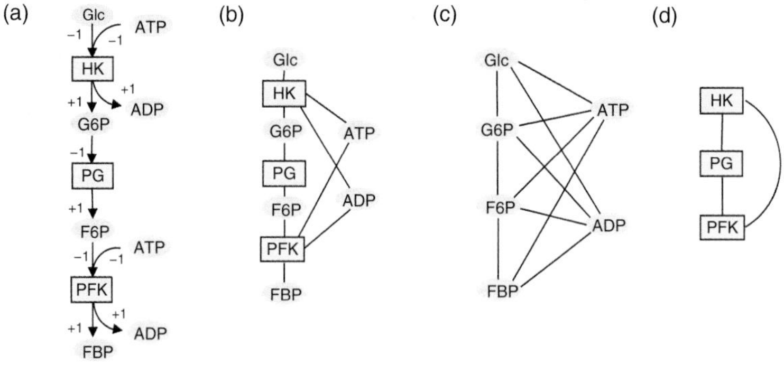

Figure 8.4 Three reactions from upper glycolysis represented by graphs. (a) Reaction network with stoichiometric coefficients. (b) Bipartite graph of metabolites and reactions. (c) Collapsed metabolite graph. (d) Collapsed reaction graph. Abbreviations: HK (hexokinase), PG (phosphoglucoisomerase), PFK (phosphofructokinase); Glc (glucose), G6P (glucose-6-phosphate), F6P (fructose-6-phosphate), FBP (fructose-1,6-bisphosphate).

Erdös–Rényi random graph with n nodes and average degree k, the diameter scales logarithmically with n: in a rough estimate, a node has approximately k neighbors, k^2 second neighbors, k^3 third neighbors, and so on. Therefore, the number of reachable nodes rises exponentially with the distance, and relatively short paths should lead to virtually any point of the network. In a clustered network with the same average degree, we would expect larger diameters because by counting the first, second, or higher neighbors, we are likely to remain in the local neighborhood of the starting point and to count the same nodes several times. Real-world networks, however, often show both properties: a clustered structure and small diameters as compared to Erdös–Rényi graphs with the same average degree. Watts and Strogatz [8] called such networks "small-world" networks and showed that they can be obtained quite easily from locally structured networks by adding relatively few global connections. Both clustering and scale-free degree distributions can be obtained in the generative *hierarchical network model* [13].

8.1.5
Network Motifs

Many real-world networks contain characteristic local patterns that recur in large numbers. If a pattern appears significantly often in a given network, it is called a *network motif* [16]. Since their discovery in transcription networks, network motifs have been found in many other kinds of real-world networks and networks can be classified according to the network motifs they contain [17]. Characteristic motifs in transcription networks, like self-inhibition and the feed-forward loop [18, 19], are discussed in Section 8.2.

To test if a given local pattern is a network motif, the original graph is compared to an ensemble of random graphs, which serves as a background model. In each realization of the random graph, the pattern appears with a certain count number, so the random graph defines a probability distribution $p(n)$ for the count number n. If the actual count number in the original network is larger than 95% of the count numbers obtained from the random graph ensemble, the motif is significant at a 5% confidence level. Tools for detection of network motifs are available [20, 21].

The test for network motifs depends on the choice of the background model. For instance, a geometric random graph contains more self-inhibition loops than a simple Erdös–Rényi graph with the same mean degree. Thus, depending on which of these two models is used as a null hypothesis, the number of self-inhibitions in a real-world graph may be either significant or not. In general, a background model should represent all structures that we expect to find anyway.

The structure of transcription networks, for instance, is determined by the binding sites for transcription factors and can evolve rather rapidly by mutation or duplication of promoter sequences [22] and by evolution of the transcription factors. By a proper arrangement of binding sites, various network topologies could be realized in principle, but there seems to be a restriction to relatively small in-degrees (numbers of regulators per gene), whereas the out-degrees (number of targets per regulator) can be rather large. For transcription networks, Milo *et al.* [10] constructed random graphs based on the original network, in which all node degrees and smaller motifs are preserved (see Section 8.1.2.3). The high frequency of motifs found with this background model cannot be explained as a mere consequence of the degree distribution. If the random graph is regarded as a realistic scenario of neutral evolution (i.e. network evolution without selection), one may conclude that the network motif has emerged by a selection pressure.

8.1.6
Structure of Metabolic Networks

The main biological function of metabolic networks is to convert metabolic substrates into products, with varying fluxes depending on supply and demand. Depending on the organism's ecological niche, metabolic networks can range from very small (in intracellular parasites) to very large sizes (e.g., in plants). Their structures depend on the laws of chemistry (e.g., atom numbers must be conserved in all reactions) and on the set of enzymes coded in the organism's genome. Theoretically, a huge number of network structures could be realized in evolution: a computational screen [23] yielded, for instance, more than 350,000 potential chemical routes from chorismate to tyrosine. It has been hypothesized, though, that existing enzymes realize thermodynamically favorable routes from substrates to products [23, 24]. Moreover, it can be assumed that enzymes that are not actually being used will disappear by mutations. Usually, metabolic pathways are highly connected by a relatively small number of cofactors, which appear in many reactions and seem to have appeared early in metabolic network evolution.

The stoichiometric matrix $\mathbf{N}$ of a chemical reaction system defines a bipartite network of metabolites and reactions with edges corresponding to the stoichiometric coefficients (see Figures 8.4(a) and (b)). For a simpler analysis, the metabolic network can be collapsed. In the metabolite graph (Figure 8.4(c)), edges indicate that metabolites participate in a common reaction. Likewise, edges in the collapsed reaction graph (Figure 8.4(d)) connect reactions that used to share a reactant in the original graph (compare Figure 3.5).

Although metabolic networks of different organisms differ strongly in their size and capabilities, they also show common characteristic structures. The collapsed metabolite graphs display a scale-free degree distribution over two orders of magnitude: such distributions have been found in 43 species [25] of various sizes and from all three kingdoms of life. A few metabolites – mostly cofactors – participate in a large number of reactions, and their order of importance (as measured by the degree) is almost identical in all organisms. The hub metabolites appeared in virtually all metabolic networks under study, and it seems that they also appeared early in evolution [7], in agreement with the model of preferential attachment.

Jeong *et al.* [25] found that metabolic networks display small-world properties: despite their very different sizes, all 43 above-mentioned networks have almost the same small diameter – which requires a higher connectivity in the larger networks. Even if a considerable percentage (8%) of the nodes are removed from the network, the diameter remains constant: there seem to be enough by-passes in the network. However, this robustness holds only for randomly selected nodes to be destroyed: if the hub metabolites are concerned (in a directed attack), then the diameter rises quickly. The collapsed metabolite graph does not distinguish between substrates and products of a reaction, so shortest paths in the graph need not correspond to routes of chemical transformations. When actual routes of chemical transformations were considered, the small-world property has not been found [26].

8.1.7
The Network Picture

Most networks are abstractions of a much more complex reality: they emphasize the structure of interactions, while neglecting the nature of the elements and the dynamics of the system. Such an abstraction can be very useful: (i) a network may be a good starting point to describe a system if little information about this system is available. (ii) Networks, especially in their graphical representation, are better understandable than very detailed quantitative descriptions. (iii) Studies of network structure may reveal similarities between seemingly unrelated systems and (iv) may explain structural features based on mathematical relationships (e.g., explain the occurrence of certain structures simply from the degree distribution). (v) Comparisons to random networks may help to decide if features could have arisen in evolution by chance or by selection. (vi) Some dynamical processes (e.g., spreading of diseases) depend rather on the network structure or its statistical properties than on the detailed quantitative properties of the nodes. However, a convincing biological explanation of network structures requires an understanding of the underlying dynamical systems and evolutionary processes.

Networks constructed from high-throughput data may hint on the structure and dynamics of the underlying dynamical systems: e.g., protein–DNA interaction (molecular) may indicate regulatory action (causal), correlated expression (statistical) may indicate a common regulator (causal), and evolutionary co-occurrence (sequence analysis) or synthetic lethality (growth measurements) may hint on common function. However, correlated fluctuations of metabolites do not necessarily imply that the metabolites participate in the same pathway. Quantitative relations between "data networks" and the layout and dynamics of biological systems can be established by modeling.

8.2 Network Motifs

Summary

Signal transduction pathways and transcription networks process biochemical signals, which are coded in the concentrations, modifications, and localization of molecules. Regulatory networks contain characteristic motifs, which may reveal small subsystems with typical dynamic behavior and specific regulatory functions. The adapation motif, for instance, translates jumps of its input signal into a transient response, but in steady-state situations, its response is completely independent of the magnitude of the input. Other typical motifs comprise negative feedback loops, which speed up response times and contribute to stability, but also to oscillations, and the feed-forward loops, which can act as filters, sign-sensitive delays, or pulse generators.

The cellular processes of life are orchestrated by complex regulatory systems including signaling pathways, the transcription network, and specialized circuits for cell cycle control, growth regulation, stress response, and many other cell functions. Signaling systems can be displayed in the form of a network, with nodes representing biochemical substances or complexes, possibly in different modifications. An arrow in the network – possibly with a sign for activation or inhibition – indicates that a substance affects another substance level, e.g., by catalyzing its production or degradation. If several arrows point to a node, their values have to be processed in qualitative models, this processing may be described by Boolean functions like logical AND or OR. Substance levels are often balanced by pairs of counteracting processes, such as synthesis and degradation or phosphorylation and dephosphorylation of proteins.

Signaling pathways sense input stimuli (e.g., extracellular ligands or intracellular metabolites) and transmit, process, and integrate this information to provide output signals to downstream processes like gene expression. Regulatory networks can be seen as information-processing devices that translate input signals into output signals. Information in signaling systems is often coded by concentrations, modifications, and localization of proteins, either in the stationary levels or in temporal patterns. On the one hand, signals are transmitted between different places in the cell (e.g., from a receptor at the cell surface to the transcription machinery in the nucleus). On the other hand, the *input–output relation* of a signaling system can realize basic

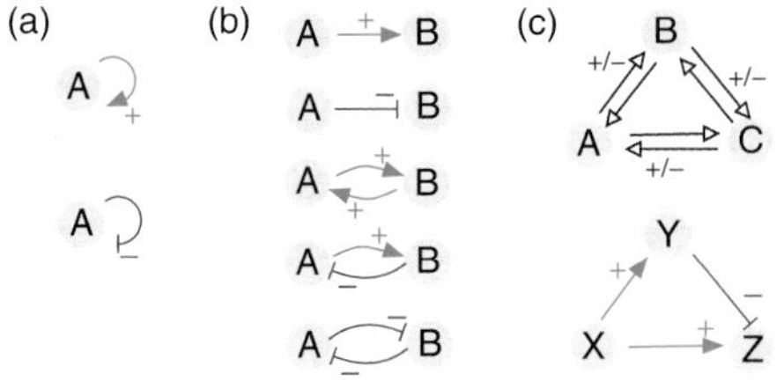

Figure 8.5 Basic regulatory patterns with one, two, or three nodes. (a) Positive (red) and negative (blue) autoregulation. (b) Two-node patterns. (c) Three-node patterns can contain up to six arrows. By selecting three arrows and signs, one obtains the incoherent feed-forward loop type I, which appears as a network motif in transcription networks (also see Figure 8.11).

information-processing tasks such as discrimination, regression, data compression, or filtering of temporal signals.

Regulation networks contain local patterns, characterized by configurations of arrows and their signs (see Figure 8.5). They represent small subsystems, possibly with characteristic dynamic behavior that allows them to exert specific functions in control and signal processing [27, 28]. Some of these patterns appear much more often than expected by chance: by definition, such subnetworks are called *network motifs* [28, 29]. Regulatory circuits have also been created artificially in synthetic biology [30–34]. In this chapter, we shall discuss how regulatory networks can be translated into dynamic models. We present a number of typical networks motifs, and discuss their dynamic behavior. For a detailed treatment of network motifs, see [29].

8.2.1
Transcription Networks and Network Motifs

Transcription networks describe the regulation of genes by transcription factors. Nodes represent proteins, and arrows indicate that a transcription factor can bind to the promoter region of a gene and possibly regulate its expression. The individual arrows can be quantified by gene input functions (see Section 6.2). The network structure is determined by binding sites in the regulatory regions of the genome. Binding site sequences of many transcription factors have been determined [35], and transcription factor binding can be detected experimentally *in vivo* on a genome-wide scale [36, 37]. Transcription networks contain several typical network motifs, like negative autoregulation or the feed-forward loop [38, 39] (see Figure 8.7). These motifs often appear in clusters, which have been described as generalized motifs [40].

The structure of transcription networks is far from random [41]. The transcription network of *E. coli* bacteria (see Figure 8.6) contains *dense overlapping regulons*, strongly interconnected subnetworks that respond to a set of input stimuli and control the expression of functionally related genes. Information flows mainly from top to bottom: many input signals are processed in the dense overlapping regulons – which,

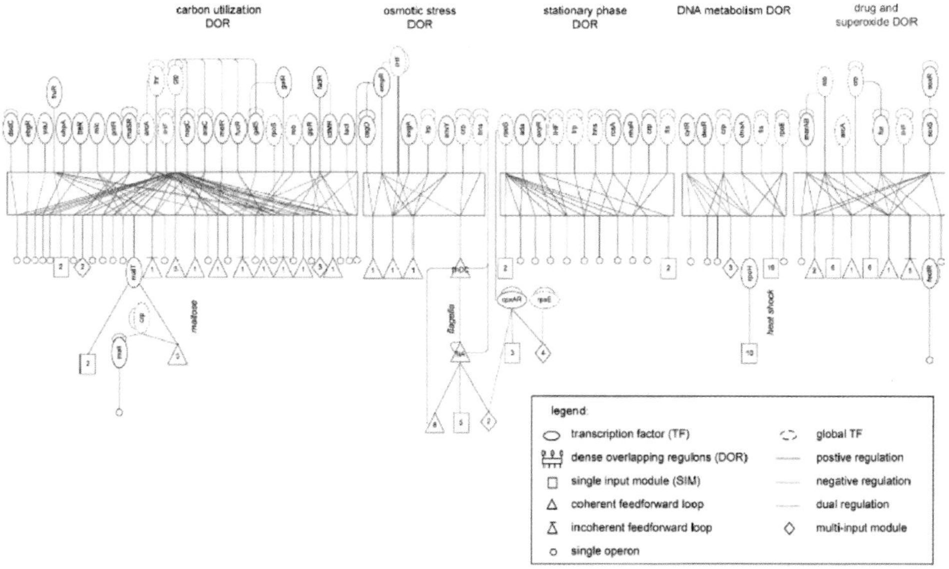

Figure 8.6 Transcription network in *E. coli* bacteria. In this arrangement, functional subsystems of the network become visible (compare Figure 8.1(b)). The network consists of several large blocks related to different cell functions, and information is processed from the top to the bottom. Feed-forward loops in the output layer are marked by triangles. Unlike in the other figures – activation is shown in blue and repression in red. From Shen-Orr *et al.* [19].

in their structure, resemble artificial neural networks – and are then distributed to an output layer, which contains a large number of feed-forward loops.

Lee *et al.* used chromatin immunoprecipitation to study the *in vivo* binding of transcription factors to DNA in the yeast *S. cerevisiae.* They identified approximately 4000 significant binding interactions between regulators and promoter regions, with an average number of 38 target promoters per regulator. The analysis also revealed six characteristic network motifs (Figure 8.7), entailing the motifs found for *E. coli.*

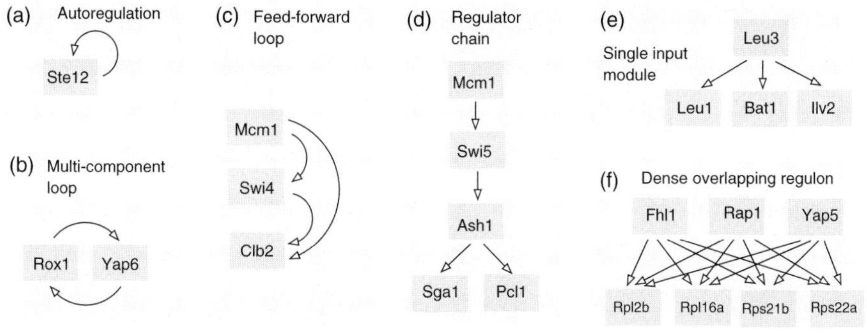

Figure 8.7 Network motifs in the transcription network of the yeast *S. cerevisiae*. Gene names refer to specific examples in the network. Redrawn from Lee *et al.* [19].

8.2.2
Single Regulation Arrows and Their Steady-State Response

Each regulatory arrow in a signaling network connects an input S (signal) to an output R (response). Possible pairs of such signal and response elements are kinase/target protein, transcription factor/target gene, and mRNA/protein. To translate a network structure into a dynamical model, we can describe the signal strength s and the response magnitude r by a rate equation

$$\frac{dr}{dt} = f(s, r). \tag{8.3}$$

By solving the steady-state equation $0 = f(s,r)$ for r, we obtain a steady-state response curve $r^{st}(s)$, the input–output relation for this individual arrow.

A single regulation arrow can symbolize different reaction patterns. Figure 8.8 shows three such patterns that can underly a regulatory arrow and may serve as building blocks for larger networks.

The steady-state response $r^{st}(s)$ in the three systems depends on their structure, but also on the kinetic laws (Table 8.2). A linear mechanism with linear kinetics leads

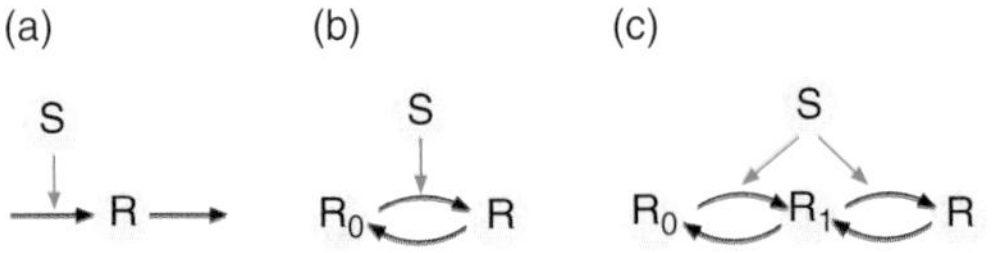

Figure 8.8 Possible regulation patterns behind a simple activation S → R. (a) Linear pattern: a substance S ("signal") regulates the production of R ("response"). (b) In a loop pattern (e.g., in a phosphorylation cycle), S converts inactive R_0 into its active form R. (c) In a double-loop pattern (e.g., double phosphorylation), two steps are necessary to activate R. Black arrows indicate chemical reactions, while red and blue arrows denote activation and inhibition, respectively.

Table 8.2 Simple signaling motifs (see Figure 8.8) with different kinetic implementations.

Structure		Kinetics	Response	$r^{st}(s)$
Linear	Linear	$dr/dt = k_0 + k_1 s - k_2 r$	Linear	$\frac{k_0 + k_1 s}{k_2}$
	MM	$dr/dt = \frac{V_1 s}{K_{M1} + s} - \frac{V_2 r}{K_{M2} + r}$	Hyperbolic	$\frac{V_1 K_{M2} s}{V_2 K_{M1} + s(V_2 - V_1)}$
Loop	Linear	$dr/dt = k_1 s(r_t - r) - k_2 r$ $r + r_0 = r_t$	Hyperbolic	$\frac{r_t k_1 s}{k_2 + k_1 s}$
	MM	$dr/dt = \frac{k_1 s(r_t - r)}{K_{M1} + r_t - r} - \frac{k_2 r}{K_{M2} + r}$ $r + r_0 = r_t$	Sigmoid	$r_t G(k_1 s, k_2, \frac{K_{M1}}{r_t}, \frac{K_{M2}}{r_t})$
Double loop	Linear	$dr/dt = k_3 s r_1 - k_4 r$ $dr_i/dt = k_1 s r_0 - (k_2 + k_3 s)\, r_1 + k_4 r$ $r + r_0 = r_t$	Sigmoid	$\frac{r_t k_1 k_3 s^2}{k_2 k_4 + k_1 s k_4 + k_1 k_3 s^2}$

The structures (left) correspond to the patterns shown in Figure 8.8. Linear kinetics and Michaelis–Menten (MM) kinetics lead to different response curves. The function $G(u, v, J, K) = 2uK/(v - u + vJ + uK + \sqrt{(v - u + vJ + uK)^2 - 4(v - u)uK})$, the so-called Goldbeter–Koshland function [42, 43], is often used to model switch-like behavior.

to a linear response. A hyperbolic response can be obtained either by a Michaelis–Menten kinetics or by the loop network structure (Figure 8.8(b)) with linear kinetics and a conservation relation $r + r_0 = r_t$ for the different forms of R. The same one-loop mechanism with Michaelis–Menten kinetics gives rise to a switch-like, sigmoid response curve. All three types of response (linear, hyperbolic, sigmoid) are gradual with respect to signal strength. Moreover, they are reversible, i.e., the steady-state output depends only on the current input signal and not on its previous history: as soon as the signal stops, the response is switched off. An overview of dynamic motifs based on such simple regulatory interactions is given in [28].

8.2.3 Adaptation Motif

Besides the steady-state response, an important property of signaling systems is their transient response to changing inputs. The system shown in Figure 8.9 shows a remarkable behavior called *precise adaptation* (see Section 7.4.1): after a jump of the input value, it shows a transient dynamics, but in the long run, it always returns to exactly the same steady state. Precise adaptation makes a system sensitive to temporal changes, but insensitive to the baseline value. It plays a vital role in the bacterial chemotaxis pathway and has been thoroughly studied in this system [44, 45].

In the *adaptation motif* shown in Figure 8.9, the input X activates the production of Z, but inhibits it again via activation of Y. With mass-action kinetics and linear activation, the levels of Y and Z follow the equations

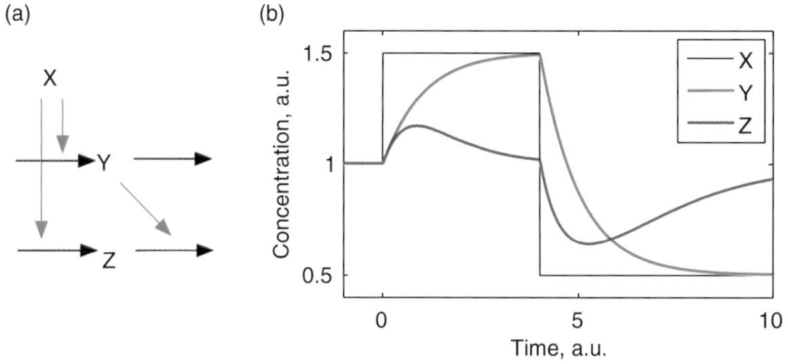

Figure 8.9 The adaptation motif. (a) A signal X catalyzes the production of Y and Z; in turn, Y catalyzes the degradation of Z. The reactions follow mass-action kinetics. (b) Temporal dynamics of the adaptation motif. A step-like input level x (black) evokes a sustained response of y (red); the output level z (blue) shows a transient response before returning to its steady-state value (all kinetic parameters set to a value of 1).

$$\begin{aligned}\frac{dy}{dt} &= \alpha_y x - \beta_y y \\ \frac{dz}{dt} &= \alpha_z x - \beta_z y\, z,\end{aligned} \tag{8.4}$$

which lead, for $x > 0$, to the steady state

$$y^{st} = \frac{\alpha_y}{\beta_y} x, \qquad z^{st} = \frac{\alpha_z \beta_y}{\beta_z \alpha_y}. \tag{8.5}$$

The steady-state level of Z depends only on the kinetic constants. In steady state, activation and inactivation cancel out, but when the input suddenly changes, the activation responds faster than the inactivation, which leads to a transient peak (Figure 8.9(b)).

8.2.4
Negative Feedback

Among the various regulatory patterns in signaling pathways, negative feedback has attracted outstanding interest. It is very common in transcription networks and it also plays an important role in the regulation of metabolic pathways. In amino acid synthesis, for instance, the first enzyme in a pathway is often inhibited by the final product. This prevents overproduction of an amino acid and stabilizes its level against fluctuations caused by varying demand.

Negative feedback can have various effects on cellular dynamics: (i) to stabilize the state of a cellular network; (ii) to reduce the variance of fluctuations and the variability of steady states [31]; (iii) to provide robustness to boundary conditions [46] (see the Bicoid model in Section 3.4.4); (iv) to produce pulse-like overshoots; (v) to induce sustained oscillations; (vi) and to speed up response times [47].

Some of these phenomena can be seen in a kinetic model for a chain of reactions (see Figure 8.10). In this model, all reactions follow irreversible mass-action kinetics $v_i = k_i\, s_{i-1}$, the external substrate level $s_0 = 1$ is kept constant, and all other metabolites start at levels $s_i = 0$. The first reaction is inhibited allosterically by one of the downstream metabolites: in our model, feedback inhibition by the jth metabolite can be implemented as $v_1 = s_1 k_1/(1 + s_j/K_I)$. Without such feedback, the metabolite concentrations reach a steady state after a short transition period (Figure 8.10(a)). If the second metabolite acts as an inhibitor, the level of the first metabolite shows an overshooting response (Figure 8.10(b)). With a long-ranging feedback involving a longer time delay, this effect becomes more pronounced. In the example, inhibition by the last metabolite leads to damped oscillations (Figure 8.10(c)).

The example also shows that negative autoregulation can speed up the system's response to external changes. The response time $\tau_{(1/2)}$, defined as the time at which the last metabolite S_r reaches its half-maximal level, decreases from (a) to (c) for the three cases shown in Figure 8.10. In the units used in the model, the values read $\tau_{(1/2)} \approx 5.68$ (no feedback), $\tau_{(1/2)} \approx 5.05$ (short-ranging feedback from second metabolite), and $\tau_{(1/2)} \approx 4.57$ (long-ranging feedback from last metabolite).

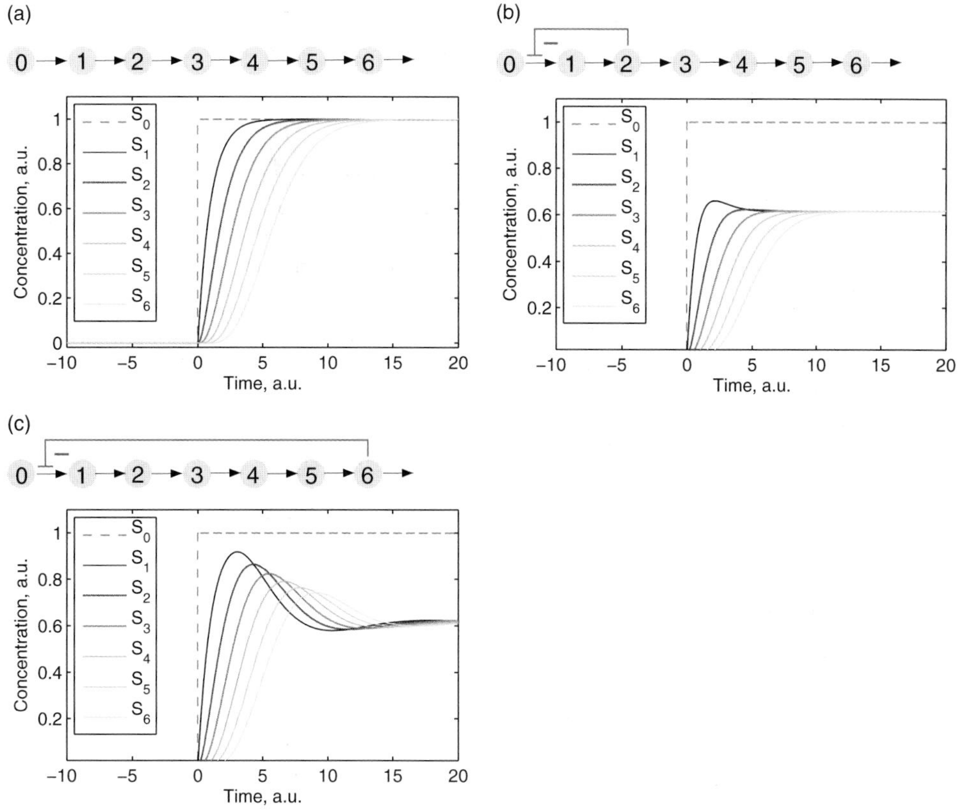

Figure 8.10 Negative feedback in an unbranched metabolic chain. (a) Concentration time series in a chain of six reactions (shown on top) after external substrate (- -) becomes available ($s_0 = 1$) at time $t = 0$. (b) Negative feedback by the second metabolite decreases the steady-state level and speeds up the response. (c) Negative feedback from the last metabolite leads to an overshoot and damped oscillations. All parameters k_i have a value of 1.

8.2.5
Feed-Forward Loops

The feed-forward loop (FFL) [37–39, 48] shown in Figure 8.11 is a common motif in transcription networks. It consists of three interacting genes: an input gene X regulates the output gene Z both directly and via an intermediate gene Y. Qualitatively, each arrow can represent activation (+) or inhibition (−), and the two inputs of Z are processed by Boolean functions, e.g., logical AND or OR (examples shown in Figure 8.11). In the feed-forward loop, eight sign combinations are conceivable, but only two of them are abundant in the transcription networks studied: the so-called *coherent FFL type 1* and the *incoherent FFL type 1* (Figure 8.11). In a coherent

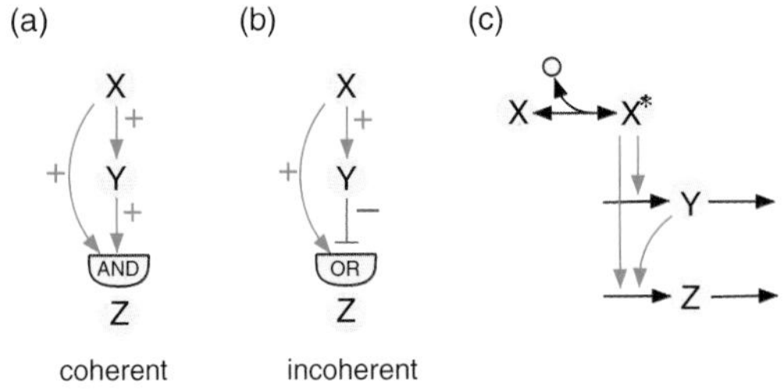

Figure 8.11 Feed-forward loops. The input gene X regulates the output gene Z directly and *via* an intermediate gene Y. (a) Coherent feed-forward loop type 1 with AND gate. (b) Incoherent feed-forward loop type 1 with OR gate. (c) Simple model of a feed-forward loop in transcription networks. The regulatory arrows represent transcriptional regulation of Y and Z; transcription and translation are modeled by a single step. X is activated by rapid ligand binding (circle denotes the ligand, X^* the active form). Red, blue, and black arrows indicate activation, inhibition, and reactions, respectively.

FFL type 1, all regulations are activating, while in an incoherent FFL type, Y inhibits Z. Other types of feed-forward loops, with different sign combinations, occur rarely and will not be considered here.

At first sight, the function of the second branch via gene Y in the feed-forward loop is not obvious: in a coherent FFL, the two branches seem redundant, and in an incoherent FFL, their effects may cancel out. But like for the adaptation motif, this argument holds only in steady-state situations. Let us consider an incoherent FFL type 1: if the input X is suddenly switched on, gene Y turns up with a delay, so Z is first activated *via* the direct branch and later inhibited again by Y. Due to the time delay on the longer branch, a step in the input X is translated into a characteristic peak of the output Z.

Mangan *et al.* [38] have suggested a biological function of feed-forward loops in the processing of temporal signals: if an external signal (e.g., a ligand concentration) changes the activity of X in time, the FFL will translate the temporal profile of X into a characteristic profile of Z, which can then serve as input for downstream processes. Dynamical models and measurements in gene circuits in *E. coli* have shown that feed-forward loops can serve as sign-sensitive delays, generate temporal pulses, and accelerate the response to input signals. Their detailed behavior depends on the kinetic parameters – or in the Boolean paradigm, on the choice of signs and the logic input function for Z.

8.2.6
Dynamic Model of the Feed-Forward Loop

To illustrate the functions of feed-forward loops in a simple dynamic model, let us assume that gene X is expressed constitutively and its activity x is controlled by the concentration of a ligand, whereas the activities of Y and Z are determined by their expression. If the processes of transcription and translation are lumped into a single step, we obtain the rate equations

$$\frac{dy}{dt} = f_y(x) - \beta_y y$$
$$\frac{dz}{dt} = f_z(x, y) - \beta_z z. \quad (8.6)$$

In this model, y and z denote protein levels, f_y and f_z are production rates, and β_y and β_z are degradation constants. For studying the qualitative dynamic behavior, it is practical to describe the transcription of Y by a simple step-like gene input function

$$f_y(x) = \alpha_y\, \Theta(x > x_0). \quad (8.7)$$

The truth function $\Theta(\cdot)$ yields a value of 1 if the inequality in the argument is satisfied, and a value of 0 otherwise. Thus, as long as x stays below the threshold value x_0, Y is not transcribed; otherwise, Y is transcribed at constant rate α_y. Piecewise constant functions like Eq. (8.7) can be seen as a rough approximation of the gene input functions discussed in Section 6.2. We shall consider two cases, a coherent FFL with a logical AND input function for the production of Z, and an incoherent FFL with a logical OR function. The corresponding input functions for gene Z read

$$\text{coherent, AND}: \quad f_z(x, y) = \alpha_z\, \Theta(x > x_0 \text{ AND } y > y_0)$$
$$\text{incoherent, OR}: \quad f_z(x, y) = \alpha_z\, \Theta(x > x_0 \text{ OR NOT } y > y_0). \quad (8.8)$$

Figure 8.12 shows simulation results from model (8.6), with input functions (8.7) and (8.8) and a predefined, pulse-like input $x(t)$. The simulations illustrate some characteristic features of the feed-forward loop: the coherent-AND FFL shows a delayed response to the onset and an immediate response to the end of pulses and as a consequence, short pulses are filtered out. The incoherent-OR FFL, on the other hand, responds immediately to an input pulse, but the response is switched off only after a while: therefore, input pulses are translated into standard pulses of similar length. The dynamics of both types of feed-forward loop has been verified experimentally in the transcription network of *E. coli* [38, 39, 48]. A combination of feed-forward loops constitutes the sporulation system in the bacterium *B. subtilis*, which upon stimulation creates several coordinated waves of expression (Figure 8.13).

8.2.7
Dynamics and Function of Network Motifs

Network motifs are structural patterns, possibly annotated with signs for activation and repression, that are more frequent than expected by chance. To explain their high abundance in regulation networks, it has been hypothesized that they are associated with characteristic dynamic behavior and can fulfill specific biological functions. Two genes that inhibit each other, for instance, can constitute a bistable genetic switch. As a switch can be useful for different purposes, it may be selected for. As instances of the switch accumulate in the network, it becomes, by definition, a network motif. It

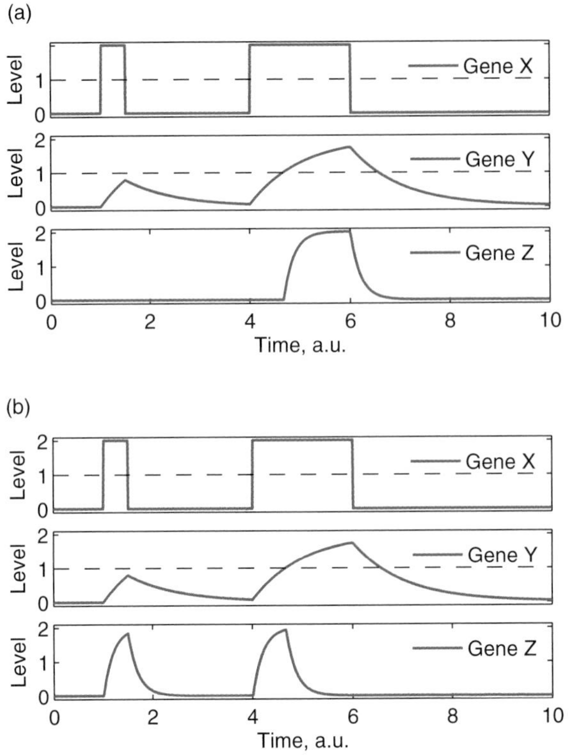

Figure 8.12 Dynamic behavior of two types of feed-forward-loop (FFL). (a) Coherent FFL type 1 with AND logic (see Figure 8.11(a)). Time curves for active input X (top), intermediate gene Y (center), and output Z (bottom) are shown (arbitrary units). The FFL filters out the short pulse; the response to the longer pulse is delayed, but the response to the end of the pulse is immediate. (b) Incoherent FFL type 1 with OR logic (see Figure 8.11(b)). The onset of each input pulse leads to a pulse of Z of fixed maximal length. Model parameters $\alpha_y = 2$, $\beta_y = 1$, $\alpha_z = 10$, $\beta_z = 5$.

has also been suggested that certain patterns can stabilize networks against dynamic perturbations, which may add another selection advantage [50, 51].

It is difficult to prove, though, that a network motif encountered has in fact been selected for its regulatory function. If we hypothesize this, we imply that the dynamics associated with this network motif is fairly robust to the details of the implementation. For specific examples, for instance, the feed-forward loop, the selection hypothesis is strongly supported by its highly significant abundance, the relatively fast rewiring of transcription networks, the high number of nonhomologous copies within networks, and the appearance in different, unrelated networks. Further support comes from the fact that these dynamical features do not depend on details of the kinetic model and that they have been confirmed in experiments with living cells.

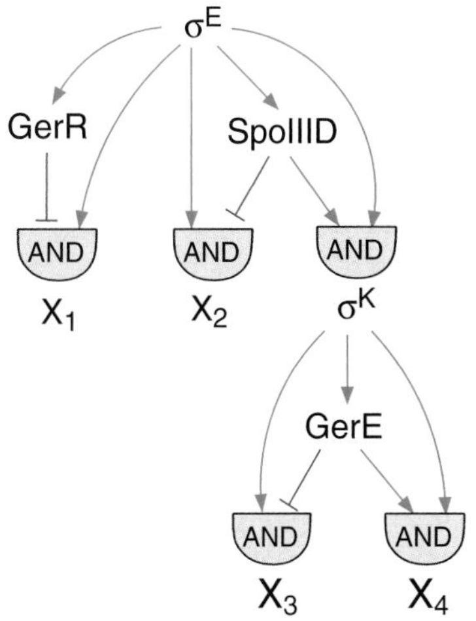

Figure 8.13 Gene regulation network coordinating sporulation in the bacterium *B. subtilis*. Some microbes can transform themselves into spores, which are much more resistant to adverse environmental conditions than the living bacteria. When sporulation is triggered in the soil bacterium *B. subtilis*, a gene regulatory network produces several waves of gene expression, in which many genes are regulated in a temporally coordinated manner. The structure of this network has been elucidated in [49]. The system contains a number of feed-forward loops that activate the downstream target genes. Activation of the Master regulator σ^E triggers waves of expression in different groups of target genes (denoted by X_1, X_2, X_3, X_4). Redrawn from Eichenberger *et al.* [49].

8.3 Modularity

Summary

Modular systems consist of subsystems that work rather autonomously and may exert specific functions. Physical modules in cells, like protein complexes, can remain functional in various contexts, sometimes even after transfection into other cell types. Cellular networks can also be dissected into modules, often called "pathways." In technical systems, a modular structure facilitates understanding, development, interoperability, and reusability. In biological networks, modularity can improve robustness and can make systems better evolvable. Moreover, the assumption of modularity also plays a vital role in modeling: if cells were not modular at all, assigning functions to genes or pathways would be difficult, and it would be virtually impossible to develop, analyze, and understand mathematical models of cells.

A system is *modular* if it can be understood in terms of subsystems ("modules") that are sparsely interconnected, show characteristic dynamics, or exert specific functions [52]. In a non-modular system, all parts of the system can be interconnected and functions are distributed over the entire system. Modular design is a common feature of many technical systems: a computer, for instance, consists of standardized parts that exert distinct and defined functions, operate more or less autonomously, communicate *via* relatively simple interfaces, and can be repeated, replaced or transferred as units. A modular design facilitates development and maintenance of complex technical devices: it makes complicated machines understandable and ensures that parts can be reused in different contexts and combinations or be replaced in case of failure.

Living systems contain physical modules such as organs, cells, organelles, or protein complexes, often with specific biological functions [52]. Such modules can even remain functional in a new context (e.g., organs can be transplanted, proteins can be transfected into different cells). Also the cellular networks can be subdivided into modules, specified by sets of enzymes or regulatory proteins; examples are metabolic pathways, signaling pathways, or the dense overlapping regulons in the transcription network of *E. coli* (see Figure 8.6). In the latter example, the network shows in fact a pronounced modular structure: theory should explain how such modules are brought about and what selection advantage they do provide.

Modularity can concern the structure, regulation, and genetics of a system at the same time. In bacterial *operons*, for instance, several functionally related proteins are encoded by a common strand of mRNA and controlled by the same promoter elements. Genes in an operon share the same expression profile, and the entire system, together with its regulatory region, can be transferred to other cells, where it may exert its function in a different biochemical context. This operon structure seems to be established and maintained in evolution because it provides a selection advantage.

8.3.1
Modularity as a Fact or as an Assumption

In a strict sense, modularity in cells is only an abstraction. Metabolic or signaling pathways are embedded in large complex networks and this can make modeling a difficult task (see Section 4.3.5). Thus, a contrary view holds that our mental models of complex systems need to be modular to be understandable, so we describe biology in terms of modules and we may even tend to pick modular systems as scientific topics. However, if biological systems were not modular at all, then our modeling approach would fail, and we would probably have noticed that in any case, the assertion that biomolecules and cellular pathways can be reasonably well understood in isolation is an important basis of molecular biology and biochemistry (see Section 4.3.2).

An aim of systems biology is to extend our understanding toward complex systems and to explore how much of this complexity needs to be modeled at the least to get a plausible dynamic picture of cells. It is an attempt to recognize simplicity in complex systems and to model complexity whenever it is necessary. The hypothesis of modularity is also routinely tested in synthetic biology [53], where existing proteins and regulatory elements are put into new contexts and used in new combinations.

8.3.2
Aspects of Modularity: Structure, Function, Dynamics, Regulation, and Genetics

Functional modules also tend to appear as modules in their regulation and genetics, as we can see in bacterial operons. If proteins operate together, for instance in an enzymatic pathway, this can have various consequences:

1. For optimal resource allocation, the enzymes should be expressed in appropriate ratios because otherwise material and energy would be wasted. Stable ratios can be obtained if the enzymes share a common regulation system, which will reduce uncorrelated fluctuations in their expression.

2. In horizontal gene transfer, bacteria can pass on pieces of DNA to each other. The entire pathway can be transferred as a unit if the respective genes are placed close to each other on the DNA. Furthermore, a transferrable pathway should be able to exert its function in changing environments and in cells with different genetic background, so its dynamics should be relatively robust against typical fluctuations of the cell state – except, of course, for fluctations that act as regulatory signals.

3. If one of the enzymes has been lost and the pathway is not functional any more, a second loss-of-function mutation will have little effect on fitness – an example of buffering epistasis (see Section 8.3.5). There is a strong selection pressure on complete pathways, but little selection pressure on the genes in an incomplete, nonfunctional pathway. Accordingly, the genes in a pathway should be either preserved together or disappear together, which will lead to correlations in phylogenetic profiles [54].

In fact, pathways in cellular networks can be defined by mathematical criteria based on network topologies [55, 56], correlated dynamics [57], regulation systems [58], correlations in high-throughput data [59], or phylogenetic profiles [54] and all these properties may be used as clues for detecting functional modules in complex biological systems.

8.3.3
Structural Modules in Cellular Networks

Metabolism is often described in terms of physiological routes between key metabolites. However, metabolic pathways can be strongly overlapping and if cofactors like ATP are taken into account, we obtain a tightly connected metabolic network, so pathways are a matter of definition.

We may use different criteria to define pathways in a given metabolic network. One possibility is to choose subgraphs with dense internal connections [56]. Another simple, but efficient way to dissect a metabolic network is to remove the hub metabolites, e.g., all metabolites participating in more than four reactions – among which are many cofactors. If enough of the hubs are disregarded in the stoichiometric matrix, the remaining metabolic network will consist of disjoint blocks [55]. To justify this simplification for kinetic models, we may regard the hub concentrations as fixed parameters. This implies that hub metabolites are very abundant (and therefore insensitive to chemical reactions), strongly buffered or stabilized (because stable concentrations are important for many biological processes), or that fluctuations average out (because the hub metabolites participate in many reactions).

Other ways to define metabolic pathways are the basic pathways [60] and the *elementary flux modes* [61] (see Section 2.2.3). An elementary mode can be seen as a module in the space of flux distributions: it converts a number of external substrates into external products and does not require any other reactions to be present. Elementary modes can be computed from the stoichiometric matrix, but for large networks, their number usually grows very fast. To avoid this combinatorial explosion, one may first decompose a network by removing the hub metabolites and then compute elementary modes for the individual modules – as it has been demonstrated for the metabolism of the bacterium *Mycoplasma pneumoniae* [55].

In contrast to traditional metabolic pathways, elementary modes are not defined by the network topology alone, but as stationary modes of operation, and they can be overlapping. All stationary flux distributions can be obtained from the linear superpositions of elementary modes, with real-valued coefficients for the nondirected modes and non-negative coefficients for the directed ones. However, this decomposition into elementary modes is not unique and, furthermore, elementary modes and linear combinations of them may violate thermodynamic constraints.

8.3.4
Modular Response Analysis

If dynamic systems are coupled, mutual interactions between them can drastically change their behavior (see Section 4.3.5); this holds both for biological systems themselves and for mathematical models describing them. The dynamic behavior of biochemical networks, which results from a coupling of many chemical reactions, is studied in metabolic control analysis. In a similar manner, modular response analysis [62, 63] tackles the coupling of entire modules: emergent global behavior can be predicted from the effective input–output behavior of modules, irrespective of the detailed internal structure.

In modular response analysis, we consider several systems that influence each other via *communicating variables* (see Figure 8.14(a)): a communicating variable is an

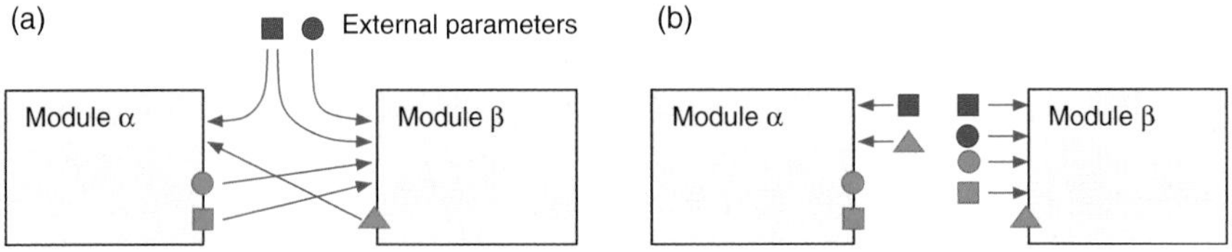

Figure 8.14 Modular response analysis. (a) Two dynamical modules interact with each other via communicating variables (red); in addition, they are influenced by external parameters (blue). (b) To study the local behavior of individual modules, the communicating variables are regarded as controllable parameters. Local response coefficients are obtained from scenario (b). Together with the wiring scheme of the communicating variables, they allow us to compute the global response coefficients for scenario (a).

output of one module and appears as a parameter in other modules. All other system parameters are collected in the external parameter vector $\boldsymbol{p}$.

We first consider the individual modules in isolation and compute local response coefficients, which will allow us, later, to calculate the global response coefficients of the coupled system. The dynamics of a module μ depends, in general, on the external parameter vector $\boldsymbol{p}$ and on the output vectors $\boldsymbol{x}_\alpha$, $\boldsymbol{x}_\beta$, ... of the other modules. The steady-state output s_μ can be written as a function $s_\mu(\boldsymbol{p}, \boldsymbol{x}_\alpha, \boldsymbol{x}_\beta, \ldots)$, where the argument list contains all module outputs except for $\boldsymbol{x}_\mu$ itself (see Figure 8.14(b)). Next, we assume that the modules are coupled and that the coupled system reaches a stable steady state, which depends on the external parameters. The steady-state values y of the output variables need to satisfy

$$\begin{aligned} y_\alpha(\boldsymbol{p}) &= s_\alpha(\boldsymbol{p}, y_\beta(\boldsymbol{p}), y_\gamma(\boldsymbol{p}), \ldots) \\ y_\beta(\boldsymbol{p}) &= s_\beta(\boldsymbol{p}, y_\alpha(\boldsymbol{p}), y_\gamma(\boldsymbol{p}), \ldots) \\ y_\gamma(\boldsymbol{p}) &= s_\gamma(\boldsymbol{p}, y_\alpha(\boldsymbol{p}), y_\beta(\boldsymbol{p}), \ldots) \end{aligned} \tag{8.9}$$

and so on. In this steady state, we define the *local response coefficients*

$$\tilde{\boldsymbol{R}}_{\mathrm{p}}^{\mathrm{S}_\mu} = \frac{\partial s_\mu}{\partial \boldsymbol{p}}, \qquad \tilde{\boldsymbol{R}}_{\mathrm{S}_\nu}^{\mathrm{S}_\mu} = \frac{\partial s_\mu}{\partial \boldsymbol{x}_\nu}\Big|_{x=y}, \qquad \tilde{\boldsymbol{R}}_{\mathrm{S}_\mu}^{\mathrm{S}_\mu} = 0. \tag{8.10}$$

The *global response coefficients* of the modules are defined as

$$\tilde{\boldsymbol{R}}_{\mathrm{p}}^{\mathrm{Y}_\mu} = \frac{\partial y_\mu}{\partial \boldsymbol{p}}. \tag{8.11}$$

We can collect the response matrices in large block matrices

$$\tilde{\boldsymbol{R}}_{\mathrm{S}}^{\mathrm{S}} = \begin{pmatrix} \tilde{\boldsymbol{R}}_{\mathrm{S}_\alpha}^{\mathrm{S}_\alpha} & \tilde{\boldsymbol{R}}_{\mathrm{S}_\beta}^{\mathrm{S}_\alpha} & \ldots \\ \tilde{\boldsymbol{R}}_{\mathrm{S}_\alpha}^{\mathrm{S}_\beta} & \tilde{\boldsymbol{R}}_{\mathrm{S}_\beta}^{\mathrm{S}_\beta} & \ldots \\ \ldots & \ldots & \ldots \end{pmatrix}, \qquad \tilde{\boldsymbol{R}}_{\mathrm{p}}^{\mathrm{S}} = \begin{pmatrix} \tilde{\boldsymbol{R}}_{\mathrm{p}}^{\mathrm{S}_\alpha} \\ \tilde{\boldsymbol{R}}_{\mathrm{p}}^{\mathrm{S}_\beta} \\ \ldots \end{pmatrix}, \qquad \tilde{\boldsymbol{R}}_{\mathrm{p}}^{\mathrm{Y}} = \begin{pmatrix} \tilde{\boldsymbol{R}}_{\mathrm{p}}^{\mathrm{Y}_\alpha} \\ \tilde{\boldsymbol{R}}_{\mathrm{p}}^{\mathrm{Y}_\beta} \\ \ldots \end{pmatrix} \tag{8.12}$$

The global response coefficients – the derivatives for the coupled system – describe the response to small external parameter changes; they can be computed by

$$\tilde{\boldsymbol{R}}_{\mathrm{p}}^{\mathrm{Y}} = -(\tilde{\boldsymbol{R}}_{\mathrm{S}}^{\mathrm{S}} - \boldsymbol{I})^{-1} \tilde{\boldsymbol{R}}_{\mathrm{p}}^{\mathrm{S}}. \tag{8.13}$$

Thus, the global behavior (at least, steady-state responses to small perturbations) can be computed without referring to the internal details of the modules; we only need to know the modules' input–output behavior for the communicating variables. Modular response analysis concerns steady-state perturbations only; in an similar approach for dynamical perturbations, modules are replaced dynamical black-box models obtained by model reduction [64].

8.3.5
Functional Modules Detected by Epistasis

Genes can be classified by categories [65] related to functions of the cell (e.g., translation, energy metabolism, mitosis, etc.) based on textbook knowledge. But can we also infer functional associations directly from deletion experiments? If two gene products can compensate for each other's loss, then deleting both of them will have a much stronger impact on cell fitness than one would expect from their single deletions. On the other hand, if two gene products are essential parts of the same pathway, a single deletion would already shut down the pathway and a double deletion would not have any further effect. Accordingly, we may try to infer functional relationships among the gene products by comparing the fitness losses caused by combined gene deletions.

Epistasis describes how the fitness loss due to a gene mutation depends on the presence of other genes. It can be quantified by comparing the fitness of a wild type organism – e.g., the growth rate of a bacteria culture – to the fitness of single and double deletion mutants. A single gene deletion (for gene i) will decrease the fitness (e.g., the growth rate) from a value f_{wt} to a value f_i, leading to a growth defect $w_i = f_i/f_{\text{wt}} \leq 1$. For a double deletion of unrelated genes i and j, we may expect a multiplicative effect[1] $w_{ij} = w_i w_j$. If the double deletion is more severe ($w_{ij} < w_i w_j$), we call the epistasis "aggravating," if it is less severe, we call it "buffering." Both cases will indicate functional associations between the genes in question.

Segrè *et al.* [66] have used flux-balance analysis (see Section 9.1.3) to predict growth rates of the yeast *Saccharomyces cerevisiae* and to calculate the epistatic effects between all metabolic genes. The model predicted relative growth defects of all single and double deletion mutants, from which they computed an epistasis measure $\hat{\varepsilon}_{ij}$

$$\hat{\varepsilon}_{ij} = \frac{w_{ij} - w_i w_j}{|\hat{w}_{ij} - w_i w_j|} \tag{8.14}$$

for each pair of genes. The growth defect $\hat{w}_{ij}$ is defined separately for buffering and aggravating interactions and either represents extreme buffering ($\hat{w}_{ij} = \min(w_i, w_j)$, the less severe deletion does not play a role) or extreme aggravation ($w_{ij} = 0$, the double mutation is lethal). The histogram of the $\hat{\varepsilon}_{ij}$ shows a strong main peak around $\hat{\varepsilon} = 0$, indicating that the growth defect is indeed multiplicative for most gene pairs. However, some pairs show either strong aggravation (lethal phenotypes) or complete buffering.

To analyze the epistasis data, genes were grouped into functional categories according to biological annotations (see Figure 8.15). The epistatic effects are strongly related to the functional groups and with only few exceptions, the epistatic effects between two functional groups are either only aggravating, or only buffering ("monochromatic interactions"). This result suggests that individual genes do not directly contribute to the biological fitness, but via their roles in distinct functional subsystems of the cell. The same kind of analysis could be employed to define functional groups from scratch based on measured growth data.

1) The multiplication for functionally unrelated genes resembles the multiplication of probabilities for independent random variables. An example: the reproduction rate depends bilinearly on (i) the probability to reach reproductional age and (ii) the mean number of offspring after this age has been reached. If a gene affects only (i) and another gene affects only (ii), they are functionally unrelated and their effect on the reproduction rate is multiplicative.

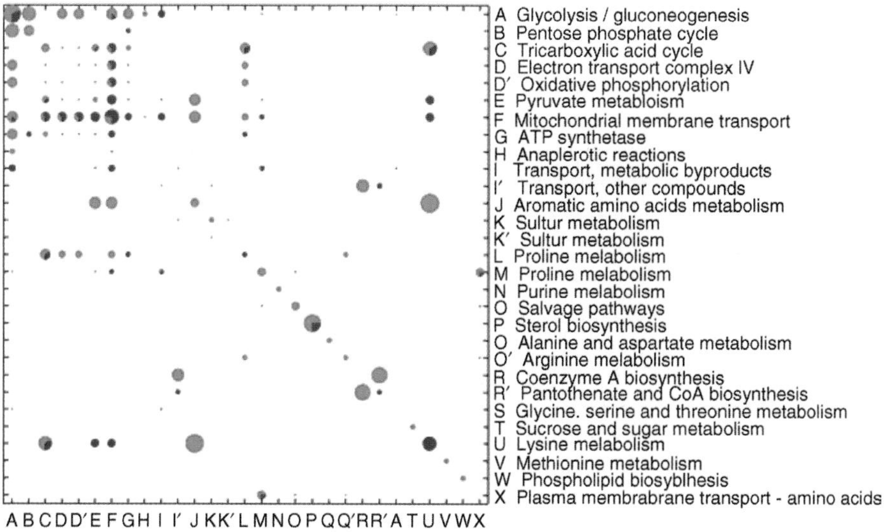

Figure 8.15 Epistatic effects reflect the shared functions of genes. Circles show the abundance of epistatic interactions between genes belonging to functional groups (rows and columns). Circle radii represent numbers of epistatic interactions. Aggravating and buffering interactions are shown as red and green pie slices, respectively. From Segrè *et al.* [66].

8.3.6 Evolution of Modularity and Complexity

Machines, computer programs, or mathematical models can be designed to be modular. In technical devices, modularity makes the design better understandable, helps to share work between developers, and facilitates repair by replacement of standard parts. As a consequence, parts of machines often serve a single defined function; sometimes there are exceptions – the wings of a plane are also used to store fuel – but it occurs rather rarely that functions of a machine are widely distributed among its parts. Such a modular design is often economically preferable even if a non-modular solution would be technically more efficient.

Biological systems, in contrast, are not designed, but shaped by mutation and selection. There is no selection advantage to understandability, so natural selection is likely to choose the solution that works best, whether it is understandable or not. Nevertheless, biological systems such as the transcription network shown in Figure 8.6 show modularity and recurrent structures. These features would not have evolved if they did not provide a selection advantage.

8.3.6.1 Tinkering and Engineering

Evolution by mutation and selection can improve existing systems and adapt them to new challenges. Existing structures can be further modified, rewired, and reused for new purposes. Optimization by iterated small modifications resembles "tinkering" [67] rather than engineering, so biological systems may look very different from the solutions that an engineer would conceive. The difference between an engineered network (a computer chip) and an evolved network (transcription network) resembles the contrast between a well-structured computer program and an artificial neural network: a trained neural network may be able to solve complex computational problems of various kinds, but we cannot expect that the logical structure of the problem is directly reflected by the network structure.

8.3.6.2 Analogy in Evolution

Despite the randomness in single mutation events, species can evolve similar, analogous traits if they are under similar selection pressure. For instance, wings have evolved independently in birds, bats, and insects under the selection pressure for the ability to fly. Due to the similar constraints (biomechanics, aerodynamics, and energy balance), they also obtained relatively similar shapes. Also in cellular networks, convergent evolution may lead to similar structural and dynamical features, for instance modules or network motifs [68–70].

The convergence toward optimal performance can also explain analogies between biological and technical systems: although both types of systems are based on very different materials (e.g., chemical reaction systems versus electronic circuits), biological and technical systems share invariant requirements like robustness and cost efficiency. Therefore, an optimization in both systems may lead to similar structures (e.g., feedback loops). Even though technical and biological systems are clearly different, technical metaphors can help to get a better functional understanding of biological systems [68, 71].

8.3.6.3 Modularity, Robustness, and Evolvability

A possible advantage of modularity is that it can contribute to robustness. Cells, for instance, are separated from each other by membranes, which allows them to undergo apoptosis without affecting the neighboring cells in a tissue. On the other hand, robustness can also be a prerequisite for modularity: if a biological module is used in various biochemical contexts (cell states or cell types), it needs to be robust against typical variations in cells, so there will be a selection pressure on robustness.

Kashtan and Alon have shown that a modular structure can contribute to evolvability, which would create a second-order selection advantage [72]. In a simulation study [70], hypothetical electronic circuits were evolved by random mutation and selection to optimally fulfill two different signal-processing tasks. In an evolution scenario with a constant task, evolution ended up with different highly optimal circuits, which turned out to be non-modular. In a second scenario, the task consisted of two subtasks that appeared in varying combinations. Although being suboptimal for each of the individual tasks, the modular circuits were able to switch from one task to the other by small genetic changes and, being better evolvable, emerged as winners in the evolution.

Exercises and Problems

1. Determine the adjacency matrices for the graphs in Figure 8.2. Compute the degrees and clustering coefficients of each node in (b) and (c). How many feed-forward loops are contained in the directed graph? Show that the topological distance in the directed graph is not a symmetric mathematical function.

2. According to Jeong *et al.* [25], the degree of metabolites, i.e., the number of reactions in which each metabolite is involved, follows to good approximation a power law. In *E. coli* bacteria, the exponent is $\gamma \approx 2.2$. About 1% of the metabolites have a degree $k = 10$. Which percentage of metabolites has a degree $k = 20$?

3. In the transcription network of *E. coli*, 42 out of 424 transcription factors show self-inhibition (Shen-Orr *et al.*, 2002). Is this number surprisingly large or would you expect it to appear by chance?

4. What are network motifs? How would you determine them for a given network? Choose a network motif that appears in transcription networks, describe its dynamic properties, and speculate about its biological function. Explain why motifs might emerge during evolution of biological networks.

5. Consider the genetic network controlling sporulation in *B. subtilis* (Figure 8.13). Find all feed-forward loops in the scheme and determine their types. Assume a dynamic model of this system with piecewise linear kinetics, all thresholds set to a value of 1/2 and all other model parameters set equal to one. Sketch the time-dependent regulator concentrations after the sigma factor σ^E exceeds its threshold value. What qualitative behavior do you expect for the four groups of target genes, X_1, X_2, X_3, X_4, in terms of pulses and delays?

6. Find examples of homology and analogy in (i) shapes or organs of animals, (ii) biochemical processes and structures on the molecular level, and (iii) biological network structures.

7. Explain why epistasis between genes may indicate functional association. State explicitly the main assumptions on which your argument is based.

8. What insights can be gained by constructing a genetic circuit (e.g., a bistable switch) if a similar system exists already in wild-type cells?

9. Derive Eq. (8.13) from the definitions (8.12).

References

1 Barabási, A.-L. and Oltvai, Z.N. (2004) Network biology: understanding the cell's functional organization. *Nature Reviews. Genetics*, **5**, 101–113.

2 Albert, R. and Barabási, A.-L. (2002) Statistical mechanics of complex networks. *Reviews of Modern Physics*, **74**, 47–97.

3 Barabási, A.-L. (2002) *Linked: The New Science of Networks*, Perseus Publishing, USA.

4 Jeong, H., Mason, S.P., Barabási, A.-L. and Oltvai, Z.N. (2001) Lethality and centrality in protein networks. *Nature*, **411**, 41–42.

5 Feist, A.M., Henry, C.S., Reed, J.L., Krummenacker, M., Joyce, A.R., Karp, P.D., Broadbelt, L.J., Hatzimanikatis, V. and Palsson, B.Ø. (2007) A genome-scale metabolic reconstruction for *Escherichia coli* K-12 MG1655 that accounts for 1260 ORFs and thermodynamic information. *Molecular System Biology*, **3**, 121.

6 Suderman, M. and Hallett, M. (2007) Tools for visually exploring biological networks. *Bioinformatics (Oxford, England)*, **23** (20), 2651–2659.

7 Wagner, A. and Fell, D.A. (2001) The small world inside large metabolic networks. *Proceedings—Biological Sciences*, **268** (1478), 1803–1810.

8 Watts, D.J. and Strogatz, S.H. (1998) Collective dynamics of 'small-world' networks. *Nature*, **393**, 440–442.

9 Itzkovitz, S. and Alon, U. (2005) Subgraphs and network motifs in geometric networks. *Physical Review E*, **71**, 026117.

10 Milo, R., Shen-Orr, S., Itzkovitz, S., Kashtan, N., Chklovskii, D. and Alon, U. (2002) Network motifs: simple building blocks of complex networks. *Science*, **298**, 824–827.

11 Barabási, A.-L. and Albert, R. (1999) Emergence of scaling in random networks. *Science*, **286**, 509.

12 Edwards, A.M. *et al.* (2007) Revisiting Levy flight search patterns of wandering albatrosses, bumblebees and deer. *Nature*, **449**, 1044–1048.

13 Ravasz, E., Somera, A.L., Mongru, D.A., Oltvai, Z.N. and Barabási, A.-L. (2002) Hierarchical organization of modularity in metabolic networks. *Science*, **297**, 1551–1555.

14 Pastor-Satorras, R., Smith, E. and Solé, R.V. (2003) Evolving protein interaction networks through gene duplication. *Journal of Theoretical Biology*, **222** (2), 199–210.

15 Wagner, A. (2003) How the global structure of protein interaction networks evolves. *Proceedings—Biological Sciences*, **270** (1514), 457–466.

16 Alon, U. (2007) Network motifs: theory and experimental approaches. *Nature Reviews. Genetics*, **8**, 450–461.

17 Milo, R., Itzkovitz, S., Kashtan, N., Levitt, R., Shen-Orr, S., Ayzenshtat, I., Sheffer, M. and Alon, U. (2004) Superfamilies of designed and evolved networks. *Science*, **303**, 1538–1542.

18 Shen-Orr, S., Milo, R., Mangan, S. and Alon, U. (2002) Network motifs in the transcriptional regulation network of *Escherichia coli*. *Nature Genetics*, **31**, 64–68.

19 Lee, T.I., Rinaldi, N.J., Robert, F., Odom, D.T., Bar-Joseph, Z., Gerber, G.K., Hannett, N.M., Harbison, C.T., Thompson, C.M., Simon, I., Zeitlinger, J., Jennings, E.G., Murray, H.L., Gordon, D.B., Ren, B., Wyrick, J.J., Tagne, J.B., Volkert, T.L., Fraenkel, E., Gifford, D.K. and Young, R.A. (2002) Transcriptional regulatory networks in *Saccharomyces cerevisiae*. *Science*, **298**, 799–804.

20 Schreiber, F. and Schwöbbermeyer, H. (2005) MAVisto: a tool for the exploration of network motifs. *Bioinformatics (Oxford, England)*, **21**, 3572–3574.

21 Wernicke, S. and Rasche, F. (2006) FANMOD: a tool for fast network motif detection. *Bioinformatics (Oxford, England)*, **22** (9), 1152–1153.

22 Dekel, E. and Alon, U. (2005) Optimality and evolutionary tuning of the expression level of a protein. *Nature*, **436**, 588–692.

23 Hatzimanikatis, V. (2005) Exploring the diversity of complex metabolic networks. *Bioinformatics (Oxford, England)*, **21** (8), 1603–1609.

24 Stephani, A., Nuño, J.C. and Heinrich, R. (1999) Optimal stoichimetric designs of ATP-producing systems as determined by

an evolutionary algorithm. *Journal of Theoretical Biology*, **199**, 45–61.

25 Jeong, H., Tombor, B., Albert, R., Oltvai, Z. and Barabási, A.-L. (2000) The large-scale organization of metabolic networks. *Nature*, **407**, 651–654.

26 Arita, M. (2004) The metabolic world of *Escherichia coli* is not small. *Proceedings of the National Academy of Sciences of the United States of America*, **101** (6), 1543–1547.

27 Mangan, S. and Alon, U. (2003) Structure and function of the feed-forward loop network motif. *Proceedings of the National Academy of Sciences of the United States of America*, **100** (21), 11980–11985.

28 Tyson, J.J., Chen, K.C. and Novak, B. (2003) Sniffers, buzzers, toggles and blinkers: dynamics of regulatory and signaling pathways in the cell. *Current Opinion in Cell Biology*, **15** (2), 221–231.

29 Alon, U. (2006) An Introduction to Systems Biology: Design Principles of Biological Circuits, *CRC Mathematical & Computational Biology*, Chapman and Hall, London.

30 Elowitz, M.B. and Leibler, S. (2000) A synthetic oscillatory network of transcriptional regulators. *Nature*, **403**, 335–338.

31 Becskei, A. and Serrano, L. (2000) Engineering stability in gene networks by autoregulation. *Nature*, **405**, 590–592.

32 Hasty, J., McMillen, D. and Collins, J.J. (2002) Engineered gene circuits. *Nature*, **420**, 224–230.

33 Elowitz, M. *et al.* (2002) Stochastic gene expression in a single cell. *Science*, **297**, 1183.

34 Pedraza, J.M. and van Oudenaarden, A. (2005) Noise propagation in gene networks. *Science*, **307**, 1965–1969.

35 Robison, K., McGuire, A.M. and Church, G.M.A., (1998) A comprehensive library of DNA-binding site matrices for 55 proteins applied to the complete *Escherichia coli K12* genome. *Journal of Molecular Biology*. **284** (2), 241–254.

36 Salgado, H., Gama-Castro, S., Martínez-Antonio, A., Díaz-Peredo, E., Sánchez-Solano, F., Peralta-Gil, M., Garcia-Alonso, D., Jiménez-Jacinto, V., Santos-Zavaleta, A., Bonavides-Martínez, C. and Collado-Vides, J. (2004) RegulonDB (version 4.0): transcriptional regulation, operon organization and growth conditions in *Escherichia coli* K-12. *Nucleic Acids Research*, 303–306.

37 Keseler, I.M., Collado-Vides, J., Gama-Castro, S., Ingraham, J., Paley, S., Paulsen, I.T., Peralta-Gil, M. and Karp, P.D. (2005) Ecocyc: A comprehensive database resource for *Escherichia coli*. *Nucleic Acids Research*.

38 Mangan, S., Zaslaver, A. and Alon, U. (2003) The coherent feedforward loop serves as a sign-sensitive delay element in transcription networks. *Journal of Molecular Biology*, **334**, 197–204.

39 Kalir, S., Mangan, S. and Alon, U. (2005) A coherent feed-forward loop with a sum input function prolongs flagella expression in *Escherichia coli*. *Molecular System Biology*, **1**, (doi: 10.1038/msb4100010).

40 Itzkovitz, S., Levitt, R., Kashtan, N., Milo, R., Itzkovitz, M. and Alon, U. (2005) Coarse-graining and self-dissimilarity of complex networks. *Physical Review E*, **71**, (1 Pt 2).

41 Guelzim, N., Bottani, S., Bourgine, P. and Képès, F. (2002) Topological and causal structure of the yeast transcriptional regulatory network. *Nature Genetics*, **31**, 60–63.

42 Goldbeter, A. and Koshland, D.E. Jr (1981) An amplified sensitivity arising from covalent modification in biological systems. *Proceedings of the National Academy of Sciences of the United States of America*, **78**, 6840–6844.

43 Goldbeter, A. and Koshland, D.E. Jr (1984) Ultrasensitivity in biological systems controlled by covalent modification. *The Journal of Biological Chemistry*, **259**, 14441–14447.

44 Barkai, N. and Leibler, S. (1997) Robustness in simple biochemical networks. *Nature*, **387**, 913–917.

45 Alon, U., Surette, M.G., Barkai, N. and Leibler, S. (1999) Robustness in bacterial chemotaxis. *Nature*, **397**, 168–171.

46 Eldar, A., Rosin, D., Shilo, B.Z. and Barkai, N. (2003) Self-enhanced ligand degradation underlies robustness of morphogen gradients. *Developmental Cell*, **5**, 635–646.

47 Rosenfeld, N., Elowitz, M.B. and Alon, U. (2002) Negative autoregulation speeds the response times of transcription networks. *Journal of Molecular Biology*, **323** (5), 785–793.

48 Mangan, S., Zaslaver, A. and Alon, U. (2006) The incoherent feed-forward loop accelerates the response time of the gal system in *E. coli*. *Journal of Molecular Biology*, **356**, 1073–1082.

49 Eichenberger, P., Fujita, M., Jensen, S.T., Conlon, E.M., Rudner, D.Z., Wang, S.T., Ferguson, C., Haga, K., Sato, T., Liu, J.S. and Losick, R. (2004) The program of gene transcription for a single differentiating cell type during sporulation in *Bacillus subtilis*. *PLoS Biology*, **2** (10), e328.

50 Prill, R.J., Iglesias, P.A. and Levchenko, A. (2005) Dynamic properties of network motifs contribute to biological network organization. *PLoS Biology*, **3** (11), 1881–1892.

51 Klemm, K. and Bornholdt, S. (2005) Topology of biological networks and reliability of information processing. *Proceedings of the National Academy of Sciences of the United States of America*, **102** (51), 18414–18419.

52 Hartwell, L.H., Hopfield, J.J., Leibler, S. and Murray, A.W. (1999) From molecular to modular cell biology. *Nature*, **402** (6761 Suppl), C47–C52.

53 Hasty, J., McMillen, D. and Collins, J.J. (2002) Engineered gene circuits. *Nature*, **420**, 224–230.

54 Pellegrini, M., Marcotte, E.M., Thompson, M.J., Eisenberg, D. and Yeates, T.O. (1999) Assigning protein functions by comparative genome analysis: Protein phylogenetic profiles. *Proceedings of the National Academy of Sciences of the United States of America*, **96** (8), 4285–4288.

55 Schuster, S., Pfeiffer, T., Moldenhauer, F., Koch, I. and Dandekar, T. (2002) Exploring the pathway structure of metabolism: decomposition into subnetworks and application to Mycoplasma pneumoniae. *Bioinformatics (Oxford, England)*, **18** (2), 351–361.

56 Guimera, R. and Nunes Amaral, L.A. (2005) Functional cartography of complex metabolic networks. *Nature*, **433**, 895.

57 Ederer, M., Sauter, T., Bullinger, E., Gilles, E. and Allgöwer, F. (2003) An approach for dividing models of biological reaction networks into functional units. *Simulation*, **79** (12), 703–716.

58 Segal, E., Shapira, M., Regev, A., Pe'er, D. and Botstein, D., Daphne Koller and Nir Friedman (2003) Module networks: identifying regulatory modules and their condition-specific regulators from gene expression data. *Nature Genetics*, **34** (2), 166–176.

59 Tanay, A., Sharan, R. and Shamir, R. (2002) Discovering statistically significant biclusters in gene expression data. *Bioinformatics (Oxford, England)*, (Suppl. 1), S136–S144.

60 Schilling, C.H. and Palsson, B.Ø. (1998) The underlying pathway structure of biochemical reaction networks. *Proceedings of the National Academy of Sciences of the United States of America*, **95** (8), 4193–4198.

61 Schuster, S., Fell, D. and Dandekar, T. (2000) A general definition of metabolic pathways useful for systematic organization and analysis of complex metabolic networks. *Nature Biotechnology*, **18**, 326–332.

62 Schuster, S., Kahn, D. and Westerhoff, H.V. (1993) Modular analysis of the control of complex metabolic pathways. *Biophysical Chemistry*, **48**, 1–17.

63 Bruggeman, F., Westerhoff, H.V., Hoek, J.B. and Kholodenko, B. (2002) Modular response analysis of cellular regulatory networks. *Journal of Theoretical Biology*, **218**, 507–520.

64 Liebermeister, W., Baur, U. and Klipp, E. (2005) Biochemical network models simplified by balanced truncation. *FEBS Journal*, **272** (16), 4034–4043.

65 Mewes, H.W., Dietmann, S., Frishman, D., Gregory, R., Mannhaupt, G., Mayer, K.F.X., Münsterkötter, M., Ruepp, A., Spannagl, M., Stümpflen, V. and Rattei, T. (2008) MIPS: analysis and annotation of genome information in 2007. *Nucleic Acids Research*, **36**, D196–D201.

66 Segrè, D., DeLuna, A., Church, G.M. and Kishony, R. (2005) Modular epistasis in yeast metabolism. *Nature Genetics*, **37**, 77–83.

67 Alon, U. (2003) Biological networks: the tinkerer as an engineer. *Science*, **301**, 1866–1867.

68 Csete, M.E. and Doyle, J.C. (2002) Reverse engineering of biological complexity. *Science*, **295** (5560), 1664–1669.

69 Conant, G.C. and Wagner, A. (2003) Convergent evolution of gene circuits. *Nature Genetics*, **34**, 264–266.

70 Kashtan, N. and Alon, U., Spontaneous evolution of modularity and network motifs. *Proceedings of the National Academy of Sciences of the United States of America*, **102**(39), 13773–13778.

71 Lazebnik, Y. (2002) Can a biologist fix a radio? or, what I learned while studying apoptosis. *Cancer Cell*, **2**, 179–182.

72 Kirschner, M. and Gerhart, J. (1998) Evolvability. *Proceedings of the National Academy of Sciences of the United States of America*, **95** (15), 8420–8427.

9
Optimality and Evolution

9.1
Optimality and Constraint-Based Models

Summary

Many observations suggest that mutation and selection can shape organisms, cells, pathways, and even kinetic constants for maximal evolutionary fitness. Theoretical optimality studies try to explain features of biological systems – e.g., structure of pathways, metabolic fluxes, values of kinetic parameters – by an optimization requirement. They can help to understand how and why biological systems have evolved the way they have, reveal nature's solutions to technical problems, and suggest how to modify cells for use in biotechnology. Flux-balance analysis, for instance, uses an optimality principle to predict stationary fluxes in metabolic networks. The basic assumption is that a certain linear function of metabolic fluxes is maximized by living cells. Other constraint-based models require thermodynamically feasible fluxes as an additional constraint.

Biological systems evolve by mutation and selection, and in many cases, this process resembles an optimization of vital biological functions. In a competition between bacteria, for instance, faster growing mutants are likely to replace the wild-type population, and after many such replacements, the bacterial genomes become enriched with genetic features that contribute to fast growth, e.g., by adjusting the performance or regulation of metabolism.

Optimization by evolution can be studied quantitatively in the laboratory: Dekel and Alon [1] measured the growth rate of *E. coli* bacteria at different extracellular lactose levels and different expression levels of the Lac operon (including the gene lacZ). They predicted that for each lactose level, there exists an optimal LacZ expression level that maximizes the growth rate and should therefore provide the highest fitness advantage in a competition between bacteria. The prediction was then tested in an evolution experiment in the lab with fixed lactose levels. Already after a few hundred generations, the wild-type population was in fact replaced by mutants with the predicted optimal LacZ expression levels.

Systems Biology: A Textbook. Edda Klipp, Wolfram Liebermeister, Christoph Wierling, Axel Kowald, Hans Lehrach, and Ralf Herwig

ISBN: 978-3-527-31874-2

9.1.1
Optimization by Evolution

Evolution is an open process without a predefined goal and does not necessarily lead to optimal phenotypes (compare Section 9.3). Nevertheless, many traits of living beings resemble a theoretical optimum or a hypothetical solution that an engineer would design. One explanation is that mutation and selection can act as an efficient search strategy in fitness landscapes (see Section 7.2.4). This view is supported by the success of numerical optimization methods like genetic algorithms [2] (see the web supplement), which are inspired by the process of evolution. Such algorithms can tackle general, not necessarily biological, optimization problems: using a biological metaphor, candidate solutions of the problem are formulated as genotypes (usually strings of numbers), and optimal solutions are found by repeated mutation and selection according to a certain (method-dependent) evolution scenario.

It is common and often helpful to use metaphors like "function" or "optimization" to describe evolved biological systems. A statement like "Cells maintain a high ATP level *in order to* use ATP as an energy source" is teleological, i.e., related to a purpose rather than to a mechanistic process. Teleological notions can help to make sense of the processes in living cells, but they need to be backed by evolutionary theory. The above statement could, for instance, be loosely rephrased as "Cells that cease to maintain high ATP levels would most likely become extinct due to lack of energy."

Optimality studies in systems biology are based on mechanistic models, but their aim is not to simulate *how* a system works (the dynamics), but to explain *why* systems look and function the way they do (the function). The dynamics concerns the system itself – given the interactions with its environment – whereas the notion of *function* emphasizes what the pathway does for the cell and moreover, how it contributes to the cell's fitness.

Optimality studies concern the theoretical limits of a system: if a known fitness function had to be maximized in evolution or biotechnology, what fitness value could be maximally achieved? And how could it be achieved? If an actual system already resembles the theoretical optimum, we may hypothesize that natural selection has optimized it according to the assumed fitness criteria. Studying a specific system, we can further ask: what in it is optimized? What features of the system could be adapted, and under what constraints?

9.1.2
Optimality Studies in Systems Biology

The concept of optimality plays an important role in physics (variational principles, see [3]), economics, and engineering. For biological questions, this concept provides valuable insights as well. The basic approach in optimality studies is as follows: different possible variants x of a biological system are scored by a fitness function $f(x)$, in order to find variants with maximal fitness values. The variants should all be mechanistically plausible, i.e., they should obey biochemical constraints. The fitness function, on the other hand, may either describe a goal to be reached in bioengineering, or some function that is presumably maximized in evolution.

In systems biology models, the variants for cellular networks can differ in their structure, kinetic parameters, or regulation. Stephani and Heinrich [4], for instance, studied the stoichiometric structure of glycolysis under the aspect of optimality: glycolysis produces two molecules of ATP per glucose molecule, but it does so by first consuming two ATP molecules and later producing four of them. In comparison to alternative stoichiometric structures, this feature was found to provide optimal thermodynamic conditions for maximizing the glycolytic flux.

9.1.2.1 The Fitness Function

If we hypothesize that cellular systems (e.g., a metabolic pathway) are optimized in evolution, which kind of fitness function should we consider for a computational model? For the evolution of competing bacterial strains, we may consider the growth rate under the experimental conditions. In nature and for higher organisms, the long-term reproduction rate may depend on complicated factors like diseases or social behavior between individuals. In either case, it cannot be written explicitly as a mathematical function scoring a metabolic pathway.

But possibly, parts of the system are at least optimized given the behavior of the other parts. In this case, we can assume that a pathway obeys a relatively simple *effective fitness function*, which scores how the pathway contributes to fitness in general. The choice of such fitness functions is not at all obvious. For example, metabolic systems might be optimized for high product fluxes or for efficient use of resources [5]. Which of these contrary objectives is relevant for evolution in a specific scenario can depend on many factors, including the social behavior of cells (see Section 9.3.7). For metabolic systems, several fitness objectives have been proposed, including (i) maximal steady-state fluxes, (ii) minimal concentrations of metabolic intermediates, (iii) minimal transition times, (iv) maximal sensitivity to external signals, and (v) optimal thermodynamic efficiency [6].

As a result of natural selection, living systems should be optimized for those situations that they encounter routinely during evolution. Optimization to variable environments poses different challenges (e.g. robustness, versatility) than adaptation to a constant environment (specialization, minimal effort). Therefore, optimization studies do not only imply assumptions about the system, but also on the statistical properties of its environment.

9.1.2.2 Optimality and Compromise

Biological behavior often results from a compromise: in the bacterial evolution experiment mentioned above, LacZ expression contributes to the cell's energy supply and thereby supports fast growth. On the other hand, high expression of LacZ also consumes energy and occupies ribosomes, which impedes growth. The trade-off between such contrary effects can be expressed by different mathematical formulations (see Figure 9.1).

9.1.2.3 Cost-Benefit Calculations

Cost-benefit calculations for metabolic systems [1, 7–9] assume, as a fitness function, the difference

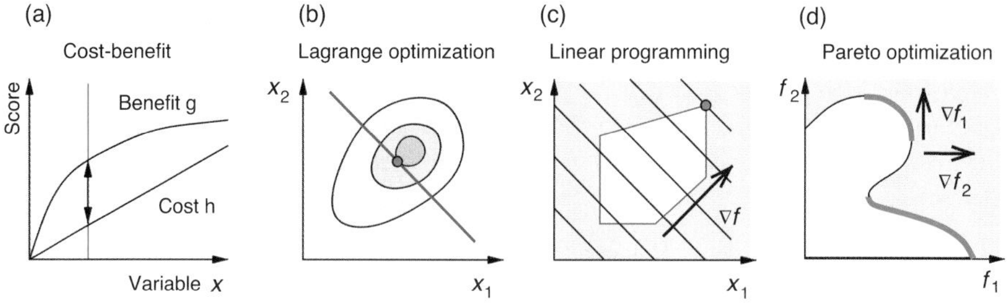

Figure 9.1 Optimization approaches. (a) Cost-benefit calculation. The fitness is the difference between benefit and cost $f(x) = g(x) - h(x)$. It is maximal at the value of x where both curves have the same slope. (b) Local optimum with equality constraint (blue line). The fitness function (as a function of two arguments x_1 and x_2) is shown by contour lines. At the constrained optimum (red circle), contour lines and constraint line (blue) are parallel. (c) Linear programming: a feasible region (white) is defined by linear inequality constraints for the arguments x_1 and x_2. The fitness function is linear, shown by contour lines and gradient (arrow). (d) Pareto (vectorial) optimization with two fitness functions f_1 and f_2. The allowed combinations (f_1, f_2) are defined (white region) by constraints on the function arguments (not visible). A state is Pareto optimal (red) if it is impossible to increase both fitness functions at the same time. Pareto optimization yields one or several continuous sets of solutions on the boundary of the feasible set. The methods depicted also apply to multidimensional problems.

$$f(x) = g(x) - h(x) \tag{9.1}$$

between a benefit term g and a cost term h (see Figure 9.1(a)). A local optimum of the variable x requires that $\mathrm{d}f/\mathrm{d}x = \mathrm{d}g/\mathrm{d}x - \mathrm{d}h/\mathrm{d}x = 0$, so the slopes (called *marginal benefit* and *marginal cost*) must be equal. In Figure 9.1(a), the benefit saturates at high x while the cost keeps increasing, which implies a local optimum.

The following quantities have been suggested as cost functions for biochemical models: the total amount of enzyme in a cell or a particular pathway [7], the total energy utilization [10], or the evolutionary effort [11] quantified as the number of mutations or events necessary to attain a certain state, and an empirical growth defect determined from measurements [1].

It is reasonable to assume that enzyme production is costly. According to cost-benefit considerations, enzymes should only be expressed if they provide a benefit, and at a local optimum, their marginal benefit (i.e., the benefit obtained from expressing one more enzyme molecule) and their marginal cost (for producing one more molecule) should be equal. However, if the marginal cost in Figure 9.1(a) exceeded the marginal benefit already at $x = 0$, then this point is a boundary optimum and the enzyme should not be expressed.

9.1.2.4 **Inequality Constraints**

Alternatively, costs can be modeled by *inequality constraints*. If a local optimum $x^{\text{opt}} = \text{argmax}_x\, g(x) - h(x)$ in a cost-benefit calculation is associated with a cost value $h^{\text{opt}} = h(x^{\text{opt}})$, we can reformulate the model with a constraint: now the system has to maximize $g(x)$ while $h(x) \leq h^{\text{opt}}$. In many cases, such an inequality can be further replaced by an equality $h(x) = h^{opt}$. Such equality constraints can be handled by the method of *Lagrange multipliers*. For instance, instead of controlling an enzyme level by a cost term, we may fix its level at a given value. In addition, there may also be physical constraints for enzymatic reactions, such as fixed equilibrium constants, limitations in the diffusive movement of compounds through the cell, or the stoichiometry of metabolic systems.

9.1.2.5 Local Optima

We can imagine the fitness function as a landscape in the space of genotypes or phenotypes. Such a landscape can have several local optima with different fitness values. If jumps between the local optima require a combination of several rare mutations, a population may remain confined to a local optimum. Therefore, it is often reasonable to consider local instead of global maxima in optimality studies.

Confinement to a local optimum has also been demonstrated experimentally: bacteria can become resistant against antibiotics by mutations which effectively make them less sensitive to a particular drug. The resistant mutants have a relative growth advantage, so resistance genes will be selected for. Chait *et al.* [12] have explored a method to prevent the emergence of resistance genes: if antibiotics are administered in combination, this can either increase or reduce their effect on cell proliferation (*synergy* or *antagonism*). There are even extreme cases of antagonism – *suppressive* drug combinations – in which the combined drugs have a weaker effect than either of the drugs alone. This has a paradoxical consequence: mutants that are resistant against one of the drugs will suffer even more strongly from the other drug and will therefore be selected against. In experiments, a suppressive combination of antibiotics prevented the emergence of resistance [12] by keeping the bacteria in a local fitness optimum.

9.1.3 Constraint-Based Flux Optimization

Flux-balance analysis, an optimality-based method for flux prediction, is one of the most popular modeling approaches for metabolic systems. Flux optimization methods do not describe *how* a certain flux distribution is realized (by kinetics or enzyme regulation), but *which* flux distribution is optimal for the cell – e.g., providing the highest rate of biomass production at a limited inflow of external nutrients. This allows us to predict flux distributions without the need for a kinetic description. From a species' genome sequence, the metabolic network can be roughly predicted [13, 14]. Even if we do not know anything about the enzyme kinetics, we can infer which metabolites the network can produce and which precursors are needed to produce biomass. Given a number of nutrients and a hypothesized optimality requirement, e.g., for fast biomass production, we can try to predict an optimal flux distribution in the network.

9.1.3.1 Flux-Balance Analysis

Flux-balance analysis [15–20] investigates the theoretical capabilities and modes of metabolism by imposing a number of constraints on the metabolic flux distributions.

A first constraint on the flux vector $\boldsymbol{v}$ is set by the assumption of a steady state $\boldsymbol{N}\boldsymbol{v}=0$, where $\boldsymbol{N}$ denotes the stoichiometric matrix. A second constraint stems from consideration of thermodynamics, assuming the irreversibility of certain reactions under physiological conditions. A third constraint acknowledges the limited capacity of enzymes and imposes upper bounds on certain reaction fluxes. For example, in the case of a Michaelis–Menten–type enzyme, the reaction rate is limited by the maximal rate set by the enzyme's concentration and turnover number. In general, the latter constraints on individual metabolic fluxes read

$$v_i^{\min} \leq v_i \leq v_i^{\max}. \tag{9.2}$$

Partial inhibition of enzymes can be modeled by tighter maximality constraints leading to reduced maximal rates [21]. Together, these constraints confine the steady-state fluxes to a feasible set, but usually do not yield a unique solution. Thus, as a fourth requirement, an optimality assumption is added: the flux distribution has to maximize an objective function $f(\boldsymbol{v})$

$$\max \stackrel{!}{=} f(\boldsymbol{v}) = \sum_{i=1}^{r} c_i v_i, \tag{9.3}$$

where the coefficients c_i represent weights for the individual rates v_i. Examples of such objective functions are maximization of ATP production, minimization of nutrient uptake, maximal yield of a desired product, maximal biomass yield, or a combination thereof. The above assumptions lead to an optimization problem with constraints

$$\begin{array}{ccc} \boldsymbol{c}^{\mathrm{T}}\boldsymbol{v} & \stackrel{!}{=} & \max \\ \boldsymbol{N}\boldsymbol{v} & = & 0 \\ \begin{pmatrix} \boldsymbol{I} \\ -\boldsymbol{I} \end{pmatrix} & \geq & \begin{pmatrix} \boldsymbol{v}^{\min} \\ -\boldsymbol{v}^{\max} \end{pmatrix} \end{array}. \tag{9.4}$$

The latter inequality represents the constraints (9.2). This is a standard problem of linear programming which can be solved by the simplex algorithm.

9.1.3.2 Geometric Interpretation of Flux-Balance Analysis

We can imagine possible flux distributions $\boldsymbol{v}$ as points in a multidimensional flux space. Each dimension in this space corresponds to a reaction in the network and represents its reaction velocity (see Figure 9.2).

The stationary fluxes, which are constrained by the linear equations $\boldsymbol{N}\boldsymbol{v}=0$, form a hyperplane. If all individual fluxes are constrained by lower and upper bounds, the resulting region of allowed flux distributions is a convex polyhedron (Figure 9.2(b)): any combination $\lambda \boldsymbol{v}_\alpha + (1-\lambda)\boldsymbol{v}_\beta$ of two allowed flux distributions $\boldsymbol{v}_\alpha$ and $\boldsymbol{v}_\beta$ with $0 \leq \lambda \leq 1$ is again an allowed flux distribution. Flux-balance analysis maximizes a linear function within this polyhedron. The optimum has to lie somewhere on the surface: depending on the direction of the fitness gradient, there is either a unique optimum in a corner of the polyhedron, or the fitness function is maximized on an entire surface.

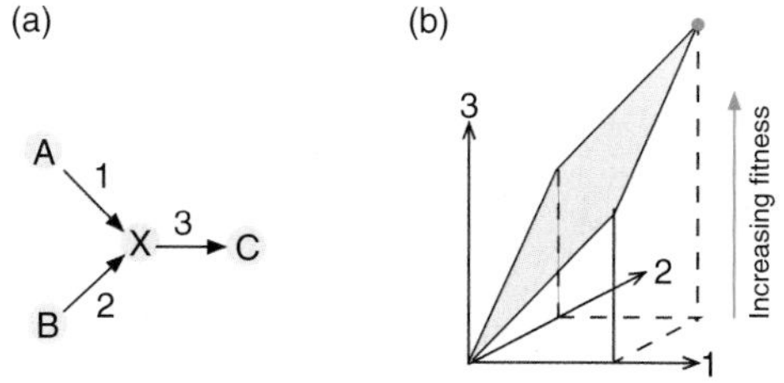

Figure 9.2 Geometric interpretation of flux-balance analysis for a simple example system. (a) Simple metabolic branch point (letters denote metabolites, numbers reactions). In stationary state, the internal metabolite X must be balanced, so $v_1 + v_2 = v_3$. (b) Geometric interpretation: the feasible fluxes form a two-dimensional rhombus in $\mathbf{R}^3$. The fitness function $f = v_3$ in this example is maximized in the upper corner (red dot).

9.1.4
Thermodynamic Constraints

Flux-balance analysis requires that flux patterns are stationary, but it does not check whether they are thermodynamically feasible. According to the second law of thermodynamics, chemical reactions at constant pressure p and temperature T need to be driven by a consumption of Gibbs free energy $G(p, T)$. The Gibbs free energy of a biochemical system is associated with the amount and types of molecules

$$G = \sum_i \mu_i n_i, \tag{9.5}$$

where μ_i and n_i, respectively, denote the chemical potential and the amount (in mol) of substance i. A chemical reaction will change the substance amounts according to the stoichiometric coefficients n_{il}, and the resulting Gibbs free energy change (in kJ per mole reaction events) can be expressed by the chemical potential difference

$$\Delta_r \mu_l = \sum_i \mu_i n_{il}. \tag{9.6}$$

The symbol Δ_r denotes changes associated with chemical reactions, and the negative value $A_l = \Delta_r \mu_l$ is also called *reaction affinity*. The vector of chemical potential differences satisfies the Wegscheider condition

$$(\Delta_r \mu)^T \boldsymbol{K} = 0, \tag{9.7}$$

where $\boldsymbol{K}$ is a right kernel matrix of the stoichiometric matrix $\boldsymbol{N}$, satisfying $\boldsymbol{NK} = 0$. According to the second law of thermodynamics, the Gibbs free energy must decrease in any occurring reaction, so for a forward reaction, the difference of chemical potentials (9.6) must be negative and the reaction affinity must be positive. In general, for a reaction l, we obtain the condition

$$\sum_i \mu_i n_{il} v_l \leq 0. \tag{9.8}$$

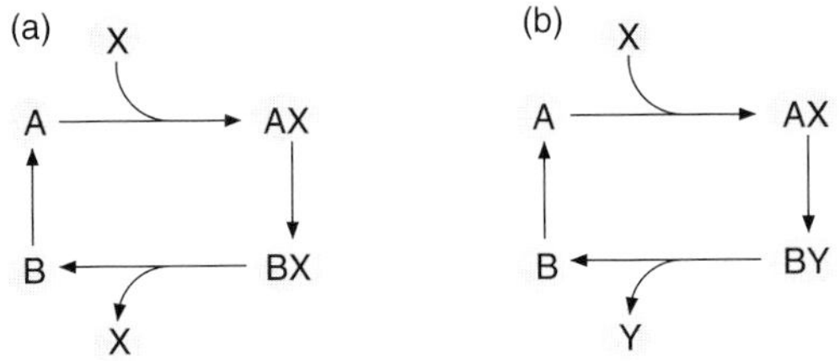

Figure 9.3 Unfeasible and feasible flux distribution. (a) The circular flux is infeasible because the total balance of all metabolite numbers in this flux is zero, and therefore no Gibbs free energy is consumed. In terms of chemical potentials, a forward flux would require $\mu_A + \mu_X > \mu_{AX} > \mu_{BX} > \mu_B + \mu_X$, as well as $\mu_B > \mu_A$, which leads to a contradiction. (b) Feasible flux distribution: with chemical potentials $\mu_X > \mu_Y$, Gibbs free energy is consumed and can drive the reactions.

Therefore, a given flux pattern $\boldsymbol{v} = (v_1, \ldots, v_n)^T$ is only feasible if condition (9.8) can be satisfied by some vector $(\mu_1, \ldots, \mu_m)^T$ of chemical potentials. This condition can be tested using the stoichiometric matrix [22]. Examples of feasible and unfeasible fluxes are shown in Figure 9.3.

Flux-balance analysis does not require that condition (9.8) is fulfilled and can therefore lead to incorrect flux signs. This problem can be avoided by predefining some of the flux directions, which will restrict the solution space in advance. *Energy-balance analysis* [22, 23], in contrast, ensures thermodynamically feasible fluxes by a joint optimization of the fluxes v_l and the chemical potential differences $\Delta_r\mu_l$. Besides the conditions (9.4), it imposes the additional requirements (9.8) and (9.7), which leads to an optimization problem with nonlinear constraints.

The chemical potentials are not only related to the flux directions, but also to the substance concentrations: for an ideal mixture (with vanishing mixing enthalpy), the chemical potential of substance i at pressure p and temperature T reads

$$\mu_i(p, T) = \mu_i^0(p, T) + RT \ln s_i, \tag{9.9}$$

where s_i denotes the concentration of metabolite i in mM. If the standard chemical potentials μ_i^0 are known (e.g., calculated by the group contribution method [24]), Eq. (9.8) translates into constraints between flux directions and substance concentrations. These constraints can be used to determine ranges possible substance concentrations or to check measured concentrations for their feasibility [25, 26].

9.1.5
Applications and Tests of Flux-Optimization Paradigm

Constraint-based methods such as flux-balance analysis allow us to predict the metabolic fluxes and the biomass production (corresponding to the maximal growth rate) under different external conditions, e.g. availability of nutrients. The predictions can be used to simulate dynamically the growth of cell populations and the consumption of nutrients [17]. By comparing the predictions of FBA (biomass production or metabolic fluxes) to experimental data, one can check the assumed network structure for errors (e.g., missing reactions) and test Boolean models of gene regulation [27]. For instance, a low predicted growth rate will indicate that the organism is not viable; by testing the networks of deletion mutants, essential genes can be predicted. The accuracy of such predictions (92% for a current *E. coli* model [14]) can be used as a quality score to check the consistency of the model structure and to point to missing reactions.

This approach implies that flux patterns in wild-type and mutant cells, under different external conditions, are optimized for the same general objective function. However, a study by Schuetz *et al.* [5] indicates that cells may optimize different objectives depending on the experimental conditions: metabolic fluxes in the central metabolism of *E. coli* cells were compared to predictions based on 11 alternative (linear and nonlinear) objective functions. Under glucose limitation in continuous cultures, cells seemed to maximize their yield of ATP or biomass per glucose consumed. Unlimited growth on glucose in respiring batch cultures, on the other hand, was best described by assuming a maximization of ATP production divided by the sum of squared reaction fluxes. This modified objective can be interpreted as a compromise between large ATP production and small enzymatic costs.

Such considerations of minimal effort had been formulated before in the *principle of minimal fluxes* [28]. Large reaction velocities require high amounts of enzymes, which puts a burden on the cell. If the cost of enzyme production plays a role, cells will profit from flux patterns that require less enzyme production, so pathways that do not contribute to biomass production (or whatever quantity is maximized) should be shut off to save energy and material. The principle of minimal fluxes assumes that the flux pattern has to meet some functional requirement – e.g., to yield a prescribed rate of biomass production – while the magnitudes of individual reaction fluxes are minimized.

Even if we accept the assumption of optimality in general, constraint-based methods (i) do not explain by which biological mechanisms changes in flux distributions are actually achieved (e.g., inherent dynamics of the metabolic network, transcriptional regulation), (ii) they do not cover the trade-off between cost and benefit of enzyme production, (iii) they rely, instead, on ad-hoc assumptions, e.g., about maximal fluxes, (iv) and they assume a steady state and do not account for dynamic objectives like fast adaption to changes of supply and demand. To address these issues, we will study the optimality of kinetic models in the following section.

9.2 Optimal Enzyme Concentrations

Summary

We exemplify how metabolic systems would be designed if they were designed according to optimality principles. We investigate the consequences of a demand for rapid conversion of substrate into product on the catalytic properties of single enzymes and on the appropriate amount of enzymes in a metabolic pathway. In the first two sections, we determine conditions on enzyme parameters and enzyme concentrations that yield maximal steady-state fluxes. The third section studies how temporal regulation of a metabolic pathway can support fast conversion of a substrate into a product.

9.2.1 Optimization of Catalytic Properties of Single Enzymes

An important function of enzymes is to increase the rate of a reaction. Therefore, evolutionary pressure should tend to maximize reaction rates: $v \rightarrow \max$ [29–32]. High reaction rates may only be achieved if the kinetic properties of the enzymes are suitably adapted. We identify the optimal kinetic parameters that maximize the rate for the reversible conversion of substrate S into product P [33].

Two constraints must be considered. First, the action of an enzyme cannot alter the thermodynamic equilibrium constant for the conversion of S to P (Section 2.1, Eqs. (2.5) and (2.10)). Changes of kinetic properties must obey the thermodynamic constraint. Second, the values of the kinetic parameters are limited by physical constraints even for the best enzymes, such as diffusion limits or maximal velocity of intramolecular rearrangments. In the following, the maximal possible values are denoted by k_{max} and all rate constants are normalized by their respective k_{max}, such that the normalized kinetic constants have a maximal value of 1. Likewise, concentrations and rates are normalized to yield dimensionless quantities. For a simple reaction

$$\mathrm{E}+\mathrm{S} \underset{k_{-1}}{\overset{k_1}{\leftrightarrows}} \mathrm{E}+\mathrm{P} \tag{9.10}$$

that can be described with mass action kinetics with the thermodynamic equilibrium constant $q = k_{eq} = k_1/k_{-1}$, the rate equation reads

$$v = E_{total} \cdot (S \cdot k_1 - P \cdot k_{-1}) = E_{total} \cdot k_{-1} \cdot (S \cdot q - P) = E_{total} \cdot k_1 \cdot \left(S - \frac{P}{q}\right). \tag{9.11}$$

It is easy to see that v is maximized for fixed values of E_{total}, S, P, and q, if k_1 and k_{-1} become maximal. This is mathematically equivalent to a minimal transition time $\tau = (k_1 + k_{-1})^{-1}$ (see Section 4.3). Note that usually only one of the two rate constants may attain its maximal value. The value of the other, submaximal constant is given by the relation to the equilibrium constant.

For a reversible reaction obeying Michaelis–Menten kinetics $v = E_{total} \cdot (Sq-P)k_{-1}k_{-2}/(Sk_1 + k_{-1} + k_2 + Pk_{-2})$ (see Eq. (2.27)) with $q = k_1k_2/(k_{-1}k_{-2})$, the optimal result depends on the value of P. For $q \geq 1$ and $P \leq 1/q$ the rate becomes maximal if k_1,k_2, and k_{-2} assume maximal values and k_{-1} is submaximal (region R_1 in Figure 9.4(a)). For $P \geq q$, we obtain submaximal values of only k_{-2} (region R_2). For $1/q < P < q$ the optimal solution is characterized by submaximal values of k_{-1} and k_{-2} with $k_{-1} = \sqrt{P/q}$ and $k_{-2} = \sqrt{1/(P \cdot q)}$ (region R_3).

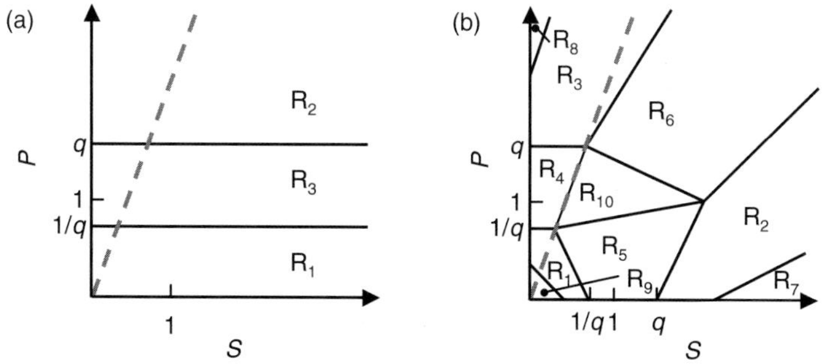

Figure 9.4 Subdivision of the plane of substrate and product concentrations (*S*, *P*) into regions of different solutions for the optimal microscopic rate constants (schematic representation). The dashed lines indicate the function $S{\cdot}q = P$. (a) Solution regions for the two-step mechanism. (b) Solution regions for the three-step mechanism.

Comparison of the optimal state with a reference state can assess the effect of the optimization. One choice for a reference state is $k_1 = k_2 = 1$ and $k_{-1} = k_{-2} = 1/\sqrt{q}$, i.e., equal distribution of the free energy difference (see Section 2.1) represented by the equilibrium constant on the first and the second step. The respective reference rate reads

$$v^{\text{ref}} = \frac{S\cdot q - P}{(S+1)\cdot q + (P+1)\cdot\sqrt{q}} \tag{9.12}$$

and the optimal rates in regions R_1, R_2, and R_3 are

$$\begin{aligned} v^{\text{opt},R_1} &= \frac{S\cdot q - P}{(S+1)\cdot q + 1 + P\cdot q}, \\ v^{\text{opt},R_2} &= \frac{S\cdot q - P}{(S+1)\cdot q + q + P}, \\ v^{\text{opt},R_3} &= \frac{S\cdot q - P}{(S+1)\cdot q + 2\sqrt{P\cdot q}}. \end{aligned} \tag{9.13}$$

For example, in the case $P = q$ and $q = 100$, the maximal rate for optimal kinetic constants is $v^{\max} = v^{\text{opt},R_3} = (S-1)/(S+3)$ and the reference rate is calculated as $v^{\text{ref}} = (S-1)/(S+11.1)$, which is lower than the maximal rate.

For the reversible three-step mechanism involving the binding of the substrate to the enzyme, the isomerization of the ES complex to an EP complex and the release of product from the enzyme,

$$\mathrm{E} + \mathrm{S} \underset{k_{-1}}{\overset{k_1}{\leftrightarrows}} \mathrm{ES} \underset{k_{-2}}{\overset{k_2}{\leftrightarrows}} \mathrm{EP} \underset{k_{-3}}{\overset{k_3}{\leftrightarrows}} \mathrm{E} + \mathrm{P} \tag{9.14}$$

the reaction rate is given as

$$v = E_{\text{total}} \cdot \frac{S\cdot k_1k_2k_3 - P\cdot k_{-1}k_{-2}k_{-3}}{k_2k_3 + k_{-1}k_3 + k_{-1}k_{-2} + S\cdot k_1(k_2 + k_3 + k_{-2}) + P\cdot k_{-3}(k_2 + k_{-1} + k_{-2})}. \tag{9.15}$$

Table 9.1 Optimal solutions for the rate constants of the three-step enzymatic reaction as functions of the concentrations of substrate and product for $q \geq 1$.

Solution	k_1	k_{-1}	k_2	k_{-2}	k_3	k_{-3}
R_1	1	$1/q$	1	1	1	1
R_2	1	1	1	$1/q$	1	1
R_3	1	1	1	1	1	$1/q$
R_4	1	$\sqrt{P/q}$	1	1	1	$\sqrt{1/Pq}$
R_5	1	$\sqrt{\frac{S+P}{q(1+P)}}$	1	$\sqrt{\frac{1+P}{q(S+P)}}$	1	1
R_6	1	1	1	$\sqrt{\frac{2P}{q(1+S)}}$	1	$\sqrt{\frac{1+S}{2Pq}}$
R_7	$\sqrt{\frac{2q(1+P)}{S}}$	1	1	$\sqrt{\frac{2(1+P)}{qS}}$	1	1
R_8	1	1	$\sqrt{\frac{2q(1+S)}{P}}$	1	1	$\sqrt{\frac{2(1+S)}{qP}}$
R_9	1	$\sqrt{\frac{2(S+P)}{q}}$	1	1	$\sqrt{2q(S+P)}$	1
R_{10}	1	a	1	$\frac{P}{qk_{-1}^2}$	1	$\frac{1}{qk_{-1}k_{-2}}$

[a] k_{-1} is solution of the equation $k_{-1}^4 + k_{-1}^3 - k_{-1}\frac{P}{q} - \frac{SP}{q} = 0$.

It turns out that the optimal solution for this mechanism depends on the values of both S and P. There are 10 different solutions, shown in Table 9.1 and Figure 9.4(b).

Among the 10 solutions, there are three solutions with a submaximal value of one backward rate constant, three solutions with submaximal values of two backward rate constants, three solutions with submaximal values of one backward and one forward rate constants, and one solution with submaximal values of all three backward rate constants. The constraint imposed by the thermodynamic equilibrium constant leads to the following effects. At very low substrate and product concentrations, a maximal rate is achieved by enhancing the binding of S and P to the enzyme (so-called high (S,P)-affinity solution). If S or P are present in very high concentrations, they should be weakly bound (low S- or P- affinity solutions). For intermediate values of S and P, only backward constants assume submaximal values. For concentrations of S and P equal to unity, the optimal solution reads

$$k_{-1} = k_{-2} = k_{-3} = q^{-1/3} \quad \text{and} \quad k_1 = k_2 = k_3 = 1. \tag{9.16}$$

This case represents an equal distribution of the drop in free energy on all three elementary steps.

9.2.2 Optimal Distribution of Enzyme Concentrations in a Metabolic Pathway

By means of regulated gene expression and protein degradation, cells can adjust the amount of enzyme allocated to the reactions of a metabolic pathway according to the current metabolic supply or demand. In many cases, the concentration of individual enzymes is regulated in such a way that the metabolic fluxes necessary to maintain cell functions are achieved while the concentration of total enzyme is maintained at a low level. A reason for keeping enzyme concentrations low is that proteins are osmotically active substances. One strategy to achieve osmotic balance is, therefore, to keep the total amount of enzyme constrained. Furthermore, enzyme synthesis is expensive for the cell, with respect to both energy and material. Therefore, it is sensible to assume that various pathways or even individual reactions compete for the available resources.

We can study theoretically how a maximal steady-state flux through a pathway is achieved with a given fixed total amount of enzyme [34]. The optimization problem is to distribute the total protein concentration $E_{\text{total}} = \sum_{i=1}^{r} E_i$ optimally among the r reactions. We will exemplify this for the simple unbranched pathway presented in Eq. (2.149). To assess the effect of optimization we will compare the optimal state to a reference state where the given total concentration of enzymes is distributed uniformly such that $E_i = E_{\text{total}}/r$.

The optimal enzyme concentrations E_i^{opt} in states of maximal steady-state flux can be determined by the variational equation

$$\frac{\partial}{\partial E_i}\left(J - \lambda\left(\sum_{j=1}^{r} E_j - E_{\text{total}}\right)\right) = 0 \quad (i = 1, \ldots, r), \tag{9.17}$$

where λ denotes the Lagrange multiplier. From this equation it follows that

$$\frac{\partial J}{\partial E_i} = \lambda \quad (i = 1, \ldots, r). \tag{9.18}$$

Equation (9.18) indicates that all nonnormalized flux response coefficients with respect to enzyme concentrations (Section 2.3) have the same value. By multiplication with E_i^{opt}/J, we find

$$\frac{E_i^{\text{opt}}}{J}\left(\frac{\partial J}{\partial E_i}\right)_{E_j = E_j^{\text{opt}}} = \frac{E_i^{\text{opt}}}{J}\lambda. \tag{9.19}$$

The left-hand term of Eq. (9.19) represents the normalized flux control coefficient (Eq. (2.114)) $(C_{v_i}^J)_{E_j = E_j^{\text{opt}}} = C_i^{\text{opt}}$ of reaction i over steady-state flux J in optimal states. Since the sum of the flux control coefficients over all reactions equals unity (summation theorem, Eq. (2.119)), it follows that

$$1 = \sum_{i=1}^{r} \frac{E_i^{\text{opt}}}{J}\lambda = \frac{E_{\text{total}}}{J}\lambda. \tag{9.20}$$

Therefore, the following equality holds:

$$C_i^{\text{opt}} = \frac{E_i^{\text{opt}}}{E_{\text{total}}}. \tag{9.21}$$

This means that the allocation of flux control coefficients in optimal states (in this case states of maximal steady-state fluxes), C_i^{opt}, is equal to the allocation of the relative enzyme concentrations along the pathway: the flux is only maximized if enzymes with higher or lower control are present in higher or lower concentration, respectively.

Example 9.1

Consider the special case that every reaction of the pathway $S_0 \overset{v_1}{\leftrightarrow} S_1 \overset{v_2}{\leftrightarrow} \cdots \overset{v_r}{\leftrightarrow} S_r$ obeys mass action kinetics, $v_i = E_i(k_i S_{i-1} - k_{-i} S_i)$ for $i = 1, \ldots r$, with the equilibrium constants $q_i = k_i/k_{-i}$. In that model, the steady-state flux reads $J = \left(S_0 \prod_{j=1}^{r} q_j - S_r\right) \cdot \left(\sum_{l=1}^{r} (E_l k_l)^{-1} \cdot \prod_{m=l}^{r} q_m\right)^{-1}$ (Eq. (2.152)). Introducing this expression into Eq. (9.18) leads to

$$E_i^{\text{opt}} = E_{\text{total}} \cdot \sqrt{Y_i} \cdot \left(\sum_{l=1}^{r} \sqrt{Y_l}\right)^{-1} \quad \text{with} \quad Y_l = \frac{1}{k_l} \prod_{m=l}^{r} q_m. \tag{9.22}$$

For the flux control coefficients (compare Eq. (2.153)) in states of maximal flux, it holds

$$C_i^{\text{opt}} = \sqrt{Y_i} \cdot \left(\sum_{l=1}^{r} \sqrt{Y_l}\right)^{-1}. \tag{9.23}$$

The effect of optimization for a chain of four consecutive reactions is discussed in Example 2.16 and shown in Figure 2.12. The larger the deviation of the value of equilibrium constant q from 1, the stronger is the effect of the optimization, i.e., the larger is the difference between maximal flux and reference flux.

The problem of maximizing the steady-state flux for a given total amount of enzyme is related to the problem of minimizing the total enzyme concentration that allows for a given steady-state flux. For an unbranched reaction pathway (Eq. (2.149)) obeying the flux equation (2.152), minimization of E_{total} results in the same optimal allocation of relative enzyme concentrations and flux control coefficients as maximization of J.

The principle of minimizing the total enzyme concentration at fixed steady-state fluxes is more general since it may be also applied to branched reaction networks. Application of the principle of maximal steady-state flux to branched networks could either lead to conflicting interests between different fluxes in different branches or the objective function must balance different fluxes by specific weights.

Special conditions hold for the flux control coefficients in states of minimal total enzyme concentration at fixed steady-state fluxes. Since the reaction rates v_i are proportional to the enzyme concentrations, i.e., $v_i = E_i \cdot f_i$, keeping fixed the steady-state fluxes $J^0 = v_i^0$ leads to the following relation between enzyme concentrations and substrate concentrations:

$$E_i = E_i(S_1, S_2, \ldots, S_{r-1}) = \frac{v_i^0}{f_i}, \tag{9.24}$$

where the function f_i expresses the kinetic part of the reaction rate that is independent of the enzyme concentration. The principle of minimal total enzyme concentration implies

$$\frac{\partial E_{\text{total}}}{\partial S_j} = \sum_{i=1}^{r} \frac{\partial E_i(S_1, \ldots, S_{r-1})}{\partial S_j} - \sum_{i=1}^{r} \frac{v_i^0}{f_i^2} \frac{\partial f_i}{\partial S_j} = 0, \tag{9.25}$$

which determines the metabolite concentrations in the optimal state. Since $f_i = v_i^0 / E_i$ it follows that

$$\sum_{i=1}^{r} \frac{E_i^{\text{opt}}}{v_i^0} \frac{\partial v_i^0}{\partial S_j} = 0 \tag{9.26}$$

and in matrix representation

$$\left(\frac{d\boldsymbol{v}}{d\boldsymbol{S}}\right)^{\mathrm{T}} (\mathrm{dg}\boldsymbol{J})^{-1} \boldsymbol{E}^{\text{opt}} = 0, \tag{9.27}$$

where $\boldsymbol{E}^{\text{opt}}$ is the vector containing the optimal enzyme concentrations. An expression for the flux control coefficients in matrix representation has been given in Eq. (2.149). Its transposed matrix reads

$$(\boldsymbol{C}^J)^{\mathrm{T}} = I - (\mathrm{dg}\boldsymbol{J})\boldsymbol{N}^{\mathrm{T}} \left(\left(\boldsymbol{N} \frac{\partial \boldsymbol{v}}{\partial \boldsymbol{S}} \right)^{-1} \right)^{\mathrm{T}} \left(\frac{\partial \boldsymbol{v}}{\partial \boldsymbol{S}} \right)^{\mathrm{T}} (\mathrm{dg}\boldsymbol{J})^{-1} \tag{9.28}$$

Postmultiplication with the vector $\boldsymbol{E}^{\text{opt}}$ and consideration of Eq. (9.27) leads to

$$(\boldsymbol{C}^J)^{\mathrm{T}} \boldsymbol{E}^{\text{opt}} = \boldsymbol{E}^{\text{opt}}. \tag{9.29}$$

This expression represents a functional relation between enzyme concentrations and flux control coefficients for enzymatic networks in states of minimal total enzyme concentration.

9.2.3
Temporal Transcription Programs

In this section, instead of considering steady-state solutions as in the previous section, we study temporal adaptation of enzyme concentrations. Consider an unbranched metabolic pathway that can be switched on or off by the cell depending on actual requirements. The product S_r of the pathway is important, but not essential for the reproduction of the cell. The faster the initial substrate S_0 can be converted into S_r the more efficiently the cell may reproduce and out-compete other individuals. If S_0 is available, then the cell produces the enzymes of the pathway to make use of the substrate. If the substrate is not available, then the cell does not synthesize the respective enzymes for economical reasons. Bacterial amino acid synthesis is organized in this way. This scenario has been studied theoretically [35] by starting with a resting pathway, i.e., although the genes for the enzymes are present, they are not expressed due to lack of the substrate. Suddenly S_0 appears in the environment (e.g. after a change in avaiable nutrients or the cell's specific location). How can the cell make use of S_0 as soon as possible and convert it into S_r?

The system of ODEs describing the dynamics of the pathway reads

$$\begin{aligned}\frac{dS_0}{dt} &= -k_1 \cdot E_1 \cdot S_0. \\ \frac{dS_i}{dt} &= k_i \cdot E_i \cdot S_{i-1} - k_{i+1} \cdot E_{i+1} \cdot S_i \quad (i = 1, \ldots, r-1) \\ \frac{dS_r}{dt} &= k_r \cdot E_r \cdot S_{r-1}.\end{aligned} \tag{9.30}$$

For sake of simplicity, we first assume that the cell can produce the enzymes instantaneously when necessary (neglecting the time necessary for transcription and translation), but that the total amount of enzyme is limited due to the limited capacity of the cell to produce and store proteins. The time necessary to produce S_r from S_0 is measured by the transition time

$$\tau = \frac{1}{S_0(0)} \int_{t=0}^{\infty} (S_0(0) - S_r(t))\mathrm{d}t. \tag{9.31}$$

The optimization problem to be solved is to find a temporal profile of enzyme concentrations that minimizes the transition time ($\tau = \min$) at a fixed value of $E_{\text{total}} = \sum_{i=1}^{r} E_i(t) = \text{const.}$

Example 9.2

For a pathway consisting of only $r = 2$ reactions with $k_i = k (i = 1, \ldots, r)$, there is an explicit solution of the above stated problem [35]. The optimal enzyme profile consists of two phases and an abrupt switch at time T_1. In the first interval $0 \le t \le T_1$, only the first enzyme is present. In the second interval $T_1 < t < \infty$ both enzymes are present with constant concentrations. The switching time is $T_1 = \ln(2/(3-\sqrt{5}))$. In the first interval holds $E_1 = E_{\text{total}}$, $E_2 = 0$, and in the second interval holds $E_1 = E_{\text{total}} \cdot (3-\sqrt{5})/2$, $E_2 = E_{\text{total}} \cdot (\sqrt{5}-1)/2$. Note, for curiosity, that in this case the ratio E_2/E_1 equals the Golden Ratio (i.e., $(1+\sqrt{5})/2 : 1$). The minimal transition time for these optimal concentrations is $\tau^{\min} = 1 + T_1 + (1-e^{-T_1})^{-1} \cong 3.58$ in units of $(k \cdot E_{\text{total}})^{-1}$. This means that in the first phase all available enzymes are used to catabolize the initial substrate; product is made only in the second phase. The fastest possible conversion of S_0 to S_2 employs a delayed onset in the formation of S_2 that favors an accelerated decay of S_0 in the initial phase and pays off in the second phase. The temporal profiles of enzyme and metabolite concentrations are shown in Figure 9.5.

To solve the above optimization problem for pathways with r enzymes, we assume the time axis to be divided into m intervals in which the enzyme concentrations are

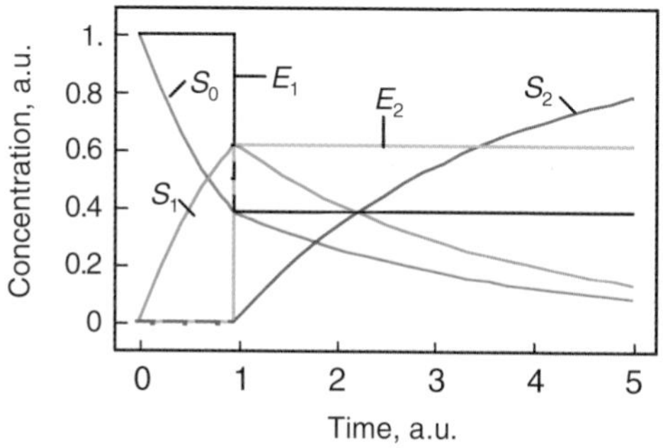

Figure 9.5 Optimal enzyme and metabolite concentration time profiles for a linear metabolic pathway as explained in Example 9.2. Parameters: $S_0(0) = 1$, $S_1(0) = S_2(0) = 0$, $E_{total} = 1$, $k = 1$.

constant. The quantities to be optimized are the switching times $T_1, T_2, \ldots$ defining the time intervals and the enzyme concentrations during these intervals. In the reference case with only one interval ($m = 0$ switches), the optimal enzyme concentrations are all equal $E_i = E_{total}/r\ (i = 1, \ldots, r)$. The optimal transition time for this case reads $\tau = r^2$ in units of $(k \cdot E_{total})^{-1}$. Permitting one switch ($m = 1$) between intervals of constant enzyme concentrations allows for a considerably lower transition time. An increasing number of possible switches ($m > 1$) leads to a decrease in the transition time until the number of switches reaches $m = r - 1$. The corresponding optimal enzyme profiles have the following characteristics: within any time interval, except for the last one, only a single enzyme is fully active whereas all others are shut off. At the beginning of the process, the whole amount of available protein is allocated exclusively to the first enzyme of the chain. Each of the following switches turns off the active enzyme and allocates the total amount of protein to the enzyme that catalyzes the following reaction. The last switch allocates finite fractions of the protein amount to all enzymes with increasing amounts from the first one to the last one (Figure 9.6).

If one compares the case of no switch (the reference case) with the case of $m = r - 1$ switches, the drop in transition time (gain in turnover speed) amplifies with increasing length r of the reaction chain.

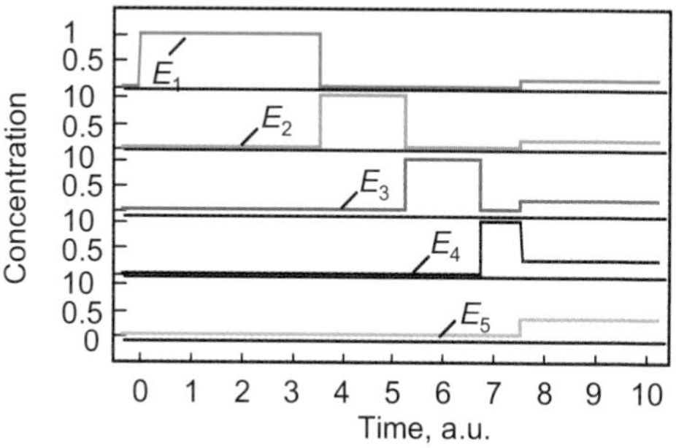

Figure 9.6 Optimal temporal enzyme profiles yielding the minimal transition time for a pathway of five reactions. The switching times are $T_1 = 3.08$, $T_2 = 5.28$, $T_3 = 6.77$, and $T_4 = 7.58$.

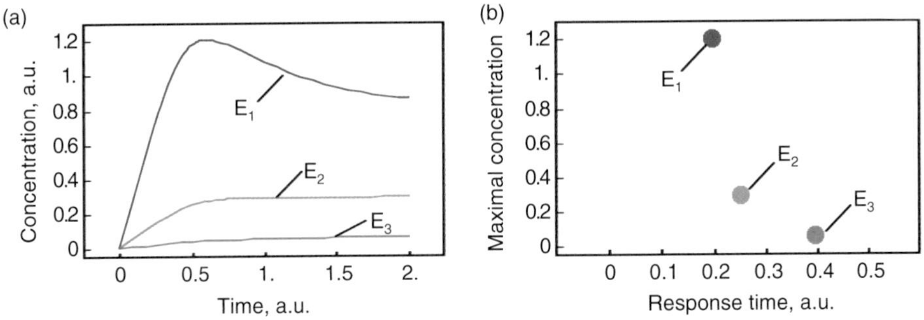

Figure 9.7 Simulation of Eq. (9.32) with $V_{max,i} = K_{m,i} = \alpha = 1$, $\beta_0 = 5$, ($\beta_1 = 3.4$, ($\beta_2 = 0.67$, ($\beta_3 = 0.1$ and $k_0 = 0.1$, $k_1 = 0.23$, $k_2 = 0.68$, $k_3 = 2.1$, $K_R = 0.0001$. (a) Time course of enzyme concentrations, (b) maximal response of enzymes versus response time, i.e., time, when enzyme concentration is half-maximal.

If we impose a weaker condition for the conversion of substrate S_0 into product S_r by demanding only conversion of 90% instead of 100%, then the optimal solution looks as follows: enzymes E_1 to E_{r-1} are switched on and off successively in the same way as in the case of 100% conversion except for the last interval, where enzyme E_r is fully activated, but none of the other enzymes. The transition time is considerably reduced compared to the strict case. In conclusion, abandonment of perfection (here demanding 90% metabolite conversion instead of 100%) may lead to incomplete, but faster metabolite conversion.

The simple example of a metabolic pathway shows that temporal adjustment of enzyme activities, for instance by regulation of gene expression, may lead to a considerable improvement of metabolic efficiency. As detailed in Example 9.3, bacterial amino acid production pathways are possibly regulated in the described manner.

Example 9.3

Zaslaver and colleagues investigated experimentally amino-acid biosynthesis systems of *Escherichia coli*. They identified the temporal expression pattern and showed a hierarchy of expression that matches the enzyme order in the unbranched pathways [36]. They included the time requirements and the costs for enzyme production in their model. For a system of three enzymes, the set of equations governing the temporal response to changes in metabolite availability is [36]

$$\begin{aligned}
\frac{dS_i}{dt} &= \frac{V_{max,i} \cdot E_i \cdot S_{i-1}}{K_{m,i} + S_{i-1}} - \frac{V_{max,i+1} \cdot E_{i+1} \cdot S_i}{K_{m,i+1} + S_i} - \alpha \cdot S_i, \quad i = 1, \ldots, 3 \\
\frac{dE_i}{dt} &= \frac{\beta_i \cdot k_i}{k_i + R(t)} - \alpha \cdot E_i, \quad i = 1, \ldots, 3 \\
\frac{dR_T}{dt} &= \frac{\beta_0 \cdot k_0}{k_0 + R(t)} - \alpha \cdot R_T \quad \text{with} \quad R(t) = \frac{R_T \cdot P(t)}{K_R + P(t)}
\end{aligned} \tag{9.32}$$

$$C = a \cdot \sum_i \int_0^T \frac{\beta_i \cdot k_i}{k_i + R(t)} dt + \int_0^T |F - F_{goal}| dt \quad \text{with} \quad F = \frac{V_{max,3} \cdot E_3 \cdot S_2}{K_{m,3} + S_2}, \tag{9.33}$$

where S_i and E_i are the concentrations of metabolites and enzymes, respectively, $V_{max,i}$ are the maximal rates, and $K_{m,i}$ are the Michaelis constants. The parameters β_i denote maximal promoter activity of gene i, and k_i are the repression coefficients, i.e., the concentration of repressor needed for 50% repression of gene i. R_T is the total repressor concentration, K_R is the dissociation constant, and $R(t)$ the active repressor level. The cost function (9.33) is composed of two terms: the cost to produce the enzymes and the rate and precision at which F approaches its goal F_{goal}. a is a weight factor and T the typical time scale of the activation of the system.

Minimization of the cost function by optimizing β_i, k_i, and K_R results in solutions with $\beta_1 > \beta_2 > \beta_3$, representing a hierarchy in the maximal promoter activity, and $k_1 > k_2 > k_3$, representing feedback strength by the repressor that is stronger the earlier the enzyme in the pathway. The time courses of the enzymes are shown in Figure 9.7.

Note that in Example 9.2 enzyme profiles have been optimized without asking how these profiles can be ensured by the cellular machinery, while in Example 9.3 the parameters of a model for the enzyme production machinery were optimized.

9.3 Evolutionary Game Theory

Summary

Simple optimality studies do not account for phenomena like competition, symbiosis, and coevolution, which involve direct and indirect interactions between individuals. Basic mechanisms of evolution can be studied by modeling the dynamics of competing subpopulations. Evolutionary game theory can explain some seemingly paradoxical findings, for instance, the fact that inefficient, selfish phenotypes can outperform more efficient, cooperative phenotypes. Nevertheless, the advantages of selfishness can be overcome by mechanisms like kin selection, which promote cooperative behavior.

Evolutionary theory suggests that mutation and selection increase the average fitness of a population and optimize the shape and behavior of organisms, given the options and restrictions of a prevailing environment. However, the optimality assumption is not always justified: genes can spread and be fixed in a population even if they do not provide a fitness advantage – a phenomenon called neutral evolution. Nonoptimal traits may also arise as by-products of other traits that are under selective pressure. But there is another caveat in the optimality assumption: by its very presence, a species can influence its own fitness landscape; paradoxically, an optimization within such a "flexible" fitness landscape may lead to an overall fitness decrease.

Let us illustrate this by an example: natural selection favors trees that grow higher and receive more light than their neighbors [37, 38]. As a consequence, the selection pressure on height becomes even stronger and trees will allocate more and more of their resources to growth, forcing other trees to do the same. Eventually, they reach a limit where growing taller would consume more resources than it generates – but the tree population as a whole does not receive more light than in the beginning. To model such phenomena, we cannot rely on simple optimization models, but we need to describe how the optimization of individuals feeds back on themselves via their own environment.

Important aspects of evolution can be understood from population dynamics models (see the web supplement). Figure 9.8 shows a simple scheme of natural selection: individuals produce offspring, but only some of the children reach an age at which they also have offspring. In a simple stochastic model, each individual has a fixed number of children: in a selection step, n children from the population are chosen at random to form the next generation. In the scenario of neutral evolution, each individual has the same number of children and the relative subpopulation sizes (blue and red in Figure 9.8) will drift randomly. Any new mutant has a fixation probability (probability to spread in the entire population) of $1/n$, where n is the population size. If subpopulations have different reproduction rates, a subpopulation that produces more offspring is more likely to outcompete the others.

To model interactions between individuals, we shall assume that the reproduction rates are not fixed, but depend on the subpopulation sizes. In a common scenario of evolutionary game theory, survival and reproduction of individuals depend on pairwise random encounters between individuals. The fitness of genotypes therefore depends on the probability to meet other genotypes or, in other words, on their frequencies, i.e., relative subpopulation sizes.

In this setting, a mutant that exploits wild-type individuals may lose its advantage when it becomes abundant. An example are "selfish" virus mutants that have lost the capability of producing certain proteins themselves and use proteins produced by the wild-type viruses instead [39]. By reducing their genome size, the mutants reach a higher fitness, but they depend on the presence of wild-type viruses: as the mutants

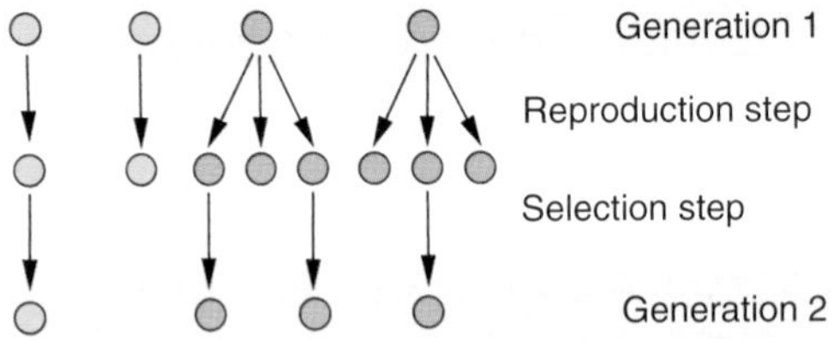

Figure 9.8 Simplified scheme of reproduction and selection. A population consists of two types (blue and red), which differ in their numbers of offspring. Generation 1 consists of two blue and two red individuals. Some of them grow up and have offspring (of the same type), which form the next generation. In a stochastic model, the number of children depends on the type of individual, and new adults are picked randomly from the previous generation of children, such that the total population size is preserved. For large population sizes, this scheme is approximated by the deterministic replicator equation Eq. (9.38).

spread in the population, their fitness decreases. On the other hand, if a mutant requires a “critical mass” of individuals to become successful, it may not emerge at all. Therefore, certain evolutionary steps (e.g., the emergence of L-amino acids as building blocks of proteins) could hardly be reverted even if a change were beneficial (“once forever selection”). Finally, different species can mutually influence their evolution: pathogens, for instance, evoke the evolution of immune responses, which in turn exerts a selection pressure on adapted pathogen strains.

9.3.1 Game Theory

Game theory [40] studies rational decisions in strategic games. In a two- player game, each of the players can choose between several strategies. Depending on their choices, each player receives a certain payoff, and they both try to maximize their own return. The payoffs are defined by a *payoff matrix* $\boldsymbol{F}$: in a game with two strategies A and B, the payoffs for the first player read

$$\begin{array}{c|cc} & 2:A & 2:B \\ \hline 1:A & f_{AA} & f_{BB} \\ 1:B & f_{BA} & f_{BB} \end{array} . \tag{9.34}$$

The rows correspond to the first player's choice, the columns to the choice of his coplayer. If a game is symmetric (as we assume here), the payoffs for the second player are given by the transposed matrix. In the following, we assume that the game is played only once, neglecting the possibility that players can respond to the coplayer's behavior in previous rounds.

9.3.1.1 Hawk–Dove Game and Prisoner's Dilemma

Figure 9.9 shows two well-studied games called *hawk–dove game* [41] (or “snow drift game”) and *prisoner's dilemma*. In both the games, a cooperative strategy is confronted by an aggressive strategy. If both players act aggressively, both of them will lose. The payoff matrix of the *hawk–dove game* has the following form:

$$\begin{array}{c|cc} & 2:\text{dove} & 2:\text{hawk} \\ \hline 1:\text{dove} & v/2 & 0 \\ 1:\text{hawk} & v & (v-c)/2 \end{array} . \tag{9.35}$$

with positive parameters v and c. The matrix $\boldsymbol{F}$ contains the payoffs for player 1 (left player in Figure 9.9); as the game is symmetric, the payoff matrix for player 2 is the transposed matrix $\boldsymbol{F}^{\mathrm{T}}$.

The elements of matrix (9.35) can be interpreted as expected payoffs that would arise from the following scenario: players compete for a common resource (for instance food) and can choose between two strategies termed “hawk” and “dove.” A hawk initiates aggressive behavior and continues until he either wins the conflict or loses and gets seriously injured, while a dove immediately retreats if the other player is aggressive. Figure 9.9 illustrates the four possible types of encounter and the

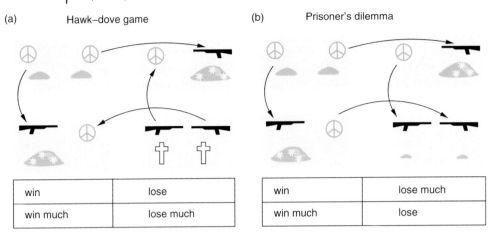

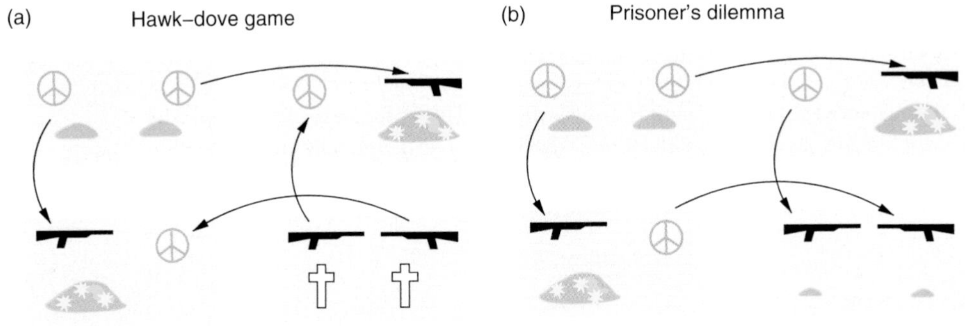

win	lose
win much	lose much

win	lose much
win much	lose

Figure 9.9 Hawk–dove game (a) and prisoner's dilemma (b). The pictures illustrate all possible choices by the two players (peaceful or aggressive behaviour) and the possible payoffs (different amounts of riches, or death). If the opponent's choice is known, players may increase their payoff by a change of strategy (arrows). If none of the players can further increase their payoff, a stable situation – a so-called Nash equilibrium – is reached. Tables on bottom: qualitative payoffs for player 1 (shown left in the pictures).

resulting payoffs: if two doves meet, the resource is shared equally and each player obtains $v/2$ as payoff. If a hawk meets a dove, the hawk obtains the full resource v and the dove gets nothing. If a hawk meets another hawk, he wins (payoff v) or becomes injured (cost c) with equal probabilities, so the expected payoff in this encounter (the element in the payoff matrix) is $(v - c)/2$. In the hawk–dove game, it is assumed that the cost of injury c exceeds the value of the resource v. The prisoner's dilemma has a similar structure as the hawk–dove game: the two strategies "cooperate" and "defect" correspond to "dove" and "hawk," respectively, and we consider the same payoff matrix (9.35). This time, however, we assume that $c < v$, so the best response to a known defector is to defect as well.

9.3.1.2 Best Choices and Nash Equilibrium

The payoff matrices directly imply a best choice of strategy if the opponent's strategy is known. In the hawk–dove game, if the coplayer plays "dove," it is advantageous to choose "hawk" to obtain the full resource. On the other hand, if the coplayer plays "hawk," it is better to avoid the possible injury and to choose "dove." Hence in this game, a player should always respond with the opposite strategy. In the prisoner's dilemma, on the other hand, it is always best to defect, no matter which strategy the coplayer will choose. Importantly, this logic need not hold if games are played repeatedly and the coplayer's choice is not known.

A situation in which neither of the players can improve his payoff by a unilateral change of strategy is called a *Nash equilibrium*. The Nash equilibria for the above games are (1: hawk/2: dove) or (1: dove/2: hawk) for the hawk–dove game and

(1: defect/2: defect) for the prisoner's dilemma. Once a Nash equilibrium has been reached, no player has a reason to deviate from his strategy – even if another state (e.g., 1: cooperate/2: cooperate) would provide a higher payoff for both players. This leads to a paradoxical situation. In the prisoner's dilemma, the players become trapped in the unfavorable "selfish" state in which they both obtain less payoff than if they cooperated. The reason is that all states besides the Nash equilibrium (including the favorable "cooperative" state) are prone to a change of strategies.

9.3.2 Evolutionary Game Theory

Initially, game theory was invented to describe rational decisions based on logical reasoning and the intention to maximize one's own profit. But it can also explain the success of traits that evolve by mutation and selection and do not involve conscious decisions. Evolutionary game theory [42] describes the evolution of biological traits in population models, assuming that evolutionary fitness depends on the success in a hypothetical game. In a common scenario, individuals encounter each other randomly. Different genotypes correspond to different strategies, and the obtained payoffs determine how fast a genotype can replicate. Based on a two-player game, we can define frequency-dependent fitness values for all strategies: assume two subpopulations playing the strategies A and B with respective frequencies x_A and x_B satisfying $x_A + x_B = 1$. With a payoff matrix $\mathbf{F}$, an individual of type A will obtain an expected payoff

$$f_A = f_{AA} x_A + f_{AB} x_B. \qquad (9.36)$$

In a direct competition, successful strategies will replicate fast and start to spread in the population. However, this will change the frequency of strategies, which may have a feedback effect on their fitness. As a successful strategy spreads, its own higher frequency may impair its further success.

In evolutionary game theory, the rational choice of a strategy (that was originally implied in game theory) is replaced by the fact that this strategy has been successful in an evolutionary process. Presumably, a strategy will only survive if it can successfully confront itself and all other prevalent strategies. We will now study such phenomena by using dynamic models.

9.3.3 Replicator Equation for Population Dynamics

Population dynamics can be described by various mathematical frameworks, including deterministic and stochastic approaches and models with spatial structure (like partial differential equations or cellular automata, see Section 3.4.1). In the following sections, we will employ the *deterministic replicator equation*, a rate equation for the relative sizes of subpopulations in a well-mixed population.

9.3.3.1 The Replicator Equation

In a simple model, the reproduction rate of a subpopulation is computed from a baseline rate plus the average payoff from pairwise random encounters between individuals. The probability to meet members of different subpopulations is given by their frequencies $x_1, x_2, \ldots$, which sum up to 1. When an individual of type i meets an individual of type j, it obtains a payoff f_{ij}. Such an encounter happens with probability x_j, so the average payoff of strategy i is

$$f_i(\mathbf{x}) = \sum_j f_{ij}\, x_j. \tag{9.37}$$

In a simple deterministic model, the frequencies x_i evolve in time according to the replicator equation

$$\frac{dx_i}{dt} = x_i(f_i(\mathbf{x}) - \langle f \rangle). \tag{9.38}$$

The term $\langle f \rangle = \Sigma_i\, x_j\, f_j(\mathbf{x})$ denotes the time-dependent mean fitness of the entire population. Within the model, it ensures that the frequencies remain normalized, that is $\Sigma_i x_i = 1$, and that the baseline fitness value cancels out in Eq. (9.38).

A competition between two subpopulations A and B can have different qualitative outcomes, including sustained oscillations (see Section 9.3.5) and convergence to a fixed point. According to Eq. (9.38), a subpopulation frequency x_i remains constant if

$$0 = x_i\,(f_i(\mathbf{x}) - \langle f \rangle), \tag{9.39}$$

i.e., either the strategy has died out ($x_i = 0$), or its fitness $f_i = f$ equals exactly the average fitness of the entire population. Thus in a fixed point of Eq. (9.38), all surviving subpopulations have the same fitness – again, given the frequencies of all subpopulations.

9.3.3.2 Outcomes of Frequency-Dependent Selection

The number and kind of fixed points depend on the payoff matrix and we can distinguish between different cases: (i) A *dominant* strategy always wins: it is a best reply to itself and to the other strategy (e.g., "defect" in the prisoner's dilemma) and its frequency approaches $x_i = 1$. (ii) Coexistence: if both strategies are best replies to each other, they can coexist in stable proportions (like in the hawk–dove game). (iii) Bistability: if each strategy is a best response to itself, it would take many individuals of the other strategy to undermine it. In the bistable case, one of the strategies eventually wins in the replicator dynamics ($x_i \rightarrow 1$) and the winner depends on their initial frequencies. A strategy A is called *risk-dominant* if it has the larger basin of attraction ($f_{AA} + f_{AB} > f_{BA} + f_{BB}$). Such a strategy will succeed if both strategies start at equal subpopulation frequencies. (iv) Neutrality: both strategies have the same expected payoff for any values of the subpopulation frequencies,

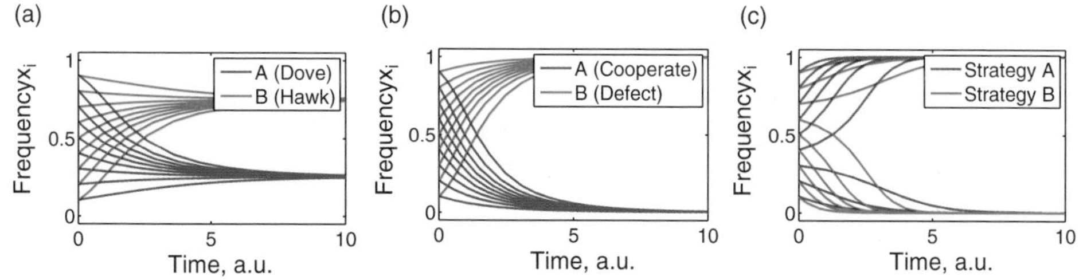

Figure 9.10 Population dynamics according to the replicator equation (9.38). Two populations playing different strategies are represented by their time-dependent frequencies (normalized population sizes x_i). The curves show simulation results with different initial frequencies. (a) The hawk–dove game leads to coexistence of individual strategies. (b) In the prisoner's dilemma, the strategy "defect" dominates "cooperate." (c) Bistability with two evolutionary stable strategies: the winner depends on the initial frequencies of the two populations.

so they are effectively identical. According to Eq. (9.38), the frequencies will remain constant in time, and in a stochastic population model, the sizes of both subpopulations would drift randomly.

Figure 9.10 shows simulations for a payoff matrix of the form (9.35) with values $v=3, c=4$ ((a), hawk–dove-game) and $v=4, c=3$ ((b), prisoner's dilemma). For each type of game, curves with different initial frequencies between 0.1 and 0.9 are shown. The hawk–dove game leads to coexistence at a frequency $x_2=c/v=3/4$ of hawks, while in the prisoner's dilemma, the cooperative strategy always dies out. In a third game (Figure 9.10(c)) with an identity payoff matrix $\boldsymbol{F}=\boldsymbol{I}$, each strategy is a best response to itself. The resulting dynamics is bistable, so different initial conditions can lead to success of either A or B.

9.3.4 Evolutionary Stable Strategies

One of the basic questions in evolutionary game theory is whether a population can be invaded by a mutant that plays a different strategy. If the resident strategy dominates all possible mutant strategies, it will outcompete the mutants under all circumstances and is called *unbeatable*. However, also other strategies can persist in evolution. The – slightly weaker – concept of *evolutionary stable strategies* (ESS) implies that the mutant initially appears in small numbers. A strategy A is evolutionary stable if a competing strategy B, starting at a very low frequency, cannot invade A. There are two cases in which A is evolutionary stable: either A dominates B, or A and B form a bistable pair and the mutant subpopulation does not manage to reach the necessary size to take over the population.

How can we tell if a strategy is evolutionary stable? Assume that A is the strategy of the resident population, while B is a new mutant strategy. With the relative frequencies x_A and x_B, the average payoffs for individuals of type A and B read, respectively,

$$\begin{aligned} f_A &= f_{AA}x_A + f_{AB}x_B \\ f_B &= f_{BA}x_A + f_{BB}x_B \end{aligned} . \tag{9.40}$$

By definition, A is evolutionary stable if it cannot be invaded by a few individuals of type B: mathematically, $f_A > f_B$ has to hold for small frequencies x_B. If x_B is very small, then an individual (of type A or B) will almost never encounter an individual of type B. Therefore, we can disregard the second terms in (9.40) and obtain the simple condition $f_{AA} > f_{BA}$. In the case of equality ($f_{AA} = f_{BA}$), however, the rare encounters with B individuals play a role, so we have to require in addition that $f_{AB} > f_{BB}$. To summarize, an evolutionary stable strategy A must perform better than B in encounters with type A individuals or, if it performs equally well, it must at least perform better in encounters with type B individuals.

Example 9.4: Evolutionary stable strategy in the prisoner's dilemma

With this criterion, we can determine evolutionary stable strategies in the prisoner's dilemma: "cooperate" is not evolutionary stable because this would require that $f_{AA} = v/2$ is larger or equal to $f_{BA} = v$, which is obviously not the case. Defection is evolutionary stable if $f_{BB} \geq f_{AB}$, or $(v - c)/2 \geq 0$, i.e., if the cost of an injury is smaller than the gain of the resource – as it is assumed in the prisoner's dilemma. Therefore, a small number of defectors can successfully invade a population of cooperators, while a small number of cooperators cannot invade an existing defector population.

9.3.5
Dynamical Behavior in the Rock-Scissors-Paper Game

Frequency-dependent selection need not always lead to stationary states, but can also evoke sustained dynamic behavior [43], like in the following example. The rock-scissors-paper game consists of the three strategies rock (A), paper (B), scissors (C), which beat each other in a circle (Figure 9.11(a)): A dominates C, B dominates A, and C dominates B. This game can describe an arms race between three strains of *E. coli* bacteria [44]. A strain K ("killer") produces the toxin colicin against other bacteria together with an immunity protein to protect itself, strain I ("immune") produces the same immunity protein, but not the toxin, and strain S ("sensitive") produces neither of them. In pairwise competitions, K kills S with its toxin, I outcompetes K because it avoids the effort of toxin production and saves resources for growth, and S outcompetes I because it does not have to produce the immunity protein.

In a direct competition between the three strategies, each strategy can invade the previous one, so the population sizes will oscillate. Figure 9.11(b) shows the dynamic behavior resulting from two different payoff matrices

$$F = \begin{pmatrix} 0 & -1 & 1 \\ 1 & 0 & -1 \\ -1 & 1 & 0 \end{pmatrix}, \quad F = \begin{pmatrix} 0 & -1 & 2 \\ 2 & 0 & -1 \\ -1 & 2 & 0 \end{pmatrix}, \tag{9.41}$$

which lead, respectively, to sustained and damped oscillations. Such ongoing arms races with several toxins have been proposed [45] as an explanation for the

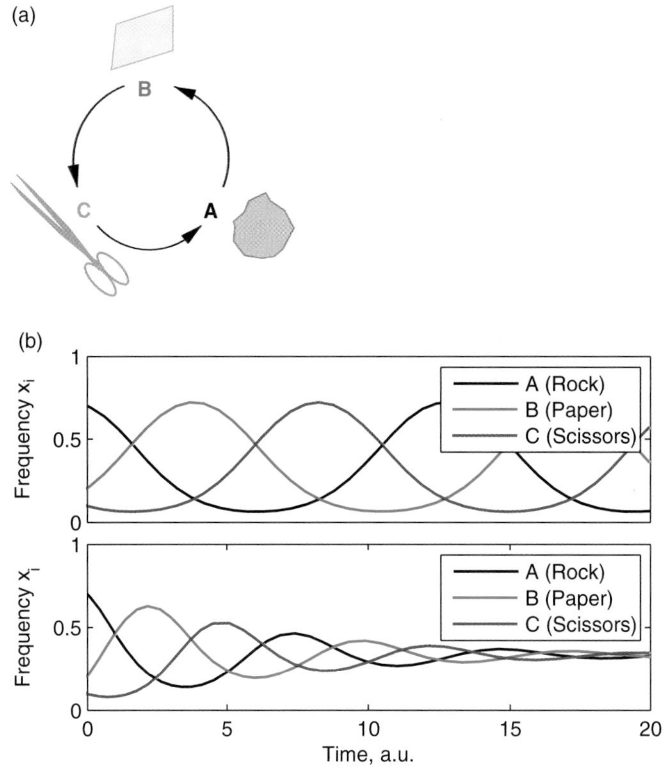

Figure 9.11 Population dynamics in the rock-scissors-paper game. (a) Each of the strategies (A: rock; B: paper; C: scissors) beats the previous one in a circle (arrowheads point to the winning strategy). (b) Simulation results from the replicator equation. The population frequencies in this game vary periodically. The subpopulations may either continue to replace each other in a periodic manner or converge to a stable mixture.

huge diversity found in microbial communities. At first sight, this diversity would contradict the *competitive exclusion principle,* which states that the number of surviving species equals the number of limited resources in a fixed environment ("*paradox of the plankton*").

9.3.6
Evolution of Cooperative Behavior

Many behavioral traits among people, animals, and even microbes can be described as forms of cooperation. From an abstract perspective, cooperation can be defined as follows: a *cooperator* C pays a cost c for another individual to receive a benefit $b > c$. A *defector* D, in contrast, does not deal out benefits and has no costs, but he can still profit from the cooperators. The corresponding payoff matrix

	2 cooperates	2 defects
1 cooperates	$f_{CC} = b - c$	$f_{CD} = -c$
1 defects	$f_{DC} = b$	$f_{DD} = 0$

(9.42)

shows that defectors will dominate cooperators because $f_{DC} > f_{CC}$ and $f_{DD} > f_{CD}$. Cooperation is not evolutionary stable in this scenario because $f_{DC} \leq f_{CC}$ is never satisfied. From this simple game, one may expect that evolution always selects for noncooperative, "selfish" traits. But obviously cooperation has evolved and evolutionary theory should thus be able to explain this fact.

9.3.6.1 Kin Selection

Altruism toward one's own genetic relatives can evolve by a mechanism called *kin selection*. For the survival of a single gene, it does not matter whether this gene is reproduced via its "host" individual or via another individual that shares the same gene. This second possibility improves chances for proliferation and leads to a selection for genes that promote altruistic behavior toward individuals that carry the same gene. If two individuals X and Y are relatives, there is a certain chance r that an arbitrarily chosen gene of X is also shared by Y. This so-called *coefficient of relatedness* has a value of $r = 1/2$ for siblings and $r = 1/8$ for cousins. Altruism toward relatives can help to reproduce some shared genes: effectively, the payoff (as seen from the perspective of a single gene) is increased by the amount of the coplayer's payoff (given by the transposed payoff matrix), multiplied by r. According to the modified payoff matrix

	2 cooperates	2 defects
1 cooperates	$(b-c)(1+r)$	$br-c$
1 defects	$b-rc$	0

(9.43)

kin selection will take place if $f_{CC} > f_{CD}$, hence $r > c/b$. This criterion is also called *Hamilton's rule*. Cooperation with relatives – and therefore kin selection – requires *kin recognition*: the plant *Cakile edentula*, for instance, grows stronger roots when it shares a pot with other plants, thus competing with them for light and nutrients. However, weaker roots are grown when groups of siblings share the same pot [46]. This finding suggests two things: that competition is weaker among siblings and that these plants recognize each other – possibly, by sensing chemicals via their roots.

9.3.6.2 Other Scenarios for Evolution of Cooperation

Cooperation can also emerge in a variety of other scenarios [47]. In spatially structured models, cooperators are less prone to exploitation by defectors if they form localized clusters. Cooperation can also emerge if individuals recompense other individuals for earlier cooperative behavior: different cooperation scenarios presuppose that individuals can remember earlier encounters (direct reciprocity), know the reputation of other individuals (indirect reciprocity), or interact locally with neighbors in a network (network reciprocity). Cooperative behavior can also evolve by a mechanism called *group selection*, which involves two levels of competition: individuals compete within groups, and groups compete with each other. In one scenario, selfish behavior within the group may be selected against because it can lead to extinction of the entire group – and therefore, of the selfish individual itself [47] (for details, see web supplement).

9.3.7 Yield and Efficiency in Metabolism

Going beyond the assumptions of the optimality approach, evolutionary game theory is highly relevant to systems biology [48]. Optimality studies suggest, for instance, that metabolic systems may maximize the speed of product formation (flux per time) or the efficiency (product yield per substrate molecule), depending on the situation [5]. Pfeiffer *et al.* [49] have added another twist to this question by relating the two strategies – maximal flux versus maximal yield – to a game-theoretical dilemma called the "tragedy of the commons."

9.3.7.1 Trade-off Between Fast and Efficient Energy Metabolism

Most cells obtain their energy from oxidation of carbohydrates, either by fermentation (without need for oxygen) or by respiration (with use of oxygen). Fermentation by glycolysis is a rather inefficient process – only two ATP molecules are produced per glucose molecule – but because of this low yield, a large amount of Gibbs free energy is released between substrates and products, and this energy difference can drive a large reaction flux. Respiration by TCA cycle and oxidative phosphorylation can be much more efficient, producing up to 36 molecules of ATP. As a consequence, only little Gibbs free energy is left for driving the reactions, and the reaction flux is slower. Altogether, the total rate of ATP production (that is, the number of molecules produced per time) is lower in respiration than in fermentation.

In an evolutionary sense, cells have the choice between two strategies: respiration leads to slow growth, but it saves glucose for later times or for other cells. Fermentation wastes sugar resources, but allows the fermenting cell to grow fast at least for a while. The competition between selfish and cooperative individuals for a shared resource leads to a game-theoretical dilemma called "tragedy of the commons." If respirators and fermentors grow separately on a constant sugar supply, the respirators will grow to a higher cell density than the fermentors, so their fitness as a population is higher. However, in a direct competition for sugar, respirers are outperformed by the fermentors, so a population of respiring cells may be invaded by fermenting mutants. In the terminology of game theory, only fermentation is evolutionarily stable.

9.3.7.2 Multicellularity Enables Cells to Profit from Respiration

Nevertheless, respiration has evolved. Unicellular organisms, which compete for external resources, tend to use fermentation, while cells in higher animals tend to use respiration, with cancer cells as an exception (Warburg effect). In a multicellular organism, ingested nutrients are shared among all cells, so there is no competition for food; the well-being of the organisms requires cooperative behavior. Pfeiffer *et al.* [49] suggested that competition between fermenting and respiring cells once triggered the evolution toward multicellularity, which appeared independently at least ten times in the tree of life [49]. In their scenario, respiration arose as a new, efficient energy source as oxygen accumulated in the atmosphere as a waste product of photosynthesis. However, single respiring cells could not turn this into a fitness advantage because they were exploited by the surrounding fermentors. By forming cell aggregates, respirators could evade this competition and profit from this new, more efficient way to use energy.

Exercises and Problems

1. Consider the branch point in Figure 9.2(a), with reactions $A \rightarrow X$, $B \rightarrow X$, $X \rightarrow C$. The concentrations of A, B, and C are fixed and the reactions are irreversible. (a) Assume upper bounds $v_1 \leq 1$, $v_2 \leq 2$ and the fitness function $f(\mathbf{v}) = v_3$. Write down the corresponding linear programming problem and compute the resulting flux distribution. (b) Assume, in addition, an upper bound $v_3 \leq 1$. Draw the allowed region in flux space and determine the optimal flux distribution.

2. (a) Show that a circular conversion flux $A \rightarrow B \rightarrow C \rightarrow A$ is thermodynamically unfeasible. (b) Consider the following reaction scheme

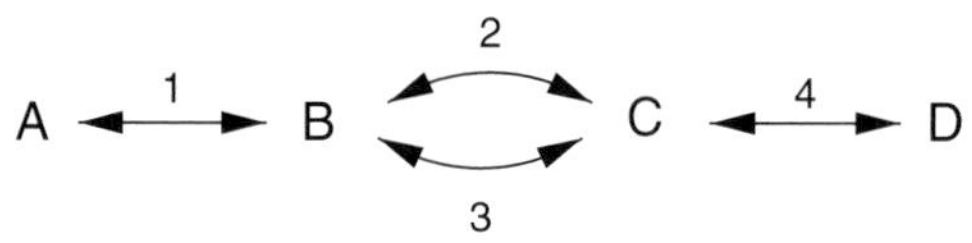

with fixed concentrations of A and B and balanced metabolites C and D. Determine all flux distributions that are both stationary and thermodynamically feasible.

3. Glycolysis from glucose to lactate effectively converts two ADP molecules into two ATP molecules.

   a. Is this process thermodynamically feasible? Assume a decrease of Gibbs free energy by 205 kJ mol^{-1} for the conversion of glucose into two lactate molecules and an increase of 49 kJ mol^{-1} for each ADP molecule converted to ATP.
   b. Imagine alternative versions of glycolysis that convert glucose into lactate and produce other numbers of ATP molecules. What are the minimal and maximal numbers possible?
   c. Assume, for simplicity, that the glycolytic flux is proportional to the total decrease of Gibbs free energy. Which number of ATP molecules produced would lead to (i) a maximal rate of ATP production and (ii) maximal efficiency, i.e., maximal ATP production per amount of glucose consumed?

4. Calculate the steady-state flux for an unbranched metabolic pathway with four reactions. Use formula (2.15). Use the parameter and concentration values $P_0 = P_r = 1$, $E_1 = E_2 = E_3 = E_4 = 1$, $q_1 = q_2 = q_3 = q_4 = 5$, $k_1 = k_2 = k_3 = k_4 = 1$.

5. Determine the maximal steady-state flux for the case that the enzyme concentrations may vary in the range from 0 to 2. Compare with the steady-state flux for the case that all enzyme concentrations are equal to 2.

6. Repeat Exercise 5 by applying the conditions (i) that the sum of enzyme concentrations is 8 and (ii) all individual enzyme concentrations are positive.

7. Calculate optimal enzyme concentrations according to formula (9.22) and the resulting steady-state flux.

8. Consider the temporal regulation of enzymatic pathways. Calculate the transition time for the case that (i) the enzyme concentrations are constant and (ii) the pathway contains only one reaction, $S_0 \leftrightarrow S_1$ and the temporal change of the reaction is given by the decay of S_0.
Note: first integrate the appropriate set of equations for the dynamics of S_1 (Eq. (9.30)) and then insert the result into Eq. (9.31). Repeat for a pathway consisting of two consecutive enzymes.

9. Consider the deterministic replicator equation with a fitness function based on the hawk–dove game (1: dove, 2: hawk). Show that the stationary frequency ratio x_1/x_2 reads $(c - \nu)/\nu$.

10. Consider the following model of competition for a common resource (from Pfeiffer *et al.*, 2001). Several microbial strains (denoted by i) compete for a shared resource S (with concentration s), which is provided at a constant rate ν. The consumption rates $J_i^S(s)$ per cell and the efficiency $\eta_i = J_i^{ATP}(s)/J_i^S(s)$ differ between the strains. Cells replicate at a rate proportional to their ATP production and die at a constant rate, with the same rate constant for all cells. Show that: (a) for a single strain (no competition with other strains), the steady-state population size is proportional to the efficiency η_i of ATP production. (b) If several strains compete for the resource, the success depends on the rate $J_i^S(S)$ of ATP production.

References

1 Dekel, E. and Alon, U. (2005) Optimality and evolutionary tuning of the expression level of a protein. *Nature*, **436**, 588–692.

2 Holland, J.H. (1975) Adaptation in natural and artificial systems: an introductory analysis with applications to biology, control, and artificial intelligence, University of Michigan Press, Ann Arbor.

3 Trigg, G.L. (ed.) (2005) *Mathematical Tools for Physicists*, Wiley-VCH, Weinheim.

4 Stephani, A., Nuño, J.C. and Heinrich, R. (1999) Optimal stoichimetric designs of ATP-producing systems as determined by an evolutionary algorithm. *Journal of Theoretical Biology*, **199**, 45–61.

5 Schuetz, R., Kuepfer, L. and Sauer, U. (2007) Systematic evaluation of objective functions for predicting intracellular fluxes in *Escherichia coli*. *Molecular Systems Biology*, **3**, 119.

6 Heinrich, R. and Schuster, S. (1996) *The Regulation of Cellular Systems*, Chapman and Hall, London.

7 Reich, J.G. (1983) Zur Ökonomie im Proteinhaushalt der lebenden Zelle. *Biomedica Biochimica Acta*, **42** (7/8), 839–848.

8 Liebermeister, W., Klipp, E., Schuster, S. and Heinrich, R. (2004) A theory of optimal differential gene expression. *BioSystems*, **76**, 261–278.

9 Kalisky, T., Dekel, E. and Alon, U. (2007) Cost-benefit theory and optimal design of gene regulation functions. *Physical Biology*, **4**, 229–245.

10 Stucki, J.W. (1980) The optimal efficiency and the economic degrees of coupling of oxidative phosphorylation. *European Journal of Biochemistry*, **109**, 269–283.

11 Heinrich, R. and Holzhütter, H. (1985) Efficiency and design of simple metabolic systems. *Biomedica Biochimica Acta*, **44**, 959–969.

12 Chait, R., Craney, A. and Kishony, R. (2007) Antibiotic interactions that select against resistance. *Nature*, 668–671.

13 Reed, J.L., Famili, I., Thiele, I. and Palsson, B.Ø. (2006) Towards multidimensional genome annotation. *Nature Reviews. Genetics*, **7**, 130–141.

14 Feist, A.M., Henry, C.S., Reed, J.L., Krummenacker, M., Joyce, A.R., Karp, P.D., Broadbelt, L.J., Hatzimanikatis, V. and Palsson, B.Ø. (2007) A genome-scale metabolic reconstruction for *Escherichia coli* K-12 MG1655 that accounts for 1260 ORFs and thermodynamic information. *Molecular Systems Biology*, **3**, 121.

15 Fell, D.A. and Small, J.R. (1986) Fat synthesis in adipose tissue: An examination of stoichiometric constraints. *The Biochemical Journal*, **238**, 781–786.

16 Varma, A. and Palsson, B.Ø. (1994) Metabolic flux balancing: basic concepts, scientific and practical use. *Biotechnology (Reading, Mass)*, **12**, 994–998.

17 Varma, A. and Palsson, B.Ø. (1994) Stoichiometric flux balance models quantitatively predict growth and metabolic by-product secretion in wild-type *Escherichia coli* W3110. *Applied and Environmental Microbiology*, **60**, 3724–3731.

18 Edwards, J.S. and Palsson, B.Ø. (2000) Metabolic flux balance analysis and the in silico analysis of *Escherichia coli* K-12 gene deletions. *BMC Bioinformatics*, **1**, 1.

19 Edwards, J.S. and Palsson, B.Ø. (2000) The *Escherichia coli* MG1655 in silico metabolic genotype: its definition, characteristics, and capabilities. *Proceedings of the National Academy of Sciences, USA*, **97**, 5528–5533.

20 Ramakrishna, R., Edwards, J.S., McCulloch, A. and Palsson, B.Ø. (2001) Flux-balance analysis of mitochondrial energy metabolism: consequences of systemic stoichiometric constraints. *American Journal of Physiology. Regulatory, Integrative and Comparative Physiology*, **280**, R695–R704.

21 Price, N.D., Schellenberger, J. and Palsson, B.Ø. (2004) Uniform sampling of steady-state flux spaces: Means to design experiments and to interpret enzymopathies. *Biophysical Journal*, **87**, 2172–2186.

22 Beard, D.A., Babson, E., Curtis, E. and Qian, H. (2004) Thermodynamic constraints for biochemical networks. *Journal of Theoretical Biology*, **228** (3), 327–333.

23 Beard, D.A., Liang, S. and Qian, H. (2002) Energy balance for analysis of complex metabolic networks. *Biophysical Journal*, **83** (1), 79–86.

24 Mavrovouniotis, M. (1990) Group contributions for estimating standard Gibbs energies of formation of biochemical compounds in aqueous solution. *Biotechnology and Bioengineering*, **36**, 1070–1082.

25 Henry, C.S., Jankowski, M.D., Broadbelt, L.J. and Hatzimanikatis, V. (2006) Genome-scale thermodynamic analysis of *E. coli* metabolism. *Biophysical Journal*, **90**, 1453–1461.

26 Kümmel, A., Panke, S. and Heinemann, M. (2006) Putative regulatory sites unraveled by network-embedded thermodynamic analysis of metabolome data. *Molecular Systems Biology*, 2006.0034.

27 Covert, M.W. and Palsson, B.Ø. (2002) Transcriptional regulation in constraint-based metabolic models of *Escherichia coli*. *The Journal of Biological Chemistry*, **277** (31), 28058–28064.

28 Holzhütter, H. (2004) The principle of flux minimization and its application to estimate stationary fluxes in metabolic networks. *European Journal of Biochemistry*, **271** (14), 2905–2922.

29 Pettersson, G. (1989) Effect of evolution on the kinetic properties of enzymes. *European Journal of Biochemistry*, **184**, 561–566.

30 Heinrich, R. and Hoffmann, E. (1991) Kinetic parameters of enzymatic reactions in states of maximal activity; an evolutionary approach. *Journal of Theoretical Biology*, **151**, 249–283.

31 Pettersson, G. (1992) Evolutionary optimization of the catalytic efficiency of enzymes. *European Journal of Biochemistry*, **206**, 289–295.

32 Wilhelm, T. Hoffmann-Klipp, E. and Heinrich, R. (1994) An evolutionary approach to enzyme kinetics; optimization of ordered mechanisms. *Bulletin of Mathematical Biology*, **56**, 65–106.

33 Klipp, E. and Heinrich, R. (1994) Evolutionary optimization of enzyme kinetic parameters; effect of constraints. *Journal of Theoretical Biology*, **171**, 309–323.

34 Klipp, E. and Heinrich, R. (1999) Competition for enzymes in metabolic pathways: implications for optimal distributions of enzyme concentrations and for the distribution of flux control. *Bio Systems*, **54**, 1–14.

35 Klipp, E.et al. (2002) Prediction of temporal gene expression. Metabolic opimization by re-distribution of enzyme activities. *European Journal of Biochemistry*, **269**, 5406–5413.

36 Zaslaver, A. *et al.* (2004) Just-in-time transcription program in metabolic pathways. *Nature Genetics*, **36**, 486–491.

37 Falster, D.S. and Westoby, M. (2003) Plant height and evolutionary games. *Trends in Ecology & Evolution*, **18**, 337–343.

38 Schuster, S., Kreft, J.-U., Schroeter, A. and Pfeiffer, T. (2008) Use of game-theoretical methods in biochemistry and biophysics. *Journal of Biological Physics*, **34**, 1–17.

39 Turner, P.E. (2005) Cheating viruses and gametheory. *American Scientist*, **93**, 428–435.

40 von Neumann, J. and Morgenstern, O. (1944) *Theory of Games and Economic Behavior*, Princeton University Press, Princeton, NJ.

41 Maynard Smith, J. and Price, G.R. (1973) The logic of animal conflict. *Nature*, **246**, 15–18.

42 Maynard Smith, J. (1982) *Evolution and the Theory of Games*, Cambridge University Press, Cambridge.

43 Nowak, A. and Sigmund, K. (2004) Evolutionary dynamics of biological games. *Science*, 303.

44 Kerr, B., Riley, M.A., Feldman, M.W. and Bohannan, B.J.M. (2002) Local dispersal promotes biodiversity in a real-life game of rock-paper-scissors. *Nature*, **418**, 171–174.

45 Czárán, T.L., Hoekstra, R.F. and Pagie, L. (2002) Chemical warfare between microbes promotes biodiversity. *Proceedings of the National Academy of Sciences of the United States of America*, **99** (2), 786–790.

46 Dudley, S.A. and File, A.L. (2007) Kin recognition in an annual plant. *Biology Letters*, **4**, 435–438.

47 Nowak, M.A. (2006) Five rules for the evolution of cooperation. *Science*, **314** (5805), 1560–1563.

48 Pfeiffer, T. and Schuster, S. (2005) Game-theoretical approaches to studying the evolution of biochemical systems. *Trends in Biochemical Sciences*, **30** (1), 20–25.

49 Pfeiffer, T., Schuster, S. and Bouhoeffer, S. (2001) Cooperation and competition in the evolution of ATP-producing pathways. *Science*, **292**, 504–507.

10
Cell Biology

Summary

A basic characteristic of life is that organisms are composed of cells that can grow, differentiate, and reproduce. Molecular interactions and molecular structures define structural and functional properties of a cell. Electrostatic interactions and different classes of biological molecules, such as carbohydrates, lipids, proteins, and nucleic acids, are the major components that govern the characteristics of biological systems such as their structural organization and physiological processes. Eukaryotic cells are compartmentalized and have organelles that fulfill specific cellular functions, e.g., the nucleus holds the cell's genome organized in chromosomes, the cytosol is the compartment where protein biosynthesis and major metabolic processes, such as glycolysis, take place, mitochondria act as cellular power plants, and the endoplasmatic reticulum and the Golgi complex are central components of protein sorting and their posttranslational modification. The expression of the genetic information in eukaryotes is a complex process that comprises gene regulation, transcription, processing, translation, posttranslational modification, and protein sorting.

10.1
Introduction

This section gives a brief overview of biology and related subjects, such as biochemistry, with a focus on molecular biology, since the latter is most relevant to current systems biology. It will review several basics and introduce fundamental knowledge of biology. The basics are required for the setup of all models for biological systems, and the meaningful interpretation of simulation results and analysis. For a broader and more detailed introduction to biology it is recommended to consult books like Alberts *et al.* [1] or Campbell and Reece [2].

Biology is the science that deals with living organisms and their interrelationships between each other and their environment in light of the evolutionary origin. Some of the main characteristics of organisms are

Systems Biology: A Textbook. Edda Klipp, Wolfram Liebermeister, Christoph Wierling, Axel Kowald, Hans Lehrach, and Ralf Herwig

ISBN: 978-3-527-31874-2

- *Physiology:* All living organisms assimilate nutrients, extract energy from these nutrients, produce substances themselves, and excrete the remains.
- *Growth and reproduction:* All living organisms grow and reproduce their own species.
- *Cellular composition:* Cells are the general building blocks of organisms.

Biology is divided into several disciplines, like physiology, morphology, cytology, ecology, developmental biology, behavioral and evolutional biology, molecular biology, biochemistry, and classical and molecular genetics. Biology tries to explain characteristics such as the shape and structure of organisms and their change during time, as well as phenomena of their regulatory, individual, or environmental relationships. This section gives a brief overview about this scientific field with a focus on biological molecules, fundamental cellular structures, and molecular biology and genetics.

10.2
The Origin of Life

The earliest development on earth began $4^1/_2$ billion years ago. Massive volcanism released water (H_2O), methane (CH_4), ammonia (NH_3), sulfur hydrogen (H_2S), and molecular hydrogen (H_2), which formed a reducing atmosphere and the early ocean. By loss of hydrogen into space and gas reactions, an atmosphere consisting of nitrogen (N_2), carbon monoxide (CO), carbon dioxide (CO_2), and water (H_2O) was formed. The impact of huge amounts of energy (e.g., sunlight with a high portion of ultraviolet radiation and electric discharges) onto the reducing atmosphere along with the catalytic effect of solid-state surfaces resulted in an enrichment of simple organic molecules such as amino acids, purines, pyrimidines, and monosaccharides in the early ocean. This is called the prebiotic broth hypothesis and is based on the experiments of Miller and Urey [3]. Another possibility is that the first forms of life formed in the deep sea utilizing the energy of hydrothermal vents, well protected from damaging UV radiation and the unstable environment of the surface [4]. Once simple organic molecules were formed in significant amounts, they presumably assembled spontaneously into macromolecules such as proteins and nucleic acids. Through the formation of molecular aggregates from these colloidally solved macromolecules, the development of simple compartmented reaction pathways for the utilization of energy sources was possible. Besides this, enzymes appeared that permitted specific reactions to take place in ordered sequences at moderate temperatures, and informational systems necessary for directed synthesis and reproduction were developed. The appearance of the first primitive cells – the last common ancestors of all past and recent organisms – was the end of the abiotic (chemical) and the beginning of the biotic (biological) evolution. Later, these first primitive cells evolved into the first prokaryotic cells (prokaryotes). About $3^1/_2$ billion years ago, the reducing atmosphere was very slowly enriched by oxygen (O_2) due to the rise of photosynthesis that resulted in an oxidative atmosphere (1.4 billion years ago: 0.2% O_2; 0.4 billion years ago: 2% O_2; today: about 21% O_2).

Table 10.1 Some important differences between prokaryotic and eukaryotic cells.

	Prokaryotes	**Eukaryotes**
Size	Mostly about 1–10 μm in length	Mostly about 10–100 μm in length
Nucleus	Nucleus is missing. The chromosomal region is called nucleolus	Nucleus is separated from the cytoplasm by the nuclear envelope
Intracellular organization	Normally, no membrane-separated compartments and no supportive intracellular skeletal framework are present in the cells' interior	Distinct compartments are present, e.g., nucleous, cytosol with a cytoskeleton, mitochondria, endoplasmatic reticulum (ER), Golgi complex, lysosomes, plastids (chloroplasts, leucoplasts)
Gene structure	No introns; some polycistronic genes	Introns and exons
Cell division	Simple cell division	Mitosis or meiosis
Ribosomes	Consists of a large 50S subunit and a small 30S subunit	Consists of a large 60S subunit and a small 40S subunit
Reproduction	Parasexual recombination	Sexual recombination
Organization	Mostly single cellular	Mostly multicellular, and with cell differentiation

Prokaryotes (eubacteria and archaebacteria) are mostly characterized by their size and simplistic structure compared to the more evolved eukaryotes. Table 10.1 summarizes several differences between these groups. The evolutionary origin of the eukaryotic cells is explained by the formation of a nucleus and several compartments, and by the inclusion of prokaryotic cells which is described by the endosymbiont hypothesis. This hypothesis states that cellular organelles, such as mitochondria and chloroplasts, are descendants of specialized cells (e.g., specialization for energy utilization) that have been engulfed by the early eukaryotes.

Prokaryotes and these early eukaryotes are single-celled organisms. Later during evolution, single-celled eukaryotes evolved further into multicellular organisms. Their cells are mostly genetically identical, but differentiate into several specialized cell types during development. Most of these organisms reproduce sexually.

The developmental process that takes place by sexual reproduction starts with a fertilized egg (zygote) that divides several times (the cell division underlying this process is discussed in more detail in Section 2.3). For instance, in the frog *Xenopus laevis* – which is a vertebrate and belongs to the amphibians – the development starts with the zygote and passes through several developmental phases, i.e., morula (64 cells), blastula (10,000 cells), gastrula (30,000 cells), and neurula (80,000 cells), before forming the tadpole (with a million cells 110 h after fertilization) that develops into the adult frog later on. This process is genetically determined, and several phases are similar between species that are related close to each other due to their identical evolutionary origin. Figure 10.1 shows a simplified tree of life that illustrates major evolutionary relations.

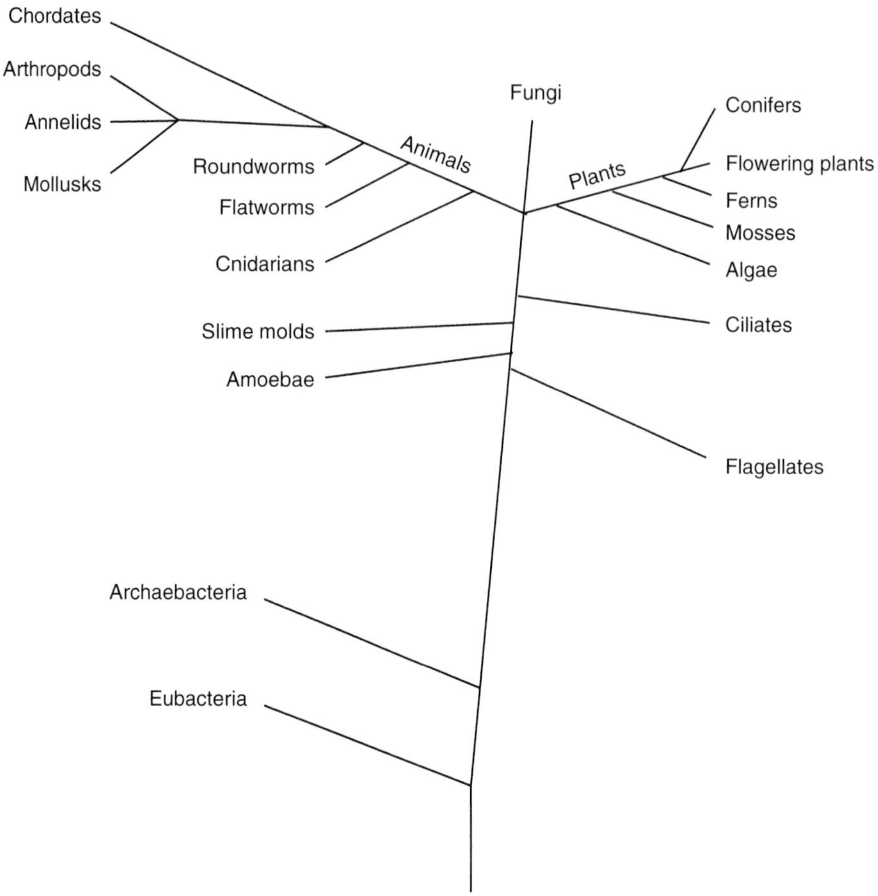

Figure 10.1 The tree of life shows phylogenetic relations between some major groups of organism.

While most places with moderate aerobic conditions were populated by eukaryotes, the prokaryotic archaebacteria in particular have specialized to survive under extreme conditions (e.g., thermophile bacteria, which propagate at temperatures of 85–105 °C in the black smokers of the deep sea, or the halobacteria, which live under conditions of high salt concentrations).

Along with organisms that have their own metabolism, parasitic viruses and viroids that utilize cells for reproduction have developed. Viruses consist of a very small genome surrounded by a protein envelope (capsid); viroids are single-stranded circular RNAs. Due to the absence of a metabolism and a cellular structure, these parasites are not regarded as living organisms.

The phenotypical diversity of organisms observed is also displayed in the structure of their hereditary information: the size of this genomic information can vary, as can its organization into different elements, i.e., plasmids and chromosomes. Table 10.2 summarizes some data acquired from commonly investigated organisms.

Table 10.2 Genome sizes of different organisms from the prokaryotic and eukaryotic kingdom[a].

Organism	Number of chromosomes (haploid genome)	Genome size (base pairs; genes)
Mycoplasma genitalium (prokaryote)	1 circular chromosome	$5.8 \cdot 10^5$ bp; 480 genes
Escherichia coli (prokaryote)	1 circular chromosome	$4.6 \cdot 10^6$ bp; 4,290 genes
Saccharomyces cerevisiae (budding yeast; eukaryote)	16 chromosomes	$12.5 \cdot 10^6$ bp; 6,186 genes
Arabidopsis thaliana (flowering plant; eukaryote)	5 chromosomes	$100 \cdot 10^6$ bp; ~25,000 genes
Drosophila melanogaster (fruit fly, eukaryote)	4 chromosomes	$180 \cdot 10^6$ bp; ~14,000 genes
Mus musculus (mouse, eukaryote)	20 chromosomes	$2.5 \cdot 10^9$ bp; ~30,000 genes
Homo sapiens (human, eukaryote)	23 chromosomes	$2.9 \cdot 10^9$; ~30,000 genes

[a]Information about further organisms can be found, e.g., at http://www.cbs.dtu.dk/services/GenomeAtlas and http://www.ensembl.org

10.3 Molecular Biology of the Cell

Cellular structures and processes result from a complex interaction network of biological molecules. The properties of these molecules determine possible interactions. Although many of these molecules are highly complex, most fall into one of the following four classes or contain substructures which belong to one of these: carbohydrates, lipids, proteins, and nucleic acids. Along with these four classes, water is highly important for all living systems. Molecules are held together by and interact through chemical bonds and forces of different types: ionic, covalent, and hydrogen bonds; nonpolar associations; and van der Waals forces. The following sections will provide a foundation for the understanding of molecular structures, functions, and interactions by giving a brief introduction to chemical bonds and forces, to the most important classes of biological molecules, and to complex macromolecular structures formed by these molecules.

10.3.1 Chemical Bonds and Forces Important in Biological Molecules

The atom model introduced by Rutherford and significantly extended by Bohr describes the atom as a positively charged nucleus being surrounded by one or more shells (or, more exactly, energy levels) that are filled with electrons. Most significant for the chemical properties of an atom is the number of electrons in its outermost shell. Atoms tend to fill up their outermost shell to obtain a stable state. The innermost or first shell is filled up by two electrons. The second and further shells are filled up by $2n^2$ electrons, where n depicts the number of the shell. However, due to reasons of energetic stability, the outermost shell will not contain more than eight electrons. For example, helium, with two electrons in its single shell, or atoms such as neon or argon, with eight electrons in their outermost shells, are essentially chemically inert. Atoms with a number of electrons near to these numbers tend to lose or gain electrons to attain these stable states. For example, sodium (one electron in its outer shell) and chlorine (seven electrons in its outer shell) can both achieve such a stable state by transferring one electron from sodium to chlorine thus forming the ions Na^+ and Cl^-. The force holding together the oppositely charged ions in solid state is called the ionic or electrostatic bond (Figure 10.2(a)). If the number of electrons in the outer shell differs by more than 1, atoms tend to share electrons by forming a so-called covalent bond (Figure 10.2(b)). Atoms held together by covalent bonds are called molecules. If the shared electron pair is equally distributed between the two involved atoms, this bond is called nonpolar (e.g., for the hydrogen molecule). If one atom has a higher attraction to the shared electron pair, it becomes partially negatively charged. Then the other atom in this polar association becomes partially positively charged, as is the case with the water molecule (H_2O), where the oxygen attracts the shared electron pairs stronger than the hydrogen atoms do. Thus, –OH and –NH groups usually form polar regions in which the hydrogen is partially positively charged. The measurement of the affinity of an atom to attract electrons in a covalent bond is given by its electronegativity, which was introduced by Linus Pauling. In addition to single covalent bonds, double and triple bonds also exist. These kinds of bonds are more exactly described by the quantum-mechanical atom model, in which the electron shells of an atom can be described by one of several differently shaped orbitals that represent the areas where the electrons are located with highest probability (electron clouds). A covalent bond is then described by molecule orbitals, which are derived from atom orbitals. Furthermore, if single and double bonds are altered in a single molecule or a double bond is in direct vicinity of an atom with a free electron pair, then one electron pair of the double bond and the free electron pair can delocalize across the participating atoms, e.g., the three electron pairs in benzol (Figure 10.2(b)) or the double bond between C and O and the free electron pair of *N* in a peptide bond (Figure 10.6(a)). Such electrons

Figure 10.2 Chemical bonds and functional organic groups. Single electrons in the outer shell are visualized by a dot; electron pairs are replaced by a dash. Shared electron pairs are represented by a dash between two atoms. (a) Single charged Na^+ and Cl^- ions are formed by the transition of the single outermost electron of sodium to chlorine. (b) In a covalent bond, electrons are shared between two atoms. If the shared electron pair is attracted more strongly by one of the participating atoms than by the other, this bond is called a polar bond. Depending on the molecule structure, double and triple bonds can occur as well. Sometimes, binding electron pairs might also be delocalized among several atoms, as it is the case in benzol. (c) Unequal electron sharing causes the formation of hydrogen bonds (shown by dotted lines) as found in water. (d) The skeleton of organic molecules essentially consists of carbon atoms bound to each other or to hydrogen. Some of these carbons are bound to or are part of functional groups with special chemical characteristics. Hence, these influence the reactivities and physicochemical properties of the molecule.

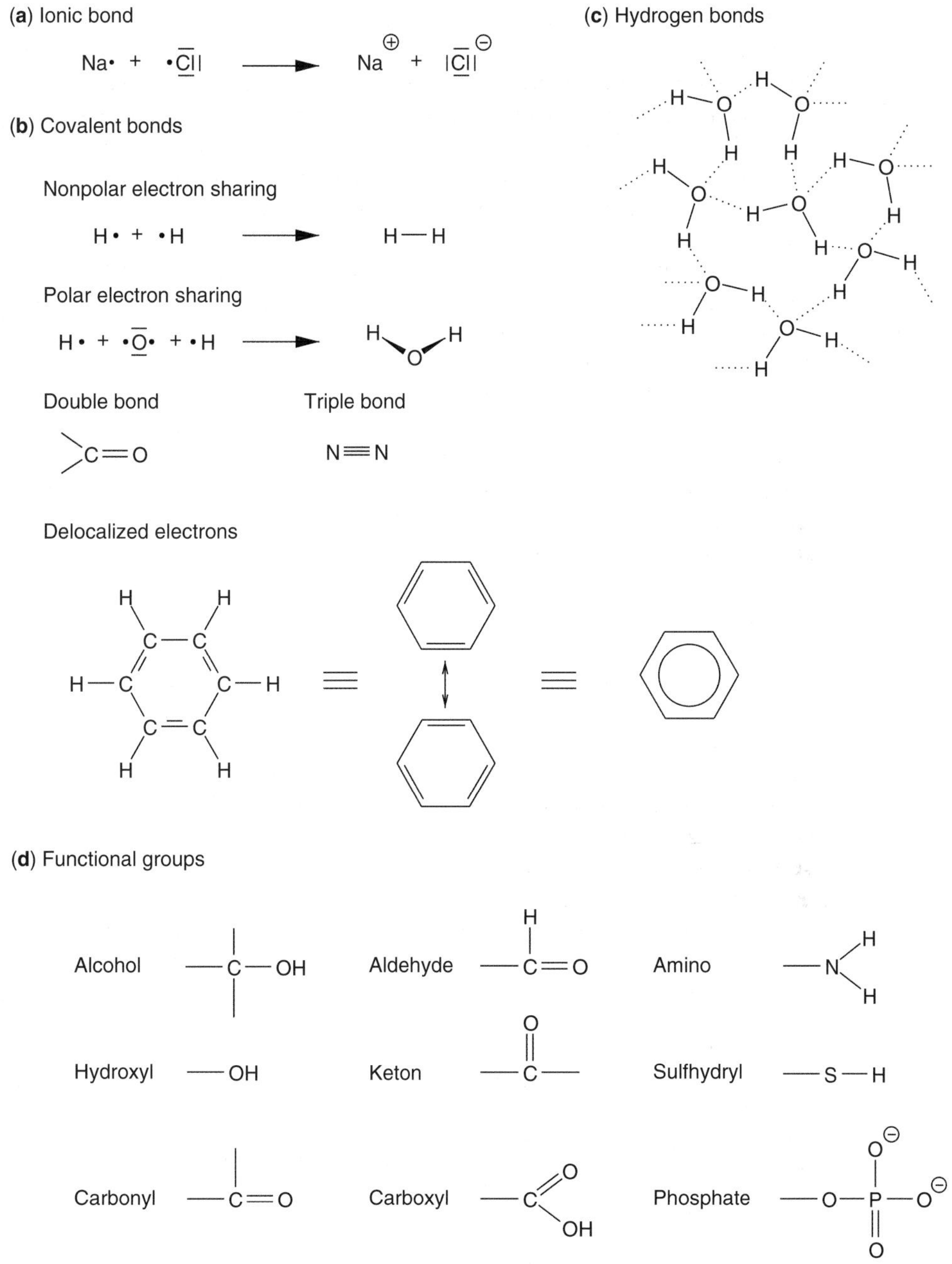

(a) Ionic bond

$$Na\bullet \ + \ \bullet\overline{\underline{C}}l| \ \longrightarrow \ \overset{\oplus}{Na} \ + \ |\overline{\underline{C}}l|^{\ominus}$$

(b) Covalent bonds

Nonpolar electron sharing

$$H\bullet \ + \ \bullet H \ \longrightarrow \ H{-}H$$

Polar electron sharing

$$H\bullet \ + \ \bullet\overline{\underline{O}}\bullet \ + \bullet H \ \longrightarrow \ H\diagdown_{O}\diagup^{H}$$

Double bond   Triple bond

$$\diagup^{\diagdown}C{=}O \qquad\qquad N{\equiv}N$$

Delocalized electrons

(c) Hydrogen bonds

(d) Functional groups

Alcohol	$-\overset{\mid}{\underset{\mid}{C}}-OH$	Aldehyde	$-\overset{H}{\underset{\ }{C}}{=}O$	Amino	$-N\diagup^{H}_{\diagdown H}$
Hydroxyl	$-OH$	Keton	$\overset{O}{\overset{\|}{-C-}}$	Sulfhydryl	$-S-H$
Carbonyl	$-\overset{\mid}{C}{=}O$	Carboxyl	$-C\diagup^{O}_{\diagdown OH}$	Phosphate	$-O-\overset{O^{\ominus}}{\underset{O}{\overset{\mid}{\underset{\|}{P}}}}-O^{\ominus}$

are called delocalized π-electrons. For a more detailed description, please consult books about general and anorganic chemistry or introductory books about biochemistry.

Hydrogen atoms with a positive partial charge that are bound to oxygen or nitrogen (as in H_2O or NH_3) are able to interact with free electron pairs of atoms with a negative partial charge. These attractions are called hydrogen bonds and are relatively weak compared to solid-state ionic bonds or covalent bonds. To break a hydrogen bond, only about 4 kJ/mol of energy is required. Therefore, hydrogen bonds separate readily at elevated temperatures, which is often the reason why proteins such as enzymes lose their function during heating. Likewise, the hydrogen bonds that hold together the double strands of nucleic acids (see Section 10.3.3.4) can be separated at high temperatures. This fact is utilized for several molecular biological methods, e.g., polymerase chain reaction (PCR) or for the radioactive labeling of DNA (deoxyribonucleic acid) fragments. Hydrogen bonds also explain why water is liquid at room temperature and boils at 100 °C. Small alcohols, such as methanol or ethanol, are fully soluble in water, due to their hydroxyl group which interacts with the hydrogen bonds of water, whereas larger alcohols, like hexanol or heptanol, are weakly soluble or insoluble in water due to their longer unpolar carbohydrate tail. As we have seen, polarized functional groups can interact with water, which is why they often are called hydrophilic (or lipophobic), while nonpolar molecules or molecule parts are called hydrophobic (or lipophilic).

Also critical to structures and interactions of biological molecules are the van der Waals forces. The electron clouds surrounding atoms that are held together by covalent bonds are responsible for these forces. Momentary inequalities in the distribution of electrons in any covalent bond, due to chance, can make one end of the covalent bond more negative or positive than the other for a short moment, which results in rapid fluctuations in the charge of the electron cloud. These fluctuations can induce opposite fluctuations in nearby covalent bonds thus establishing a weak attractive force. This attractive force is stronger the closer the electron clouds are, but if the outermost electron orbitals begin to overlap, the negatively charged electrons strongly repel each other. Thus, van der Waals forces can be either attractive or repulsive. Their binding affinity is, at 0.4 kJ mol^{-1} in water, even lower than hydrogen bonds. The optimal distance for maximum van der Waals forces of an atom is called its van der Waals contact radius. The van der Waals repulsions have an important influence on the possible conformations of a molecule.

10.3.2
Functional Groups in Biological Molecules

As outlined before, one major characteristic of life is physiological processes in which nutrients from the outside are converted by the organism to maintain a thermodynamically open system with features such as development or behavior. These physiological processes are realized on the metabolic level by myriads of reactions in which specific molecules are converted into others. These intra- or intermolecular rearrangements often take place at specific covalent bonds that can more readily be disturbed than others. Such covalent bonds are often formed by certain intramolecular substructures that are called functional groups. Thus, functional groups often serve as reaction centers converting some molecules into others or link some molecular subunits to form larger molecular assemblies, e.g., polypeptides or nucleic acids. The functional groups most relevant in biological molecules are hydroxyl, carbonyl, carboxyl, amino, phosphate and sulfhydryl groups (Figure 10.2(d)).

Hydroxyl groups (−OH) are strongly polar and often enter into reactions that link subunits to larger molecular assemblies in which a water molecule is released. These reactions are called condensations. The reverse reaction in which a water molecule enters a reaction by which a larger molecule is split into two subunits is called hydrolysis. The formation of a dipeptide from two amino acids is an example of a condensation, and its reverse reaction is the hydrolysis of the dipeptide (Figure 10.6(a)). If the hydroxyl group is bound to a carbon atom, which in turn is bound to other hydrogen and/or carbon atoms, it is called an alcohol. Alcohols can easily be oxidized to form aldehydes or ketones, which are characterized by their carbonyl group (Figure 10.2(d)). Aldehydes and ketones are particularly important for carbohydrates (such as sugars) or lipids (such as fats). In aldehydes, the carbonyl group occurs at the end of a carbon chain, whereas in ketones it occurs in its interior. A carboxyl group is strongly polar and formed by an alcohol group and an aldehyde group. The hydrogen of the hydroxyl part can easily dissociate as H^+ due to the influence of the nearby carbonyl oxygen. In this way, it acts as an organic acid. The carboxyl group (−COOH) is the characteristic group of organic acids such as fatty acids and amino acids. Amino acids are further characterized by an amino group. Amino groups ($-NH_2$, Figure 10.2(d)) have a high chemical reactivity and can act as a base in organic molecules. They are, for instance, essential for the linkage of amino acids to form proteins and for the establishment of hydrogen bonds in DNA double strands. Moreover, amino acids carrying NH_2 in their residual group often play a crucial role as part of the catalytic domain of enzymes. Another group that has several important roles is the phosphate group (Figure 10.2(d)). As part of large organic molecules, this group acts as a bridging ligand connecting two building blocks to each other, as is the case in nucleic acids (DNA, RNA; see Section 10.3.3.4) or phospholipids. Furthermore, the di- and triphosphate forms in conjunction with a nucleoside serve as a universal energy unit in cells, e.g., adenosine triphosphate (ATP, Figure 10.7(a). Phosphate groups are also involved in the regulation of the activity of enzymes, e.g., MAP kinases, which participate in signal transduction. Sulfhydryl groups (Figure 10.2(d)) are readily oxidized. If two sulfhydryl residues participate in an oxidization, a so-called disulfid bond is created (Figure 10.6(d)). These linkages often occur between sulfhydryl residues of amino acids that form a protein. Thus, they are responsible for the stable folding of proteins, which is required for their correct functioning.

10.3.3 Major Classes of Biological Molecules

The structural and functional properties of an organism are based on a vast number of diverse biological molecules and their interplay. The physicochemical properties of a molecule are determined through their functional groups. In the following sections, four major classes of biological molecules that are ubiquitously present and are responsible for fundamental structural and functional characteristics of living organisms will be introduced: carbohydrates, lipids, proteins, and nucleic acids.

10.3.3.1 **Carbohydrates**

Carbohydrates function as energy storage molecules and furthermore can be found as extracellular structure mediators, e.g., in plants. The chemical formula of carbohydrates is mostly $C_n(H_2O)_n$. The individual building blocks of all carbohydrates are the monosaccharides, which consist of a chain of three to seven carbon atoms. Depending on the number of carbon atoms, they are categorized as trioses, tetroses, pentoses, hexoses, or heptoses (cf. Figure 10.3(a)). All monosaccharides can occur in linear form, and with more than four carbons, they exist in equilibrium with a ring form. In the linear form, all carbons of the chain, except for one, carry a hydroxyl group (polyalcohol), which makes the carbohydrates hydrophilic. The remaining carbon carries a carbonyl group, and depending on its position – whether it is an aldehyde or ketone – it is called an aldose or a ketose. The circular configuration is attained by an intramolecular reaction between the carbonyl group and one of the hydroxyl groups. Such a compound is called a hemiacetal. An example of the ring formation for the six-carbon monosaccharide glucose is given in Figure 10.3(b), in which it forms a so-called glucopyranose ring. Depending on the orientation of the hydroxyl group at the 1-carbon, i.e., whether it points downward (α-glucose) or upward (β-glucose), two alternate conformations exist. Glucose is one of the most important energy sources for organisms. It is metabolized during glycolysis into ATP and reduction equivalents (e.g., NADH, NADPH, or $FADH_2$).

The hydroxyl group at the 1-carbon position of the cyclic hemiacetal can react via a condensation with the hydroxyl group of another monosaccharide. This linkage forms a disaccharide from two monosaccharides (Figure 10.3(c)). If this happens subsequently for several carbohydrates, polysaccharides that occur as linear chains or branching structures are formed.

10.3.3.2 **Lipids**

Lipids are a very diverse and heterogeneous group. Since they are made up mostly of nonpolar groups, lipids can be characterized by their higher solubility in nonpolar solvents, such as acetone. Due to their hydrophobic character, lipids tend to form

Figure 10.3 Carbohydrates. (a) Some examples of carbohydrates with a backbone of three to seven carbon atoms. (b) Glucose, like other monosaccharides with more than four carbons in their backbone, can form a circular structure, known as hemiacetal, by an intramolecular condensation reaction that can occur in two different conformations. (c) By further condesation reactions, such sugar monomers can form disaccharides or even larger linear or branched molecules called oligomers or polymers depending on the number of monomers involved.

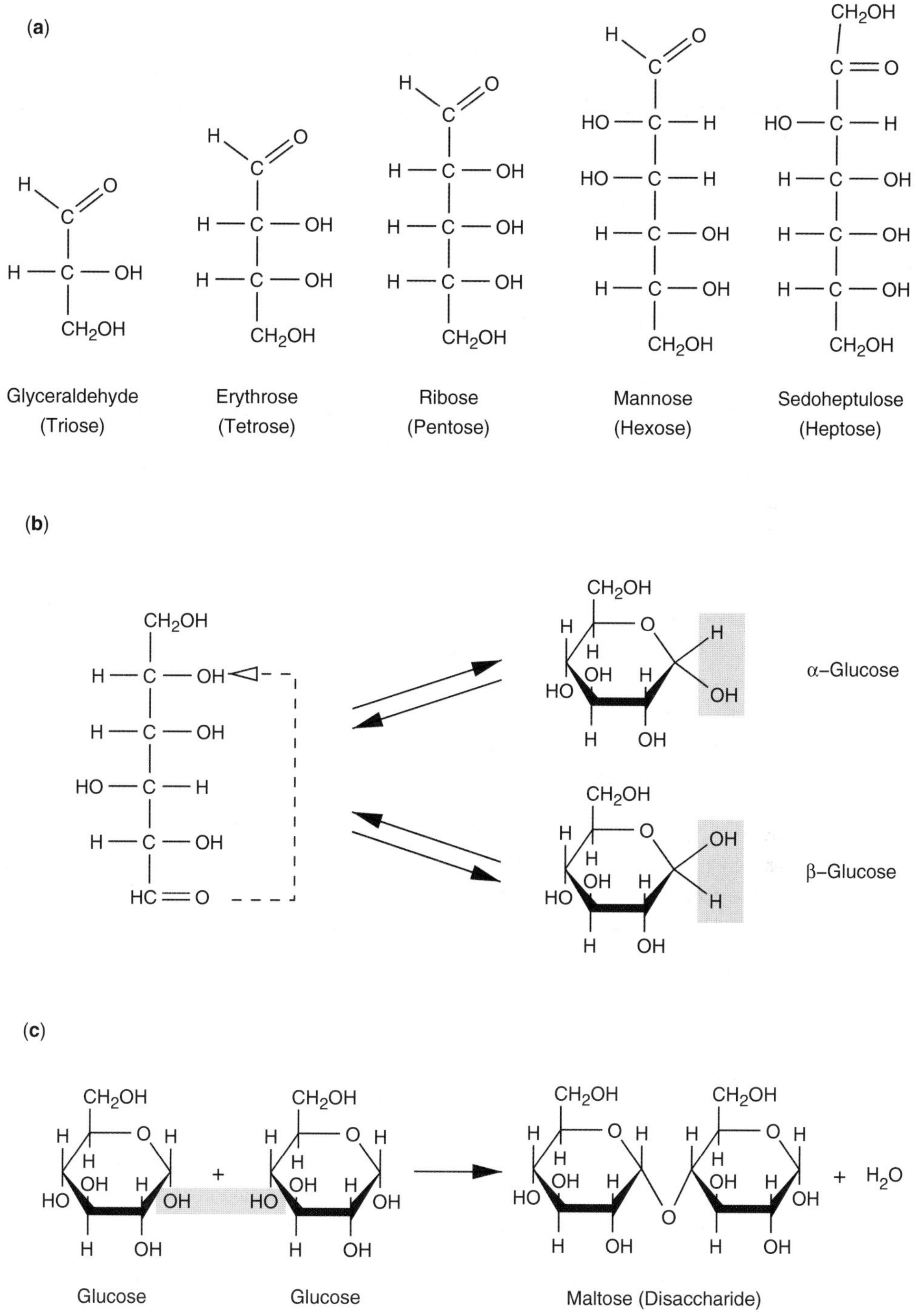
(a)
Glyceraldehyde
(Triose)
Erythrose
(Tetrose)
Ribose
(Pentose)
Mannose
(Hexose)
Sedoheptulose
(Heptose)
(b)
α–Glucose
β–Glucose
(c)
Glucose
Glucose
Maltose (Disaccharide)
+ H_2O

nonpolar associations or membranes. Eventually, these membranes form cellular hydrophilic compartments. Furthermore, such hydrophobic regions offer a local area for reactions that require a surrounding deprived of water. Three different types of lipids are present in various cells and tissues: neutral lipids, phospholipids, and steroids. Lipids can also be linked covalently to proteins or carbohydrates to form lipoproteins or glycolipids, respectively.

Neutral lipids are generally completely nonpolar and are commonly found as storage fats and oils in cells. They are composed of the alcohol glycerol (an alcohol with three hydroxyl groups), which is covalently bound to fatty acids. A fatty acid is a linear chain of 4 to 24 or more carbon atoms with attached hydrogens (molecules like this are well known as hydrocarbons) and a carboxyl group at one end (Figure 10.4(a)). Most frequent are chains with 16 or 18 carbons. Fatty acids can be either saturated or unsaturated (polyunsaturated). Unsaturated fatty acids contain one or more double bonds in their carbon chain and have more fluid character than do saturated ones. Linkage of the fatty acids to glycerol results from a condensation reaction of the carboxyl group with one of the alcohol groups of glycerol; this is called an ester binding. If all three sites of the glycerol bind a fatty acid, it is called a triglyceride, which is the most frequent neutral lipid in living systems. Triglycerides – in the form of fats or oils – mostly serve as energy reserves.

Phospholipids are the primary lipids of biological membranes (cf. Section 10.4.1). Their structure is very similar to the neutral lipids. However, the third carbon of glycerol binds a polar residue via a phosphate group instead of a fatty acid. Polar subunits commonly linked to the phosphate group are ethanolamine, choline, glycerol, serine, threonine, or inositol (Figure 10.4(c)). Due to their polar and unpolar parts, phospholipids have dual-solubility properties termed amphipathic or amphiphilic. This property enables phospholipids to form a so-called bilayer in an aqueous environment, which is the fundamental design principle of biological membranes (Figure 10.9(a)). Polar and nonpolar parts of the amphipathic molecules are ordered side by side in identical orientation and form a one molecule thick layer (monolayer) with a polar and a nonpolar side; the aqueous environment forces the lipophilic sides of two such layers to each other, thus creating the mentioned bilayer.

Steroids are based on a framework of four condensed carbon rings that are modified in various ways (Figure 10.4(d)). Sterols – the most abundant group of steroids – have a hydroxyl group linked to one end of the ring structure, representing the slightly polar part of the amphiphilic molecule; a nonpolar carbon chain is attached to the opposite end. The steroid cholesterol plays an important part in the plasma membrane of animal cells. Among other things, cholesterol loosens the packing of membrane phospholipids and maintains membrane fluidity at low temperatures. Other steroids act as hormones (substances that regulate biological processes in tissues far away from their own place of production) in animals, and they are, e.g., involved in regulatory processes concerning sexual determination or cell growth.

In glycolipids, the lipophilic part is constituted of fatty acids bound to the 1-carbon and 2-carbon of glycerol, as is the case with phospholipids. The 3-carbon is covalently attached to one or more carbohydrate groups that confer an amphiphilic character to

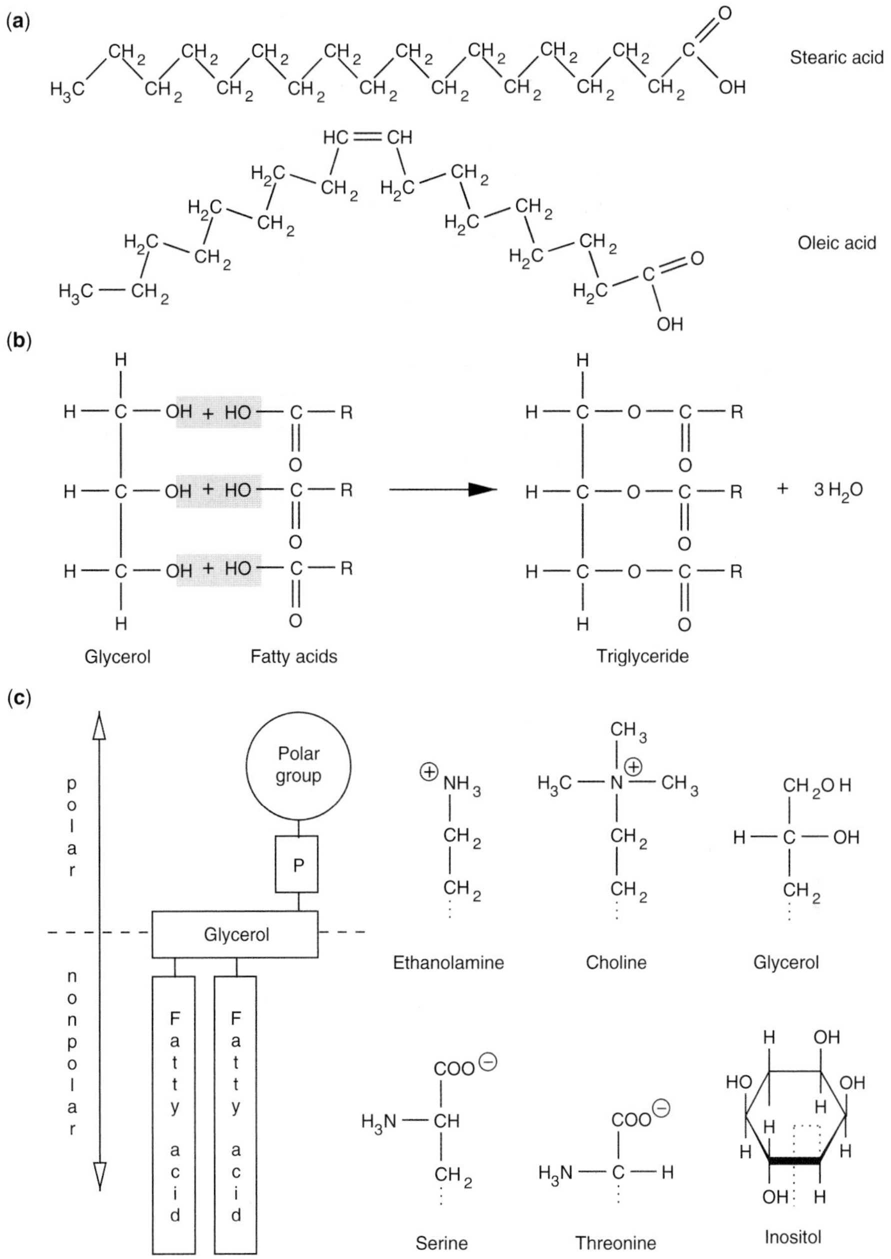

Figure 10.4 (a) Fatty acids represent one part of fats and phospholipids. They are either saturated or unsaturated. (b) Triglycerides are formed by condensation reactions of glycerol and three fatty acids. (c) In phospholipids, the third carbon of glycerol is bound to a polar group via a phosphate group (P), which usually is ethanolamine, choline, glycerol, serine, threonine, or inositol. (d) Steroids constitute another major lipid class. They are formed by four condensed carbon rings. Cholesterol, shown here, is important, e.g., for membrane fluidity of eukaryotic cells.

(d)

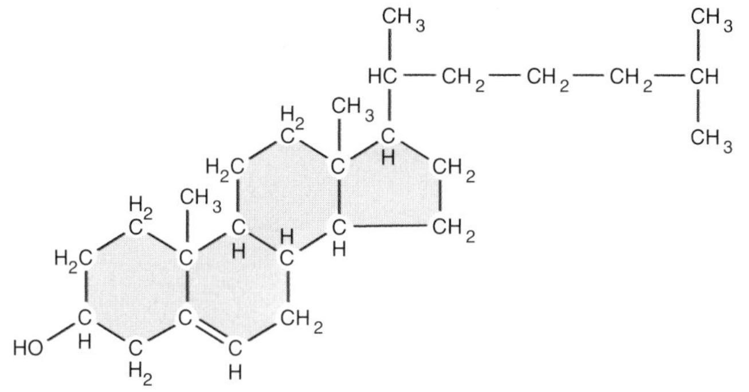

Figure 10.4 (*Continued*).

the molecule. Glycolipids do occur, e.g., in the surface-exposed parts of the plasma membrane bilayer of animal cells that are subject to physical or chemical stress. Furthermore, among several other things, they are responsible for the AB0 blood system of humans.

10.3.3.3 **Proteins**

Proteins fulfill numerous highly important functions in the cell, only a few of which can be mentioned here. They build up the cytoskeletal framework, which forms the cellular structure and is responsible for cell movements (motility). Proteins are also part of the extracellular supportive framework (extracellular matrix), e.g., as collagen in animals. As catalytic enzymes for highly specific biochemical reactions, they rule and control the metabolism of a single cell or whole organism. Furthermore, proteins regulated by transient modifications are relevant for signal transduction, e.g., proteins controlling cell division such as cyclin-dependent protein kinases (CDK). A further highly important function of proteins is their ability to control the transcription and translation of genes as well as the degradation of proteins (see Section 10.5).

Proteins consist of one or more polypeptides. Each polypeptide is composed of covalently linked amino acids; these covalent bonds are called peptide bonds. Such a bond is formed by a condensation reaction between the amino group of one amino acid and the carboxyl group of another (Figure 10.6(a)). The primary structure of a polypeptide is coded by the genetic information that defines in which order amino acids – chosen from a set of 20 different ones – do appear. Figure 10.5 shows the chemical structures of these amino acids. Common to all amino acids is a central carbon (α-carbon), which carries an amino group (except for proline where this is a ring-forming imino group), a carboxyl group, and a hydrogen. Furthermore, it carries a residual group with different physicochemical properties, due to which the amino acids can be divided into different groups, such as amino acids that carry (i) nonpolar residues that can grant lipophobic characteristics, (ii) uncharged polar residues, (iii) residues containing a carboxyl group, which is negatively charged at physiological pH and thus act as acids, and (iv) residues, which are usually positively charged at common pH ranges of living cells and thus show basic characteristics. Due to the

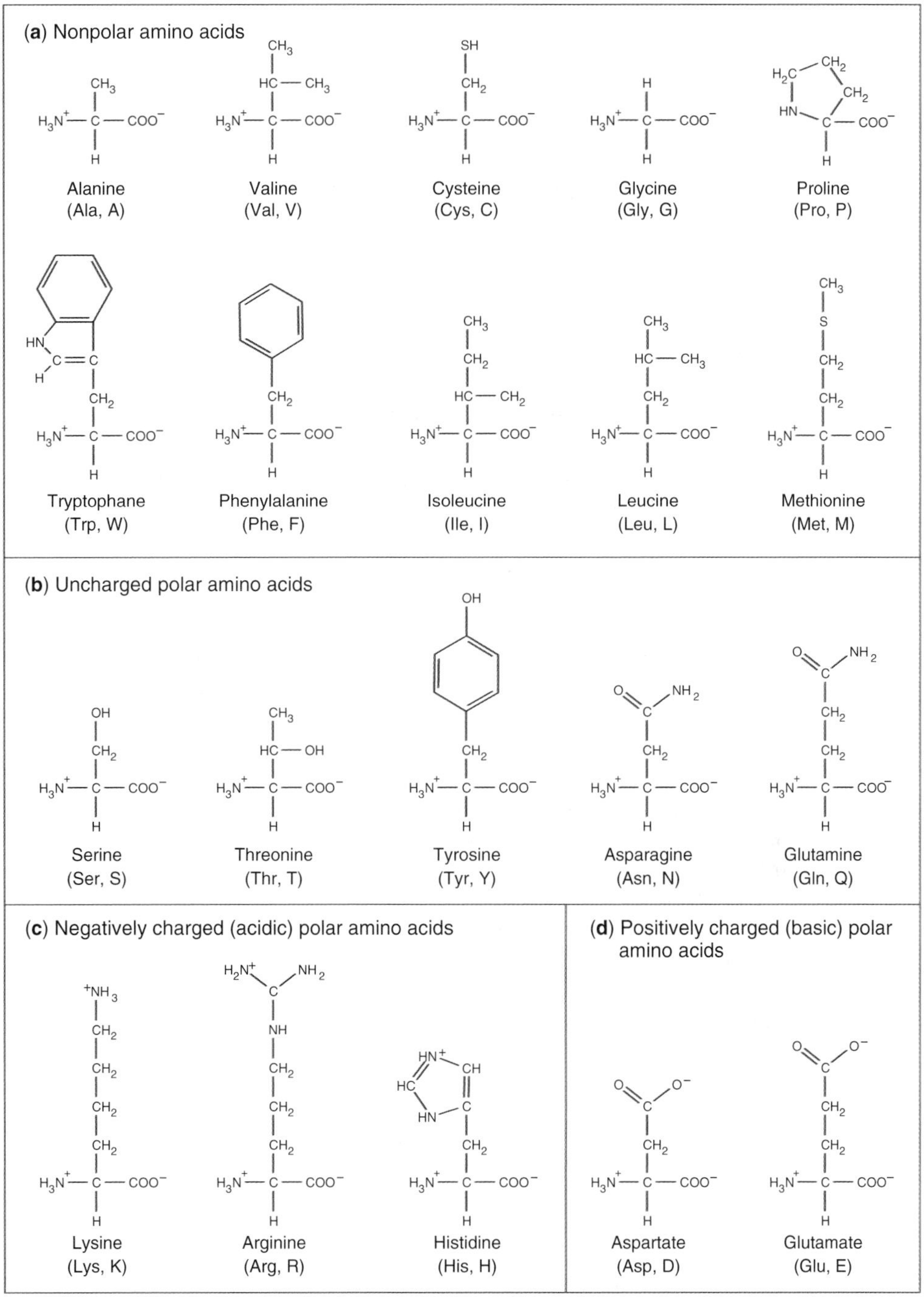

Figure 10.5 Amino acids are formed by carbon that is bound to an amino group, a carboxy group, a hydrogen, and a residual group. Depending on the physicochemical characteristics of the residual group, they can be categorized as (a) nonpolar, (b) uncharged polar, (c) acidic, or (d) basic amino acids.

combination of possibilities of these amino acids, proteins are very diverse. Usually proteins are assembled from about 50 to 1,000 amino acids, but they might be much smaller or larger. Except for glycin, the α-carbon of amino acids binds four different residues and therefore amino acids can occur in two different isoforms that behave like an image and its mirror image. These two forms are called the L- isoform and the D-isoform, of which only the L-isoform is used in naturally occurring proteins. Furthermore, amino acids of proteins are often altered posttranslational. For instance, proline residues in collagen are modified to hydroxyproline by addition of a hydroxyl group.

The primary structure of a protein is given by the sequence of the amino acids linked via peptide bonds. This sequence starts at the N-terminus of the polypeptide and ends at its C-terminus (cf. Figure 10.6(a)). In the late 1930s, Linus Pauling and Robert Corey elucidated the exact structure of the peptide bond. They found that the hydrogen of the substituted amino group almost always is in opposite position to the oxygen of the carbonyl group, so that both together with the carbon of the carbonyl group and the nitrogen of the amino group build a rigid plane. This is due to the fact that the bond between carbon and nitrogen does have a partial double-bond character. In contrast to this, both the bonds of the α-carbon with the nitrogen of the substituted amino group and the carbon of the carbonyl group are flexible since they are pure single bonds. The free rotation around these two bonds is limited only by steric interactions of the amino acid residuals. Based on this knowledge, Pauling and Corey proposed two very regular structures: the α-helix and the β-strand. Both are very common in proteins. They are formed by the polypeptide backbone and are supported and stabilized by a specific local amino acid sequence composition. Such regular arrangements are called secondary structures. An α-helix (Figure 10.6(b)) has a cylindrical helical structure in which the carbonyl oxygen atom of each residue (n) accepts a hydrogen bond from the amide nitrogen four residues further in sequence ($n + 4$). Amino acids often found in α-helices are Glu, Ala, Leu, Met, Gln, Lys, Arg, and His. In a β-sheet, parallel peptide strands – β-strands that may be widely separated in the linear protein sequence – are linked side by side via hydrogen bonds between hydrogen and oxygen atoms of their backbone (Figure 10.6(c)). The sequence direction (always read from the amino/N-terminal to the carboxy/C-terminal of the polypeptide) of pairing β-strands can be either parallel or antiparallel. The residual groups of the amino acids point up and down from the β-sheet. Characteristic amino acids of β-sheets are Val, Ile, Tyr, Cys, Trp, Phe, and Thr. The regular secondary structure elements fold into a compact form that is

Figure 10.6 (a) Formation of a peptide linkage by a reaction between the carboxyl group of one amino acid and the amino group of a second. (b) The molecular structure of an α-helix, as shown in the upper part of the image, is often illustrated by a simple helical structure as shown below. (c) An antiparallel β-sheet. (d) A disulfide bridge is formed by oxidation of the SH groups of cysteine residues belonging to either the same or different polypeptides. (e) Three-dimensional illustration of the copper zinc superoxide dismutase (CuZnSOD) of *E. coli* (PDB: 1EOS). α-helices are depicted as helical structures and β-strands illustrated by arrows. The two metal ions are shown as spheres.

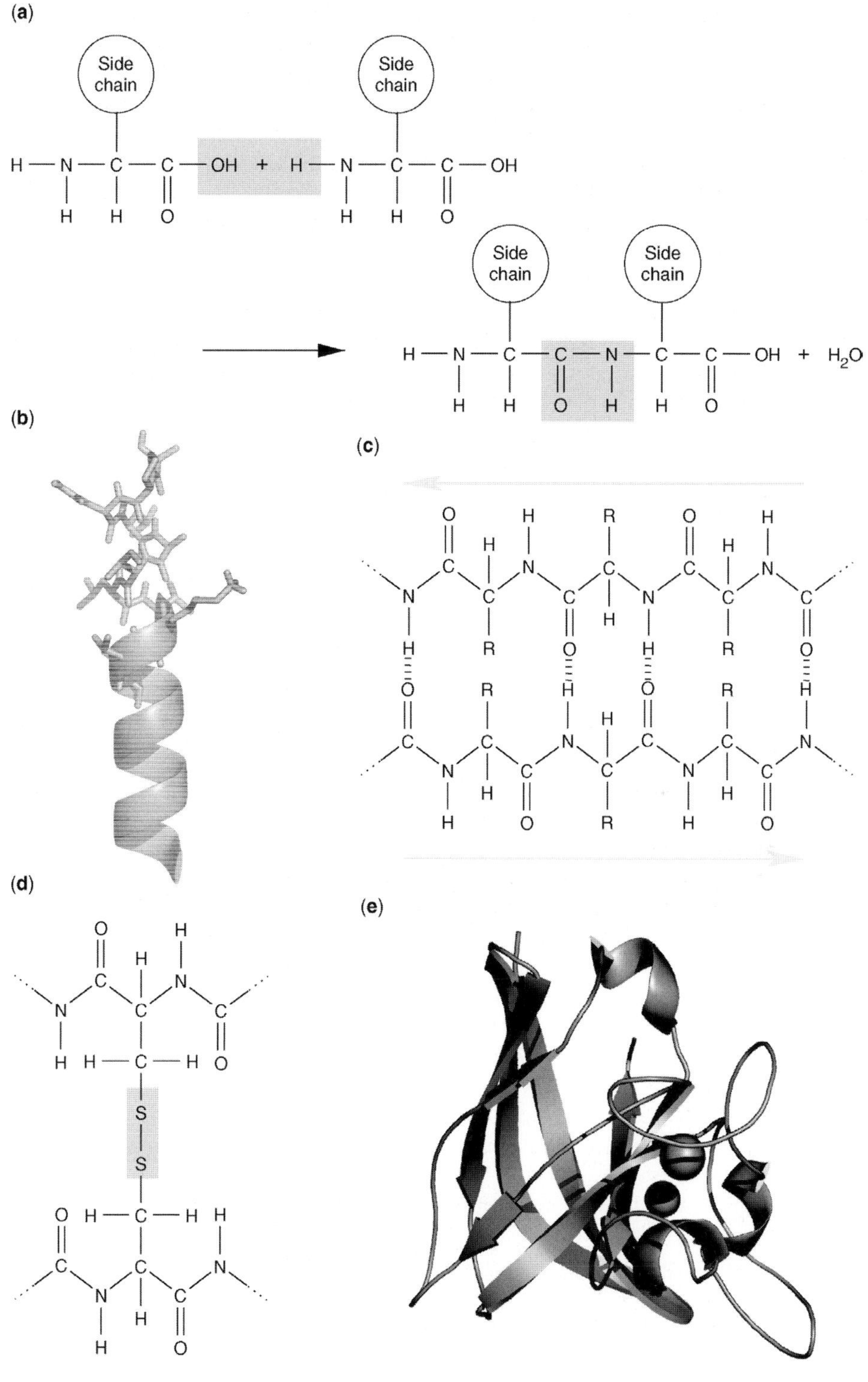
(a)
Side chain
Side chain
H — N — C — C — OH + H — N — C — C — OH
Side chain
Side chain
H — N — C — C — N — C — C — OH + H₂O
(b)
(c)
(d)
(e)

called the tertiary structure of a protein. Its surface topology enables specific interactions with other molecules. Figure 10.6(e) shows a model of the three-dimensional structure of the superoxide dismutase (SOD), which detoxifies aggressive superoxide radicals ($O_2^{\bullet-}$). Sometimes the tertiary structure is stabilized by posttranslational modifications like disulfide bridges (Figure 10.6(d)) or metal ions like calcium (Ca^{2+}) or zinc (Zn^{2+}). Some proteins are fibrous, i.e., they form filamentous structures (e.g., the keratin of hair). But most proteins fold into globular, compact shapes. Larger proteins often fold into several independent structural regions: the domains. Domains frequently consist of 50 to 350 residues and are often capable of folding stably enough to exist on their own. Often proteins are composed of assemblies of more than one polypeptide chain. Such a composition is termed the quarternary structure. The subunits can either be identical or different in sequence, and the protein is thus referred to as a homo- or heteromer, e.g., a protein composed of four identical subunits such as the *lac* repressor is called a homotetramer.

10.3.3.4 **Nucleic Acids**

Deoxyribonucleic acid (DNA) is present in all living organisms and is the molecule storing the heredity information, i.e., the genes. Another molecule, the ribonucleic acid (RNA), takes part in a vast number of processes. Amongst these, the transfer of the hereditary information leading from DNA to protein synthesis (via transcription and translation; see Section 10.5) is the most important. Both DNA and RNA are nucleic acids. Nucleic acids are polymers built up of covalently bound mononucleotides. A nucleotide consists of three parts: (i) a nitrogen-containing base, (ii) a pentose, and (iii) one or more phosphate groups (Figure 10.7(a)). Bases are usually pyrimidines such as cytosine (C), thymine (T) or uracil (U), or purines like adenine (A) or guanine (G) (Figure 10.7(b)). In RNA the base is covalently bound to the first carbon (1′-carbon) of the circular pentose ribose. In DNA it is bound to the 1′-carbon of deoxyribose, a pentose that lacks the hydroxyl group of the 2′-carbon. A unit consisting of these parts – a base and a pentose – is named nucleo*side*. If it furthermore carries a mono-, di-, or triphosphate, it is called a nucleo*tide*. Nucleotides are named according to their nucleoside, e.g., adenosine monophosphate (AMP), adenosine diphosphate (ADP), or adenosine triphosphate (ATP); prepending *deoxy* to the name (or *d* in the abbreviation) indicates the deoxy form (e.g., deoxyguanosine triphosphate or dGTP). Nucleotides are not only relevant for nucleic acid construction but also are responsible for energy transfer in several metabolic reactions (e.g., ATP and ADP) or play certain roles in signal transduction pathways, such as 3′–5′-cyclic AMP (cAMP), which is synthesized by the adenylate cyclase and is involved, for instance, in the activation of certain protein kinases.

In DNA and RNA, the 3′-carbon of a nucleotide is linked to the 5′-carbon of the next nucleotide in sequence via a single phosphate group. These alternating sugar and phosphate groups form the backbone of the nucleic acids. Both DNA and RNA can carry the bases adenine, guanine, and cytosine. In DNA thymine can also be present, which is replaced by uracil in RNA. The sequence of

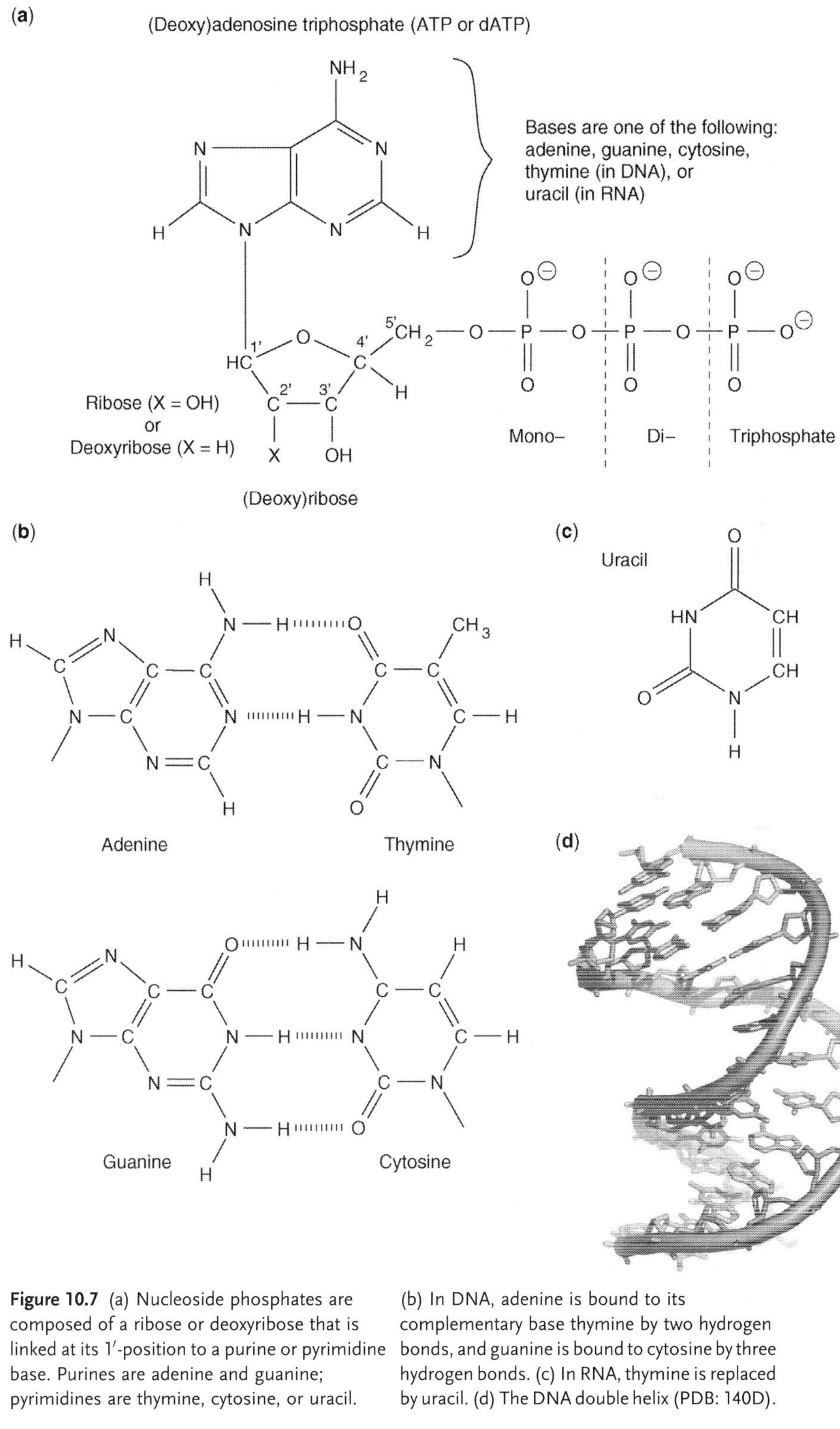

Figure 10.7 (a) Nucleoside phosphates are composed of a ribose or deoxyribose that is linked at its 1′-position to a purine or pyrimidine base. Purines are adenine and guanine; pyrimidines are thymine, cytosine, or uracil. (b) In DNA, adenine is bound to its complementary base thymine by two hydrogen bonds, and guanine is bound to cytosine by three hydrogen bonds. (c) In RNA, thymine is replaced by uracil. (d) The DNA double helix (PDB: 140D).

different bases has a direction – because of the 5′–3′-linkage of its backbone – and is used in living organisms for the conservation of information. DNA contains millions of nucleotides, e.g., a single DNA strand of human chromosome 1 is about 246 million nucleotides long. Each base of the sequence is able to pair with a so-called complementary base by hydrogen bonds. Due to the number and steric arrangement of hydrogen bonds, only two different pairing types are possible (Figure 10.7(b)): adenine can bind thymine (A-T, with two hydrogen bonds) and guanine can bind cytosine (G-C, with three hydrogen bonds). In RNA, thymine is replaced by uracil. In 1953, Watson and Crick proposed a double strand for the DNA, with an antiparallel orientation of the backbones. Each of the bases of one strand binds to its complementary base on the other strand, and together they form a helical structure (Figure 10.7(d)). This so-called double helix is the usual conformation of DNA in cells. RNA usually occurs as a single strand. Occasionally it is paired to a DNA single strand, as during the mRNA synthesis (Section 10.5.1), or complementary bases of the same molecule are bound to each other, e.g., as in tRNA.

10.4 Structural Cell Biology

This section gives a general introduction to the structural elements of eukaryotic cells. Fundamental differences between prokaryotic and eukaryotic cells have already been mentioned and are summarized in Table 10.1.

The first microscopic observations of cells were done in the 17th century by Robert Hooke and Anton van Leeuwenhoek. The general cell theory was developed in the 1830s by Theodor Schwann and Matthias Schleiden. It states that all living organisms are composed of nucleated cells, which are the functional units of life and that cells arise only from preexisting cells by a process of division. Today we know that this is true not only for nucleated eukaryotic cells but also for prokaryotic cells lacking a nucleus. The interior of a cell is surrounded by a membrane that separates it from its external environment. This membrane is called the cell membrane or plasma membrane and it is semipermeable, i.e., the traffic of substances across this membrane in either orientation is restricted to some specific molecule species or specifically controlled by proteins of the membrane that handle the transport. Fundamental to eukaryotic cells – in contrast to prokaryotic cells – is their subdivision by intracellular membranes into distinct compartments. Figure 10.8 illustrates the general structure of a eukaryotic cell as it is found in animals. Generally, one distinguishes between the storage compartment of the DNA, the nucleus, and the remainder of the cell interior that is located in the cytoplasm. The cytoplasm contains further structures that fulfill specific cellular functions and which are surrounded by the cytosol. Among these cytoplasmatic organelles are the endoplasmatic reticulum (ER), which forms a widely spread intracellular membrane system; the mitochondria, which are the cellular power plants; the Golgi complex; transport vesicles; peroxisomes; and,

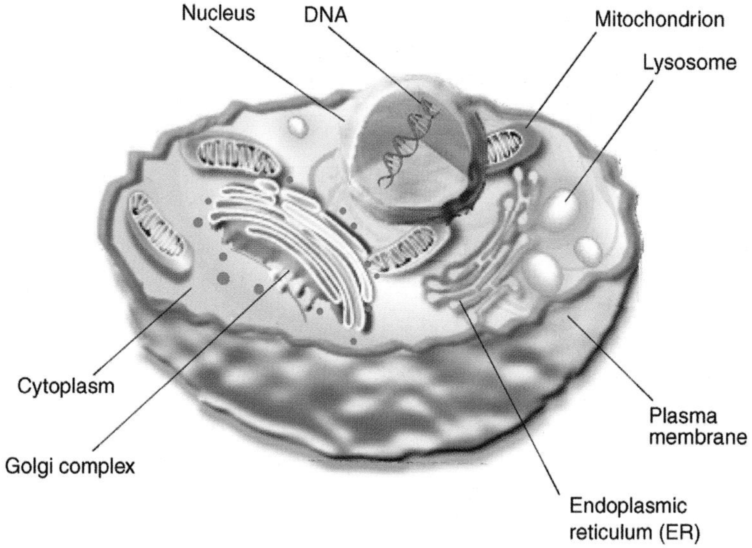

Figure 10.8 Schematic illustration of an animal cell with its major organelles.

additionally in plant cells, chloroplasts, which act as sunlight harvesting systems performing photosynthesis, and the vacuole. In the following sections, we will describe the structure and function of biological membranes and the most important cellular compartments that are formed by them.

10.4.1 Structure and Function of Biological Membranes

All cells are surrounded by a plasma membrane. It not only separates the cell plasma from its surrounding environment but also acts as a selective filter for nutrients and byproducts. By active transport of ions, for which the energy source ATP is usually utilized, a chemical and/or electrical potential can be established across the membrane that is essential, e.g., for the function of nerve cells. Furthermore, receptor proteins of the plasma membrane enable the transmission of external signals that enable the cell to react to its environment. As already mentioned, eukaryotes additionally possess an intracellular membrane system acting as a boundary for different essential compartments.

The assembly of a bilayer, which is the fundamental structure of all biological membranes, is described in the section about lipids (Section 10.3.3.2; cf. also Figure 10.9(a)). Biological membranes are composed of this molecular bilayer of lipids (mainly phospholipids, but also cholesterol and glycolipids) and membrane proteins that are inserted and held in the membrane by noncovalent forces. Besides integral membrane proteins, proteins can also be attached to the surface of the membrane (peripheral proteins). This model of biological membranes is known as

(**a**)

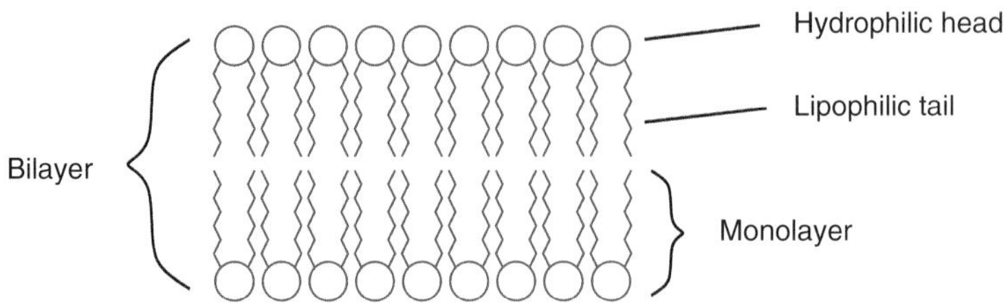
Hydrophilic head
Lipophilic tail
Bilayer
Monolayer

(**b**)

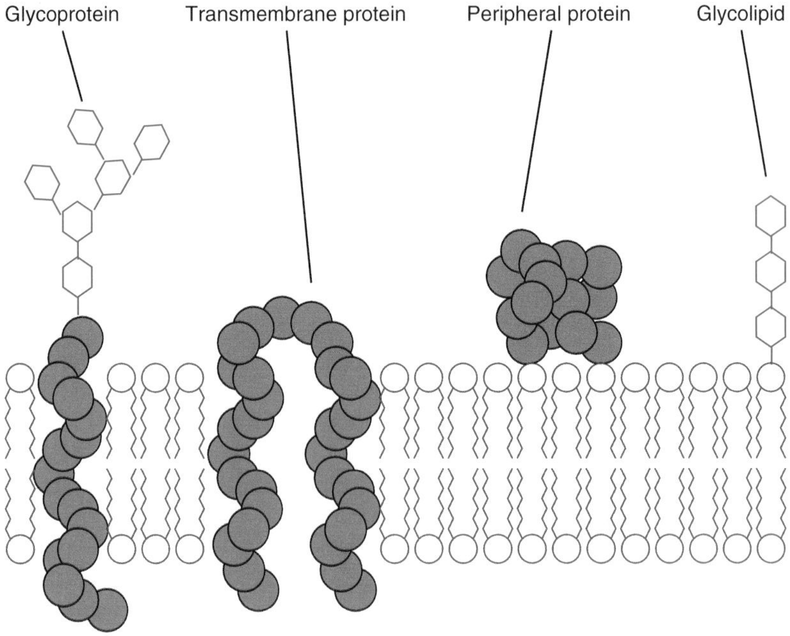
Glycoprotein
Transmembrane protein
Peripheral protein
Glycolipid

(**c**)

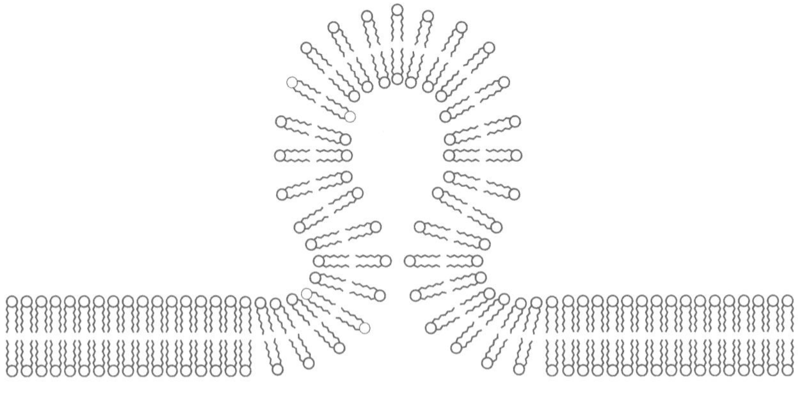

the fluid mosaic model and was introduced by Singer and Nicolson [5] (Figure 10.9(b)). Furthermore, they proposed a possible asymmetric arrangement of adjoining monolayers caused by different lipid composition and orientation of integral proteins, as well as specific occurrence of peripheral proteins in either of the monolayers. In the plasma membrane, for example, glycolipids always point to the exterior. While an exchange of lipid molecules between the two monolayers – a so-called flip-flop – very seldom occurs by mere chance, lateral movement of lipid molecules takes place frequently. This can also be observed with proteins as long as their movement is not prevented by interaction with other molecules. Lateral movement of lipids depends on the fluidity of the bilayer. The fluidity is strongly enhanced if one of the hydrocarbon chains of the phospholipids is unsaturated and the membrane contains a specific amount of cholesterol.

An important feature of biological membranes is their ability to form a cavity that pinches off as a spherical vesicle, and the reverse process in which the membrane of a vesicle fuses with another membrane and becomes a part of it (Figure 10.9(c)). This property is utilized by eukaryotic cells for vesicular transport between different intracellular compartments and for the exchange of substances with the exterior. The latter process is termed exocytosis when proteins produced by the cell are secreted to the exterior and endocytosis or phagocytosis when extracellular substances are taken up by the cell.

There are two different kinds of exocytoses. The first one is a constitutive secretion: synthetized proteins packed into transport vesicles at the Golgi complex move to the plasma membrane and fuse with it, thereby delivering their payload to the exterior. This happens, e.g., with proteins intended for the extracellular matrix. In the second case termed regulated exocytosis, the proteins coming from the Golgi complex via transport vesicles are enriched in secretory vesicles that deliver their content usually due to an external signal recognized by a receptor and further transmitted via second messengers (e.g., Ca^{2+}). This pathway is common, for example, to neurotransmitters secreted by neurons or digestive enzymes produced by ascinus cells of the pancreas.

Vesicular transport is important for large molecules like proteins. For smaller molecules (e.g., ions or glucose) there are alternative mechanisms. In the case of passive transport, the flux takes place along an osmotic or electrochemical concentration gradient and requires no expenditure of cellular energy. Therefore, either the molecules can diffuse through the membrane or, since especially polar and charged substances cannot pass this hydrophobic barrier, transport is mediated selectively by integral transmembrane proteins. Other transmembrane proteins enable an active transport against a concentration gradient that requires cellular energy (e.g., ATP).

Figure 10.9 (a) In a lipid bilayer, the amphipathic lipids are orientated to both aqueous compartments with their hydrophilic parts. The hydrophobic tails point to the inner membrane space. (b) The fluid mosaic model of a cellular membrane. (c) Formation of a spherical vesicle that is in the process of either pinching off from or fusing with a membrane. Such vesicles are formed during endo- or exocytosis by peripheral proteins inducing the process.

Sensing of exterior conditions and communication with other cells are often mediated by receptors of the cell membrane that tackle the signal transmission. Alternatively, mostly hydrophobic substances like steroid and thyroid hormones can cross the cell membrane directly and interact with receptors in the cell's interior. Signal transduction is discussed in more detail in Chapter 3. A general overview of biochemistry of signal transduction is given, e.g., in Krauss [6].

Besides the plasma membrane, plant cells are further surrounded by a cell wall with cellulose, a polysaccharide, as main polymer forming the fundamental scaffold. Prokaryotes also often have a cell wall where different monosaccharides act as building blocks for the polymer.

10.4.2 Nucleus

Prokaryotes store their hereditary information – their genome – in a single, circular, double-stranded DNA (located in a subregion of the cell's interior called the nucleoid) and optionally in one or several small, circular DNAs (the plasmids), which code for further genes. The genome of eukaryotes is located in the cell nucleus and forms the chromatin that is embedded into the nuclear matrix and has dense regions (heterochromatin) and less dense regions (euchromatin). The nucleus occupies about 10% of the cellular volume and is surrounded by the nuclear envelope formed by an extension of the ER that creates a double membrane. The nuclear envelope has several protein complexes that form nuclear pores and that are responsible for the traffic between the nucleus and the cytosol. A subregion of the chromatin in which many repeats of genes encoding ribosomal RNAs are located appears as a roughly spherical body called nucleolus.

The structure of the chromatin usually becomes optically clearer during cell division, when the DNA strands condense into chromosomes, each consisting of two DNA double strands called chromatids. Both chromatids are joined at the centromere. The ends of the chromatids are called telomeres. At the molecular level, the DNA of a chromosome is highly ordered: the double strand is wound around protein complexes, the histones; each DNA/histone complex is called a nucleosome.

10.4.3 Cytosol

The cytosol fills the space between the organelles of the cytoplasm. It represents about half of the cell volume and contains the cytoskeletal framework. This fibrous network consists of different protein filaments that constitute a general framework and are responsible for the coordination of cytoplasmatic movements. These activities are controlled by three major types of protein filaments: the actin filaments (also called microfilaments), the microtubules, and the intermediate filaments.

The long stretched actin filaments, with a diameter of about 5–7 nm, are built up of globular actin proteins. One major task of actin filaments is the generation of motility during muscle contraction. For the generation of movement, actin filaments slide along another filament type called myosin. This ATP-consuming process is driven by a coordinated interaction of these proteins. Together with other proteins involved in the regulation of muscle activity, these filaments form very regular structures in muscle cells. Furthermore, in many animal cells, actin filaments associated with other proteins are often located directly under the plasma membrane in the cell cortex and form a network that enables the cell to change its shape and to move.

Another filament type found in eukaryotes is the microtubles. They consist of heterodimers of the proteins α- and β-tubulin, which form unbranched cylinders of about 25 nm in diameter with a central open channel. These filaments are involved, e.g., in rapid motions of flagella and cilia, which are hair-like cell appendages. Flagella are responsible for the movement of, e.g., sperm and many single-celled eukaryotic protists. Cilia occur, for instance, on epithelial cells of the human respiratory system. The motion of a cilia or flagella is due to the bending of a complex internal structure called axoneme. Almost all kinds of cilia and eukaryotic flagella have nearly the same characteristic structure of the axoneme. This is called the $9 + 2$ structure because of its appearance: nine doublets that look like two condensed microtubles form a cylinder together with other associated proteins, the center of which contains two further single microtubles. The flexibility of the axoneme is also an ATP-consuming process that is further assisted by the protein dynein.

The third major filament type of the cytoskeleton is the intermediate filament. In contrast to actin filaments and microtubles, which are built of globular proteins, intermediate filaments consist of fibrous proteins. Several subtypes of these filaments are known, e.g., keratin filaments in the cytosol of epithelial cells, which make these cells resistant against mechanical influence, or lamin filaments, which are involved in the formation of the nuclear lamina.

Furthermore, the cytosol contains ribosomes responsible for protein synthesis (see Section 10.5.3), and it is filled with thousands of metabolic enzymes. A central metabolic pathway that is catalyzed by some of these enzymes is the glycolysis. Substrates of this pathway are glucose or some similar six-carbon derivatives of it. These substrates are converted by several reactions into two molecules of the three-carbon compound pyruvate. Each metabolized glucose molecule generates two molecules of ATP, and one NAD^+ (the oxidized form of nicotinamide adenine dinucleotide) is reduced to NADH. But via this pathway – which does not involve molecular oxygen – only a small amount of the energy that can be gained through oxidation of glucose is made available. In aerobic organisms, the bulk of ATP is produced from pyruvate in the mitochondria (see the following section).

10.4.4 Mitochondria

Mitochondria have a spherical or elongated shape and are about the size of a bacterium. Their interior is surrounded by two membranes: a highly permeable outer membrane and a selective inner membrane. Therefore, mitochondria have two internal compartments, the intermembrane space and the matrix. The outer membrane is permeable for ions and most of the small molecules due to several transmembrane channel proteins called porins. The inner membrane's surface area is strongly increased by numerous folds and tabular projections into the mitochondrial interior, which are called cristae. Mitochondria are partially autonomous: they possess their own DNA and enzymatic complexes required for protein expression (such as ribosomes and mRNA polymerase). Nevertheless, they depend on the symbiosis with their cell since most genes of mitochondrial proteins left the mitochondrial chromosome during evolution and are encoded by the nuclear DNA today. These mitochondrial proteins are synthesized in the cytoplasm and are later imported into the organelle.

As mentioned above, the bulk of ATP (34 out of 36 molecules per metabolized glucose molecule) is gained in mitochondria; thus, they can be termed the "power plants" of eukaryotic cells. The underlying oxidative process that involves molecular oxygen and yields CO_2 and ATP is driven mainly by pyruvate from the glycolysis and fatty acids. Both pyruvate and fatty acids can be converted into acetyl-CoA molecules. Acetyl-CoA has an acetyl group (CH_3CO^-, a two-carbon group consisting of a methyl group and a carbonyl group) that is covalently liked to coenzyme A (CoA). Cytosolic pyruvate can pass the outer mitochondrial membrane and enter the mitochondrial matrix via a transporter of the inner membrane. Pyruvate is then converted into acetyl-CoA by a huge enzyme complex called pyruvate dehydrogenase. Acetyl-CoA reacts with oxaloacetate and thus enters the citrate cycle, a sequence of several reactions during which two CO_2 molecules and energetic reduction equivalents (mainly NADH, but also $FADH_2$) are produced. Finally, oxaloacetate is regenerated and thus the cycle is closed. The electrons provided by the reduction equivalents are further transferred step by step onto O_2, which then reacts together with H^+ ions to form water. The huge amount of energy provided by this controlled oxyhydrogen reaction is used subsequently for the transfer of H^+ ions out of the mitochondrial matrix, thus establishing an H^+ gradient across the inner membrane. The energy provided by this very steep gradient is used by another protein complex of the inner mitochondrial membrane – the ATP synthetase – for the production of ATP inside the mitochondrial matrix by a flux of H^+ from the intermembrane space back into the matrix. This coupled process of an oxidation and phosphorylation is called the oxidative phosphorylation. The complete aerobic oxidation of glucose produces as many as 36 molecules of ATP:

$$C_6H_{12}O_6 + 6O_2 + 36P_i^- + 36ADP^{3-} + 36H^+ + 6CO_2 + 36ATP^{4-} + 42H_2O$$

10.4.5 Endoplasmatic Reticulum and Golgi Complex

The endoplasmatic reticulum (ER) is a widely spread cytosolic membrane system that forms tubular structures and flattened sacs. Its continuous and unbroken membrane encloses a lumen that stays in direct contact with the perinuclear space of the nuclear envelope. The ER occurs in two forms: the rough ER and the smooth ER. The rough ER forms mainly flattened sacs and has many ribosomes that are attached to its cytosolic surface; the smooth ER lacks ribosomes and forms mostly tubular structures. Secretory proteins and proteins for the ER itself, the Golgi complex, the lysosomes or the outer plasma membrane enter the lumen of the ER directly after being synthesized by ribosomes of the rough ER. The total amount of ER membranes of a cell as well as the ratio of smooth and rough ER varies strongly depending on species and cell type. All enzymes required for biosynthesis of membrane lipids, such as phosphatidylcholine, phosphatidylethanolamine, or phosphatidylinositol, are located in the ER membrane, their active centers facing the cytosol. Membrane lipids synthesized by these enzymes are integrated into the cytosolic part of the ER bilayer. Since this would result in an imbalance of lipids in the two layers of the membrane, phospholipid translocators can increase the flip-flop rate for specific membrane lipids; thus the lipid imbalance can be compensated and the membrane asymmetry concerning specific membrane lipids can be established. Furthermore, the ER can form transport vesicles responsible for the transfer of membrane substance and proteins to the Golgi complex.

The Golgi complex (also called Golgi apparatus), usually located in vicinity of the nucleus, consists of piles of several flat membrane cisternae. ER transport vesicles enter these piles at its *cis*-side. Substances leave the Golgi complex at the opposite *trans*-site. Transport between the different cisternae is mediated by Golgi vesicles. Some modifications of proteins by the addition of a specific oligosaccharide happen in the ER, but further glycosylations of various types take place in the lumen of the Golgi complex. Since such modified membrane proteins and lipids point to the organelles' inner space, they will be exposed to the cell's outer space when they are transported to the plasma membrane. The synthesis of complex modifications by several additions of carbohydrates requires a special enzyme for each specific addition. Therefore, these reaction pathways become very complex.

10.4.6 Other Organelles

Eukaryotic cells have further compartments for certain functions. Some of these organelles and their major functions will be mentioned briefly here.

Lysosomes are responsible for the intracellular digestion of macromolecules. These vesicular organelles contain several hydrolyzing enzymes (hydrolases), e.g., proteases, nucleases, glycosidases, lipases, phosphatases, and sulfatases. All of them have their optimal activity at pH 5. This pH value is maintained inside the lysosomes via ATP dependent H^+ pumps (for comparison, the pH of the cytosol is about 7.2).

Peroxisomes (also called microbodies) contain enzymes that oxidize organic substances (R) and use therefore molecular oxygen as an electron acceptor. This reaction produces hydrogen peroxide (H_2O_2).

$$RH_2 + O_2 \rightarrow R + H_2O_2.$$

H_2O_2 is used by peroxidase to further oxidize substances like phenols, amino acids, formaldehyde, and ethanol, or it is detoxified by catalase ($2H_2O_2 \rightarrow 2H_2O + O_2$).

In contrast to the ER, the Golgi-cisternae, lysosomes, peroxisomes, and vesicles, which are surrounded by a single membrane, chloroplasts, as well as mitochondria, have a double membrane of which the inner one is not folded into cristae as in mitochondria. Instead, a chloroplast has a third membrane that is folded several times and forms areas that look like piles of coins. This membrane contains light harvesting complexes and ATP synthases that utilize the energy of the sunlight for the production of cellular energy and reduction equivalents used for the fixation of carbon dioxide (CO_2) into sugars, amino acids, fatty acids, or starch. Chloroplasts, as well as mitochondria, have own circular DNA and ribosomes.

10.5
Expression of Genes

Classically, a gene is defined as the information encoded by the sequence of a DNA region that is required for the construction of an enzyme or – more generally – of a protein. We will see that this is a simplified definition, since, e.g., mature products of some genes are not proteins but RNAs with specific functions; eukaryotic gene sequences in particular also contain noncoding information. The term gene expression commonly refers to the whole process during which the information of a particular gene is translated into a particular protein. This process involves several steps. First, during transcription (Figure 10.10 ①, the DNA region encoding the gene is transcribed into a complementary messenger RNA (mRNA). In eukaryotic cells this mRNA is further modified ② inside the nucleus and transferred to the cytosol ③. In the cytosol, the mRNA binds to a ribosome that uses the sequence as a template for the synthesis of a specific polypeptide that can fold into the three-dimensional protein structure ④. In prokaryotic cells the mRNA is not further modified and ribosomes can bind to the nascent mRNA during transcription.

In eukaryotic cells the synthesized proteins can either remain in the cytosol ⑤ or, if they have a specific signaling sequence, be synthesized by ribosomes of the rough ER and enter its lumen ⑦. However, there are several mechanisms of directing each protein to its final destination. During this sorting ⑤–⑩, proteins are often modified, e.g., by cleavage of signaling peptides or by glycosylations.

All the genes of a single organism make up its genome. But only a subset of these genes will be expressed at a particular time or in a specific cell type. Some genes fulfill basic functions of the cell and are always required; these are called constitutive or housekeeping genes. Others are expressed only under certain conditions. The amount of a gene product, e.g., a protein, depends mainly on its stability and the number of its mRNA templates. The number of the latter depends on the transcription rate, which is influenced by regulatory regions of the gene and transcription factors that control the initialization of transcription. Thus, quantitative changes in gene expression can be monitored by mRNA and protein concentrations (see Chapter 11 on experimental techniques used for this purpose). Rate changes in any production or degradation step of a specific gene, which might happen in different cell types or developmental stages, can lead to differential gene expression.

The whole procedure of gene expression, protein sorting, and posttranslational modifications is summarized in Figure 10.10 and will be described in more detail in the following sections.

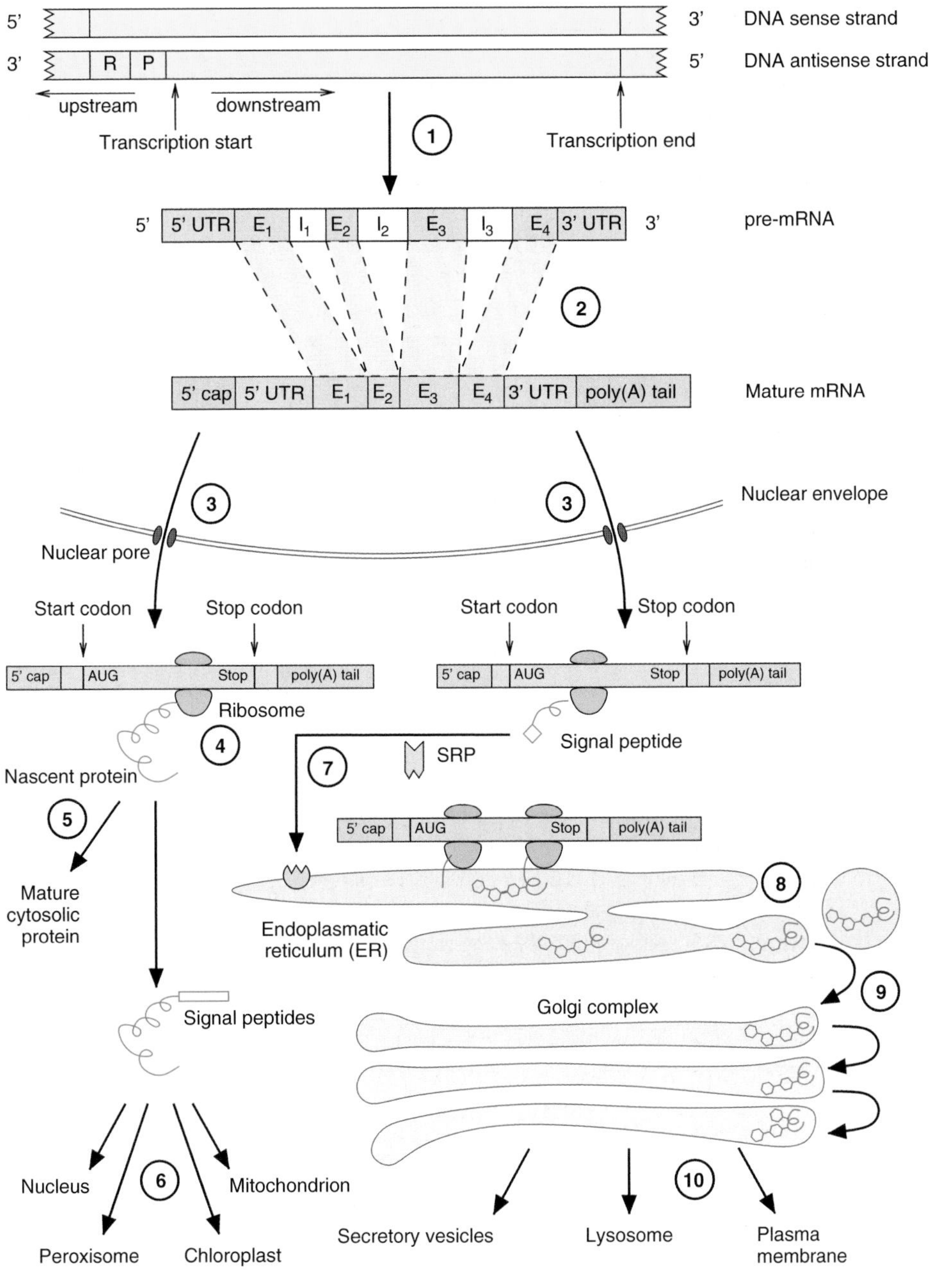

Figure 10.10 Gene expression in eukaryotic cells comprises several steps from the DNA to the mature protein at its final destination. This involves the ① transcription of the gene, ② splicing and processing of the pre-mRNA, ③ export of the mature mRNA into the cytosol, ④ translation of the genetic code into a protein, and ⑤–⑩ several steps of sorting and modification. More details are given in the text.

10.5.1 Transcription

The synthesis of an RNA polymer from ATP, GTP, CTP, and UTP employing a DNA region as a template is called transcription. RNA synthesis is catalyzed by the RNA polymerase. In eukaryotic cells there are different types of this enzyme that are responsible for the synthesis of different RNA types, including messenger RNA (mRNA), ribosomal RNA (rRNA), or transfer RNA (tRNA). In prokaryotic cells all these different RNA types are synthesized by the same polymerase. This enzyme has an affinity to a specific DNA sequence, the promoter, that also indicates the first base to be copied. During initiation of transcription, the RNA polymerase binds to the promoter with a high affinity that is supported by further initiation factors. Complete formation of the initiation complex causes the DNA to unwind in the promoter region. Now the enzyme is ready to add the first RNA nucleoside triphosphate to the template strand of the opened DNA double strand. In the subsequent elongation phase, the RNA polymerase moves along the unwinding DNA and extends the newly developing mRNA continuously with nucleotides complementary to the template strand. During this phase a moving transient double stranded RNA–DNA hybrid is established. As the polymerase moves along, the DNA rewinds again just behind it. As RNA synthesis always proceeds in the $5' \rightarrow 3'$ direction, only one of the DNA chains acts as template, the so-called antisense (−) strand. The other one, the sense (+) strand, has the same sequence as the transcribed RNA, except for the thymine nucleotides that are replaced by uracil nucleotides in RNA. As much as the promoter is responsible for initiation of transcription, the terminator – another specific DNA sequence – is responsible for its termination. For the bacterium *E. coli*, two different termination mechanisms are described: the Rho-independent and the Rho-dependent termination. In Rho-independent termination, the transcribed terminator region shows two short GC-rich and self-complementary sequences that can bind to each other and thus form a so-called hairpin structure. This motif is followed by a block of uracil residues that bind the complementary adenine residues of the DNA only weakly. Presumably, this RNA structure causes the RNA polymerase to terminate and release the RNA. In Rho-dependent termination, a protein – the Rho factor – can bind the newly synthesized RNA near the terminator and mediate the RNA release. Termination in eukaryotic cells shows both similarities to and differences from the mechanisms found in bacteria.

10.5.2 Processing of the mRNA

In eukaryotic cells the primary mRNA transcript (precursor mRNA or pre-mRNA) is further processed before being exported into the cytosol and entering translation (Figure 10.10 ②). The protein-coding sequence lies internally in the mRNA and is flanked on both sides by nucleotides that are not translated. During processing, a so-called 5′ cap is attached to the flanking 5′ untranslated region (5′ UTR, about 10 to 200 nucleotides) preceding, or lying upstream of, the coding sequence. This 5′ cap consists of three nucleotides that are further modified. The 3′ untranslated region (3′ UTR) of most mRNAs is also modified after transcription by addition of a series of about 30 to 200 adenine nucleotides that are known as the poly(A) tail. Furthermore, the pre-mRNA is often much longer than the mature RNA because the coding sequence is often interrupted by one or several intervening sequences called introns, which do not occur in the mature mRNA exported to the cytosol. These intron sequences are removed during processing by a mechanism called splicing. The remaining sequences are called exons. The final coding sequence thus consists of a series of exons joined together. It starts with AUG, which is the first triplet being translated into an amino acid, and it stops with a stop codon (UGA, UAA, or UAG). Via the pores of the nuclear envelope, the mature mRNA is finally exported to the cytoplasm, where the translation process takes place.

10.5.3 Translation

Translation of the genetic information encoded by the mRNA into the amino acid sequence of a polypeptide is done by ribosomes in the cytosol. To encode 20 different amino acids occurring in polypeptides, at least three bases out of the four possibilities (G, U, T, C) are necessary ($4^3 = 64 > 20$). During evolution a code developed that uses such triplets of exactly three bases, which are called codons, to code the amino acids and signals for start and end of translation. By using three bases for each codon, more than 20 amino acids can be coded, and hence some amino acids are encoded by more than one triplet. The genetic code is shown in Table 10.3. It is highly conserved across almost all prokaryotic and eukaryotic species except for some mitochondria or chloroplasts. For translation of the genetic information, adapter molecules are required. These are the transfer RNAs (tRNAs). They consist of about 80 nucleotides and are folded into a characteristic form similar to an "L." Each tRNA can recognize a specific codon by a complementary triplet, called an anticodon, and it can also bind the appropriate amino acid. For each specific tRNA, a certain enzyme (aminoacyl-tRNA synthetase) attaches the right amino acid to the tRNAs 3′ end. Such a loaded tRNA is called an aminoacyl-tRNA.

During translation (Figure 10.11), the genetic information of the mRNA is read codon by codon in the 5′ → 3′ direction of the mRNA, starting with an AUG codon. AUG codes for methionine, and therefore newly synthesized proteins always begin with this amino acid at their amino terminus. Protein biosynthesis is catalyzed by ribosomes. Both eukaryotic and prokaryotic ribosomes consist of a large and a small subunit, and both subunits are composed of several proteins and rRNAs. In eukaryotic cells, the small ribosomal subunit first associates with an initiation tRNA (Met-$tRNA_i$) and binds the mRNA at its 5′ cap. Once attached, the complex scans along the mRNA until reaching the start AUG codon. In most cases this is the first AUG codon in the 5′ → 3′ direction. This position indicates the translation start and determines the reading frame. Finally, during initiation the large ribosomal subunit is added to the complex and the ribosome becomes ready for protein synthesis. Each ribosome has three binding sites: one for the mRNA and

Table 10.3 The genetic code[a].

	Position 2				
Position 1 (5′ end)	**U**	**C**	**A**	**G**	**Position 3 (3′ end)**
	Phe	Ser	Tyr	Cys	U
U	Phe	Ser	Tyr	Cys	C
	Leu	Ser	Stop	Stop	A
	Leu	Ser	Stop	Trp	G
	Leu	Pro	His	Arg	U
C	Leu	Pro	His	Arg	C
	Leu	Pro	Gln	Arg	A
	Leu	Pro	Gln	Arg	G
	Ile	Thr	Asn	Ser	U
A	Ile	Thr	Asn	Ser	C
	Ile	Thr	Lys	Arg	A
	Met	Thr	Lys	Arg	G
	Val	Ala	Asp	Gly	U
G	Val	Ala	Asp	Gly	C
	Val	Ala	Glu	Gly	A
	Val	Ala	Glu	Gly	G

[a]Each codon of the genetic code – read in the 5′ → 3′ direction along the mRNA – encodes a specific amino acid or a starting or termination signal of translation.

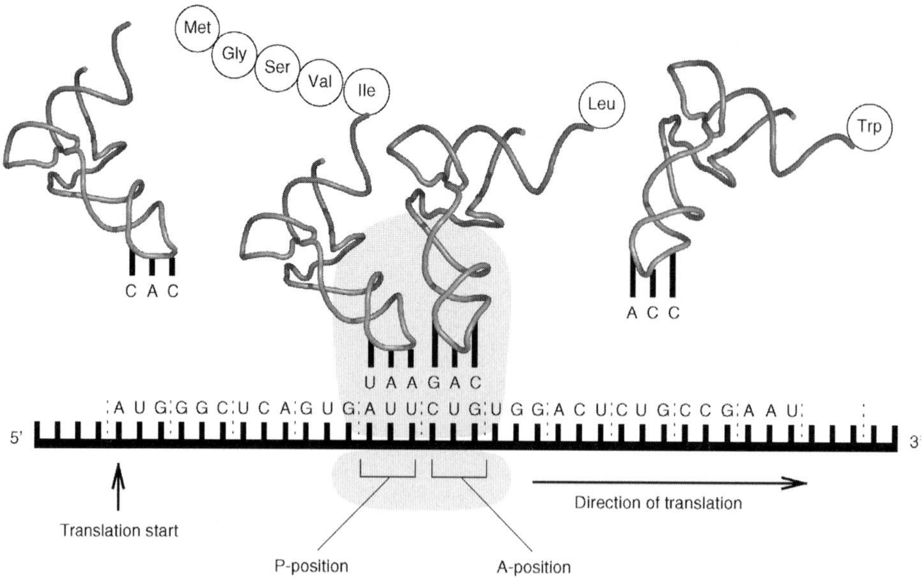

Figure 10.11 During translation, the genetic information of the mRNA is converted into the corresponding polypeptide. More details are given in the text.

two for tRNAs. In the beginning the first tRNA binding site, also called P site, contains the initiation tRNA. The second or A site is free to be occupied by an aminoacyl tRNA that carries an anticodon complementary to the second codon. Once the A site is filled, the amino acid at the P site, which is the methionine, establishes a peptide bond with the amino group of the amino acid at the A site. Now the unloaded tRNA leaves the P site, and the ribosome moves one codon further downstream. Thus, the tRNA carrying the dipeptide enters the P site and the A site is open for another aminoacyl tRNA, which is complementary to the third codon in sequence. This cycle is repeated until a stop codon (UAA, UAG, or UGA) is reached. Then the newly synthesized polypeptide detaches from the tRNA and the ribosome releases the mRNA. It is obvious that the addition or alteration of nucleotides of a gene can lead to changes in the reading frame or to the insertion of false amino acids, which might result in malfunctioning proteins. Such changes can happen by mutations, which are random changes of the genomic sequence of an organism that either occur spontaneously or are caused by chemical substances or radiation. A mutation can be either an exchange of a single nucleotide by another or some larger rearrangement. Even the exchange of a single nucleotide by another might severely influence the function of an enzyme, if it occurs, e.g., in the sequence coding for its active site.

10.5.4
Protein Sorting and Posttranslational Modifications

Cells possess a sorting and distribution system that routes newly synthesized proteins to their intra- or extracellular destination. This is mediated by signal peptides – short sequences of the polypeptide occurring at diverse positions. The sorting begins during translation when the polypeptide is synthesized either by a free ribosome or by one that becomes attached to the ER membrane. The latter occurs if the nascending polypeptide has a signal sequence at its amino terminus that can be recognized by a specific signal-recognition particle (SRP) that routes it to a receptor located in the ER membrane (Figure 10.10 ⑦). Such polypeptides are transferred into the ER lumen, where the signal peptide is cleaved off.

Peptides synthesized in the cytosol (Figure 10.10④) either remain in the cytosol (⑤), if not possessing a specific signal sequence, or are routed further to a mitochondrion, chloroplast, peroxisome, or the nucleus (⑥). The nuclear localization sequence (NLS) is usually located inside the primary sequence of the protein and is not found terminally; thus it is not cleaved from the protein as happens with many other signal peptides. Similarly, some transmembrane proteins synthesized by ribosomes of the rough ER have internal signal peptides that are required for correct routing to the membrane.

Polypeptides entering the ER after synthesis are usually further modified by glycosylations, where oligosaccharides are bound to specific positions of the newly synthesized proteins (⑧). Most proteins entering the ER do not remain in the ER but are transferred via transport vesicles to the Golgi complex (⑨), where further modifications of the bound oligosaccharids and additional glycosylations take place. If the proteins are not intended to remain in the Golgi complex, they are further transferred into lysosomes or secretory vesicles or they become transmembrane protein complexes of the plasma membrane (⑩).

10.5.5
Regulation of Gene Expression

The human genome presumably contains about 30,000–35,000 protein-coding genes, with an average coding length of about 1400 basepairs (bp) and an average genomic extend of about 30 kb (1 kb = 1,000 bp). This would mean that only about 1.5% of the human genomes consist of coding sequences and only one-third of the genome would be transcribed in genes [7,8]. Besides coding sequences also regulatory sequences are known, which play important roles, in particular through control of replication and transcription. The remaining noncoding genomic DNA, which does not yet appear to have any function, is often referred to as "junk DNA."

Since only a small subset of all the genes of an organism must be expressed in a specific cell (e.g., detoxification enzymes produced by liver cells are not expressed in epidermal cells), there must be regulatory mechanisms that repress or specifically induce the expression of genes. This includes mechanisms that control the level of gene expression.

In 1961, François Jacob and Jacques Monod proposed a first model for the regulation of the *lac* operon, a genetic region of the *E. coli* genome that codes for three genes required for the utilization of the sugar lactose by this bacterium. These genes are activated only when glucose is missing but lactose, as an alternative carbon source, is present in the medium. The transcription of the *lac* genes is under the control of a single promoter, which overlaps with a regulatory region laying downstream called operator to which a transcription factor, a repressor, can bind. Jacob and Monod introduced the term operon for such a polycistronic gene. (The term cistron is defined as the functional genetic unit within which two mutations cannot complement. The term is often used synonymous with gene and describes the region of DNA that encodes a single polypeptide [or functional RNA]. Thus, the term polycistronic refers to a DNA region encoding several polypeptides. Polycistronic genes are known only for prokaryotes.)

Besides the negative regulations or repressions mediated by a repressor, positive regulations or activations that are controlled by activators are also known. An activator found in *E. coli* that is also involved in the catabolism of alternative carbon sources is the catabolite activator protein (CAP). Since the promoter sequence of the *lac* operon shows only low agreement to the consensus sequence of normal *E. coli* promoters, the RNA polymerase has only a weak affinity to it. (The consensus sequence of a promoter is a sequence pattern that shows highest sequence similarity to all promoter sequences to which a specific RNA polymerase can bind.) The presence of CAP, which indicates the lack of glucose, enhances the binding affinity of RNA polymerase to the *lac* promoter and thus supports the initiation of transcription.

The regulation of gene expression in eukaryotic cells is more complicated than that in prokaryotic cells. In contrast to the bacterial RNA polymerase that recognizes specific DNA sequences, the eukaryotic enzymes require a protein/DNA complex that is established by general transcription factors. One of these transcription factors (TFIIB) binds the so-called TATA box – a promoter sequence occurring in most protein-coding genes with the consensus sequence TATAAA. Besides these general transcription factor-binding sites, most genes are further regulated by a combination of sequence elements lying in the vicinity of the promoter and enhancer sequence elements located up to 1000 nucleotides or more upstream of the promoter.

Regulation of gene expression is not only carried out by transcriptional control but can also be controlled during processing and export of the mRNA into the cytosol, by the translation rate, by the decay rates of the mRNA and the protein, and by control of the protein activity.

Exercises and Problems

1. What are the different structures and conformations a protein can have and by which properties is the protein conformation defined?
2. Why is it necessary that the protein sequences are encoded in the DNA by nucleotide triplets and not by nucleotide duplets?
3. Why are proteins of thermophilic bacteria not rapidly denatured by the high temperatures these organisms are exposed to?
4. What is the purpose of posttranslational modifications? List six functional groups that are used for posttranslational modifications.
5. What is the purpose of introns and why do eukaryotes have introns but prokaryotes do not?
6. What is the benefit of cellular compartments?
7. Why do most transmembrane proteins have their N-terminus outside and the C-terminus inside?
8. If a eukaryotic cell has lost all its mitochondria (lets say during mitosis one daughter cell got none), how long does it take to regrow them?

References

1 Alberts, B. *et al.* (2008) *Molecular Biology of the Cell,* 5th edn, Garland Science, UK.

2 Campbell, N.A. and Reece, J.B. (2007) *Biology,* 8th edn, Benjamin Cummings, New York.

3 Miller, S.L. and Urey, H.C. (1959) Organic compound synthesis on the primitive earth. *Science,* **130**, 245–251.

4 Wächtershäuser, G. (1988) Before enzymes and templates: theory of surface metabolism. *Microbiological Reviews,* **52**, 452–484.

5 Singer, S.J. and Nicolson, G.L. (1972) The fluid mosaic model of the structure of cell membranes. *Science,* **175**, 720–731.

6 Krauss, G. (2003) *Biochemistry of Signal Transduction and Regulation,* 3rd edn, Wiley-VCH, Weinheim.

7 Lander, E.S. *et al.* (2001a) Initial sequencing and analysis of the human genome. *Nature,* **409**, 860–921.

8 Venter, J.C. *et al.* (2001b) The sequence of the human genome. *Science,* **291**, 1304–1351.

11
Experimental Techniques in Molecular Biology

Summary

The development of experimental techniques for the purification, amplification, and investigation of biologically relevant molecules is of crucial importance for our understanding how living cells and organisms work.

With the discovery of restriction endonucleases and ligases in the 1960s and 1970s, it was possible to cut DNA at specific positions and join pieces together in new combinations. Since then, a large collection of methods has been developed to manipulate DNA in almost arbitrary ways. With the help of the polymerase chain reaction (PCR) and cloning vectors, pieces of DNA can be amplified billion-fold and capillary electrophoresis combined with fluorescence detection makes high-throughput sequencing possible.

The separation and analysis of mixtures of proteins is also of great importance, and the researcher can nowadays choose from a diverse variety of gel and chromatographic techniques. A technologically very advanced and demanding method for the identification of peptides and proteins is mass spectrometry (MS). Using a database approach, it is possible to identify known proteins and also to characterize posttranslational modifications.

An important driving force of current developments is miniaturization, leading to high-throughput methods. Prominent representatives of this approach are DNA and protein chips. DNA microarrays allow us to simultaneously measure the expression of thousands of different genes, and protein chips can be used to study interactions of proteins with antibodies, other proteins, DNA, or small molecules. Large numbers of transcription factor (TF) binding sites can be measured *in vivo* using ChIP-on-Chip and also binding constants can be obtained in a semi-high-throughput fashion using the surface plasmon resonance (SPR) technique.

Systems Biology: A Textbook. Edda Klipp, Wolfram Liebermeister, Christoph Wierling, Axel Kowald, Hans Lehrach, and Ralf Herwig

ISBN: 978-3-527-31874-2

11.1
Introduction

In this chapter, we will give a brief description of the experimental techniques used in modern molecular biology. In the same way that Chapters 10 and 12 are only introductions into biology and mathematics, this chapter is only an introduction into the large arsenal of experimental techniques that are used and is not meant to be a comprehensive overview. We felt, however, that for readers without experimental background, it might be interesting and helpful to get a basic idea of the techniques that are used to actually acquire the immense biological knowledge that is nowadays available. A basic understanding of the techniques is also indispensable for understanding experimental scientific publications or simply discussing experiments with colleagues.

The order in which the different techniques are presented corresponds roughly to their historical appearance and complexity. Some of these techniques are of special interest, because they are able to generate large quantities of data (high-throughput techniques) that can be used for quantitative modeling in systems biology.

11.2
Restriction Enzymes and Gel Electrophoresis

We have seen in Chapter 10 that the genes, which code for the proteins of a cell, are all located on very long pieces of DNA, the chromosomes. To isolate individual genes, it is, therefore, necessary to break up the DNA and isolate the fragment of interest. However, until the early 1970s, this was a very difficult task. DNA consists only of four different nucleotides, making it a very homogeneous and monotonous molecule. In principle, the DNA can be broken into smaller pieces by mechanical shear stress. However, this results in random fragments, which are not useful for further processing.

This situation began to change when the first restriction endonucleases were isolated from bacteria at the end of the 1960s. These enzymes recognize specific short sequences of DNA and cut the molecule only at these positions (type II restriction enzymes). Restriction enzymes are part of a bacterial defense system against bacteriophages (prokaryote-specific viruses). The recognition sequences are typically between 4 and 8 bp long. Methylases form the second part of this defense system. They modify DNA molecules at specific sequences by adding methyl groups to the nucleotides of the target sequence. The DNA of the bacterium is methylated by the methylase, and this protects it against the nuclease activity of the restriction enzyme. But the DNA of a phage that enters the cell is not methylated and hence degraded by the restriction enzyme.

Most restriction enzymes cut the double helix in one of three different ways, as depicted by Figure 11.1. Some produce blunt ends, but others cut the DNA in a staggered way resulting in short stretches (here 4 bp) of single-stranded DNA, called sticky ends. Sometimes the cutting site is some distance away from the recognition

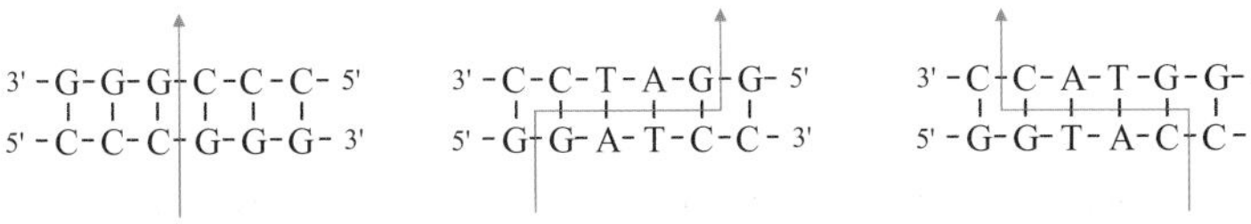

Figure 11.1 Restriction enzymes recognize short stretches of DNA that often have a palindromic structure. The enzyme then cuts the DNA in one of three different ways producing either blunt ends or sticky ends. This behavior is shown here for the type II enzymes Sma I, Bam HI, and Kpn I. The red line indicates where the enzymes cut the double helix.

site (18 bp in case of MmeI), which is the basis for recent experimental techniques (see Section 11.12).

Restriction enzymes generate reproducibly specific fragments from large DNA molecules. This is a very important advantage over the random fragments that can be generated by shear forces. If the restriction fragments that result from an enzymatic digestion are separated according to size, they form a specific pattern, which represents a fingerprint of the digested DNA. Changes of this fingerprint indicate that the number or position of the recognition sites of the used restriction enzyme has changed. Restriction enzyme patterns can, therefore, be used to characterize mutational changes or to compare orthologous genes from different organisms.

The size separation of digested DNA is also a prerequisite to isolate clone-specific fragments. If the sequence of the DNA is known, the number and size of the restriction fragments for a given restriction enzyme can be predicted. By choosing the right enzyme from the large number of available restriction enzymes, it is often possible to produce a fragment that contains the gene, or region of DNA, of interest. This fragment can then be separated from the others and cloned into a vector (see Section 11.3) for further investigation.

Electrophoresis is one of the most convenient and most often used methods of molecular genetics to separate molecules that differ in size or charge. Many different forms of electrophoresis exist, but they all work by applying an electrical field to the charged molecules. Since each nucleotide of DNA (or RNA) carries a negative charge, nucleic acids move from the anode to the cathode. The separation is carried out in a gel matrix to prevent convection currents and present a barrier to the moving molecules, which causes a sieving effect. Size, charge, and shape of the molecules decide how fast they move through the gel. Generally it holds that the smaller the molecule, the faster it moves. For a typical restriction fragment, which is between 0.5 and 20 kb, agarose gels are used. Agarose is a linear polysaccharide that is extracted from seaweed. For DNA fragments smaller than 500 bp, agarose gels are not suited. In this case, polyacrylamide gels are used that have smaller pores. For such small molecules, size differences of a single basepair can be detected. Another problem represent very large DNA molecules that are completely retarded by the gel matrix. Those fragments are not separated by the usual type of electrophoresis. In this case, a special form of electrophoresis, the so-called pulse-field electrophoresis,

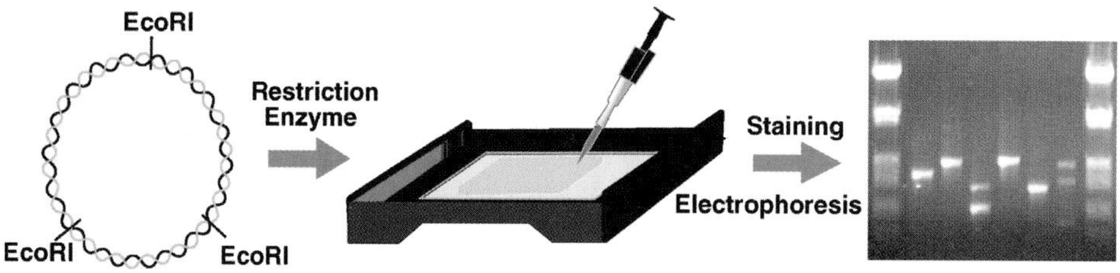

Figure 11.2 Agarose gel electrophoresis of DNA restriction fragments. A plasmid containing several recognition sites for a restriction enzyme (here Eco RI) is digested with the enzyme and the resulting fragments are placed on an agarose gel (middle). An applied electrical field moves the charged molecules through the gel (here from top to bottom) and separates them according to size. After staining, the individual fragments appear under UV light as bright bands (right). Courtesy of Dr. P. Weingarten, Protagen AG.

can be used, which allows the separation of DNA molecules of up to 10^7 bp. This technique varies the direction of the electric field periodically so that the molecules follow a zigzag path through the gel. Very long DNA fragments move head-on through the gel, which results in a velocity that is independent of size. Because of the oscillating field, the molecules have to reorientate themselves. This is easier for the smaller fragments so that the larger ones lag behind. A typical application of this technique is the separation of whole chromosomes of microorganisms (mammalian chromosomes are even too large for this technique).

Whatever type of electrophoresis or gel is used, the DNA is invisible unless it is especially labeled or stained. A commonly used dye for staining is ethidiumbromide that intercalates between DNA bases. In the intercalated state, ethidium exposed to UV light is fluorescing in a bright orange.

Figure 11.2 sketches the different processing steps from the DNA to the size-separated restriction fragments on an agarose gel. On the gel (right part Figure 11.2), different lanes can be seen, where different DNA probes are separated in parallel. The concentrated solution of DNA fragments is filled in the pockets at the top of the gel and the fragments migrate during electrophoresis to the bottom. The smallest fragments move fastest and appear at the bottom of the gel. The lanes on the left and right side contain fragments of known length that serve as size markers.

11.3
Cloning Vectors and DNA Libraries

In the last section, we discussed how restriction enzymes generate DNA fragments by cutting the DNA at short, specific recognition sites. In this section, we will see how the generated fragments can be used to generate billions of identical copies (clones).

For the actual cloning (amplification) step, a restriction fragment has to be inserted into a self-replicating genetic element. This can, for instance, be a virus or a plasmid. Plasmids are small circular rings of DNA that occur naturally in many bacteria. They often carry a few genes for resistance to antibiotics or to enable the degradation of

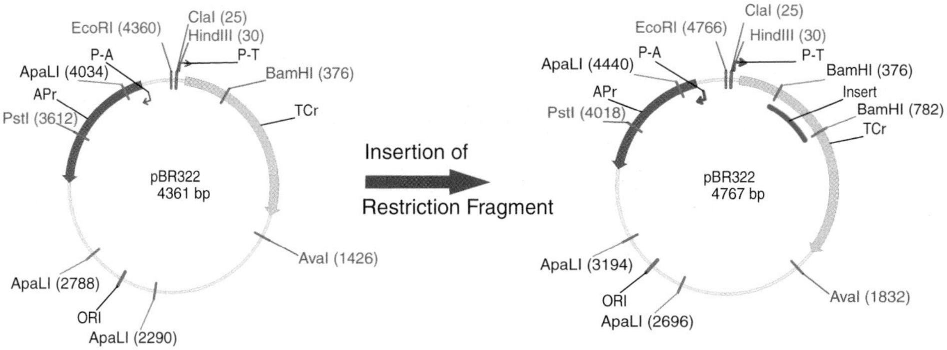

Figure 11.3 pBR322 is a circular plasmid of 4.3 kb that is often used as cloning vector. The diagram on the left shows several important genetic elements of the plasmid. *ORI* marks a region of DNA that controls the replication of the plasmid. It is the origin of replication. The boxes represent genes that confer resistance to the plasmid for the antibiotics ampicillin (APr) and tetracycline (TCr). P-A and P-R are the promoters of the resistance genes and the lines and text mark recognition sites for the corresponding restriction enzyme. The right part shows pBR322 after a restriction fragment has been inserted into the Bam HI restriction site.

unusual carbon sources and are normally only a few thousand basepairs long (Figure 11.3). Genetic elements that are used in the laboratory to amplify DNA fragments of interest are called cloning vectors, and the amplified DNA is said to be cloned. In the following, we will concentrate on the use of plasmids as vectors. The actual insertion process requires that the DNA to be cloned and the vector are being cut with the same restriction enzyme and that the vector has only one recognition site for this enzyme. That gives a linearized plasmid that has the same type of sticky ends as the DNA that is to be cloned. If the linearized vector and the digested DNA are now mixed at the right concentration and temperature, the complementary sticky ends basepair and form a new recombinant DNA molecule. Initially, the resulting molecule is only held together by hydrogen bonds. This is made permanent using the enzyme DNA ligase that forms covalent bonds between the phosphodiester backbones of the DNA molecules. This procedure enables the combination of DNA from arbitrary sources.

Finally, the vector is introduced into bacterial cells, which are then grown in culture. Every time the bacteria double (approx. every 30 min), the recombinant plasmids also double. Each milliliter of the growth medium can finally contain up to 10^7 bacteria! The actual process of introducing the vector into the bacteria is called transformation. For this end, the cells are especially treated so that they are temporarily permeable for the DNA molecules.

But loss occurs at all steps of this genetic engineering. Not all vector molecules will have received an insert, because it is possible that the sticky ends of some vectors self-ligate without insert. Furthermore, not all bacteria used in the transformation step will have received a vector molecule. It can, therefore, be that there is only a small proportion of cells that contain a vector with insert in the growing cell population. Normally, selection markers are used to cope with this problem. Figure 11.3 shows pBR322, a typical cloning vector. Apart from a DNA sequence that enables the cell machinery to replicate the plasmid (ori), it also contains two genes for resistance against the antibiotics ampicillin and tetracycline. If the DNA fragment is cloned into a restriction site that lies within one of the resistance genes, for instance the Bam HI site, simple selection steps can be used to end up with cells that contain the desired construct. For this purpose, the bacteria are grown in a medium that contains ampicillin so that only cells carrying the plasmid can survive. The next step is more complicated since we are interested in all those bacteria that contain a vector with a nonfunctional tetracycline gene (caused by an insert). The cells are plated in high dilution on the surface of an agar plate, where each individual cell forms a colony. After the colonies become visible, some bacteria of each colony are copied onto a second agar plate by a stamping technique (which preserves the spatial arrangement of colonies). This second plate contains tetracycline and so only those cells with intact resistance gene can grow. By comparing the colony pattern of the two plates, it is now possible to identify those colonies that exist on the first plate, but not on the second. These are the colonies that we are interested in.

Unfortunately, there is an upper size limit for the DNA one can clone into a plasmid vector. Above 10 kb, the cloning efficiency declines so much that other vectors are required. Lambda is a linear bacteriophage of approx. 48 kb, and up to 20 kb of the original phage DNA can be replaced by foreign DNA. Cosmids are artificial constructs that combine some features of the phage lambda and of classical plasmids. The advantage is that fragments up to 45 kb can be cloned. For really large fragments of up to one million basepairs, yeast artificial chromosomes (YACs) have been developed [1], which are now gradually replaced by bacterial artificial chromosomes (BACs) [2]. BACs are based on the naturally occurring F-plasmid, which itself is around 100 kb in length. While the copy number per cell of most of the smaller plasmids is rather large, the F-plasmid and the derived BACs are maintained at only one to two copies per cell. This reduces the risk of unwanted recombination events between different copies and contributes to the stability of such large inserts.

Since the average fragment size of restriction enzymes is much smaller than 1 Mb, the enzyme reaction is only allowed to proceed for a very short time. This time is not long enough to cut all recognition sites and, therefore, the resulting fragments are much longer. This technique is called a partial digest.

So far we have discussed the situation where we wanted to clone a specific fragment after a restriction digest. The DNA was separated on an agarose gel, and the desired fragment was excised from the gel and cloned into an appropriate vector. However, often the situation is different insofar that we do not know in advance the fragment that contains our gene of interest. In this case, we can construct a DNA library by simply cloning all fragments that result from a digest into vectors. Such a library is maintained in a population of bacteria that contain vectors with many different inserts. Bacteria with different inserts are either kept together or are separated so that the library consists of thousands of clones (each kept in a separate plastic tube) each carrying a specific fragment. This is for instance important for the construction of DNA chips (see Section 11.7). This strategy is also known as shotgun cloning.

There are two basic types of DNA libraries that are extensively used in molecular genetics. The first type is genomic DNA libraries that were described in the last section. They are directly created from the genetic material of an organism. But restriction enzymes cut DNA irrespective of the start and end points of genes, and hence there is no guarantee that the gene of interest does completely fit on a single clone. Furthermore, in Chapter 10 we have seen that the genome of most higher organisms contains large amounts of junk DNA. These sequences also end up in the genomic DNA library, which is not desired.

A different type of library, the cDNA library, circumvents these problems. This technique does not use DNA as source material, but starts from the mRNA pool of the cells or tissue of interest. The trick is that the mRNA molecules are a copy of exactly those parts of the genome that are normally the most interesting. They represent the coding regions of the genes and contain neither introns nor intergene junk DNA. Using the enzyme reverse transcriptase that exists in some viruses, mRNA can be converted into cDNA. The resulting DNA is called complementary DNA (cDNA) because it is complementary to the mRNA. cDNA libraries are different from genomic libraries in several important points: (i) they contain only coding regions, (ii) they are tissue-specific since they represent a snapshot of the current gene expression pattern, and (iii) because they are an image of the expression pattern, the frequency of specific clones in the library is an indicator of the expression level of the corresponding gene. cDNA libraries have many different applications. By sequencing cDNA libraries, it is possible to experimentally determine the intron–exon boundaries of eukaryotic genes. Constructing cDNA libraries from different tissues helps to understand which genes are expressed in which parts of the body. A derivative of the cDNA library is the expression library. This type of library is constructed in such a way that it contains a strong promoter in front of the cloned cDNAs. This makes it possible not only to amplify the DNA of interest, but also to synthesize the protein that is encoded by this DNA insert.

11.4
1D and 2D Protein Gels

The basic principle of electrophoresis works for all charged molecules. That means not only nucleic acids, but also other kinds of cellular macromolecules, like proteins, can be separated by electrophoresis. But the distribution of charges in a typical protein is quite different from the distribution in nucleic acids. DNA molecules carry a negative charge that is proportional to the length of the DNA, since the overall charge is controlled by the phosphodiester backbone. The net charge of proteins, however, varies from protein to protein, since it depends on the amount and type of charged amino acids that are incorporated into the polypeptide chain. If proteins are separated in this native form, their velocity is controlled by a function of charge, size, and shape that is difficult to predict.

It was a major improvement when Shapiro *et al.* [3] introduced the detergent sodium dodecylsulfat (SDS) to protein electrophoresis. SDS has a hydrophilic sulfate group and a hydrophobic part that binds to the hydrophobic backbone of polypeptides. This has important consequences: (i) the negative charge of the protein–detergent complex is now proportional to the protein size because the number of SDS molecules that bind to a protein is proportional to the number of its amino acids, (ii) all proteins denature and adopt a linear conformation, and (iii) even very hydrophobic, normally insoluble, proteins can be separated by gel electrophoresis. Under those conditions, the separation of proteins is reduced to a function of their size, as in the case of nucleic acids.

For proteins, a different gel matrix is used than for nucleic acids. Acrylamide monomers are polymerized to give a polyacrylamide gel. During the polymerization step, the degree of cross-linking and thus the pore size of the network can be controlled to be optimal for the size range of interest. Over the past years, SDS polyacrylamide gel electrophoresis (SDS-PAGE) has become an easy-to-use standard technique for separating proteins by size. As in the case of DNA, the gel has to be stained to make the protein bands visible (for instance using coomassie blue or silver staining). Figure 11.4(a) sketches the basic steps required for SDS-PAGE. In this example, the right lane contains protein size markers (large proteins at top, small ones at the bottom) and the other lanes different samples of interest.

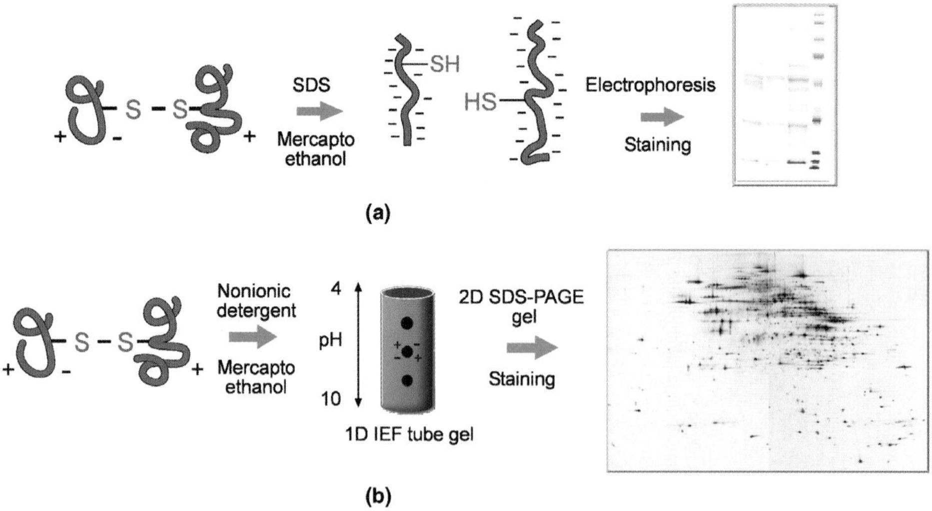

Figure 11.4 (a) *SDS-PAGE*: Native proteins are treated with the negatively charged detergent SDS and the reducing agent mercapto ethanol to break up disulfide bridges and unfold the protein. After this treatment, even extremely hydrophobic proteins can be separated on a polyacrylamide gel according to their size. Courtesy of Dr. P. Weingarten, Protagen AG. (b) *2D Gel Electrophoresis*: For the first dimension, proteins are separated in a tube gel according to their isoelectric point. To preserve the native charge of the proteins, a nonionic detergent is used to unfold the polypeptides. For the second dimension, the tube gel is placed on top of a standard SDS-PAGE slab gel and the proteins are now separated by size. Up to 2000 proteins can be separated with this technique. Courtesy of Dr. L. Mao & Prof. J. Klose, Charité Berlin.

On the gel shown in Figure 11.4(a), only a few protein bands can be seen. This will be the case after several protein purification steps. However, a cell or subcellular fraction contains hundreds or thousands of different proteins. If such a mixture is used for SDS-PAGE, individual bands overlap and proteins cannot be separated clearly. The solution to this problem is the two-dimensional (2D) polyacrylamide gel electrophoresis [4]. The idea is to separate the proteins in a second dimension according to a property different than size.

Isoelectric focusing (IEF) is such a separation technique. The net charge of a protein depends on the number of charged amino acids, but also on the pH of the medium. At a very low pH, the carboxy groups of aspartate and glutamate are uncharged ($-COOH$), while the amino groups of lysine and arginine are fully ionized ($-NH_3^+$), conferring a positive net charge to the protein. At a very basic pH, by contrast, the carboxy groups are charged ($-COO^-$) and the amino groups are neutral ($-NH_2$), resulting in a negative net charge. Accordingly, for each protein, there exists a pH that results in an equal amount of negative and positive charges. This is the isoelectric point of the protein where it has no net charge. For IEE, the proteins are treated with a nonionic detergent so that the proteins unfold, but retain their native charge distribution (Figure 11.4(b)). Then they are placed onto a rodlike tube gel, which has been prepared such that it has a pH gradient from one end to the other. After a voltage is applied, the proteins travel until they reach the pH that corresponds to their isoelectric point.

For the second dimension, the tube gel is soaked in SDS and then placed on top of a normal SDS slab gel. A voltage is applied perpendicular to the direction of the first dimension and the proteins are now separated according to size. The result is a 2D distribution of proteins in the gel as shown in Figure 11.4(b).

Difference gel electrophoresis (DIGE) is a recently developed variation of this technique that makes 2D gels available for high-throughput experiments [5]. Before the protein samples are separated electrophoretically, they are labeled with fluorescent dyes. Up to three samples are marked with different dyes and the total mixture is then separated on one 2D gel. Three different images are generated from this gel by using different, dye-specific, excitation wavelengths for the scanning process. This approach ensures that identical protein species from the different samples are located at the same gel position, avoiding the error-prone spot matching step that is necessary when comparing two different 2D gels.

11.5
Hybridization and Blotting Techniques

Hybridization techniques are based on the specific recognition of a probe and target molecule. The aim is to use such techniques to detect and visualize only those molecules in a complex mixture that are of interest to the researcher. The basepairing of complementary single-stranded nucleic acids is the source of specificity for Southern Blotting, Northern Blotting, and *in situ* hybridization, which are described in the following sections. A short fragment of DNA, the probe, is labeled in such a way that it can later easily be visualized. Originally, radioactive labeling has been used, but in recent years, it is often been replaced by fluorescent labels. The probe is incubated with the target sample and after the recognition of probe and target molecules is completed, the location of the probe shows the location and existence of the sought for target molecule. In principle, 16 nucleotides are sufficient to ensure that the sequence is unique in a typical mammalian genome ($4^{16} \approx 4.29 \times 10^9$), but in practice much longer probes are used. The Western Blot is not a hybridization technique, since it is not based on the formation of double-stranded DNA, RNA, or DNA/RNA hybrids by complementary basepairing. Instead, it is based on the specific interaction between antibody and antigen.

11.5.1
Southern Blotting

The technique of Southern Blotting is used to analyze complex DNA mixtures [6]. Normally, the target DNA is digested by restriction enzymes and separated by gel electrophoresis. If the DNA is of genomic origin, the number of resulting fragments will be so large that no individual bands are visible. If we are interested in a certain gene and know its sequence, small DNA fragments can be synthesized, which are complementary to the gene. However, before the actual hybridization step, the digested DNA has to be transferred from the gel onto the surface of a nitrocellulose or nylon membrane so that the DNA molecules are accessible for hybridization. This is achieved with the help of a blotting apparatus, as shown in Figure 11.5. Originally the transfer was achieved by placing the nitrocellulose filter between the gel and a stack of blotting paper. Capillary forces lead to a flow of water and DNA fragments from the gel into the blotting paper. On this way, the DNA gets trapped by a nitrocellulose or nylon filter. Nowadays, more sophisticated blotting machines are used that transfer the DNA by applying a voltage across the gel and membrane. Once the DNA is blotted, the membrane is placed into a plastic bag and incubated

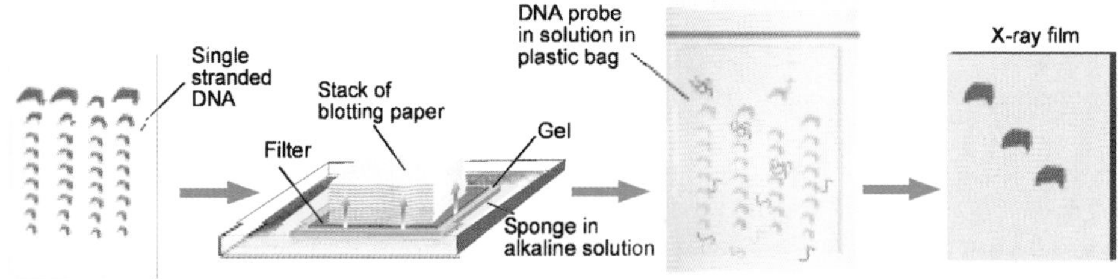

Figure 11.5 Elementary steps required for Southern Blotting. Following gel electrophoresis, the DNA fragments are treated with an alkaline solution to make them single stranded. The nitrocellulose or nylon membrane is sandwiched between the gel and a stack of blotting paper, and the DNA is transferred onto the membrane through capillary forces. Finally, the membrane is incubated with the labeled DNA probe (here radioactive labeling) and the bands are then visualized by X-ray film exposure. Courtesy of Dr. P. Weingarten, Protagen AG.

for several hours with a solution containing the labeled DNA probe. In case of a radioactive label, the membrane is finally placed against an X-ray film. The radioactive DNA fragments expose the film and form black bands that indicate the location of the target DNA.

With this technique, the presence of the gene of interest can be tested, but also modifications of the gene structure (in case of a mutation) can be studied. By performing several Southern Blots with DNA probes that correspond to different regions of the gene, modifications like deletions and insertions can be detected. Point mutations, however, cannot be identified with Southern Blotting.

11.5.2 Northern Blotting

Northern Blotting is very similar to Southern Blotting. The only difference is that here mRNA is used for blotting, not DNA. Although the experimental technique is very similar, Northern Blotting can be used to answer different questions than Southern Blotting. Even though mRNA is only an intermediate product on the way from the gene to the protein, it is normally a reasonable assumption that the amount of mRNA is correlated to the amount of the corresponding protein in the cell. Northern hybridization is, therefore, not only used to verify the existence of a specific mRNA, but also to estimate the amount of the corresponding protein via the amount of mRNA. Since the expression profile of genes varies among tissues, Northern Blotting gives different results for different organs in contrast to Southern Blotting, which is based on genomic DNA.

11.5.3 Western Blotting

So far we have seen techniques for blotting different types of nucleic acids. The same type of technique exists for proteins, called Western Blot. Depending on the problem at hand, 1D or 2D protein gels can be used for blotting. It is more difficult to obtain specific probes for proteins than for nucleic acids. Apart from special cases, antibodies are used that are directed against the desired protein.

Once the proteins are transferred to the nitrocellulose membrane, they are incubated with the primary antibody. In a further step, the membrane is incubated with the so-called secondary antibody, which is an antibody against the primary antibody. If the primary antibody was obtained by immunizing a rabbit, the secondary antibody could be a goat-anti-rabbit antibody. This is an antibody from a goat, which recognizes all rabbit antibodies. The secondary antibody is chemically linked to an enzyme, like horseradish peroxidase that catalyzes a chemiluminescence reaction, and exposure of an X-ray film finally produces bands, indicating the location of the protein–antibody complex. The intensity of the band is proportional to the amount of protein. The secondary antibody serves as signal amplification step.

11.5.4 *In Situ* Hybridization

The described blotting and hybridization techniques are applied to mixtures of nucleic acids or proteins that have been extracted from cells or tissues. During this process, all information about the spatial location is lost. *In situ* hybridization avoids this problem by applying DNA probes directly to cells or tissue slices.

One common application is the location of specific genes on chromosomes. For this purpose, metaphase chromosomes, which have been exposed to a high pH to separate the double strands, are incubated with labeled DNA probes. This makes it possible to directly see where and how many copies of the gene are located on the chromosome. If the label is a fluorescent dye, the technique is called fluorescent *in situ* hybridization (FISH). Not only chromosomes but also slices of whole tissues and organisms can be hybridized to DNA probes. This can be used to study the spatial and temporal expression pattern of genes by using probes specific to certain mRNAs. This method is often used to study gene expression patterns during embryogenesis. Immunostaining, finally, uses antibodies to localize proteins within cells. Knowledge about the subcellular localization often helps to better understand the functioning or lack of functioning of the studied proteins.

11.6 Further Protein Separation Techniques

11.6.1 Centrifugation

One of the oldest techniques for the separation of cell components is centrifugation. This technique fractionates molecules (and larger objects) according to a combination of size and shape. However, in general it is true that the larger the object, the faster it moves to the bottom. A typical low-speed centrifugation collects cell fragments and nuclei in the pellet, at medium speeds cell organelles and ribosomes are collected, and at ultrahigh speeds even typical enzymes end up in the pellet. The sedimentation rate for macromolecules is measured in Svedberg units (S). The ribosomal subunits for instance got their name from their sedimentation coefficient (40 S subunit and 60 S subunit). Because the friction is controlled not only by the size of the particle, but also by its shape, S values are not additive. The complete ribosome sediments at 80 S and not at 100 S.

If the density of the particle and surrounding medium are identical, the sedimentation rate is zero. This is the basis for the equilibrium centrifugation method in which the medium forms a stable density gradient caused by the gravitational forces. If the centrifugation is run long enough, the particles move to the position where the density of the medium and particle are identical and form stable bands there. Thus equilibrium centrifugation separates the molecules by density, independent of their size.

11.6.2
Column Chromatography

Other classical separation techniques include different forms of column chromatography (Figure 11.6). A column is filled with a solid carrier material and the protein mixture is placed on top of it. Then buffer is slowly washed through the column and takes along the protein mixture. Different proteins are held back to a different degree by the column material and arrive after different times at the bottom of the column. The eluate is fractionated and tested for the presence of the desired protein. The ratio of desired protein to total protein is a measure of purity. Different column materials are available and the success of a separation often depends critically on the choice of the appropriate material.

The material for ion exchange chromatography (Figure 11.6(a)) contains negatively or positively charged beads that can be used to separate hydrophilic proteins according to charge. The binding between the proteins and the beads is also controlled by the salt concentration and pH of the elution buffer. Some proteins possess hydrophobic surfaces, which can be used to separate proteins by hydrophobic interaction chromatography (Figure 11.6(b)). For this purpose, short aliphatic side chains are attached to the surface of the column material. Gel filtration chromatography (Figure 11.6(c)) is often used as well to separate proteins according to size. The beads contain a range of pores and channels that allow small molecules to enter, which increases their retention times. This not only allows their separation by size, but also to estimate the absolute size of a protein or protein complex. A more recent development is affinity chromatography (Figure 11.6(d)) that makes use of highly specific interactions between a protein and the column material. This can for

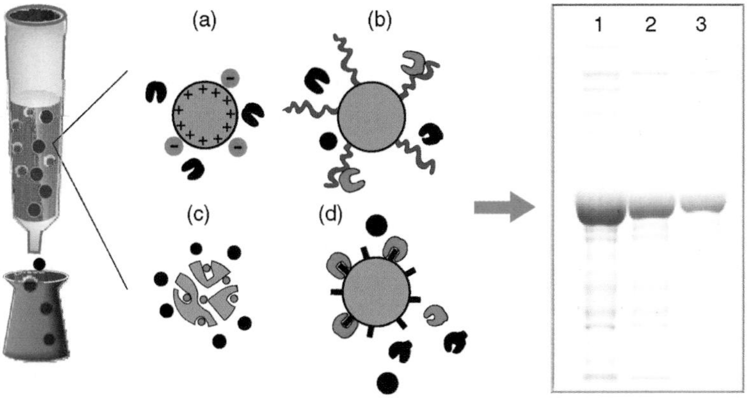

Figure 11.6 In column chromatography a protein mixture is placed on top of the column material and then eluted with buffer. Different types of material are available that separate the proteins according to charge (a), hydrophobicity (b), size (c), or affinity to a specific target molecule (d). Often different chromatographic steps have to be used successively to purify the desired protein to homogeneity (lane 1 to 3 of the gel). Courtesy of Dr. P. Weingarten, Protagen AG.

instance be achieved by chemically linking antibodies to the column material. The proteins of interest bind, while the other proteins pass through the column. In a second step, the elution process is started by using a high salt or pH buffer that recovers the bound protein from the column.

A major improvement regarding speed and separating power was achieved through the development of high-performance liquid chromatography (HPLC). The columns are much smaller and the carrier material is packed more densely and homogenously. To achieve reasonable buffer flow rates, very high pressures (up to several hundred atmospheres) are needed that are generated using special pumps.

The enrichment factor of a single chromatographic step is normally between 10- and 20-fold. However, since many proteins represent only a tiny fraction of the total protein content of a cell, often different chromatographic columns have to be used consecutively. A notable exception is affinity chromatography, which can achieve enrichments up to 10^4 in a single step. In combination with modern recombinant DNA techniques, affinity chromatography has many applications. Recombinant proteins can be designed to contain special short sequences of amino acids that do not compromise the functionality of the protein but can serve as molecular tags. A short stretch of histidine residues is called a His-tag and is specifically be recognized by a nickel surface or special His-antibodies.

11.6.3 Polymerase Chain Reaction

The PCR allows the billion-fold amplification of specific DNA fragments (typically up to 10 kbp) directly from genomic DNA [7]. A pair of short oligonucleotides (15–25 bp), the primers, are synthesized chemically such that they are complementary to an area upstream and downstream of the DNA of interest. DNA is made single stranded by heating, and during the cooling phase primers are added to the mixture, which then hybridize to the single-stranded DNA. In a next step, a DNA polymerase extends the primers, doubling the copy number of the desired DNA fragment. This concludes one PCR cycle. Each additional cycle (denaturation, annealing, and amplification) doubles the existing amount of the DNA, which is located between the primer pair. Thus, 30 cycles correspond to a $2^{30} = \sim 10^9$-fold amplification step (25–35 cycles are typically used). Today, the different steps of the PCR reaction do not have to be performed manually. Small, automated PCR machines, also called thermal cycler, can perform dozens of PCR reactions in parallel and a single cycle is finished in 3–4 min.

In the last years, sequence information for many complete genomes has become available, which allows the use of PCR to clone genes directly from genomic DNA without the use of DNA libraries. PCR has revolutionized modern molecular genetics and has many applications. For instance, by combining reverse transcriptase (which makes a DNA copy from RNA) with PCR, it is also possible to clone mRNA with this technique. Furthermore, the extreme sensitivity of PCR makes it the method of choice for forensic studies. Highly variable tandem repeats are amplified and used to test if genetic material that comes from hair follicle cells, saliva, or blood stains belongs to a certain suspect. This is possible because different individuals have tandem repeats of different length, which results in amplified DNA fragments of different length. By looking at a large number of different tandem repeats, the chances of a false positive result can be made arbitrarily small. This principle is also the basis of paternity tests.

An important, more recent, development is real-time PCR that is especially suited to quantify the amount of template that was initially present. Classical PCR is normally unable to give quantitative results because of saturation problems during the later cycles. Real-time PCR circumvents these problems by using fluorescent dyes that either intercalate in double-stranded DNA or are bound to sequence-specific oligonucleotides (TaqMan® probe). The increase of fluorescence with time is used in real-time, as an indicator of product generation during each PCR cycle.

11.7 DNA and Protein Chips

11.7.1 DNA Chips

DNA chips, also called DNA microarrays, are a high-throughput method for the analysis of gene expression [8]. Instead of looking at the expression of a single gene, microarrays make it possible to monitor the expression of several thousand genes in a single experiment, resulting in a global picture of the cellular activity.

A microarray experiment starts with the construction of the chip from a DNA library (see Section 11.2). The inserts of individual clones are amplified by PCR (a single primer pair can be used, which is specific for the vector that was used to construct the library) and spotted in a regular pattern on a glass slide or nylon membrane. These steps are normally automated and performed by robots. Then total mRNA is extracted from two samples that we would like to compare (e.g., yeast cells before and after osmotic shock). Using reverse transcriptase, the mRNA is transcribed into cDNA and labeled with a fluorescent dye. It is important that the dyes emit light at different wavelength. Red and green dyes are commonly used. The cDNAs are now incubated with the chip where they hybridize to the spot that contains the cDNA fragment. After washing, the ratio of the fluorescence intensities for red and green are measured and displayed as false color picture. Red or green spots indicate a large excess of mRNA from one or the other sample, while yellow spots show that the amount of this specific mRNA was roughly equal in both samples. Very low amounts of both mRNA samples result in dark spots. These ratios can of course also be quantified numerically and used for further calculations, like the generation of a clustergram. For this analysis, a complete linkage cluster of the genes that were spotted on the chip is generated and the mRNA ratio is displayed as color. This helps to test if groups of related genes (maybe all involved in fatty acid synthesis) also show a similar expression pattern.

A variant of DNA chips, oligonucleotide chips, are based on an alternative experimental design. Instead of spotting cDNAs, short oligonucleotides (25–50 mer) are used. Approximately a dozen different and specific oligonucleotides are used per gene. In this case, only one probe of mRNA is hybridized per chip and the ratio of fluorescence intensity of different chips is used to estimate the relative abundance of each mRNA. Most commonly chips from the companies Affimetrix or Agilent are used for this approach.

In the last years, this technique was used to study such diverse problems as the effects of caloric restriction and aging in mice [9], influence of environmental changes on yeast [10], or the consequences of serum withdrawal on human fibroblasts [11].

11.7.2
Protein Chips

Despite the large success of DNA chips, it is clear that the function of genes is realized through proteins and not by mRNAs. Therefore, efforts are under way to construct chips that consist of spotted proteins instead of DNA. In this case, the starting point is an expression library for obtaining large quantities of the recombinant proteins. The proteins are spotted and fixed on a coated glass slide and can then be incubated with interaction partners. This could be (i) other proteins to study protein complexes, (ii) antibodies to quantify the spotted proteins or to identify the recognized antigens, (iii) DNA to find DNA-binding proteins, or (iv) drugs to identify compounds of pharmaceutical interest [12].

However, the generation of protein chips poses more problems than DNA chips because proteins are not as uniform as DNA. One challenge is to express sufficient amounts of recombinant proteins in a high-throughput approach. Another problem is that the optimal conditions (temperature, ionic strength, etc.) for the interaction with the reaction partner are not identical for different proteins. But academic groups and companies like Protagen, Invitrogen, or Procognia are constantly improving the technique, and chips with several hundred different proteins are now used successfully [13].

The main advantage of DNA and protein chips is the huge amount of data that can be gathered in a single experiment. However, this is also a feature that needs careful consideration. The quality of an expression profile analysis based on array data is highly dependent on the number of repeated sample measurements, the array preparation and hybridization as well as signal quantification procedure [14]. The large number of samples on the chip also pose a problem regarding multiple testing. If care is not taken, a large number of false positives is to be expected.

11.8
Yeast Two-Hybrid System

The yeast two-hybrid (Y2H) system is a technique for the high-throughput detection of protein–protein interactions. It rests on the fact that some transcription factors

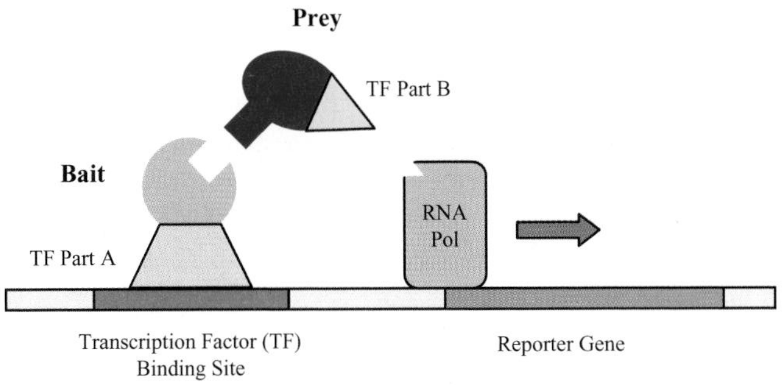

Figure 11.7 The yeast two-hybrid system identifies protein–protein interactions. The genes of the bait and prey proteins are fused to parts of a yeast TF. If bait and prey interact, the different parts of the TF come close enough together to activate the expression of a reporter gene.

(TF), like the yeast *Gal4* gene, have a modular design, with the DNA-binding domain separated from the activating domain. To test if two proteins, called bait and prey, interact, their genes are fused to the DNA-binding or DNA-activating domain, respectively, of the TF (Figure 11.7). The bait binds to the DNA via its TF fragment. If bait and prey do interact, the two domains of the TF come close enough together to stimulate the expression of a reporter gene. If bait and prey do not interact, the reporter gene is silent. This technique can be used to find all interacting partners of the bait protein. For this purpose, yeast cells are transformed with an expression library containing prey proteins fused to the activating part of the TF. Although the detection occurs in yeast, the bait and prey proteins can come from any organism. This single-bait multiple-prey system can even be extended to a multiple-bait multiple-prey approach, which made it possible to obtain the complete protein interactome of yeast [15]. However, as with most high-throughput techniques, the two-hybrid system is prone to false positives, as indicated by the fact that a second study using the same technique derived a quite dissimilar yeast interactome [16]. To corroborate the interactions obtained with Y2H, affinity chromatography or co-immunoprecipitation can be used.

11.9 Mass Spectrometry

The identification of individual proteins of a cell is an essential part of studying biological processes. The first step toward identification involves often a separation of the protein broth. 2D gels (see Section 11.3) or the different forms of chromatography (see Section 11.5.2) are frequently used for this task. The separated proteins can then be identified by cleaving them enzymatically into specific peptides and determining the exact size and sequence of these fragments using different types of mass spectrometry (MS).

MS has been used for the past 50 years to measure the masses of small molecules with high accuracy. But its application to large biomolecules has been limited by the fragility and low volatility of these materials. However, the situation changed in the late 1980s with the emergence of the matrix-assisted laser desorption/ionization mass spectrometry (MALDI-MS) [17] technique and the electrospray ionization (ESI) [18]. For MALDI, the polypeptide is mixed with solvent and an excess of low-molecular-weight matrix material. Polypeptide and matrix molecules cocrystallize and are placed in the spectrometer under vacuum conditions. The probe is then targeted with a laser beam that transfers most of its energy to the matrix material, which heats up and is vaporized. During this process, the intact polypeptide is charged and carried into the vapor phase. ESI is, in contrast to MALDI, a continuous method that can be used together with chromatographic separation techniques, such as HPLC. In this case, a spray of small droplets is generated that contains solvent and charged macromolecules. Evaporation of the solvent leads to individual, charged protein molecules in the gas phase.

For both methods, the following steps are very similar. An electrical field accelerates the molecules, and the time-of-flight (TOF) for a specific distance is measured, which depends on the ratio of mass and charge ($\text{TOF} \sim \sqrt{m/z}$). The mass accuracy depends strongly on the used MS technique and type of probe, but accuracies around 1 ppm (part per million) are often achievable. In addition to measure peptide masses, MS can also be used to obtain sequence information. Specific peptide ions are selected and subjected to further fragmentation through collision with gas molecules. The sequence information obtained by this tandem mass spectrometry (MS/MS) is then used to identify the protein using powerful search engines like Mascot (www.matrixscience.com), Sequest (fields.scripps.edu/sequest), Phenyx (www.phenyx-ms.com), or the free X! Tandem engine (www.thegpm.org/TANDEM). Many different types of MS machines and techniques exist for specialized applications, and a good review is available by Domon and Aebersold [19].

11.10 Transgenic Animals

Genetic material can be introduced into single-cell organisms (bacteria, yeast) by transformation (see Section 11.2) and is then automatically passed down to the offspring during each cell division. To achieve the same in a multicellular organism is much more complicated.

The first method that was applied successfully to mammals is DNA microinjection [20]. It is based upon the observation that in mammalian cells, linear DNA fragments are rapidly assembled into tandem repeats, which are then integrated into the genomic DNA. This integration occurs at a single random location within the genome. A linearized gene construct is, therefore, injected into the pronucleus of a fertilized ovum. After introduction into foster mothers, embryos develop that contain the foreign DNA in some cells of the organism; it is a chimera. If the construct is also present in germ-line cells, some animals of the daughter generation (F_1 generation) will carry the transgene in all of its body cells. A transgenic animal has been created. The advantage of DNA microinjection is that it is applicable to a wide range of species. The disadvantage is that the integration is a random process and so the genomic neighborhood of the insert is unpredictable. This often means that the expression of the recombinant DNA is suppressed by silencers or an unfavorable chromatin structure. If a mutant form of an endogenous gene has been introduced, it has to be considered that in general the wild type is also present, which restricts this approach to the investigation of dominant mutants.

This problem can be overcome by using the method of embryonic stem cell (ES-cell) mediated transfer [21]. In rare cases (approx. 0.1%), the integration of a gene variant into the genome does not occur randomly, but actually replaces the original gene via homologous recombination. This paves the way to modify or inactivate any gene. In the latter case, this results in knockout animals. For this technique, the gene construct is introduced into ES-cells, which are omnipotent and can give rise to any cell type. With the help of PCR or Southern Blotting, the few ES-cells that underwent homologous recombination can be identified. Some of these cells are then injected into an early embryo at the blastocyst stage, which leads to chimeric animals that are composed of wild-type cells and cells derived from the manipulated ES-cells. As in the case of DNA microinjection, an F_1 generation of animals has to be bred to obtain genetically homogeneous animals. ES-cell mediated transfer works particularly well in mice and is the method of choice to generate knockout mice, which are invaluable in deciphering the function of unknown genes.

11.11 RNA Interference

We have seen that the generation of transgenic animals and the use of homologous recombination to produce knockout animals is one way to elucidate the function of a gene. However, this approach is time consuming, technically demanding, and expensive. A new convenient method for transiently downregulating arbitrary genes makes use of the phenomenon of RNA interference (RNAi). In 1998, it was discovered that the injection of double-stranded RNA (dsRNA) into the nematode *Caenorhabditis elegans* led to a sequence-specific downregulation of gene expression [22]. It turned out that this effect is a part of a natural defense system of eukaryotes against viruses and selfish genetic elements that propagate via long double-stranded RNA intermediates.

The dsRNA is recognized by a cellular endoribonuclease of the RNase III family, called DICER. This cuts the dsRNA into short pieces of 21–23 bp length with a 2-bp single-stranded overhang at the 3′ end. These short fragments are called short interfering RNAs (siRNAs). After phosphorylation, they are assembled (as single strands) into a riboprotein complex called RISC (RNA-induced silencing complex). If RISC encounters an mRNA complementary to its siRNA, the mRNA is enzymatically cut at a position that corresponds to the middle of the siRNA (Figure 11.8). In mammals, long dsRNA also induces the interferon response that causes unspecific

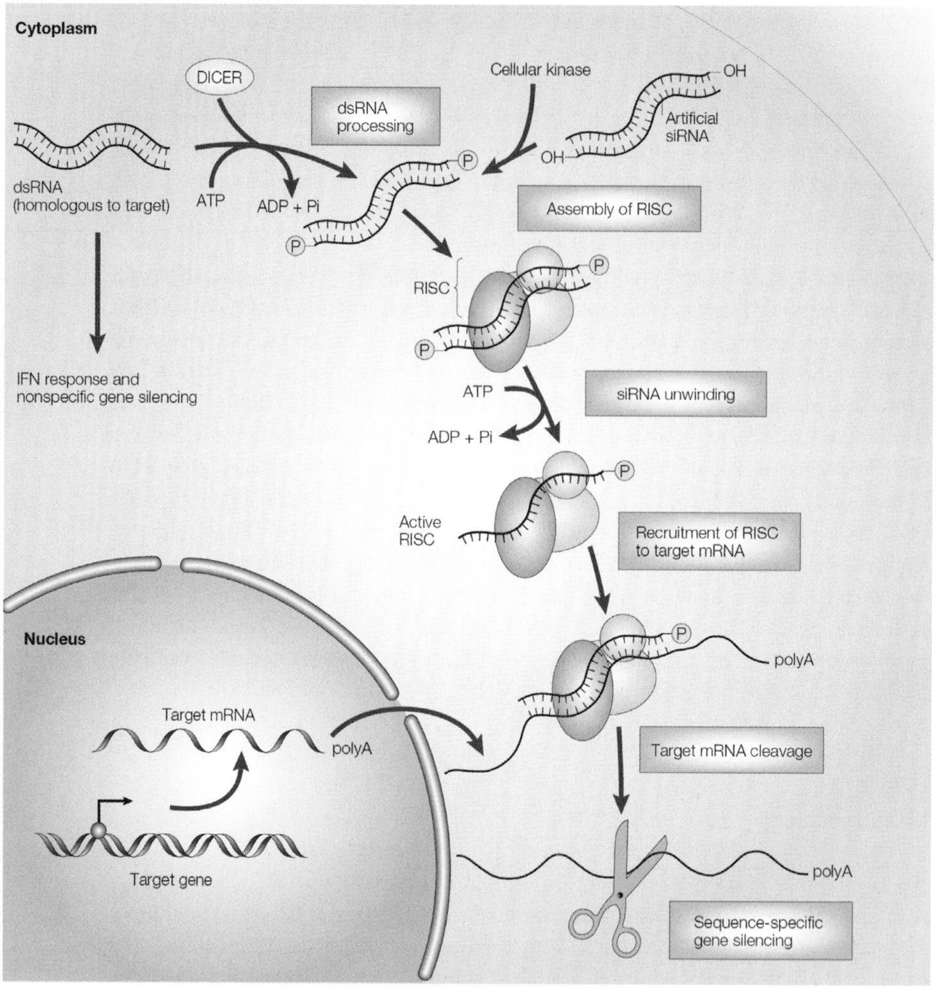

Figure 11.8 Mechanism of RNA interference (RNAi). Double-stranded RNA (dsRNA) is cleaved by the endoribonuclease DICER into small fragments of 21–23 nucleotides, which are subsequently phosphorylated at the 5′ end. To become functional, these small interfering RNAs (siRNAs) form an RNA-induced silencing complex (RISC) with cellular proteins. If the RISC complex encounters an mRNA that is complementary to the siRNA, this mRNA is cleaved in the middle of the complementary sequence, leading to gene silencing (From [25]). Exogenously added siRNAs are also functional in triggering RNAi.

degradation of mRNA and a general shutdown of translation. This would severely hamper the use of RNA interference as research tool, but luckily artificial siRNAs can also be used to activate the RNA interference machinery [23].

Artificial siRNAs are synthesized chemically and can in principle be targeted against any mRNA. However, currently there are no clear design rules that would yield the most effective siRNAs and positional effects can lead to suppression levels that vary between 10% and 70% [24]. Because the transfection of siRNA is only transient (it only lasts a few days in mammals), there might also be problems to silence genes that encode for long-lived proteins.

If siRNAs are expressed from plasmids or viral vectors, their effects are more persistent and they can be used as therapeutic agents by downregulating specific disease genes. Applications to HIV and other targets have been discussed [23, 25]. They can also be used to study regulatory interactions among proteins by targeting individual components and then measuring the effects on the global gene expression. Following this approach makes it possible to study the structure of a signaling pathway involved in the immune response of *Drosophila melanogaster* [26]. Finally, RNA interference would also be very useful for the model building of metabolic or gene networks. After a network has been formulated by a set of equations, it can be tested by silencing genes individually or in combination and then measuring the resulting new expression levels. This type of network perturbation can be used to iteratively improve the agreement of the model predictions with the experimental data.

11.12 ChIP on Chip and ChIP-PET

We have already discussed several techniques that produce various types of high-throughput data, such as protein–protein interactions (Y2H, Section 11.8) or gene expression levels (DNA chips, Section 11.7.1). Now that more and more whole eukaryotic genomes are being sequenced, another type of information that becomes increasingly interesting are all the recognition sites that exist for DNA-binding proteins. Of particular interest is this for TFs, which are of crucial importance for gene regulation (but the same strategy can also be applied to all other types of DNA-binding proteins). TF-binding sites are notoriously difficult to determine using computational approaches since they often represent degenerate motifs of 5–10 nucleotides that appear far too often in genomic DNA as to be specific. It seems that additional factors and specific conditions that exist *in vivo* provide the required additional specificity.

Chromatin immunoprecipitation (ChIP) is an experimental technique that can be used to identify TF-binding sites under *in vivo* conditions. In a first step, the TF of interest is cross-linked with the DNA it binds to using formaldehyde fixation. Then the cells are lysed and the DNA is broken down mechanically (sonication) or enzymatically (nucleases), leading to double-stranded pieces of DNA around 1 kb in length. The next step is the purification of the TF–DNA complexes using immunoprecipitation. For this, either an antibody specific for the studied TF is necessary or an antibody against a tag (His-tag or c-myc) that is fused to the TF. At this point, the DNA fragments are released from the TF–DNA complexes by heat treatment and are finally amplified by PCR (see Section 11.6).

The problem with classical ChIP is that prior knowledge of the target DNA sequence is required to synthezise the PCR primers. The combination of ChIP

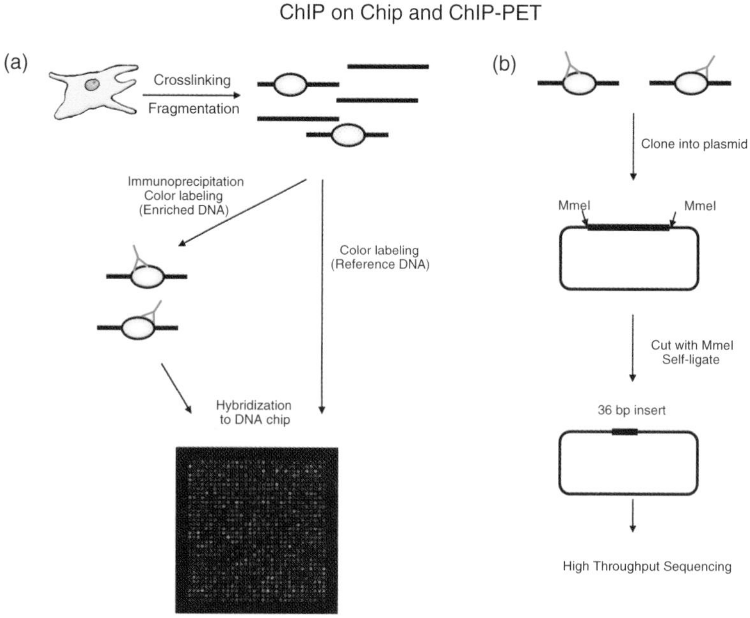

Figure 11.9 (a) ChIP on Chip is a high-throughput technique that provides information about DNA-binding sites of proteins under *in vivo* conditions. After formaldehyde cross-linking, DNA protein complexes are immunoprecipitated followed by fluorescent labeling of the DNA and hybridization to a DNA microarray. (b) ChIP-PET also looks after DNA binding sites, but uses a high-throughput sequencing method to identify precipitated DNA sequences.

with array techniques overcomes this limitation, resulting in the ChIP-on-Chip method [27] (Figure 11.9(a)). The initial steps of both the methods are identical, but for ChIP-on-Chip, all amplified DNA fragments are labeled with one type of fluorescent dye and a reference DNA sample (DNA nonenriched in TF-binding sites) is labeled with a different dye. A mixture of enriched and control DNA is then hybridized to a DNA-chip for identification and quantification of TF-binding sites. The resolution, coverage, and density of the DNA-chip are important factors that control the quality and quantity of the identified binding sites. The method has been used successfully to determine the genome-wide locations of TFs in yeast [28] and Drosophila [29]. It has also been applied to recombination [30], replication [31], and studies of chromatin structure [32].

An important limitation of ChIP-on-Chip is that the parts of the genome that contain the DNA-binding sites have to be represented on the microarray. For DNA-binding proteins, these are normally intergenic regions, which make up a large fraction of the DNA of higher eukaryotes. ChIP-PET (Paired End diTag) avoids these problems by combining ChIP with a high-throughput sequencing approach [33,34] (Figure 11.9(b)). The precipitated DNA sequences are cloned into a vector with flanking *MmeI* restriction sites. The corresponding restriction enzyme cuts 18 bp away from its recognition site so that restriction followed by re-ligation results in a 36-bp-ditag insert, consisting of the 5′ and 3′ ends of the isolated DNA fragment. High-throughput sequencing of a large number of ditags (to improve the signal-to-noise ratio) is finally used to identify different genomic binding sites.

This technique allows in principle to identify arbitrary sequences that are not present on any DNA chip. Although currently hampered by high costs for sequencing, this problem might be overcome by future technological advances.

11.13 Surface Plasmon Resonance

One major aim of Systems Biology is to model large and complex biological systems using mathematical equations. An important and necessary resource for this kind of quantitative modeling are kinetic data. The SPR technique provides this type of data in the form of binding constants (k_{on}, k_{off}) for biochemical reactions [35,36].

The underlying principles of the method are in detail rather intricate, but a simplified overview is given in Figure 11.10(a). Polarized light is directed onto a gold-coated glass carrier. When a light beam traveling in a medium of high refractive index meets the interface to a medium of lower refractive index below a certain critical angle, the beam experiences total internal reflection and is directed back into the medium with higher refractive index. During this process, the light beam generates an electrical field (called an evanescent field wave) in the medium of low refractive index. Under the right angle, it also excites surface plasmons (oscillating electrons) in the thin gold layer, which enhance the evanescent wave by extracting energy from the light beam. The angle required for inducing surface plasmons depends strongly on the refractive index of the sample medium close to the surface since the strength of the evanescing wave decays rapidly with its distance from this surface. Thus, the more material is bound to the surface, the higher the refractive index and the stronger the change of the SPR angle.

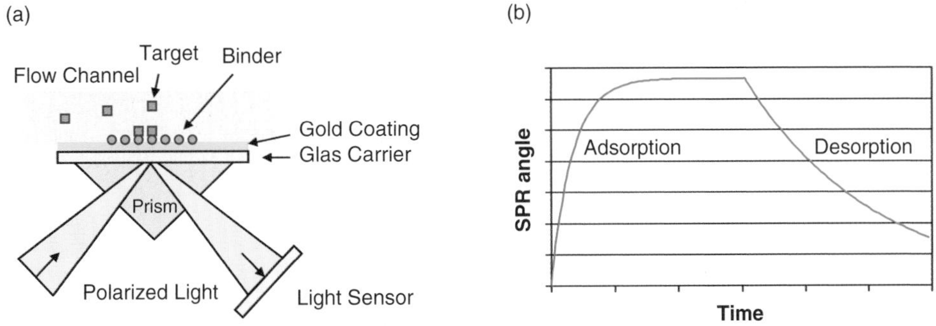

Figure 11.10 (a) Schematic diagram of the SPR technique. If target and binder form a complex, the refractive index near the gold surface increases, causing a change in the amount of reflected light. (b) Typical result of an SPR experiment. Initially the flow channel contains target molecules, leading to the formation of target/binder complexes. Later, a washing solution is applied, leading to the desorption of target molecules.

The sensitivity of SPR depends on the studied biomolecule, and ranges from 10 fmol for single-stranded DNA 18-mers [37] to 1 fmol for the specific binding of antibodies to peptide arrays [38]. By enzymatically amplifying the SPR signal, it was even possible to detect 5 amol of a single-stranded DNA 18-mer [39]. A typical result of an SPR experiment consists of an adsorption phase during which the carrier is exposed to a solution containing target molecules and a desorption phase during which the surface is exposed to washing fluid (Figure 11.10(b)).

How are k_{on} and k_{off} values calculated from SPR curves? On the surface, the binding of target and binder ($T + B \underset{k_{off}}{\overset{k_{on}}{\rightleftharpoons}} TB$) takes places, leading to the following differential equation for the time-dependent accumulation of TB complexes. It is assumed that target molecules exist in excess so that their concentration remains unchanged at T_0, while the concentration of binder molecules is given by the total concentration minus those in the complex TB. Equation (11.1) can be solved analytically and is given by Eq. (11.2) (assuming that the initial concentration of TB is zero). Once the washing fluid is applied, desorption starts and the TB complexes are decaying according to Eq. (11.3).

$$\frac{dTB}{dt} = k_{on} \cdot (B_0 - TB) \cdot T_0 - k_{off} \cdot TB \tag{11.1}$$

$$TB(t) = \frac{k_{on} \cdot T_0 \cdot B}{k_{on} \cdot T_0 + k_{off}} \cdot \left(1 - e^{-(k_{on} \cdot T_0 + k_{off})t}\right) \tag{11.2}$$

$$TB(t) = TB_0 \cdot e^{-k_{off} \cdot t} \tag{11.3}$$

By fitting (11.3) to the desorption curve, it is immediately possible to determine k_{off}. The calculation of k_{on}, however, is more difficult. Because k_{on} always appears together with T_0 in Eq. (11.2), it is not possible to obtain this value from a single measurement as shown in Figure 11.10(b). Instead, a series of such experiments has to be performed with different target concentrations. By fitting Eq. (11.2) to each of these adsorption curves, we obtain estimates of $(k_{on} \cdot T_0 + k_{off})$ for different values of T_0. The linear slope of these data represents k_{on} and the intercept corresponds to k_{off}.

The SPR phenomenon can be measured using two different approaches, "SPR imaging" as implemented in the instruments of GWC Technologies or HTS Biosystems and "SPR angle shift," which is the most popular method and used by Biacore and Texas Instruments. While SPR imaging is an array format method, naturally applicable to high-throughput measurements, the latest instruments of Biacore (Biacore Flexchip) are also able to measure up to 400 interactions in parallel.

11.14
Population Heterogeneity and Single Entity Experiments

For the understanding of complex biological processes, a quantitative description of the participating components is necessary. Traditionally, purification and quantification methods of molecules, proteins, or organelles start with a large number of cells, and the finally obtained rate or concentration represents an average value for the initial cell population. However, several situations exist where this value is misleading and obscures the underlying structure at the single-cell level. This can occur when the cellular process depends on a small number of molecules and is thus subject to stochastic noise [40–42].

In this case, single-cell studies are necessary to reveal individual variability. A high-throughput method that has recently been presented, combines flow cytometry with a library of green fluorescent protein (GFP) tagged yeast strains to measure the amount of more than 2500 different proteins in individual yeast cells [43]. GFP is a small protein (27 kDa) found in jellyfish [44]. GFP and its variants are widely used as a reporter of expression by fusing it to target proteins or cloning it after a promoter of interest. Using this approach, the fluorescence of approx. 350,000 cells can be measured per minute. Analysis of these data shows that there is considerably inter-cell variability of different proteins, which is inversely correlated with protein abundance. The data are in good agreement with the hypothesis that the variation arises from the stochastic production and degradation of mRNA molecules that exist in very small numbers (1–2) per cell. But variability is also controlled by biological function and cellular location. Furthermore, cell-cycle-regulated proteins showed a bimodal distribution, which is very instructive because it reveals that the population of cells was not homogeneous, but consisted of two subpopulations (in different cell-cycle phases). This could not be seen if the measurements were taken on a population of cells.

A similar phenomenon was observed in the field of aging research. It has been known for a long time that cells accumulate mutations in the mitochondrial DNA (mtDNA) with age. However, this phenomenon was regarded as not relevant since the fraction of defective mtDNA is only around 1% [45, 46]. However, it turned out that the underlying assumption that mitochondrial damage is distributed homogeneously within a tissue is wrong. Single-cell studies revealed that muscle tissue displays a mosaic pattern of mitochondrial damage. While in old individuals most cells harbor little or no damaged mitochondria, there are a few cells that contain such a large proportion of mitochondrial mutants that the affected cells show physiological deficits [47, 48].

Problems of hidden heterogeneity not only occur at the cellular level, but also in populations of individuals. In many species, age-specific mortality levels off at advanced ages and one explanation is that the population consists of subgroups exhibiting different aging rates. To test this idea, Wu *et al.* [49] coupled GFP to the endogenous heat shock protein HSP-16.2 in the nematode *C. elegans*. After application of a heat shock, worms were sorted according to fluorescence (HSP-16.2 activity) and it was found that the lifespan of worms correlated with the amount of individual HSP-16.2 activity. This is a strong indication that population heterogeneity contributes to the flattening of mortality rates at advanced ages.

Exercises and Problems

1. The restriction enzyme Bam HI recognizes a sequence of 6 bp. How many restriction sites do you expect to find in the bacteriophage λ (48,502 bp)?

How many would you find in *Escherichia coli* (4.6 Mb) if the recognition sequence is 8-bp long ?

2. Bacteria can reach concentrations of up to 10^7 per milliliter in culture media. How long does it take to reach this concentration if 100 ml medium is inoculated with a single bacterium and the generation time is 20 min?

3. For DNA and protein gels, the pore size can be adjusted. When would you use a small pore size, and when a large one?

4. What is the isoelectric point of a protein?

5. What is the purpose of the secondary antibody in Western blotting?

6. What is a His-tag?

7. Is it possible that a 100-kDa protein has a smaller sedimentation coefficient, S, than a 70-kDa protein?

8. What are the advantages of HPLC over conventional chromatography?

9. Why are protein chips more difficult to generate and use than DNA chips?

10. What accuracy in ppm is necessary for a mass spectrometer to be able to separate the following two peptides according to mass? Consider that each peptide bond releases one molecule of water. We further assume that the peptides carry no net charge and that the atomic masses are given by the mass of the most frequent isotope rounded to the next dalton (i.e., C = 12 Da).

    Asp-Gly-Asn-Lys-Ile-His

    Leu-Gly-Asp-Gln-Leu-His

11. If a transgenic animal is heterozygous for a transgene, what is the proportion of offspring that are homozygous for the transgene if the animal is crossed (a) with another heterozygous animal or (b) with wild-type animals?

12. What are the advantages and disadvantages of the RNAi technique in contrast to knockout animals?

13. The analysis of binding curves of SPR experiments is based on the assumption that one binder molecule reacts with one target molecule ($T + B \underset{k_{off}}{\overset{k_{on}}{\rightleftarrows}} TB$). Try to develop the differential equations that would result if one binder reacts with two targets ($2T + B \underset{k_{off}}{\overset{k_{on}}{\rightleftarrows}} T_2B$), as could be expected if the binder were antibodies. Try to solve the differential equations for the washing period.

References

1 Burke, D.T. *et al.* (1987) Cloning of large segments of exogenous DNA into yeast by means of artificial chromosome vectors. *Science*, **236**, 806–812.

2 Shizuya, H. *et al.* (1992) Cloning and stable maintenance of 300-kilobase-pair fragments of human DNA in *Escherichia coli* using an F-factor-based vector. *Proceedings of the National Academy of Sciences of the United States of America*, **89**, 8794–8797.

3 Shapiro, A.L. *et al.* (1967) Molecular weight estimation of polypeptide chains by electrophoresis in SDS-polyacrylamide gels. *Biochemical and Biophysical Research Communications*, **28**, 815–820.

4 O'Farrell, P.H. (1975) High resolution two-dimensional electrophoresis of proteins. *The Journal of Biological Chemistry*, **250**, 4007–4021.

5 Tonge, R. *et al.* (2001) Validation and development of fluorescence two-dimensional differential gel electrophoresis proteomics technology. *Proteomics*, **1**, 377–396.

6 Southern, E.M. (1975) Detection of specific sequences among DNA fragments separated by gel electrophoresis. *Journal of Molecular Biology*, **98**, 503–517.

7 Saiki, R.K. *et al.* (1985) Enzymatic amplification of beta-globin genomic sequences and restriction site analysis for diagnosis of sickle cell anemia. *Science*, **230**, 1350–1354.

8 DeRisi, J.L. *et al.* (1997) Exploring the metabolic and genetic control of gene expression on a genomic scale. *Science*, **278**, 680–686.

9 Lee, C.-K. *et al.* (1999) Gene expression profile of aging and its retardation by caloric restriction. *Science*, **285**, 1390–1393.

10 Causton, H.C. *et al.* (2001) Remodeling of yeast genome expression in response to environmental changes. *Molecular Biology of the Cell*, **12**, 323–337.

11 Eisen, M.B. *et al.* (1998) Cluster analysis and display of genome-wide expression patterns. *Proceedings of the National Academy of Sciences of the United States of America*, **95**, 14863–14868.

12 Cahill, D.J. and Nordhoff, E. (2003) Protein arrays and their role in proteomics. *Advances in Biochemical Engineering/Biotechnology*, **83**, 177–187.

13 Feyen, O. *et al.* (2008) Off-target activity of TNF-alpha inhibitors characterized by protein biochips. *Analytical and Bioanalytical Chemistry*, **391**, 1713–1720.

14 Wierling, C.K. *et al.* (2002) Simulation of DNA array hybridization experiments and evaluation of critical parameters during subsequent image and data analysis. *BMC Bioinformatics*, **3**, 29.

15 Uetz, P. *et al.* (2000) A comprehensive analysis of protein–protein interactions in Saccharomyces cerevisiae. *Nature*, **403**, 623–627.

16 Ito, T. *et al.* (2001) A comprehensive two-hybrid analysis to explore the yeast protein interactome. *Proceedings of the National Academy of Sciences of the United States of America*, **98**, 4569–4574.

17 Karas, M. and Hillenkamp, F. (1988) Laser desorption ionization of proteins with molecular masses exceeding 10,000 daltons. *Analytical Chemistry*, **60**, 2299–2301.

18 Fenn, J.B. *et al.* (1989) Electrospray ionization for mass spectrometry of large biomolecules. *Science*, **246**, 64–71.

19 Domon, B. and Aebersold, R. (2006) Mass spectrometry and protein analysis. *Science*, **312**, 212–217.

20 Gordon, J.W. and Ruddle, F.H. (1981) Integration and stable germ line transmission of genes injected into mouse pronuclei. *Science*, **214**, 1244–1246.

21 Gossler, A. *et al.* (1986) Transgenesis by means of blastocyst-derived embryonic stem cell lines. *Proceedings of the National Academy of Sciences of the United States of America*, **83**, 9065–9069.

22 Fire, A. *et al.* (1998) Potent and specific genetic interference by double-stranded RNA in Caenorhabditis elegans. *Nature*, **391**, 806–811.

23 Dykxhoorn, D.M. *et al.* (2003) Killing the messenger: short RNAs that silence gene expression. *Nature Reviews. Molecular Cell Biology*, **4**, 457–467.

24 Holen, T. *et al.* (2002) Positional effects of short interfering RNAs targeting the human coagulation trigger tissue factor. *Nucleic Acids Research*, **30**, 1757–1766.

25 Stevenson, M. (2003) Dissecting HIV-1 through RNA interference. *Nature Reviews. Immunology*, **3**, 851–858.

26 Boutros, M. *et al.* (2002) Sequential activation of signaling pathways during innate immune responses in Drosophila. *Developmental Cell*, **3**, 711–722.

27 Buck, M.J. and Lieb, J.D. (2004) ChIP-chip: considerations for the design, analysis, and application of genome-wide chromatin immunoprecipitation experiments. *Genomics*, **83**, 349–360.

28 Lee, T.I. *et al.* (2002) Transcriptional regulatory networks in Saccharomyces cerevisiae. *Science*, **298**, 799–804.

29 Zeitlinger, J. *et al.* (2007) Whole-genome ChIP-chip analysis of Dorsal, Twist, and Snail suggests integration of diverse patterning processes in the Drosophila embryo. *Genes and Development*, **21**, 385–390.

30 Gerton, J.L. *et al.* (2000) Inaugural article: global mapping of meiotic recombination hotspots and coldspots in the yeast Saccharomyces cerevisiae. *Proceedings of the National Academy of Sciences of the United States of America*, **97**, 11383–11390.

31 Wyrick, J.J. *et al.* (2001) Genome-wide distribution of ORC and MCM proteins in S. cerevisiae: high-resolution mapping of replication origins. *Science*, **294**, 2357–2360.

32 Robyr, D. *et al.* (2002) Microarray deacetylation maps determine genome-wide functions for yeast histone deacetylases. *Cell*, **109**, 437–446.

33 Hudson, M. E. and Snyder, M. (2006) High-throughput methods of regulatory element discovery. *Biotechniques*, **41**, 673, 675, 677 passim.

34 Wei, C.L. *et al.* (2006) A global map of p53 transcription-factor binding sites in the human genome. *Cell*, **124**, 207–219.

35 Wegner, G.J. *et al.* (2004) Real-time surface plasmon resonance imaging measurements for the multiplexed determination of protein adsorption/desorption kinetics and surface enzymatic reactions on peptide microarrays. *Analytical Chemistry*, **76**, 5677–5684.

36 Lee, H.J. *et al.* (2005) Quantitative functional analysis of protein complexes on surfaces. *The Journal of Physiology*, **563**, 61–71.

37 Lee, H.J. *et al.* (2001) SPR imaging measurements of 1-D and 2-D DNA microarrays created from microfluidic channels on gold thin films. *Analytical Chemistry*, **73**, 5525–5531.

38 Wegner, G.J. *et al.* (2002) Characterization and optimization of peptide arrays for the study of epitope–antibody interactions using surface plasmon resonance imaging. *Analytical Chemistry*, **74**, 5161–5168.

39 Goodrich, T.T. *et al.* (2004) Enzymatically amplified surface plasmon resonance imaging method using RNase H and RNA microarrays for the ultrasensitive detection of nucleic acids. *Analytical Chemistry*, **76**, 6173–6178.

40 Ferrell, J.E. Jr and Machleder, E.M. (1998) The biochemical basis of an all-or-none cell fate switch in Xenopus oocytes. *Science*, **280**, 895–898.

41 Biggar, S.R. and Crabtree, G.R. (2001) Cell signaling can direct either binary or graded transcriptional responses. *EMBO Journal*, **20**, 3167–3176.

42 Lahav, G. *et al.* (2004) Dynamics of the p53-Mdm2 feedback loop in individual cells. *Nature Genetics*, **36**, 147–150.

43 Newman, J.R. *et al.* (2006) Single-cell proteomic analysis of *S. cerevisiae* reveals the architecture of biological noise. *Nature*, **441**, 840–846.

44 Tsien, R.Y. (1998) The green fluorescent protein. *Annual Review of Biochemistry*, **67**, 509–544.

45 Cortopassi, G.A. *et al.* (1992) A pattern of accumulation of a somatic deletion of mitochondrial DNA in aging human tissues. *Proceedings of the National Academy* *of Sciences of the United States of America*, **89**, 7370–7374.

46 Randerath, K. *et al.* (1996) Genomic and mitochondrial DNA alterations in aging, in *Handbook of The Biology of Aging* (eds L.E. Schneider and J.W. Rowe), Academic Press, London, pp. 198–214.

47 Khrapko, K. *et al.* (1999) Cell by cell scanning of whole mitochondrial genomes in aged human heart reveals a significant fraction of myocytes with clonally expanded deletions. *Nucleic Acids Research*, **27**, 2434–2441.

48 Cao, Z. *et al.* (2001) Mitochondrial DNA deletion mutations are concomitant with ragged red regions of individual, aged muscle fibers: Analysis by laser-capture microdissection. *Nucleic Acids Research*, **29**, 4502–4508.

49 Wu, D. *et al.* (2006) Visualizing hidden heterogeneity in isogenic populations of C. elegans. *Experimental Gerontology*, **41**, 261–270.

12
Mathematics

Summary

Mathematics is the *conditio sine qua non* of systems biology. Even for a user who only wants to apply existing tools and programs, a basic understanding of the underlying mathematics is very helpful to judge the meaning and reliability of the simulation results. For a developer of systems biological analysis tools a much deeper understanding of equations, matrices and networks is, of course, necessary. In this chapter we sum up necessary and basic concepts and methods, which may be well known to some readers and hard to recall for others. We will avoid long derivations and proofs, but present proven tools and recipes. References to further reading are given.

12.1
Linear Modeling

In the modeling of biochemical systems, many relations do not hold just for a single quantity but for several. For example, all metabolites of a pathway have concentrations that may be concisely represented in a vector of concentrations. These metabolites are involved in a subset of the reactions occurring in this pathway; the respective stoichiometric coefficients may be presented in a matrix. Using techniques of linear algebra helps us to understand properties of biological systems. In Section 12.1.1 we will briefly recall the classical problem of how to solve a system of linear equations. Afterward we will introduce our notions for vectors, matrices, rank, nullspace, eigenvalues, and eigenvectors.

12.1.1
Linear Equations

A linear equation in n variables $x_1, x_2, \ldots, x_n$ is an equation of the form

$$a_1x_1 + a_2x_2 + \cdots + a_nx_n = b. \tag{12.1}$$

Systems Biology: A Textbook. Edda Klipp, Wolfram Liebermeister, Christoph Wierling, Axel Kowald, Hans Lehrach, and Ralf Herwig

ISBN: 978-3-527-31874-2

We assume that $a_1, a_2, \ldots, a_n, b$ are real numbers. For example, $2x_1 + 5x_2 = 10$ describes a line passing through the points $(x_1, x_2) = (5, 0)$ and $(x_1, x_2) = (0, 2)$. A *system* of m linear equations in n variables $x_1, x_2, \ldots, x_n$ is a system of linear equations as follows:

$$\begin{aligned} a_{11}x_1 + a_{12}x_2 + \cdots + a_{1n}x_n &= b_1 \\ a_{21}x_1 + a_{22}x_2 + \cdots + a_{2n}x_n &= b_2 \\ &\vdots \\ a_{m1}x_1 + a_{m2}x_2 + \cdots + a_{mn}x_n &= b_m \end{aligned} \quad . \tag{12.2}$$

If $b_1 = b_2 = \cdots b_m = 0$, the system is *homogeneous*. We wish to determine whether the system in Eq. (12.2) has a solution, i.e., if there exist numbers $x_1, x_2, \ldots, x_n$, which satisfy each of the equations simultaneously. We say that the system is *consistent* if it has a solution. Otherwise the system is called *inconsistent*.

In order to find a solution, we employ the matrix formalism (Section 12.1.2). The matrix $\mathbf{A}_c$ is the coefficient matrix of the system and has the dimension $m \times n$, while the matrix $\mathbf{A}_a$ of dimension $m \times (n + 1)$ is called the augmented matrix of the system:

$$\mathbf{A}_c = \begin{pmatrix} a_{11} & a_{12} & \ldots & a_{1n} \\ a_{21} & a_{22} & \ldots & a_{2n} \\ \vdots & \vdots & \ddots & \vdots \\ a_{m1} & a_{m2} & \ldots & a_{mn} \end{pmatrix} \quad \mathbf{A}_a = \left(\begin{array}{cccc|c} a_{11} & a_{12} & \ldots & a_{1n} & b_1 \\ a_{21} & a_{22} & \ldots & a_{2n} & b_2 \\ \vdots & \vdots & \ddots & \vdots & \vdots \\ a_{m1} & a_{m2} & \ldots & a_{mn} & b_m \end{array}\right) . \tag{12.3}$$

The solution of a single linear equation with one unknown is easy. A system of linear equations can be solved using the Gaussian elimination algorithm. A matrix is said to be in the row-echelon form if (1) all zero rows (if any) are at the bottom of the matrix and (2) if two successive rows are nonzero, the second row starts with more zeros than the first (moving from left to right).

Example 12.1

Matrix $\mathbf{B}_r$ is in the row-echelon form and matrix $\mathbf{B}_n$ in non row-echelon form:

$$\mathbf{B}_r = \begin{pmatrix} 3 & 0 & 0 & 1 \\ 0 & 2 & 2 & 3 \\ 0 & 0 & 0 & 4 \\ 0 & 0 & 0 & 0 \end{pmatrix} \quad \mathbf{B}_n = \begin{pmatrix} 3 & 0 & 0 & 1 \\ 0 & 2 & 2 & 3 \\ 0 & 0 & 0 & 4 \\ 0 & 1 & 2 & 0 \end{pmatrix} . \tag{12.4}$$

A matrix is said to be in the reduced row-echelon form if (1) it is in the row-echelon form, (2) the leading (leftmost nonzero) entry in each nonzero row is 1, and (3) all other elements of the column in which the leading entry 1 occurs are equal to zero.

Example 12.2

A_1 and A_2 are matrices in the reduced row-echelon form, A_3 is not:

$$\mathbf{A}_1 = \begin{pmatrix} 1 & 4 & 0 & 7 \\ 0 & 0 & 1 & 2 \end{pmatrix} \quad \mathbf{A}_2 = \begin{pmatrix} 1 & 0 & 0 & -2 \\ 0 & 1 & 0 & 4 \\ 0 & 0 & 1 & -5 \\ 0 & 0 & 0 & 0 \end{pmatrix} \quad \mathbf{A}_3 = \begin{pmatrix} 1 & 0 \\ 0 & 0 \\ 0 & 1 \end{pmatrix}. \tag{12.5}$$

The zero matrix of any size is always in the reduced row-echelon form.

The following operations can be applied to systems of linear equations and do not change the solutions.

There are three types of *elementary row operations* that can be performed on matrices:

1. Interchanging two rows: $R_i \leftrightarrow R_j$
2. Multiplying a row by a real number: $R_i \longrightarrow \alpha \cdot R_i$
3. Adding a multiple of one row to another row: $R_j \longrightarrow R_j + \alpha \cdot R_i$.

A matrix $\mathbf{A}$ is row equivalent to matrix $\mathbf{B}$ if $\mathbf{B}$ is obtained from $\mathbf{A}$ by a sequence of elementary row operations.

Example 12.3

Elementary row operations

$$\mathbf{A} = \begin{pmatrix} 2 & 4 \\ 7 & 5 \\ 1 & 2 \end{pmatrix} \underset{R_1 \leftrightarrow R_3}{\longrightarrow} \begin{pmatrix} 1 & 2 \\ 7 & 5 \\ 2 & 4 \end{pmatrix} \underset{R_2 \longrightarrow R_2 - 7R_1}{\longrightarrow} \begin{pmatrix} 1 & 2 \\ 0 & -9 \\ 2 & 4 \end{pmatrix} \underset{R_3 \longrightarrow 1/2 \cdot R_3}{\longrightarrow} \begin{pmatrix} 1 & 2 \\ 0 & -9 \\ 1 & 2 \end{pmatrix} = \mathbf{B}. \tag{12.6}$$

Thus, $\mathbf{A}$ and $\mathbf{B}$ are row equivalent.

If $\mathbf{A}$ and $\mathbf{B}$ are row-equivalent augmented matrices of two systems of linear equations, then the two systems have the same solution sets – a solution of one system is a solution of the other.

12.1.1.1 The Gaussian Elimination Algorithm

The Gaussian elimination algorithm is a method for solving linear equation systems by transforming the systems augmented matrix $\mathbf{A}$ into its row-equivalent reduced row-echelon form $\mathbf{B}$ by elementary row operations. $\mathbf{B}$ is simpler than $\mathbf{A}$, and it allows one to read off the consistency or inconsistency of the corresponding equation system and even the complete solution of the equation system.

1. Sort the rows such that the upper rows always have less or equal zero entries before the first nonzero entry (counting from the left) than the lower rows. Perform the following row operations. If the mentioned matrix element is zero continue with its next nonzero right neighbor.
2. Divide the first row by a_{11} (or in case, by its next nonzero right neighbor a_{1C_1}) and subtract then $a_{i1}\cdot R_1$ (or $a_{iC_1}\cdot R_1$) from all other rows i. Now all elements of the first (C_1th) column apart from the first are zero.
3. Divide the second row by the new value of a_{22} (or a_{2C_2}); subtract $a_{i2}\cdot R_2$ (or $a_{iC_2}\cdot R_2$) from all other rows i. Now all elements of the second (C_2th) column apart from the second are zero.
4. Repeat this for all lower rows until the lowest row or all lower rows contain only zeros.

Example 12.4

$$\begin{pmatrix} 2 & 2 & 2 \\ 1 & 0 & -1 \\ 3 & 2 & 1 \end{pmatrix} \underset{R_1\to R_1/2}{\rightarrow} \begin{pmatrix} 1 & 1 & 1 \\ 1 & 0 & -1 \\ 3 & 2 & 1 \end{pmatrix} \underset{\substack{R_2\to R_2-R_1 \\ R_3\to R_3-3R_1}}{\rightarrow} \begin{pmatrix} 1 & 1 & 1 \\ 0 & -1 & -2 \\ 0 & -1 & -2 \end{pmatrix} \underset{R_2\to R_2/-1}{\rightarrow} \begin{pmatrix} 1 & 1 & 1 \\ 0 & 1 & 2 \\ 0 & -1 & -2 \end{pmatrix} \underset{\substack{R_1\to R_1-R_2 \\ R_3\to R_3+R_2}}{\rightarrow} \begin{pmatrix} 1 & 0 & -1 \\ 0 & 1 & 2 \\ 0 & 0 & 0 \end{pmatrix}. \qquad (12.7)$$

The reduced row-echelon form of a given matrix is unique.

12.1.1.2 Systematic Solution of Linear Systems

Suppose a system of m linear equations in n unknowns $x_1, x_2, \ldots, x_n$ has the augmented matrix $\boldsymbol{A}$ and $\boldsymbol{A}$ is row equivalent to the matrix $\boldsymbol{B}$, which is in the reduced row-echelon form. $\boldsymbol{A}$ and $\boldsymbol{B}$ have the dimension $m \times (n+1)$. Suppose that $\boldsymbol{B}$ has r nonzero rows and that the leading entry 1 in row i occurs in column number C_i for $1 \le i \le r$. Then

$$1 \le C_1 < C_2 < \cdots < C_r \le n+1. \qquad (12.8)$$

The system is inconsistent, if $C_r = n+1$. The last nonzero row of $\boldsymbol{B}$ has the form $(0, 0, \ldots, 0, 1)$. The corresponding equation is

$$0x_1 + 0x_2 + \cdots + 0x_n = 1. \qquad (12.9)$$

This equation has no solution. Consequently, the original system has no solution. The system of equations corresponding to the nonzero rows of $\boldsymbol{B}$ is consistent if $C_r \leq n$. It holds that $r \leq n$. If $r=n$ then $C_1=1,\ C_2=2,\ \ldots,\ C_n=n$ and the corresponding matrix is

$$B = \begin{pmatrix} 1 & 0 & \ldots & 0 & d_1 \\ 0 & 1 & \ldots & 0 & d_2 \\ \vdots & & & \vdots & \vdots \\ 0 & 0 & \ldots & 1 & d_n \\ 0 & 0 & \ldots & 0 & 0 \\ \vdots & \vdots & \ddots & \vdots & \vdots \\ 0 & 0 & \ldots & 0 & 0 \end{pmatrix}. \tag{12.10}$$

There is a unique solution $x_1=d_1,\ x_2=d_2,\ \ldots,\ x_n=d_n$, which can be directly read off from $\boldsymbol{B}$. If $r<n$, the system is underdetermined. There will be more than one solution (in fact, infinitely many solutions). To obtain all solutions take $x_{C_1}, \ldots, x_{C_r}$ as *dependent* variables and use the r equations corresponding to the nonzero rows of $\boldsymbol{B}$ to express these variables in terms of the remaining *independent* variables $x_{C_{r+1}}, \ldots, x_{C_n}$, which can assume arbitrary values:

$$\begin{aligned} x_{C_1} &= b_{1n+1} - b_{1C_{r+1}} x_{C_{r+1}} - \cdots - b_{1C_n} x_{C_n} \\ &\vdots \\ x_{C_r} &= b_{rn+1} - b_{rC_{r+1}} x_{C_{r+1}} - \cdots - b_{rC_n} x_{C_n} \end{aligned}. \tag{12.11}$$

In particular, taking $x_{C_{r+1}} = 0, \ldots, x_{C_{n-1}} = 0$ and $x_{C_n} = 0$ or $x_{C_n} = 1$ produces at least two solutions.

Example 12.5

Solving the system

$$\begin{aligned} x_1 + x_2 + x_3 &= 0 \\ x_1 - x_2 - x_3 &= 1 \end{aligned}, \tag{12.12}$$

with the following augmented and the reduced row-echelon-form matrices:

$$\boldsymbol{A} = \left(\begin{array}{ccc|c} 1 & 1 & 1 & 0 \\ 1 & -1 & -1 & 1 \end{array}\right) \quad \boldsymbol{B} = \left(\begin{array}{ccc|c} 1 & 0 & 0 & 1/2 \\ 0 & 1 & 1 & -1/2 \end{array}\right), \tag{12.13}$$

leads with the choice $x_3=1$ to the solution $x_2=-3/2$ and $x_1=1/2$.

A system of linear equations (12.2) with $b_1=0,\ \ldots,\ b_m=0$ (i.e., a homogeneous system) is always consistent as $x_1=0, \ldots, x_n=0$ is always a solution, which is called the *trivial* solution. Any other solution is called a *nontrivial* solution. It holds that a homogeneous system of m linear equations in n unknowns always has a nontrivial solution if $m<n$.

12.1.2
Matrices

12.1.2.1 Basic Notions

Let us consider the space of real numbers $\Re$. A *scalar* is a quantity whose value can be expressed by a real number, i.e., by an element of $\Re$. It has a magnitude, but no direction. A *vector* is an element of the space $\Re^n$. It contains numbers for each coordinate of this space, e.g., $\boldsymbol{x} = \begin{pmatrix} x_1 \\ x_2 \\ \vdots \\ x_n \end{pmatrix}$.

A *matrix* is a rectangular array of $m \times n$ elements of real or complex numbers in m rows and n columns, like

$$\boldsymbol{A} = \begin{pmatrix} a_{11} & a_{12} & \dots & a_{1n} \\ a_{21} & a_{22} & \dots & a_{2n} \\ \vdots & \vdots & \ddots & \vdots \\ a_{m1} & a_{m2} & \dots & a_{mn} \end{pmatrix} = [a_{ik}]. \tag{12.14}$$

Here and below holds $i = 1, \dots, m$ and $k = 1, \dots, n$. For our purpose, a vector can be regarded as a matrix comprising only one column ($m \times 1$). In a *zero* matrix **o**, all elements are zero ($a_{ik} = 0$ for all i, k). The matrix is a *square* matrix if $m = n$ holds. A square matrix is a *diagonal* matrix if $a_{ik} = 0$ for all $i \neq k$.

A diagonal matrix is called *identity* matrix $\boldsymbol{I}_n$ if it holds that $a_{ik} = 1$, for $i = k$, so

$$\boldsymbol{I}_n = \begin{pmatrix} 1 & 0 & \dots & 0 \\ 0 & 1 & & 0 \\ \vdots & & \ddots & \vdots \\ 0 & 0 & \dots & 1 \end{pmatrix}$$

12.1.2.2 Linear Dependency

The vectors $\boldsymbol{x}_1, \dots, \boldsymbol{x}_m$ of type $n \times 1$ are said to be *linearly dependent* if there exist scalars $\alpha_1, \dots, \alpha_m$, not all zero, such that $\alpha_1 \boldsymbol{x}_1 + \cdots + \alpha_m \boldsymbol{x}_m = 0$. In other words, one of the vectors can be expressed as a sum over certain scalar multiples of the remaining vectors, i.e., one vector is a linear combination of the remaining vectors. If $\alpha_1 \boldsymbol{x}_1 + \cdots + \alpha_m \boldsymbol{x}_m = 0$ has only the trivial solution $\alpha_1 = \cdots = \alpha_m = 0$, the vectors are linearly independent. A set of m vectors of type $n \times 1$ is linearly dependent if $m > n$. Equivalently, a linearly independent set of m vectors must have $m \leq n$.

12.1.2.3 Basic Matrix Operations

The *transpose*$\boldsymbol{A}^{\mathrm{T}}$ of a matrix $\boldsymbol{A}$ is obtained by interchanging the rows and columns:

$$\boldsymbol{A}^{\mathrm{T}} = [a_{ik}]^{\mathrm{T}} = [a_{ki}]. \tag{12.15}$$

The sum of two matrices $\boldsymbol{A}$ and $\boldsymbol{B}$ of the same size $m \times n$ is

$$\boldsymbol{A} + \boldsymbol{B} = [a_{ik}] + [b_{ik}] = [a_{ik} + b_{ik}]. \tag{12.16}$$

The matrix product of matrix $\boldsymbol{A}$ with sizes $m \times n$ and matrix $\boldsymbol{B}$ with size $n \times p$ is

$$\boldsymbol{A}\,\boldsymbol{B} = \left[\sum_{j=1}^{n} a_{ij} \cdot b_{jk}\right]. \tag{12.17}$$

A scalar multiple of a matrix $\boldsymbol{A}$ is given by

$$\alpha \cdot \boldsymbol{A} = \alpha \cdot [a_{ik}] = [\alpha \cdot a_{ik}]. \tag{12.18}$$

Subtraction of matrices is composed of scalar multiplication with –1 and summation:

$$\boldsymbol{A} - \boldsymbol{B} = \boldsymbol{A} + (-1) \cdot \boldsymbol{B}. \tag{12.19}$$

Division of two matrices is not possible. However, for a square matrix $\boldsymbol{A}$ of size $n \times n$ one may in some cases find the *inverse* matrix $\boldsymbol{A}^{-1}$ fulfilling

$$\boldsymbol{A}\,\boldsymbol{A}^{-1} = \boldsymbol{A}^{-1}\,\boldsymbol{A} = I_n. \tag{12.20}$$

If the respective inverse matrix $\boldsymbol{A}^{-1}$ exists, then $\boldsymbol{A}$ is called *nonsingular* (*regular*) and *invertible*. If the inverse matrix $\boldsymbol{A}^{-1}$ does not exist, then $\boldsymbol{A}$ is called *singular*. The inverse of an invertible matrix is unique. For invertible matrices it holds

$$(\boldsymbol{A}^{-1})^{-1} = \boldsymbol{A}. \tag{12.21}$$

$$(\boldsymbol{A}\,\boldsymbol{B})^{-1} = \boldsymbol{B}^{-1}\,\boldsymbol{A}^{-1} \tag{12.22}$$

$$(\boldsymbol{A}^{\mathrm{T}})^{\mathrm{T}} = \boldsymbol{A} \tag{12.23}$$

$$(\boldsymbol{A}\,\boldsymbol{B})^{\mathrm{T}} = \boldsymbol{B}^{\mathrm{T}}\,\boldsymbol{A}^{\mathrm{T}}. \tag{12.24}$$

Matrix inversion: for the inverse of a 1×1 matrix it holds that $(a_{11})^{-1} = (a_{11}^{-1})$. The inverse of a 2×2 matrix is calculated as

$$\begin{pmatrix} a & b \\ c & d \end{pmatrix}^{-1} = \frac{1}{ad-bc} \begin{pmatrix} d & -b \\ -c & a \end{pmatrix}. \tag{12.25}$$

In general, the inverse of a $n \times n$ matrix is given as

$$\boldsymbol{A}^{-1} = \frac{1}{\mathrm{Det}\,A} \begin{pmatrix} A_{11} & A_{21} & \dots & A_{n1} \\ A_{12} & A_{22} & \dots & A_{n2} \\ \vdots & \vdots & & \vdots \\ A_{1n} & A_{2n} & \dots & A_{nn} \end{pmatrix}, \tag{12.26}$$

where A_{ik} are the adjoints of $\boldsymbol{A}$. The determinant $\mathrm{Det}\,\boldsymbol{A}$ is explained below:

If a square matrix $\boldsymbol{A}$ is invertible, its rows (or columns) are linearly independent. In this case, the linear equation system $\boldsymbol{Ax}=0$ with $\boldsymbol{x}=(x_1,\ldots,x_m)^{\mathrm{T}}$ has only the trivial solution $\boldsymbol{x}=0$. If $\boldsymbol{A}$ is singular, i.e., rows (or columns) are linearly dependent, and the linear equation system $\boldsymbol{Ax}=0$ has a nontrivial solution.

The *determinant* of $\boldsymbol{A}$ (Det $\boldsymbol{A}$) is a real or complex number that can be assigned to every square matrix. For the 1×1 matrix (a_{11}) holds Det $\boldsymbol{A}=a_{11}$. For a 2×2 matrix, it is calculated as

$$\mathrm{Det}\begin{pmatrix} a_{11} & a_{12} \\ a_{21} & a_{22} \end{pmatrix} = \begin{vmatrix} a_{11} & a_{12} \\ a_{21} & a_{22} \end{vmatrix} = a_{11}a_{22}-a_{12}a_{21}. \tag{12.27}$$

The determinant of a larger square matrix can be obtained by an iterative procedure, i.e., by expanding the determinant with respect to one row or column: sum up every element of this row (or column) multiplied by the value of its adjoint. The *adjoint* A_{ik} of element a_{ik} is obtained by deleting the ith row and the kth column of the matrix (called the (i, k) minor of $\boldsymbol{A}$), computing the determinant and multiplying by $(-1)^{i+k}$. For example, the determinant of a 3×3 matrix is

$$\begin{aligned}\begin{vmatrix} a_{11} & a_{12} & a_{13} \\ a_{21} & a_{22} & a_{23} \\ a_{31} & a_{32} & a_{33} \end{vmatrix} &= a_{11}A_{11}+a_{12}A_{12}+a_{13}A_{13} \\ &= a_{11}\cdot(-1)^2\cdot\begin{vmatrix} a_{22} & a_{23} \\ a_{32} & a_{33} \end{vmatrix} + a_{12}\cdot(-1)^3\cdot\begin{vmatrix} a_{21} & a_{23} \\ a_{31} & a_{33} \end{vmatrix} \\ &\quad + a_{13}\cdot(-1)^4\cdot\begin{vmatrix} a_{21} & a_{22} \\ a_{31} & a_{32} \end{vmatrix} \\ &= a_{11}\cdot(a_{22}a_{33}-a_{23}a_{32})-a_{12}\cdot(a_{21}a_{33}-a_{23}a_{31}) \\ &\quad + a_{13}\cdot(a_{21}a_{32}-a_{22}a_{31}). \end{aligned} \tag{12.28}$$

The value of a determinant is zero if (a) the matrix contains a zero row or a zero column or if (b) one row (or column) is a linear combination of the other rows (or columns). In this case the respective matrix is singular. The trace of a square matrix is defined as the sum of the diagonal elements.

12.1.2.4 Dimension and Rank

Subspace of a vector space: Let us further consider the vector space V^n of all n-dimensional column vectors $(n\times 1)$. A subset S of V^n is called a *subspace* of V^n if (a) the zero vector belongs to S, (b) with two vectors belonging to S, their sum belongs to S, and (c) with one vector belonging to S, also its scalar multiples belong to S. A set of vectors $\boldsymbol{x}_1,\ldots,\boldsymbol{x}_m$ belonging to a subspace S forms a *basis* of a vector subspace S if they are linearly independent and if S is the set of all linear combinations of $\boldsymbol{x}_1,\ldots,\boldsymbol{x}_m$. A subspace where at least one vector is nonzero has a basis. In general, a subspace will have more than one basis. The number of vectors forming a basis is called the dimension of S (dim S). For an n-dimensional vector space it holds that dim $S \leq n$.

The *rank* of a matrix is an integer number associated with a matrix $\boldsymbol{A}$ of size $m \times n$: Rank $\boldsymbol{A}$ is equal to the number of linearly independent columns or rows in $\boldsymbol{A}$ and equal to the number of nonzero rows in the reduced row-echelon form of the matrix $\boldsymbol{A}$. It holds that Rank $\boldsymbol{A} \leq m, n$.

Example 12.6

The matrix

$$\mathbf{A} = \begin{pmatrix} 2 & 1 & 1 \\ 4 & 2 & 2 \end{pmatrix} \quad \text{with} \quad R_2 \rightarrow R_2 - 2R_1 \begin{pmatrix} 2 & 1 & 1 \\ 0 & 0 & 0 \end{pmatrix},$$

has $m = 2$ rows, $n = 3$ columns, and Rank $\mathbf{A} = 1$.

Null space of a vector space: The solution of a homogeneous linear equation system, $\boldsymbol{Ax} = 0$, leads to the notion *null space* (or *kernel*) of matrix $\boldsymbol{A}$. Nontrivial solutions for the vector $\boldsymbol{x}$ exist if Rank $\boldsymbol{A} < n$, i.e., if there are linear dependences between the columns of $\boldsymbol{A}$. A kernel matrix $\boldsymbol{K}$ with

$$AK = 0, \tag{12.29}$$

can express these dependences. The n-Rank $\boldsymbol{A}$ columns, $\boldsymbol{k}_i$, of $\boldsymbol{K}$ are particular, linear independent solutions of the homogeneous linear equation system and span the null space of matrix $\boldsymbol{A}$. $\boldsymbol{K}$ is not uniquely determined: all linear combinations of the vectors $\boldsymbol{k}_i$ constitute again valid solutions. In other words, postmultiplying the matrix $\boldsymbol{K}$ by a nonsingular square matrix $\boldsymbol{Q}$ of matching type gives another null-space matrix $\boldsymbol{K}'$.

12.1.2.5 Eigenvalues and Eigenvectors of a Square Matrix

Let $\boldsymbol{A}$ be a $(n \times n)$ square matrix. If λ is a complex number and $\boldsymbol{b}$ a nonzero complex vector satisfying

$$\boldsymbol{Ab} = \lambda \boldsymbol{b}, \tag{12.30}$$

then $\boldsymbol{b}$ is called an *eigenvector* of $\boldsymbol{A}$, while λ is called the corresponding *eigenvalue*. Equation (12.30) can be rewritten as $(\boldsymbol{A} - \lambda \boldsymbol{I}_n)\boldsymbol{b} = 0$. This equation has nontrivial solutions only if

$$\text{Det}(\boldsymbol{A} - \lambda \boldsymbol{I}_n) = 0. \tag{12.31}$$

In this case there are at most n distinct eigenvalues of $\boldsymbol{A}$. Equation (12.31) is called the *characteristic equation* of $\boldsymbol{A}$ and Det$(\boldsymbol{A} - \lambda \boldsymbol{I}_n)$, a polynomial in λ, is the *characteristic polynomial* of $\boldsymbol{A}$. The eigenvalues are the roots, i.e., solutions for λ of the characteristic equation.

For a (2×2) matrix $A = \begin{pmatrix} a_{11} & a_{12} \\ a_{21} & a_{22} \end{pmatrix}$ the characteristic polynomial is $\lambda^2 - \lambda \cdot \text{Trace}\, A + \text{Det}\, A$, where $\text{Trace}\, A = a_{11} + a_{22}$ is the sum of the diagonal elements of A.

Example 12.7

For the matrix $A = \begin{pmatrix} 2 & 1 \\ 1 & 2 \end{pmatrix}$ the characteristic equation reads $\lambda^2 - \lambda \cdot 4 + 3 = (\lambda - 1) \cdot (\lambda - 3) = 0$ and the eigenvalues are $\lambda_1 = 1$, $\lambda_2 = 3$. The eigenvector equation reads $\begin{pmatrix} 2-\lambda & 1 \\ 1 & 2-\lambda \end{pmatrix} \begin{pmatrix} b_1 \\ b_2 \end{pmatrix} = \begin{pmatrix} 0 \\ 0 \end{pmatrix}$. Taking $\lambda_1 = 1$ results in the equation system $\begin{cases} b_1 + b_2 = 0 \\ b_1 + b_2 = 0 \end{cases}$. Thus it holds that $b_1 = -b_2$ with arbitrary values $b_1 \neq 0$. The eigenvectors corresponding to λ_1 are the vectors $\begin{pmatrix} b_1 \\ -b_1 \end{pmatrix}$. For $\lambda_2 = 3$ the corresponding eigenvectors are $\begin{pmatrix} b_1 \\ b_1 \end{pmatrix}$.

12.2 Ordinary Differential Equations

An important problem in the modeling of biological systems is to characterize how certain properties vary with time and space. A common strategy is to describe the change of state variables by differential equations. If only temporal changes are considered, ordinary differential equations (ODEs) are used. For changes in time and space, partial differential equations are appropriate. In this chapter we will deal with the solution, analysis, and numerical integration of ordinary differential equations and with basic concepts of dynamical systems theory such as state space, trajectories, steady states, and stability.

The temporal behavior of biological systems in a continuous, deterministic approach can be described by a set of differential equations

$$\frac{dx_i}{dt} = \dot{x}_i = f_i(x_1, \ldots, x_n, p_1, \ldots, p_l, t), \quad i = 1, \ldots, n, \tag{12.32}$$

where x_i are the variables, e.g., concentrations, p_j are the parameters, (e.g., constant enzyme concentrations or kinetic constants) and t is time. We will use the notations $\frac{dx}{dt}$ and $\dot{x}$ interchangeably. In vector notation Eq. (12.32) reads

$$\frac{d}{dt}\boldsymbol{x} = \dot{\boldsymbol{x}} = \boldsymbol{f}(\boldsymbol{x}, \boldsymbol{p}, t), \tag{12.33}$$

with $\boldsymbol{x} = (x_1, \ldots, x_n)^T$, $\boldsymbol{f} = (f_1, \ldots, f_n)^T$, and $\boldsymbol{p} = (p_1, \ldots, p_l)^T$.

Example 12.8

The linear pendulum is a classical example of a problem that can be described by differential equations: the restoring force, which is proportional to acceleration $\ddot{s} = \frac{d^2 s}{dt^2}$, is proportional to the deviation s or $\ddot{s}(t) = \omega^2 s(t)$

An important example for metabolic modeling is substance degradation: the concentration change $\dot{c}$ is proportional to the current concentration c: $\dot{c}(t) = -k \cdot c(t)$

12.2.1 Notions Regarding Differential Equations

Ordinary differential equations (ODEs) describe functions of one independent variable (e.g., time t). Partial differential equations (PDEs) that describe functions of several variables are not considered here.

An *implicit* ODE

$$F(t, x, x', \ldots, x^{(n)}) = 0 \tag{12.34}$$

includes the variable t, the unknown function x, and its derivatives up to nth order. An *explicit* ODE of nth order has the form

$$x^{(n)} = f(t, x, x', \ldots, x^{(n-1)}). \tag{12.35}$$

The highest derivative (here n) determines the order of the ODE. Studying the time behavior of our system, we are normally interested in finding solutions of the ODE, i.e., finding an n times differentiable function $x(t)$ fulfilling Eq. (12.35). This solution may depend on parameters, so-called integration constants, and represents a set of curves. A solution of an ODE of nth order depending on n integration parameters is a *general* solution. Specifying the integration constants, for example by specifying n initial conditions (for $n = 1$: $x(t = 0) = x^0$) leads to a special or *particular* solution. We will not show here all possibilities of solving ODEs, instead we will focus on specific cases that are relevant for the following chapters.

If the right-hand sides of the explicit ODEs are not explicitly dependent on time t ($\dot{\boldsymbol{x}} = \boldsymbol{f}(\boldsymbol{x}, \boldsymbol{p})$), the system is called *autonomous*. Otherwise it is *nonautonomous*. The nonautonomous case will not be considered here. The *system state* is a snapshot of the system at a given time that contains enough information to predict the behavior of the system for all future times. The set of variables describes the state of the system. And the set of all possible states is the *state space*. Finally, the number n of independent variables is equal to the *dimension* of the state space. For $n = 2$ the two-dimensional state space is also called *phase plane*. A particular solution of the ODE system $\dot{\boldsymbol{x}} = \boldsymbol{f}(\boldsymbol{x}, \boldsymbol{p}, t)$, determined from the general solution by specifying parameter values $\boldsymbol{p}$ and initial conditions $\boldsymbol{x}(t_0) = \boldsymbol{x}^0$, describes a path through the state space and is called *trajectory*.

Stationary (or steady) states are points $\boldsymbol{x}^{st}$ in the phase space, where the condition $\dot{\boldsymbol{x}} = 0$ ($x_1 = 0, \ldots, x_n = 0$) is met. At steady state, the system of n differential equations is represented by a system of n algebraic equations for n variables. The equation $\dot{\boldsymbol{x}} = 0$ can have multiple solutions referring to multiple steady states. The change of number or type (12.2.4) of steady states upon changes of parameter values $\boldsymbol{p}$ is called a *bifurcation*.

Linear systems of ODEs have linear functions of the variables as right-hand sides, like

$$\begin{aligned} \frac{dx_1}{dt} &= a_{11}x_1 + a_{12}x_2 + z_1 \\ \frac{dx_2}{dt} &= a_{21}x_1 + a_{22}x_2 + z_2 \end{aligned}, \qquad (12.36)$$

or in general $\dot{\boldsymbol{x}} = \boldsymbol{Ax} + \boldsymbol{z}$. The matrix $\boldsymbol{A} = \{a_{ik}\}$ is the system matrix containing the system coefficients $a_{ik} = a_{ik}(\boldsymbol{p})$ and the vector $\boldsymbol{z} = (z_1, \ldots, z_n)^T$ contains the inhomogeneities. The linear system is *homogeneous* if $\boldsymbol{z} = 0$ holds. Linear systems can be solved analytically. Although in real-world problems the differential equations are usually nonlinear, linear systems are important as linear approximations for the investigation of steady states.

Example 12.9

The simple linear system

$$\begin{aligned} \frac{dx_1}{dt} &= a_{12}x_2 \\ \frac{dx_2}{dt} &= -x_1 \end{aligned}, \qquad (12.37)$$

has a general solution

$$\begin{aligned} x_1 &= \frac{1}{2}e^{-i\sqrt{a_{12}}t}\left(1 + e^{2i\sqrt{a_{12}}t}\right)C_1 - \frac{1}{2}ie^{-i\sqrt{a_{12}}t}\left(-1 + e^{2i\sqrt{a_{12}}t}\right)\sqrt{a_{12}}C_2 \\ x_2 &= \frac{i}{2\sqrt{a_{12}}}e^{-i\sqrt{a_{12}}t}\left(1 + e^{2i\sqrt{a_{12}}t}\right)C_1 + \frac{1}{2}e^{-i\sqrt{a_{12}}t}\left(1 + e^{2i\sqrt{a_{12}}t}\right)C_2 \end{aligned},$$

with the integration constants C_1, C_2. Choosing $a_{12} = 1$ simplifies the system to

$$x_1 = C_1\cos(t) + C_2\sin(t), x_2 = C_2\cos(t) - C_1\sin(t).$$

Specification of the initial conditions to $x_1(0) = 2$, $x_2(0) = 1$ gives the particular solution

$$x_1 = 2\cos(t) + \sin(t), x_2 = \cos(t) - 2\sin(t).$$

The solution can be displayed in the phase plane or directly as functions of time (Figure 12.1):

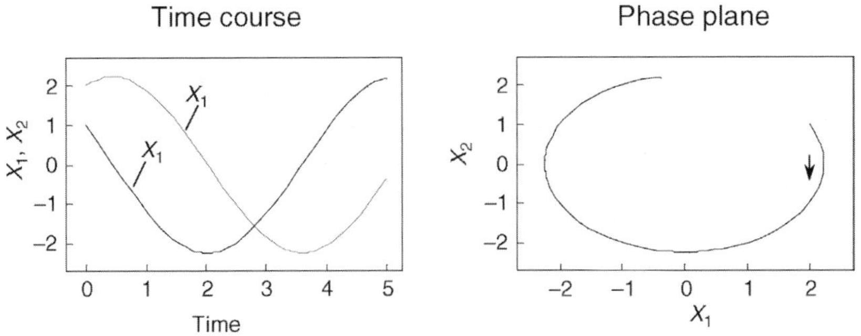

Figure 12.1 Phase plane and time course for the linear system of ODEs represented in Eq. (12.37). In time course panel: gray line $x_1(t)$, black line $x_2(t)$. Parameters: $a_{12} = 1$, $x_1(0) = 1$, $x_2(0) = 2$.

12.2.2
Linearization of Autonomous Systems

In order to investigate the behavior of a system close to steady state, it may be useful to linearize it. Starting with the deviation $\xi(t)$ from steady state with $\boldsymbol{x}(t) = \boldsymbol{x}^{\mathrm{st}} + \xi(t)$. It follows that

$$\dot{\boldsymbol{x}} = \frac{\mathrm{d}}{\mathrm{d}t}(\boldsymbol{x}^{\mathrm{st}} + \xi(t)) = \frac{\mathrm{d}}{\mathrm{d}t}\xi(t). \tag{12.38}$$

Taylor expansion of the temporal change of the deviation, $\frac{\mathrm{d}}{\mathrm{d}t}\xi_i = f_i(x_1^{\mathrm{st}} + \xi_1, \ldots, x_n^{\mathrm{st}} + \xi_n)$, gives

$$\frac{\mathrm{d}}{\mathrm{d}t}\xi_i = f_i(x_1^{\mathrm{st}}, \ldots, x_n^{\mathrm{st}}) + \sum_{j=1}^{n} \frac{\partial f_i}{\partial x_j}\xi_j + \frac{1}{2}\sum_{j=1}^{n}\sum_{k=1}^{n} \frac{\partial^2 f_i}{\partial x_j \partial x_k}\xi_j\xi_k + \ldots. \tag{12.39}$$

Since we consider steady state, it holds that $f_i(x_1^{\mathrm{st}}, \ldots, x_n^{\mathrm{st}}) = 0$. Neglecting terms of higher order, we have

$$\frac{\mathrm{d}}{\mathrm{d}t}\xi_i \approx \sum_{j=1}^{n} \frac{\partial f_i}{\partial x_j}\xi_j = \sum_{j=1}^{n} a_{ij}\xi_j. \tag{12.40}$$

The coefficients a_{ij} are calculated at steady state and are constant. They form the so-called *Jacobian* matrix:

$$J = \{a_{ij}\} = \begin{pmatrix} \frac{\partial f_1}{\partial x_1} & \frac{\partial f_1}{\partial x_2} & \cdots & \frac{\partial f_1}{\partial x_n} \\ \frac{\partial f_2}{\partial x_1} & \frac{\partial f_2}{\partial x_2} & \cdots & \frac{\partial f_2}{\partial x_n} \\ \vdots & \vdots & \ddots & \vdots \\ \frac{\partial f_n}{\partial x_1} & \frac{\partial f_n}{\partial x_2} & \cdots & \frac{\partial f_n}{\partial x_n} \end{pmatrix}. \tag{12.41}$$

For linear systems $\dot{\boldsymbol{x}} = \boldsymbol{A}\boldsymbol{x} + \boldsymbol{z}$ it holds $\boldsymbol{J} = \boldsymbol{A}$.

12.2.3 Solution of Linear ODE Systems

Often we are interested in two different types of problems: describing the temporal evolution of the system and finding its steady state. The problem of finding the steady state $\boldsymbol{x}^{st}$ of a linear ODE system $\dot{\boldsymbol{x}} = 0$ implies $\boldsymbol{A}\boldsymbol{x}^{st} + \boldsymbol{z} = 0$. The solution necessitates inversion of the system matrix $\boldsymbol{A}$:

$$\boldsymbol{x}^{st} = -\boldsymbol{A}^{-1}\boldsymbol{z}. \tag{12.42}$$

The time course solution of homogeneous linear ODEs is described in the following. The systems can be solved with an exponential ansatz. In the case $n = 1$ we have

$$\frac{dx_1}{dt} = a_{11}x_1. \tag{12.43}$$

Substituting the ansatz $x_1(t) = b_1 e^{\lambda t}$ with constant b_1 into Eq. (12.43) yields

$$b_1 \lambda e^{\lambda t} = a_{11} b_1 e^{\lambda t}. \tag{12.44}$$

Equation (12.44) is true if $\lambda = a_{11}$. This leads to a general solution

$$x_1(t) = b_1 e^{a_{11}t}. \tag{12.45}$$

To find a particular solution, we must specify the initial conditions $x_1(t = 0) = x_1^0 = b_1 e^{a_{11}t}|_{t=0} = b_1$. Thus, the solution is

$$x_1(t) = x_1^0 e^{a_{11}t}. \tag{12.46}$$

For a linear homogeneous system of n differential equations, $\dot{\boldsymbol{x}} = \boldsymbol{A}\boldsymbol{x}$, the ansatz is $\boldsymbol{x} = \boldsymbol{b}e^{\lambda t}$. This gives $\dot{\boldsymbol{x}} = \boldsymbol{b}\lambda e^{\lambda t} = \boldsymbol{A}\boldsymbol{b}e^{\lambda t}$. The scalar factor $e^{\lambda t}$ can be cancelled out, leading to $\boldsymbol{b}\lambda = \boldsymbol{A}\boldsymbol{b}$ or the characteristic equation

$$(\boldsymbol{A} - \lambda \boldsymbol{I}_n)\boldsymbol{b} = 0. \tag{12.47}$$

The solution of this equation is described in Section 12.1.2.

For homogeneous linear systems holds the *superposition principle*: if $\boldsymbol{x}_1$ and $\boldsymbol{x}_2$ are solutions of this ODE system, then their linear combination is also a solution. This leads in most cases (if the eigenvalues have identical algebraic and geometric multiplicities) to the general solution of the homogeneous linear ODE system:

$$\boldsymbol{x}(t) = \sum_{i=1}^{n} c_i \boldsymbol{b}^{(i)} e^{\lambda_i t}, \tag{12.48}$$

where $\boldsymbol{b}^{(i)}$ are the eigenvectors of the system matrix $\boldsymbol{A}$ corresponding to the eigenvalues λ_i. A particular solution specifying the coefficients c_i can be found considering the initial conditions $\boldsymbol{x}(t = 0) = \boldsymbol{x}^0 = \sum_{j=1}^{n} c_i \boldsymbol{b}^{(i)}$. This constitutes an inhomogeneous linear equation system to be solved for c_i.

For the solution of inhomogeneous linear ODEs, the system $\dot{\boldsymbol{x}} = \boldsymbol{A}\boldsymbol{x} + \boldsymbol{z}$ can be transformed into a homogeneous system by the coordination transformation $\hat{\boldsymbol{x}} = \boldsymbol{x} - \boldsymbol{x}^{st}$. Since $\frac{d}{dt}\boldsymbol{x}^{st} = \boldsymbol{A}\boldsymbol{x}^{st} + \boldsymbol{z} = 0$ it holds $\frac{d}{dt}\hat{\boldsymbol{x}} = \boldsymbol{A}\hat{\boldsymbol{x}}$. Therefore, we can use the solution algorithm for homogeneous systems for the transformed system.

12.2.4
Stability of Steady States

If a system is at steady state it stays there – until an external perturbation occurs. Depending on the behavior of the system after a perturbation steady states are either

- *stable* – the system returns to this state
- *unstable* – the system leaves this state
- *metastable* – the system behavior is indifferent.

A steady state is *asymptotically* stable if it is stable and nearby initial conditions tend to this state for $t \to \infty$. *Local* stability describes the behavior after small perturbations, *global* stability after any perturbation.

To investigate whether a steady state $\boldsymbol{x}^{st}$ of the ODE system $\dot{\boldsymbol{x}} = \boldsymbol{f}(\boldsymbol{x})$ is asymptotically stable, we consider the linearized system $\dot{\xi} = A\xi$ with $\xi(t) = \boldsymbol{x}(t) - \boldsymbol{x}^{st}$. The steady state $\boldsymbol{x}^{st}$ is asymptotically stable if the Jacobian $\boldsymbol{A}$ has n eigenvalues with strictly negative real parts each. The steady state is unstable, if at least one eigenvalue has a positive real part. This will be explained in more detail for one- and two-dimensional systems.

We start with one-dimensional systems, i.e., $n = 1$. Be without loss of generality $x_1^{st} = 0$, i.e., $x_1 = \xi_1$. To the system $\dot{x}_1 = f_1(x_1)$ belongs the linearized system $\dot{x}_1 = \frac{\partial f_1}{\partial x_1}\big|_{\bar{x}_1} x_1 = a_{11}x_1$. The Jacobian matrix $\boldsymbol{A} = \{a_{11}\}$ has only one eigenvalue $\lambda_1 = a_{11} = \frac{\partial f_1}{\partial x_1}\big|_{\bar{x}_1}$. The solution is $x_1(t) = x_1^0 e^{\lambda_1 t}$. It is obvious that $e^{\lambda_1 t}$ increases for $\lambda_1 > 0$ and the system deviates from the steady state. For $\lambda_1 < 0$ the distance from steady state decreases and $x_1(t) \to x_1^{st}$ for $t \to \infty$. For $\lambda_1 = 0$ consideration of the linearized system allows no conclusion about stability of the original system.

Consider a two-dimensional case $n = 2$ with $\boldsymbol{x}^{st} = 0$. To the system

$$\begin{aligned}\dot{x}_1 &= f_1(x_1, x_2)\\ \dot{x}_2 &= f_2(x_1, x_2)\end{aligned} \tag{12.49}$$

belongs the linearized system

$$\begin{aligned}\dot{x}_1 &= \frac{\partial f_1}{\partial x_1}\bigg|_{x^{st}} x_1 + \frac{\partial f_1}{\partial x_2}\bigg|_{x^{st}} x_2\\ \dot{x}_2 &= \frac{\partial f_2}{\partial x_1}\bigg|_{x^{st}} x_1 + \frac{\partial f_2}{\partial x_2}\bigg|_{x^{st}} x_2\end{aligned} \quad \text{or} \quad \dot{\boldsymbol{x}} = \begin{pmatrix} \frac{\partial f_1}{\partial x_1}\big|_{x^{st}} & \frac{\partial f_1}{\partial x_2}\big|_{x^{st}} \\ \frac{\partial f_2}{\partial x_1}\big|_{x^{st}} & \frac{\partial f_2}{\partial x_2}\big|_{x^{st}} \end{pmatrix} \boldsymbol{x} = \begin{pmatrix} a_{11} & a_{12} \\ a_{21} & a_{22} \end{pmatrix} \boldsymbol{x} = \boldsymbol{A}\boldsymbol{x}. \tag{12.50}$$

To find the eigenvalues of $\boldsymbol{A}$, we have to solve the characteristic equation

$$\lambda^2 - \underbrace{(a_{11} + a_{22})}_{\text{Trace}\,A}\lambda + \underbrace{a_{11}a_{22} - a_{12}a_{21}}_{\text{Det}\,A} = 0 \tag{12.51}$$

and get

$$\lambda_{1/2} = \frac{\text{Trace}\,\boldsymbol{A}}{2} \pm \sqrt{\frac{(\text{Trace}\,\boldsymbol{A})^2}{4} - \text{Det}\,\boldsymbol{A}}. \tag{12.52}$$

The eigenvalues are either real for $((\text{Trace}\,\boldsymbol{A})^2/4 - \text{Det}\,\boldsymbol{A} \geq 0)$ or complex (otherwise). For complex eigenvalues, the solution contains oscillatory parts.

For stability it is necessary that Trace $\boldsymbol{A} < 0$ and Det $\boldsymbol{A} > 0$. Depending on the sign of the eigenvalues, steady states of a two-dimensional system may have the following characteristics:

1. $\lambda_1 < 0$, $\lambda_2 < 0$, both real: stable node
2. $\lambda_1 > 0$, $\lambda_2 > 0$, both real: unstable node
3. $\lambda_1 > 0$, $\lambda_2 < 0$, both real: saddle point, unstable
4. $\text{Re}(\lambda_1) < 0$, $\text{Re}(\lambda_2) < 0$, both complex with negative real parts: stable focus
5. $\text{Re}(\lambda_1) > 0$, $\text{Re}(\lambda_2) > 0$, both complex with positive real parts: unstable focus
6. $\text{Re}(\lambda_1) = \text{Re}(\lambda_2) = 0$, both complex with zero real parts: center, unstable.

A graphical representation of stability depending on trace and determinant is given in Figure 12.2.

Up to now we considered only the linearized system. For the stability of the original system holds:

If the steady state of the linearized system is asymptotically stable, then the steady state of the complete system is also asymptotically stable. If the steady state of the

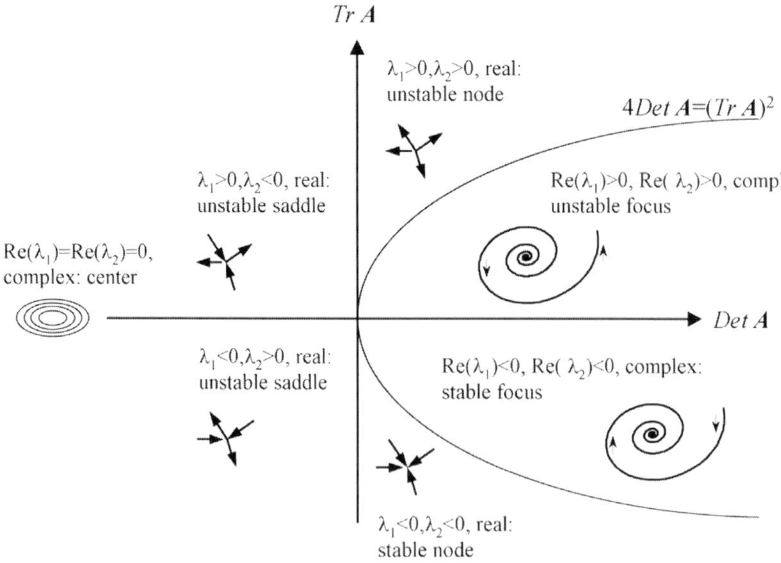

Figure 12.2 Stability of steady states in two-dimensional systems: the character of steady-state solutions is represented depending on the value of the determinant (*x*-axis) and the trace (*y*-axis) of the Jacobian matrix. Phase plane behavior of trajectories in different cases is schematically represented.

linearized system is a saddle, an unstable node or an unstable focus, then the steady state of the complete system is also unstable. This means that statements about the stability remain true, but the character of the steady state is not necessarily kept. About the center no statement is possible.

Routh–Hurwitz theorem [1]: For systems with $n > 2$ differential equations holds that the characteristic polynomial

$$a_n\lambda^n + a_{n-1}\lambda^{n-1} + \cdots + a_1\lambda + a_0 = 0, \tag{12.53}$$

is a polynomial of degree n and the characteristic equation often cannot be solved analytically (for $n > 4$). We can use the Hurwitz criterion to test whether the real parts of all eigenvalues are negative. We have to form the Hurwitz matrix $\boldsymbol{H}$, containing the coefficients of the characteristic polynomial:

$$\boldsymbol{H} = \begin{pmatrix} a_{n-1} & a_{n-3} & a_{n-5} & \cdots & 0 \\ a_n & a_{n-2} & a_{n-4} & \cdots & 0 \\ 0 & a_{n-1} & a_{n-3} & \cdots & 0 \\ 0 & a_n & a_{n-2} & \cdots & 0 \\ \vdots & \vdots & \vdots & \ddots & \vdots \\ 0 & 0 & 0 & \cdots & a_0 \end{pmatrix} = \{h_{ik}\}, \tag{12.54}$$

where the h_{ik} follow the rule

$$h_{ik} = \begin{cases} a_{n+i-2k}, & \text{if } 0 \le 2k-i \le n \\ 0, & \text{else} \end{cases}. \tag{12.55}$$

It can be shown that all solutions of the characteristic polynomial have negative real parts if all coefficients a_i of the polynomial and all principal leading minors of $\boldsymbol{H}$ have positive values.

12.2.4.1 Global Stability of Steady States

A state is globally stable if the trajectories for all initial conditions approach it for $t \to \infty$. The stability of a steady state of an ODE system can sometimes be proven with a method of Lyapunov.

Transfer the steady state into the point of origin by coordination transformation $\hat{x} = \boldsymbol{x} - \boldsymbol{x}^{\text{st}}$.

Find a Lyapunov function $V_L(x_1, \ldots, x_n)$ with the following properties:

1. $V_L(x_1, \ldots, x_n)$ has steady derivatives with respect to all variables x_i.
2. $V_L(x_1, \ldots, x_n)$ is positive definite, i.e., $V_L(x_1, \ldots, x_n) = 0$ for $x_i = 0$ and $V_L(x_1, \ldots, x_n) > 0$ for $x_i \neq 0$.

The time derivative of $\mathrm{d}V_L(x(t))/\mathrm{d}t$ is given by

$$\frac{\mathrm{d}V_L}{\mathrm{d}t} = \sum_{i=1}^{n} \frac{\partial V_L}{\partial x_i}\frac{\mathrm{d}x_i}{\mathrm{d}t} = \sum_{i=1}^{n} \frac{\partial V_L}{\partial x_i} f_i(x_1, \ldots, x_n). \tag{12.56}$$

It holds that a steady state $x^{\text{st}} = 0$ is stable if the time derivative of V_L in a certain region around this state has no positive values. The steady state is asymptotically stable if the time derivative of V_L in this region is negative definite, i.e., $dV_L/dt = x(t) = 0$ for $x_i = 0$ and $dV_L/dt < 0$ for $x_i \neq 0$.

Example 12.10

The system $\dot{x}_1 = -x_1$, $\dot{x}_2 = -x_2$ has a solution $x_1(t) = x_1^0 e^{-t}$, $x_2(t) = x_2^0 e^{-t}$ and the state $x_1 = x_2 = 0$ is asymptotically stable.

The global stability can also be shown using the positive definite function $V_L = x_1^2 + x_2^2$ as Lyapunov function. It holds $dV_L/dt = x(t) = (\partial V_L/\partial x_1)\dot{x}_1 + (\partial V_L/\partial x_2)\dot{x}_2 = 2x_1(-x_1) + 2x_2(-x_2)$, which is negative definite.

12.2.5 Limit Cycles

Oscillatory behavior is a typical phenomenon in biology. The cause of the oscillation may be different; either externally imposed or internally implemented. Internally caused stable oscillations as a function of time can be found if a limit cycle exists in the phase space.

A *limit cycle* is an isolated closed trajectory for which all trajectories in its vicinity are periodic solutions winding toward (stable limit cycle) or away from (unstable) the limit cycle for $t \to \infty$.

Example 12.11

The nonlinear system $\dot{x}_1 = x_1^2 x_2 - x_1$, $\dot{x}_2 = p - x_1^2 x_2$ has a steady state at $x_1^{st} = p$, $x_2^{st} = 1/p$

Choosing, e.g., $p = 0.98$ this steady state is unstable since Trace $\mathbf{A} = 1 - p^2 > 0$ (Figure 12.3).

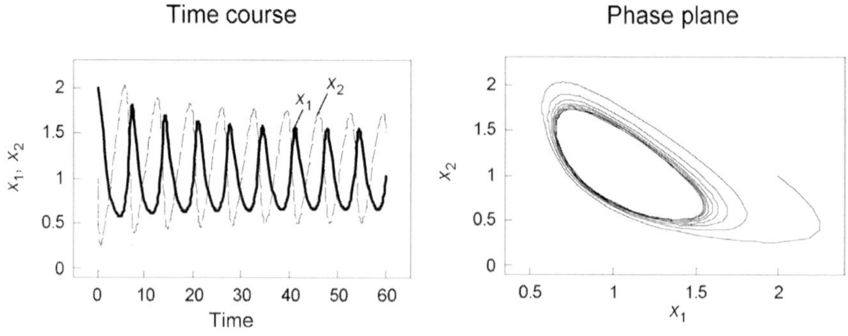

Figure 12.3 Solution of the equation system of Example 12.11 represented as time course (left panel) and as phase plane (right panel). Initial conditions $x_1(0) = 2$, $x_2(0) = 1$.

For two-dimensional systems there are two criteria to check whether a limit cycle exists. Consider a system of differential equations

$$\begin{aligned} \dot{x}_1 &= f_1(x_1, x_2) \\ \dot{x}_2 &= f_2(x_1, x_2) \end{aligned} . \tag{12.57}$$

The *negative criterion of Bendixson* states: if the trace of the Jacobian Trace $J = \frac{\partial f_1}{\partial x_1} + \frac{\partial f_2}{\partial x_2}$ does not change its sign in a certain region of the phase plane, then there is no closed trajectory in this area. Hence, a necessary condition for the existence of a limit cycle is the change of the sign.

Example 12.12

In Example 12.11 it holds that Trace $= (2x_1x_2 - 1) + (-x_1^2)$. Therefore, Trace $= 0$ is fulfilled at $x_2 = \frac{x_1^2 + 1}{2x_1}$ and Trace may assume positive or negative values for varying x_1, x_2, and the necessary condition for the existence of a limit cycle is met.

The *criteria of Poincaré--Bendixson* states that if a trajectory in the phase plane remains within a finite region without approaching a singular point (a steady state), then this trajectory is either a limit cycle or it approaches a limit cycle. This criterion gives a sufficient condition for the existence of a limit cycle. However, the limit cycle trajectory can be computed analytically only in very rare cases.

12.3 Difference Equations

Modeling with difference equations employs a discrete time scale, compared to the continuous time scale in ODEs. In some models the value of the variable x at a discrete time point t depends directly on the value of this variable at a former time point. For instance, the number of individuals in a population of birds in one year can be related to the number of individuals that existed last year.

A general (first-order) difference equation takes the form

$$x_i = f(x_{i-1}) \quad \text{for} \quad \text{all } i. \tag{12.58}$$

We can solve such an equation by successive calculation: given x_0 we have

$$\begin{aligned} x_1 &= f(x_0) \\ x_2 &= f(x_1) = f(f(x_0)) \\ &\vdots \end{aligned} . \tag{12.59}$$

In particular, given any value x_0, there exists a unique solution path $x_1, x_2, \ldots$. For simple forms of the function f we can also find general solutions.

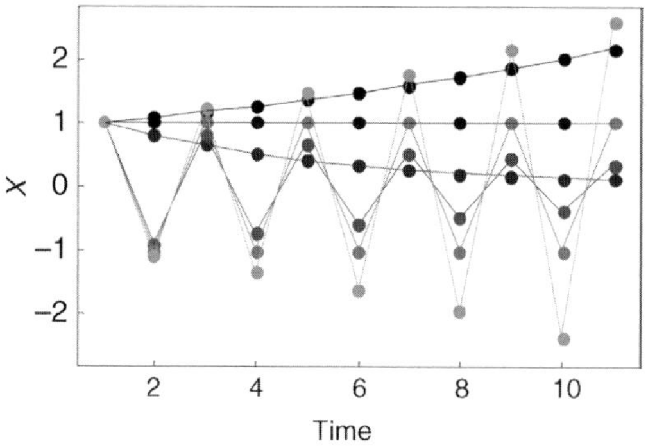

Figure 12.4 Temporal behavior of a difference equation describing exponential growth for various values of parameter r. (r drops with the gray level).

Example 12.13

Consider the exponential growth of a bacterial population with a doubling of the population size x_i in each time interval. The recursive equation $x_i = 2x_{i-1}$ is equivalent to the explicit equation $x_i = x_0 \cdot 2^i$ and also to the difference equation $x_i - x_{i-1} = \Delta x = x_{i-1}$.

The difference equation expresses the relation between values of a variable at discrete time points. We are interested in the dynamics of the variable (Figure 12.4). For the general case $x_i = rx_{i-1}$ it can be easily shown that $x_i = r^i x_0$. This corresponds to the law of exponential growth (Malthus law). The dynamic behavior depends on the parameter r:

$1 < r$:	exponential growth
$r = 1$:	x remains constant, steady state
$0 < r < 1$:	exponential decay
$-1 < r < 0$:	alternating decay
$r = -1$:	periodic solution
$r < -1$:	alternating increase

A difference equation of the form

$$x_{i+k} = f(x_{i+k}, \ldots, x_{i+1}, x_i), \qquad (12.60)$$

is a kth order difference equation. Like ODEs, difference equations may have stationary solutions that might be stable or unstable, which are defined as follows.

The value x^{st} is a stationary solution or *fixed point* of the difference equation (12.60) if $x^{st} = f(x^{st})$. A fixed point is stable (or unstable), if there is a neighborhood $N = \{x: |x - x^{st}| < \varepsilon\}$ such that every series that begins in N converges against x^{st} (leaves N). Practically applicable is the following sentence: The fixed point is stable under the condition that f is continuously differentiable, if $\left|\frac{df(x)}{dx}\right|_{x^{st}} < 1$.

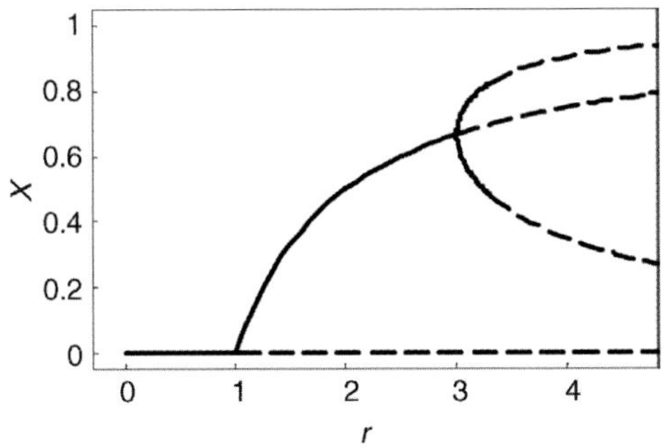

Figure 12.5 Bifurcation diagram of the logistic equation. For increasing parameter r the number of steady states increments. At the points $r = 1$, $r = 3$, and $r = 3.3$ occur stability changes from stable (solid lines) to unstable (dashed lines). Only the constant solution and the solution of period 1 and 2 are shown.

Example 12.14

The simplest form of the logistic equation, which plays a role in population dynamics, is $x_{n+1} = rx_n(1 - x_n)$ with $f(x) = rx(1 - x)$, where r is a positive valued parameter. This difference equation has two fix points, $x_1^{st} = 0$ and $x_2^{st} = 1 - \frac{1}{r}$. Stability analysis yields that fix point x_1^{st} is stable, if $\left|\frac{df(x)}{dx}\right|_{x_1^{st}} = r < 1$ and fix point x_2^{st} is stable, if $\left|\frac{df(x)}{dx}\right|_{x_2^{st}} = |2 - r| < 1$, hence $1 < r < 3$.

For $r > 3$ there are stable oscillations of period 2, i.e., successive generations alternate between two values. Finding the steady states x_1^{st} and x_2^{st} is enabled by a new function $g(x) = f(f(x))$. The equation $g(x) = x$ has two solutions $x_{1,2}^{st} = \frac{r+1 \pm \sqrt{(3-r)(r+1)}}{2r}$. They are stable if $\left|\frac{dg(x)}{dx}\right|_{x_i^{st}} < 1$ holds for $i = 1, 2$ or $\left|\left(\frac{df(x)}{dx}\right)\Big|_{x_1^{st}} \cdot \left(\frac{df(x)}{dx}\right)\Big|_{x_2^{st}}\right| < 1$, i.e., for $3 < r < 3.3$. For $r > 3.3$ oscillations occur of higher period, which can be treated in an analogous manner as oscillations of period 2. For $r > r_{crit}$ chaos arises, i.e., albeit deterministic description the system trajectories cannot in fact be reliably predicted and may differ remarkably for close initial conditions. The points $r = 1$, $r = 3$, and $r = 3.3$ are bifurcation points since the number and stability of steady states changes. A graphical representation is given in Figure 12.5.

12.4 Graph and Network Theory

Many kinds of structures described in systems biology, such as metabolic pathways, signaling pathways, or gene-regulatory networks, can be represented as graphs. Other examples are taxonomies, e.g., of enzymes or organisms (directed acyclic graphs), protein interaction networks (undirected graphs), DNA, RNA or protein sequences (linear graphs), chemical structure graphs (undirected graphs), gene coexpression (undirected graphs). In this section we give a brief overview of the calculus and formalization of graph problems, describe basic algorithms underlying some of the practical problems and introduce specifically into the framework of gene-regulatory networks that are essential in analyzing transcriptome data.

A *graph*, $G(V, E)$, is composed of a set of *vertices* (or nodes), V, and a binary relation, E, on V. A visual representation of a graph consists of a set of vertices, whereby each pair is connected by an edge whenever the binary relation holds. If the edges have a specific direction, then $G(V, E)$ is called a *directed graph* otherwise it is called an *undirected graph*.

Computationally, a graph containing n vertices can be represented in two ways: as an adjacency list or as an adjacency matrix [2]. An *adjacency list* stores for each vertex i the list of vertices connected to vertex i. An *adjacency matrix* is an $n \times n$ binary matrix defined as $\mathbf{A} = [a_{ij}]$, where $a_{ij} = \begin{cases} 1 & \text{there is an edge from vertex } i \text{ to vertex } j \\ 0 & \text{else} \end{cases}$.

In the case of an undirected graph, $\mathbf{A}$ is symmetric. Commonly, the adjacency-list presentation is preferred if the graph structure is sparse and there are not many edges compared to the number of vertex pairs, i.e., $|E| \ll |V|^2$, because then the amount of memory is far less than using a matrix representation. If there is an edge from vertex i to j we denote it by $(i, j) \in E$. A *weighted graph* consists of a graph, $G(V, E)$, together with a real-valued weight function $w: E \to \Re$. Weighted graphs are used, for example, to represent gene-regulatory networks.

The *degree* of a vertex i, $d(i)$, in an undirected graph is the number of edges connected to i, $d(i) = |\{(i, j) \in E; j = 1, \ldots, n\}|$. The degree of a vertex i in a directed graph is defined as the sum of its in-degree and out-degree. The *in-degree* of vertex i is defined as the number of edges entering vertex i and the *out-degree* is the number of edges leaving it. The degree of a vertex i can be computed from the adjacency matrix as the sum of the ith row (out-degree) and the ith column sums (in-degree).

Topological properties of interaction graphs are commonly used in applications to characterize biological function [3–5]. For example, lethal mutations are defined by highly connected parts of a protein interaction graph whose removal disrupts the graph structure.

A *path* of length l from a vertex v_0 to a vertex v_l in a graph $G(V, E)$ is a sequence of vertices $v_0, \ldots, v_l$ such that $(v_{i-1}, v_i) \in E$ for $i = 1, \ldots, l$. A path is a *cycle* if $l \geq 1$ and $v_0 = v_l$. A directed graph that contains no cycle is called a *directed acyclic graph*. The *weight of a path* in a weighted directed graph is the sum of the weights of all edges constituting the path. The *shortest path* from vertex v_0 to vertex v_l is the path with the minimal weight. If all weights are equal, then the shortest path is the path from vertex v_0 to vertex v_l with the minimal number of edges. An important practical problem consists of the identification of substructures of a given graph. An undirected graph is *connected* when there exists a path for each pair of vertices. If a subset of a graph is connected it is called a *connected component*.

Gene-regulatory networks are graph-based models for a simplified view on gene regulation. Transcription factors are stimulated by upstream signaling cascades and bind on cis-regulatory positions of their target genes. Bound transcription factors promote or inhibit RNA polymerase assembly and thus determine, if and to what abundance the target gene is expressed. The modeling of gene regulation via genetic networks has been widely used in practice (for a review see de Jong [6]). Here we use this biological problem as an example to introduce networks.

12.4.1
Linear Networks

A nonlinear dynamic model of gene regulation assumes that the change of gene expression of gene x_i at time t can be described by the following equation:

$$\frac{\mathrm{d}x_i(t)}{\mathrm{d}t} = r_i f\left(\sum_{j=1}^{n} w_{ij}x_j(t) + \sum_{k=1}^{m} v_{ik}u_k(t) + b_i\right) - \lambda_i x_i(t), \tag{12.61}$$

where

f is the activation function,
$x_i(t)$ is the gene expression of gene i at time t (for instance measured as mRNA concentration),
r_i is the transcription rate of gene i,
w_{ij} is the weights that determines the influence of gene j on gene i,
$u_k(t)$ are the external inputs (e.g., the concentration of a chemical compound) at time t,
v_{ik} is the weights that determines the influence of external compound k on gene i,
b_i is a lower base level of gene i,
λ_i is the degradation constant for gene i.

The activation function, f, is a monotonic function, assuming that the concentration of the gene product is monotonically dependent on the concentrations of its regulators. Often, these functions have sigmoidal form, such as $f(z) = (1 + e^{-z})^{-1}$. If this function is the identity, i.e., $f(z) = z$ then the network is linear. Additionally, common simplifications include constancy in the reaction rates, no external influence, and linear activation so that formula (12.61) reduces to

$$\frac{\mathrm{d}x_i(t)}{\mathrm{d}t} = \sum_{j=1}^{n} w'_{ij}x_j(t) + b_i. \tag{12.62}$$

The degradation term is incorporated in the matrix $w' = w - \mathrm{diag}(\lambda)$. These models have been investigated, for example, by D'Haeseleer *et al.* (1999). The parameters of interest are the weights w_{ij}, which are estimated by statistical methods.

12.4.2
Boolean Networks

Boolean networks are qualitative descriptions of gene-regulatory interactions. Gene expression in such models has two states on (1) and off (0) [7–10]. Let $\boldsymbol{x}$ be an n-dimensional binary vector representing the state of a system of n genes. Thus, the state space of the system consists of 2^n possible states. Each component, x_i, determines the expression of the ith gene. With each gene i we associate a Boolean rule, b_i. Given the input variables for gene i at time t this function determines whether the regulated element is active or inactive at time $t + 1$, i.e.,

$$x_i(t+1) = b_i(\mathbf{x}(t)), \quad 1 \leq i \leq n. \tag{12.63}$$

Equation (12.63) describes the dynamics of the Boolean network. The practical feasibility of Boolean network models is heavily dependent on the number of input variables, k, for each gene. The number of possible input states of k inputs is 2^k. For each such combination a specific Boolean function must determine whether the next state would be on or off. Thus, there are 2^{2^k} possible Boolean functions (or rules). This number rapidly increases with the connectivity. For $k = 2$ we have four possible input states and 16 possible rules, for $k = 3$, we have eight possible input states and 256 possible rules, etc.

In a Boolean network each state has a deterministic output state. A series of states is called a *trajectory*. If no change occurs in the transition between two states, i.e., output state equals input state then the system is in a *point attractor*. Point attractors are analogous to steady states of differential equation models. If the system is in a cycle of states then we have a *dynamic attractor*.

Example 12.15: Boolean network

Consider three genes where each gene has connectivity 2, i.e., $n = 3$ and $k = 2$. Then we have $2^{2^2} = 16$ possible Boolean rules. These can be listed as follows:

Input	Output rules															
	1	2	3	4	5	6	7	8	9	10	11	12	13	14	15	16
00	0	1	0	0	0	1	1	1	0	0	0	1	1	1	0	1
01	0	0	1	0	0	1	0	0	1	1	0	1	1	0	1	1
10	0	0	0	1	0	0	1	0	1	0	1	1	0	1	1	1
11	0	0	0	0	1	0	0	1	0	1	1	0	1	1	1	1

The rules include all possible combinations of Boolean logic such as *AND* (rule 5) and *OR* (rule 15). Figure 12.6 illustrates a simple Boolean network. Node 1 and node 2 follow the *OR* rule and node 3 follows the *AND* rule. Thus, for example if a state of the system is $\mathbf{x(t)} = (101)$, then the Boolean functions would be $b_1(101) = 1$, $b_2(101) = 1$, $b_3(101) = 0$ and we would get $\mathbf{x(t + 1)} = (110)$.

The system has two point attractors, (0 0 0) and (1 1 1). The trajectory starting with (0 0 0) ends in the first attractor, all trajectories starting from other states end in the second attractor, except for the cycle (0 1 0) $\leftrightarrow$ (1 0 0).

Several algorithms have been developed to reconstruct or *reverse engineer* Boolean networks from time series of gene-expression data, i.e., from a limited number of states. Among the first was *REVEAL* developed by Liang *et al.* [11]. Additionally, properties of random Boolean networks were intensively investigated by Kauff-

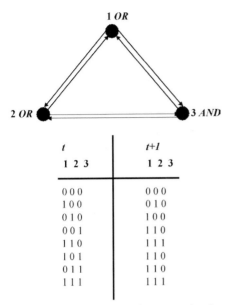

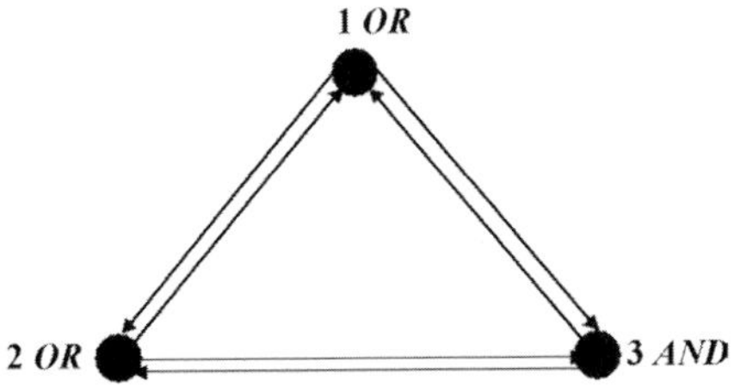

t (1 2 3)	$t+1$ (1 2 3)
0 0 0	0 0 0
1 0 0	0 1 0
0 1 0	1 0 0
0 0 1	1 1 0
1 1 0	1 1 1
1 0 1	1 1 0
0 1 1	1 1 0
1 1 1	1 1 1

Figure 12.6 Example of a Boolean network with $n=3$ nodes and connectivity $k=2$. Node 1 and 2 follow the OR rule, i.e., whenever one of the two inputs is on, the resulting output of the function is on, node 3 follows the AND rule, i.e., only if both inputs are on, the output would be on. The table displays the eight possible states of the system and the corresponding output states.

man [7]; for example, global dynamics, steady states, connectivity, and the specific types of Boolean functions.

12.4.3
Bayesian Networks

Bayesian networks describe the conditional dependences between random variables [12–14]. Bayesian networks necessitate the notion of a *directed acyclic graph*, $G(V, E)$. The vertices correspond to n genes each corresponding to a random variable x_i, $1 \leq i \leq n$. In gene-regulatory networks the random variables describe the gene expression level of the respective gene. For each x_i there is defined a conditional probability $p(x_i|\mathrm{L}(x_i))$, where $L(x_i)$ denotes the *parents* of gene i, i.e., the set of genes that have a direct regulatory influence on gene i. Figure 12.7 gives an example.

The set of conditional distributions for each gene and the graph define a joint probability distribution via

$$p(x) = \prod_{i=1}^{n} p(x_i|L(x_i)). \tag{12.64}$$

The central assumption for the above formula is that for each gene we have a *conditional independence* of x_i from its nondescendants given the parent set of x_i. Here,

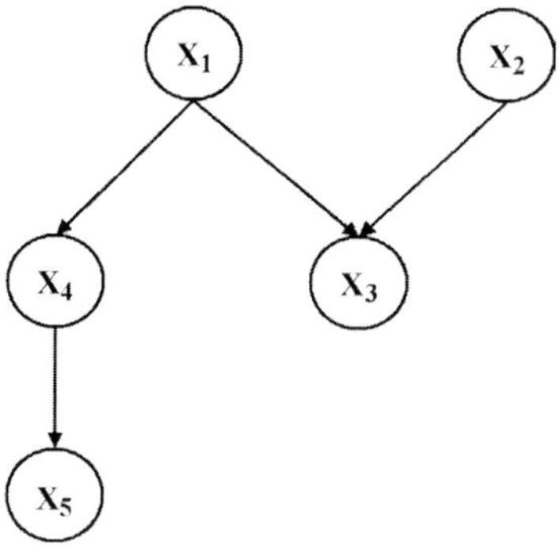

Figure 12.7 Bayesian network. The graph determines the conditional independences.

conditional independence of two random variables x_i and x_j given a random variable x_k means that $p(x_i, x_j|x_k) = p(x_i|x_k)p(x_j|x_k)$ or, equivalently, $p(x_i|x_j, x_k) = p(x_i|x_k)$.

References

1 Bronstein, I.N. and Semendjajew, K.A. (1987) *Taschenbuch der Mathematik*, 23rd Edition, Nauka, Moscow.

2 Cormen, T.H. *et al.* (2001) *Introduction to algorithms*, 2nd Edition MIT Press, Cambridge, MA.

3 Jeong, H. *et al.* (2001) Lethality and centrality in protein networks. *Nature*, **411**, 41–42.

4 Stelling, J. *et al.* (2002) Metabolic network structure determines key aspects of functionality and regulation. *Nature*, **420**, 190–193.

5 Przulj, N. *et al.* (2004) Functional topology in a network of protein interactions. *Bioinformatics*, **20**, 340–348.

6 de Jong, H. (2002) Modeling and simulation of genetic regulatory systems: a literature review. *J Comput Biol*, **9**, 67–103.

7 Kauffman, S.A. (1993) The origins of order: Self-organization and selection in evolution, Oxford University Press, New York.

8 Akutsu, T. *et al.* (1999) 'Identification of genetic networks from a small number of gene expression patterns under the Boolean network model', in: R. B. A. a. others, (ed.), Singapore, pp. 17–28.

9 Akutsu, T. *et al.* (2000) Inferring qualitative relations in genetic networks and metabolic pathways. *Bioinformatics*, **16**, 727–734.

10 TH, C. *et al.* (2001) *Introduction to algorithms*. 2nd Edition, MIT Press, Cambridge, MA.

11 Liang, S. *et al.* (1999) REVEAL, a general reverse engineering algorithm for inference of genetic network architecture in R. B. A. a. others, ed. *Proceedings of the Pacific Symposium on Biocomputing '98, Singapore*, pp. 18–28.

12 Heckerman, D. (1998) *A tutorial on learning with Bayesian networks* (ed. M.I. Jordan), Learning in Graphical Models, Kluwer, Dordrecht, The Netherlands.

13 Friedman, N. *et al.* (2000) Using Bayesian networks to analyze expression data. *J Comput Biol*, **7**, 601–620.

14 Jensen, F.V. (2001) *Bayesian networks and decision graphs*, Springer, New York.

13
Statistics

Summary

In this section we give an introduction to basic concepts of probability theory and statistics. In practice, experimental measurements are afflicted with some uncertainty (concentrations, RNA level, etc.) and statistical concepts give us a framework to quantify this uncertainty. Concepts of *probability theory* (Section 13.1) provide the necessary mathematical models for computing the significance of the experimental outcome. The focus of *elementary statistics* (Section 13.2) is to describe the underlying probabilistic parameters by functions on the experimental sample, the sample statistics, and provide tools for visualization of the data. *Statistical test theory* (Section 13.3) provides a framework for judging the significance of statements (hypotheses) with respect to the data. *Linear Models* (Section 13.4) are one of the most prominent tools to analyze complex experimental procedures.

13.1
Basic Concepts of Probability Theory

The quantification and characterization of uncertainty is formally described by the concept of a probability space for a random experiment. A *random experiment* is an experiment that consists of a set of possible outcomes with a quantification of the possibility of such an outcome. For example, if a coin is tossed one cannot deterministically predict the outcome of heads or tails but rather assign a probability that either of the outcomes will occur. Intuitively, one will assign a probability of 0.5 if the coin was fair (both outcomes are equally likely). Random experiments are described by a set of probability axioms.

A *probability space* is a triplet (Ω, A, P), where Ω is a nonempty set, A is a σ-algebra of subsets of Ω and P is a probability measure on A. A *σ-algebra* is a family of subsets of Ω that (i) contains Ω itself, (ii) contains for every element $B \in A$ the complementary element $B^c \in A$, and (iii) contains for every series of elements $B_1, B_2, \ldots \in A$ their union, i.e., $\cup_{i=1}^{\infty} B_i \in A$. The pair (Ω, A) is called a *measurable space*. An element

Systems Biology: A Textbook. Edda Klipp, Wolfram Liebermeister, Christoph Wierling, Axel Kowald, Hans Lehrach, and Ralf Herwig

ISBN: 978-3-527-31874-2

of A is called an *event*. If Ω is discrete, i.e., it has at most countable many elements then a natural choice of A would be the *power set* of Ω, i.e., the set of all subsets of Ω.

A *probability measure* $P{:}A \to [0,1]$ is a real-valued function that has the properties

$$P(B) \geq 0 \text{ for all } B \in A \text{ and } P(\Omega) = 1,$$

and

$$P(\cup_{i=1}^{\infty} B_i) = \sum_{i=1}^{\infty} P(B_i) \text{ for all series of disjoint sets } B_1, B_2, \ldots \in A(\sigma\text{-additivity}). \tag{13.1}$$

Example 13.1: Urn models

Many practical problems can be described with *urn models*. Consider an urn containing N balls out of which K are red and $N-K$ are black. The random experiment consists of n draws from that urn. If the ball is replaced in the urn after each draw we call the experiment *drawing with replacement* otherwise *drawing without replacement*. Here, Ω is the set of all n-dimensional binary sequences, $\Omega = \{(x_1, \ldots, x_n); x_n \in \{0,1\}\}$ where "1" means that a red ball was drawn and "0" means that a black ball was drawn. Since Ω is discrete, a suitable σ-algebra is the power set of Ω. Of practical interest is the calculation of the probability of having exactly k red balls among the n balls drawn. This is given by $P(k) = \binom{n}{k} p^k (1-p)^{n-k}$, with $p = \frac{K}{N}$, if we draw with replacement and $P(k) = \frac{\binom{K}{k}\binom{N-K}{n-k}}{\binom{N}{n}}$ if we draw without replacement. Here, for all numbers $a, b \geq 0$ it is defined

$$\binom{a}{b} = \frac{a!}{(a-b)!b!}. \tag{13.2}$$

We can define the concept of *conditional dependency*. Let (Ω, A, P) be a probability space. Let $B_1, B_2 \in A$ be two events. In general, there will be some dependency between the two events that influence the probability that both events will occur simultaneously. For example, consider B_1 being the event that a randomly picked person has lung cancer and let B_2 be the event that the person is a smoker. If both events were independent on each other, then the joint event, $B_1 \cap B_2$would be the product of the probabilities, i.e., $P(B_1 \cap B_2) = P(B_1)P(B_2)$. That would mean the probability that a randomly picked person has lung cancer is independent on the fact that he is a smoker. Otherwise, the probability of B_1would be higher conditioned on B_2.

We can generalize this to define another probability measure with respect to any given event C with positive probability. For any event $B \in A$ define $P(B|C) = \frac{P(B \cap C)}{P(C)}$,

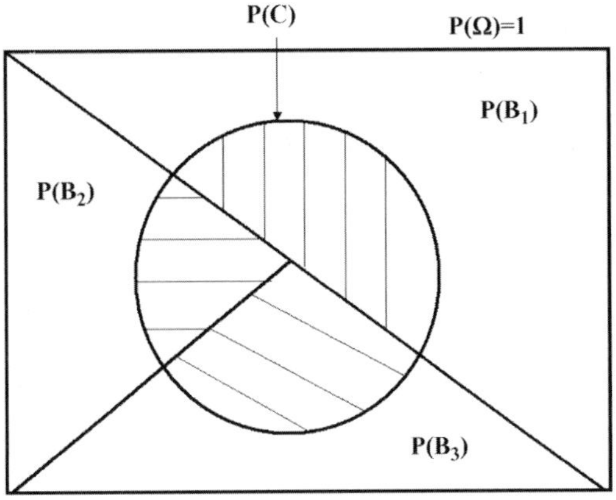

Figure 13.1 Illustration of conditional probabilities. Three events B_1, B_2, B_3 build a partition of the probability space Ω with *a priori* probabilities $P(B_1) = 0.5$, $P(B_2) = P(B_3) = 0.25$. Any event C defines a conditional probability measure with respect to C. Here, the *a posteriori* probabilities given C are $P(B_1) = 0.5$, $P(B_2) = 0.17$, $P(B_3) = 0.33$, respectively.

the *conditional probability* of B given C (Figure 13.1). The measure $P(.|C)$ is a probability measure on the measurable space (Ω, A).

If we have a decomposition of Ω into disjoint subsets $\{B_1, B_2, \ldots\}$ with $P(B_i) > 0$ then the probability of any event C can be retrieved by the sum of probabilities with respect to the decomposition, i.e.,

$$P(C) = \sum_i P(C|B_i)P(B_i). \tag{13.3}$$

Conversely, if $P(C) > 0$ the probability for each B_i conditioned on C can be calculated by *Bayes' rule*, i.e.,

$$P(B_i|C) = \frac{P(C|B_i)P(B_i)}{\sum_j P(C|B_j)P(B_j)}. \tag{13.4}$$

In the Bayesian set up, the probabilities $P(B_i)$ are called *a priori* probabilities. These describe the probability of the events with no additional information. If we now consider an event C with positive probability one can ask about the *a posteriori* probabilities $P(B_i|C)$of the events in the light of event C. In practice, formula (13.4) is very important since many problems do not allow a direct calculation of the probability of an event but rather the probability of the event conditioned on another event or series of other events.

Example 13.2: Power of diagnostics

Consider a specific disease affecting 0.5% of the population. A diagnostic test with a false positive rate of 5% and a true positive rate of 90% is conducted with a randomly picked person. The test result is positive. What is the probability that this person has the disease? Let B_1 be the event that a person has the disease (B_1^c is the complementary event). Let B_2 be the event that the test is positive. Thus, we are asking for the conditional probability that the person has the disease given that the test is positive, i.e., $P(B_1|B_2)$. From Eq. (13.4) we get

$$P(B_1|B_2) = \frac{P(B_2|B_1)P(B_1)}{P(B_2|B_1)P(B_1) + P(B_2|B_1^c)P(B_1^c)} = \frac{0.9 \cdot 0.005}{0.9 \cdot 0.005 + 0.05 \cdot 0.995} = 0.083.$$

It means that only 8% of the persons with a positive test result will actually have the disease!

The above effect is due to the fact that the disease is rare and thus that a randomly picked person will have a low chance *a priori* to have the disease. The diagnostic test, however, will produce a high number of false positives on this sample. The diagnostic power of the test can be improved by decreasing the error rate. For example, decreasing the false positive rate to 1% would give a predictive success of 31.142% (0.5% would give 47.493%).

13.1.1
Random Variables, Densities, and Distribution Functions

Let (Ω, A) and (Ω', A') be two measurable spaces, then a function $f{:}\Omega \to \Omega'$ is called *measurable*, if $f^{-1}(B') \in A$ for all $B' \in A'$. A measurable function defined on a probability space is called a *random variable*. Random variables are used to describe outcomes of random experiments. A particular result of a random experiment will occur with a given probability.

Of practical interest are real- or vector-valued random variables, i.e., $\Omega' = \Re$ or $\Omega' = \Re^n$. In this case a σ-algebra can be defined straightforwardly. Let $\Im$ be the family of all n-dimensional intervals $Q = (a_1, b_1] \times \ldots \times (a_n, b_n]$ then there exists a minimal σ-algebra that contains $\Im$, the *Borel-σ-algebra*. This σ-algebra contains all sets that one can typically imagine such as all open, closed, semiopen intervals, and arbitrary mixtures of these. Indeed, it is not straightforward to define sets in $\Re^n$ that are not contained in the Borel-σ-algebra! A random variable is commonly denoted as $x : \Omega \to \Re$ in order to point to the outcomes (or realizations) of x. The probability measure P defined on Ω induces a probability measure, P_x, on the Borel-σ-algebra on $\Re$ through the equality $P_x(B') = P(x \in B') = P(x^{-1}(B'))$.

If $\boldsymbol{x}$ is a random vector, then the distribution of $\boldsymbol{x}$ is uniquely defined by assigning a probability to each n-dimensional vector $\boldsymbol{z}$ by $\boldsymbol{F}(\boldsymbol{z}) = P(\boldsymbol{x} \le \boldsymbol{z}) = P(x_1 \le z_1, \ldots, x_n \le z_n)$. F is called the *cumulative distribution function* of $\boldsymbol{x}$. If F admits the nth order mixed partial derivative, then the *density function* of $\boldsymbol{x}$ is defined as $f(\boldsymbol{z}) = f(z_1, \ldots, z_n) = \frac{\partial^n}{\partial z_1 \ldots \partial z_n} F(z_1, \ldots, z_n)$ and the relation holds

$$F(\boldsymbol{z}) = F(z_1, \ldots, z_n) = \int_{-\infty}^{z_1} \ldots \int_{-\infty}^{z_n} f(t_1, \ldots, t_n) \mathrm{d}t_1 \ldots \mathrm{d}t_n. \tag{13.5}$$

If $\boldsymbol{x}$ is a discrete random vector, i.e., if $\boldsymbol{x}$ can adopt only countable many outcomes, then the density function can be denoted as $f(\boldsymbol{z}) = P(\boldsymbol{x} = \boldsymbol{z}) = P(x_1 = z_1, \ldots, x_n = z_n)$. In the discrete case f is often called the probability mass function of $\boldsymbol{x}$.

Example 13.3

In the one-dimensional case, the distribution function of a random variable is defined by $F(t) = P(x \leq t) = P_x((-\infty, t])$. If x is a continuous random variable, the density function f is defined as $P_x((-\infty, t]) = \int_{-\infty}^{t} f(z)dz$, if x is a discrete random variable, then we have $Px((-\infty, t]) = \sum_{x \leq t} f(x)$.

Important characteristics of a probability distribution are the mean outcome that one would expect if all possible outcomes together with their respective probabilities were considered (expectation) and the mean squared deviation of the outcomes from the mean outcome (variance). The *expectation* of a random variable, x, is defined as

$$E(x) = \int_{-\infty}^{\infty} tf(t)dt = \mu, \tag{13.6}$$

and the *variance* as

$$\mathrm{Var}(x) = \int_{-\infty}^{\infty} (t-\mu)^2 f(t)dt. \tag{13.7}$$

The variance is equal to $\mathrm{Var} = E(x^2) - E(x)^2$. The *covariance* of two random variables x and y is defined as

$$\mathrm{Cov}(x, y) = E((x-E(x))(y-E(y))). \tag{13.8}$$

Note that $\mathrm{Var}(x) = \mathrm{Cov}(x, x)$ If $x_1, \ldots, x_n$ are random variables with means $E(x_i) = \mu_i$, variances $\mathrm{Var}(x_i) = c_{ii}$ and covariances $\mathrm{Cov}(x_i, x_j) = c_{ij} = c_{ji}$, then the random vector $\boldsymbol{x} = (x_1, \ldots, x_n)^{\mathrm{T}}$ has expectation $E(\boldsymbol{x}) = \boldsymbol{\mu}$, where $\boldsymbol{\mu} = (\mu, \ldots, \mu_n)^{\mathrm{T}}$, and *covariance matrix*

$$\mathrm{Cov}(\boldsymbol{x}) = E((\boldsymbol{x}-\boldsymbol{\mu})(\boldsymbol{x}-\boldsymbol{\mu})^{\mathrm{T}}) = \begin{pmatrix} c_{11} & \ldots & c_{n1} \\ \ldots & \ldots & \ldots \\ c_{n1} & \ldots & c_{nn} \end{pmatrix} \tag{13.9}$$

A random vector is called *nonsingular* (*singular*) when its covariance matrix is nonsingular (singular).

If $\boldsymbol{x}$ is an n-dimensional random vector, $\boldsymbol{A}$ is a $p \times n$ matrix, and $\boldsymbol{b}$ is a p-dimensional vector, we get the following transformation rules:

$$E(\boldsymbol{Ax} + \boldsymbol{b}) = \boldsymbol{A}E(\boldsymbol{x}) + \boldsymbol{b} \quad \text{and} \quad \mathrm{Cov}(\boldsymbol{Ax} + \boldsymbol{b}) = \boldsymbol{A}\mathrm{Cov}(\boldsymbol{x})\boldsymbol{A}^{\mathrm{T}}. \tag{13.10}$$

Equation (13.10) gives the expectation of a random vector under an affine transformation. Under general transformations the expectation cannot be calculated straightforwardly from the expectation of $\boldsymbol{x}$. However, one can give a lower bound for the expectation of the transformation in some cases that is useful in practice. Let $\boldsymbol{x}$ be a random vector and let g be a real-valued *convex function*, i.e., a function for which $g(\sum_{i=1}^{n} \lambda_k x_k) \leq \sum_{i=1}^{n} \lambda_k g(x_k)$, where $0 \leq \lambda_k \leq 1$ and $\sum_{i=1}^{n} \lambda_k = 1$ (if the inequality is reversed we call g a *concave function*). Then the inequality holds (*Jensen's inequality*)

$$g(E(x)) \leq E(g(x)). \tag{13.11}$$

Example 13.4

The variance of a random variable is always nonnegative, because $g(x) = x^2$ is a convex function and thus it follows from Eq. (13.11): $E(x)^2 \leq E(x^2)$.

Example 13.5

The *normal distribution* is the most important distribution in probability theory. Numerous methods in test theory and multivariate statistics rely on calculus with the normal distribution (compare also Sections 13.3 and 13.4). x has a one-dimensional normal (or Gaussian) distribution with parameters μ, σ^2 if the density of x is equal to

$$f(t) = \frac{1}{\sqrt{2\pi\sigma^2}} \exp^{\frac{-(t-\mu)^2}{2\sigma^2}}. \tag{13.12}$$

This is also denoted as $x \sim N(\mu, \sigma^2)$. The special case $\mu = 0$, $\sigma^2 = 1$ is called the standard normal distribution. The expectation and the variance of the standard normal distribution can be calculated as $E(x) = 0$ and $\mathrm{Var}(x) = 1$. If z is standard normally distributed, then the random variable $x = \sigma z + \mu$ is distributed with parameters $x \sim N(\mu, \sigma^2)$. From Eq. (13.10) it follows that $E(x) = \mu$ and $\mathrm{Var}(x) = \sigma^2$. The normal distribution can be easily generalized. Let $\boldsymbol{x}$ be an n-dimensional random vector that follows a normal distribution, then the density of $\boldsymbol{x}$ is

$$f(z) = \frac{1}{(2\pi)^{n/2}(\det(\Sigma))^{1/2}} \exp\left(-\frac{1}{2}(z-\mu)^{\mathrm{T}} \Sigma (z-\mu)\right), \tag{13.13}$$

where μ is the mean vector and Σ is covariance matrix composed of the components $x_1, \ldots, x_n$ of $\boldsymbol{x}$.

Example 13.6

The *exponential distribution* is important in modeling decay rates and in characterization of stochastic processes. A random variable is exponentially distributed with parameter $\lambda > 0$ if the density of $\boldsymbol{x}$ is equal to

$$f(t) = \lambda e^{-\lambda t}, \tag{13.14}$$

where $t \geq 0$. Expectation and variance of $\boldsymbol{x}$ are equal to $\frac{1}{\lambda}$.

Example 13.7

An example for a discrete distribution is the *binomial distribution*. The binomial distribution is used to describe urn models with replacement (cf., Example 13.1, Urn models), where we ask specifically after the number of successes in n independent repetitions of a random experiment with binary outcomes (a *Bernoulli experiment*). If x_i is the random variable that describes the outcome of the ith experiment, then the random variable $x = \sum_{i=1}^{n} x_i$ has a binomial distribution with probability mass function

$$f(x = k) = \binom{n}{k} p^k (1-p)^{n-k}. \tag{13.15}$$

The expectation and the variance are $E(\boldsymbol{x}) = np$ and $\mathrm{Var}(x) = np(1-p)$.

13.1.2 Transforming Probability Densities

Let x be a random variable with probability density f then for each measurable function h, $y = h(x)$ $Y = h(x)$ is a random variable too. The *transformation rule* states that if h is a function with strictly positive (negative) derivative and inverse function h^{-1} then y has the density $g(y) = \frac{f(h^{-1}(y))}{|h'(h^{-1}(y))|}$. More generally, let $\boldsymbol{x}$ be an n-dimensional random vector, let $\boldsymbol{h}$ be a vector-valued function $\boldsymbol{h} : \Re^n \rightarrow \Re^n$ that is differentiable, i.e., $\boldsymbol{h}$ admits the partial derivatives. Let $\boldsymbol{h}^{-1}$ be the inverse function with $\det(J_{h^{-1}}(\boldsymbol{y})) \neq 0$ for all $\boldsymbol{y} \in \Re^n$, where $J_{h^{-1}}$ is the Jacobi matrix of $\boldsymbol{h}^{-1}$. Then, the density of the random vector $\boldsymbol{y} = \boldsymbol{h}(\boldsymbol{x})$ is given by

$$g(\boldsymbol{y}) = f(\boldsymbol{h}^{-1}(\boldsymbol{y}))|\det(J_{h^{-1}}(\boldsymbol{y}))|. \tag{13.16}$$

Example 13.8: Affine transformations of a probability density

Let $\boldsymbol{x}$ be a random vector with density function f, let $\boldsymbol{h}$ be a vector-valued affine function $\boldsymbol{h} : \Re^n \rightarrow \Re^n$, i.e., $\boldsymbol{h}(\boldsymbol{x}) = \boldsymbol{A}\boldsymbol{x} + \boldsymbol{\mu}$ for an $n \times n$ matrix $\boldsymbol{A}$ and an n-dimensional vector $\boldsymbol{\mu}$, then the density function of the random vector $\boldsymbol{y} = \boldsymbol{h}(\boldsymbol{x})$ is equal to $g(\boldsymbol{y}) = f(\boldsymbol{A}^{-1}(\boldsymbol{y} - \boldsymbol{\mu}))|\det(\boldsymbol{A}^{-1})|$. In particular, in the one-dimensional case we have the transformation $h(x) = ax + b$ and the corresponding probability density $g(\boldsymbol{y}) = f\left(\frac{y-b}{a}\right)\frac{1}{|a|}$.

Example 13.9: The density function of a log-normal distribution

A random variable y is log-normally distributed, if the random variable $\ln(y) = x$ is Gaussian distributed with parameters $x \sim N(\mu, \sigma^2)$. The density of y can be calculated according to the transformation rule, we have $y = h(x) = e^x$ and $h^{-1}(y) = \ln(y)$ and we get the density function of y as $g(y) = \frac{1}{\sqrt{2\pi\sigma^2}} e^{\frac{-(\ln(y)-\mu)^2}{2\sigma^2}} \frac{1}{y}$.

13.1.3
Product Experiments and Independence

Consider n different probability spaces (Ω_i, A_i, P_i). In many applications the actual interesting probability space would be the *product space*$(\otimes\Omega_i, \otimes A_i, \prod P_i)$. Here, the product set and the product σ-algebra denote the *Cartesian products*. The product measure is defined as the product of the individual probability measures. Implicitly, we have used this definition before, for example, an experiment described by the binomial distribution is the product experiment of individual Bernoulli experiments.

Let $\boldsymbol{x} = (x_1, \ldots, x_n)^{\mathrm{T}}$ and $\boldsymbol{y} = (y_1, \ldots, y_m)^{\mathrm{T}}$ be two n- and m-dimensional random vectors, respectively, then the *joint probability density* of the vector $(\boldsymbol{x}^{\mathrm{T}}, \boldsymbol{y}^{\mathrm{T}})^{\mathrm{T}}$ is defined as $f_{xy}(x_1, \ldots, x_n, y_1, \ldots, y_m)$ and the *marginal density* f_x of x can be written as

$$f_x(\boldsymbol{x}) = f_x(x_1, \ldots, x_n) = \int_{-\infty}^{+\infty} \cdots \int_{-\infty}^{+\infty} f_{xy}(x_1, \ldots, x_n, y_1, \ldots, y_m) \mathrm{d}y_1 \ldots \mathrm{d}y_m. \tag{13.17}$$

Two random vectors $\boldsymbol{x}$ and $\boldsymbol{y}$ are *independent* on each other, when the joint probability function is the product of the marginal probability functions, i.e.,

$$f_{xy}(\boldsymbol{x}, \boldsymbol{y}) = f_x(\boldsymbol{x}) f_y(\boldsymbol{y}). \tag{13.18}$$

Let x_1, x_2 be two independent real-valued random variables with probability densities f_1, f_2. Many practical problems require the distribution of the sum of the random variables, $y = g(x_1, x_2) = x_1 + x_2$. For each realization c of y we have $g^{-1}(c) = \{(a,b);\ a + b = c\}$ and we get $p(y \leq c) = \int\int_{\{(a,b);a+b\leq c\}} f_1(a) f_2(b) \mathrm{d}a\, \mathrm{d}b = \int_{-\infty}^{c} \left(\int_{-\infty}^{+\infty} f_1(u-b) f_2(b) \mathrm{d}b \right) \mathrm{d}u = \int_{-\infty}^{c} (f_1 {}^* f_2)(u) \mathrm{d}u$. The function $f_1 {}^* f_2$ is called the *convolution* of f_1, f_2.

Example 13.10: Convolution rule of the normal distribution

Let $x_1, \ldots, x_n$ be independent random variables that are Gaussian distributed with $x_i \sim N(\mu_i, \sigma_i^2)$. Then, $y = x_1 + \cdots + x_n$ is Gaussian distributed $y \sim N(\mu_i, + \cdots + \mu_n, \sigma_i^2 + \cdots + \sigma_n^2)$.

13.1.4
Limit Theorems

In this subsection we list some fundamental theorems of probability theory that describe the convergence properties of series of random variables. The first theorem states that the empirical distribution function (compare Section 13.2) is converging against the true underlying (but unknown) distribution function. The second tells us that the mean and the variance (Section 13.2) are estimators for the first distribution moments and the third states that distributions for series of random variables converge asymptotically against a Gaussian distribution if they are transformed conveniently.

All convergence properties are defined *almost everwhere*. This technical term of measure theory is introduced to indicate that a result for a probability space is valid everywhere except on subsets of probability zero.

Theorem of Glivenko–Cantelli. Let $x_1, \ldots, x_n$ be random variables that are independently and identically distributed with distribution function F. Then the empirical distribution function $F_n(t)$ converges (almost everywhere) to the true distribution function, i.e.,

$$\sup_{t\in\Re}|F_n(t)-F(t)| \rightarrow_{n\rightarrow+\infty} 0 \text{ (almost everywhere)}. \tag{13.19}$$

Strong Law of the Large Numbers. Let $x_1, x_2, \ldots$ be a series of uncorrelated real-valued random variables with $\mathrm{Var}(x_i) \leq M < +\infty$ for all i, then the series of random variables

$$z_n = \frac{1}{n}\sum_{i=1}^{n}(x_i - E(x_i)), \tag{13.20}$$

converges to zero (almost everywhere)

Central Limit Theorem. Let Φ be the distribution function of the standard Gaussian distribution. Let $x_1, x_2, \ldots$ be a series of independently identically distributed random variables with finite and nonzero variance, i.e., $0 < \mathrm{Var}(x_i) < +\infty$. Define the series of random variables $z_n = \frac{\sum_{i=1}^{n} x_i - nE(x_1)}{\mathrm{Var}(x_1)\sqrt{n}}$, then z_n converges to Φ (almost everywhere), i.e.,

$$\sup_{t\in\Re}|z_n(t)-\Phi(t)| \rightarrow_{n\rightarrow+\infty} 0. \tag{13.21}$$

13.2
Descriptive Statistics

The basic object of descriptive statistics is the *sample*. A sample is a subset of data measured from an underlying population, for example, repeated measurements of expression levels from the same gene. A numerical function of a sample is called a *statistic*. Commonly, a statistic is used to compress the information inherent in the sample and to describe certain properties of the sample. Interesting features that characterize the sample are

- statistics for sample location
- statistics for sample variance
- statistics for sample distribution.

In the following sections the main concepts are introduced.

13.2.1
Statistics for Sample Location

Measures of location describe the center or gravity of the sample. The most commonly used measures of location are the mean and the median. Let $x_1, \ldots, x_n$ be a sample of n values, then the *mean* of the sample is defined as

$$\bar{x} = \frac{1}{n}\sum_{i=1}^{n} x_i, \tag{13.22}$$

and the *median* is defined as the value that is greater than or equal to 50% of the sample elements. For the proper definition of the median it is necessary to introduce the definition of a *percentile*: Consider the ordered sample $x^{(1)} \leq \ldots \leq x^{(n)}$ derived from $x_1, \ldots, x_n$ by sorting the sample in increasing order, then the pth percentile is the smallest value that is larger or equal than p% of the measurements. It is clear that the 0th-percentile and the 100th-percentile are the minimum and the maximum of the sample, respectively. The median is the 50th percentile. If the sample size is odd then the median is defined as $x^{\left(\frac{n+1}{2}\right)}$, if the sample size is even the median is not unique. It can be any value between $x^{\left(\frac{n}{2}\right)}$ and $x^{\left(\frac{n}{2}+1\right)}$, for example, the average of both values $\left(x^{\left(\frac{n}{2}\right)} + x^{\left(\frac{n}{2}+1\right)}\right)/2$. An important characteristic of the median is its robustness against outlier values. In contrast, the mean value is biased to a large extent by outlier values. In order to robustify the mean value, we define the *α-trimmed mean*. Here, simply the α% lowest and highest values are deleted from the data set and the mean is calculated of the remaining sample values. Common values of α are between 10% and 20%.

Example 13.11

Consider the measurements of gene expression for a particular gene in a certain tissue in 12 individuals. These individuals represent a common group (disease type) and we want to derive the mean expression level.

Sample	x_1	x_2	x_3	x_4	x_5	x_6	x_7	x_8	x_9	x_{10}	x_{11}	x_{12}
Value	2434	2289	5599	2518	1123	1768	2304	2509	14820	2489	1349	1494

We get the following values for the mean, $\bar{x} = 3391.33$ and for the median, $x_{med} = 0.5(2304 + 2434) = 2369$. If we look more deeply into the sample we would rather prefer the median as sample location since most values scatter around the median. The overestimation of the sample location by the mean results from the high values of the outlier value x_9 (and probably x_3). The 10%-trimmed mean of the sample is $\bar{x}_{10} = 2475.3$, which is comparable with the median.

Another measure of location that is preferably used if the sample values represent proportions rather than absolute values is the *geometric mean*. The geometric mean is defined as

$$\bar{x}_g = \sqrt[n]{\prod_{i=1}^{n} x_i}. \tag{13.23}$$

Note that it always holds that $\bar{x} \geq \bar{x}_g$.

13.2.2
Statistics for Sample Variability

Once we have determined the center of the sample, another important bit of information is how the sample values scatter around that center. A very simple way of measuring sample variability is the *range*, the difference between the maximum and the minimum values, $x_{max} - x_{min}$. The most common statistic for sample variability is the *standard deviation*,

$$s_n = \sqrt{\frac{1}{n-1}\sum_{i=1}^{n}(x_i - \bar{x})^2}, \tag{13.24}$$

where s_n^2 is called the *variance* of the sample. The standard deviation measures the individual difference of each sample value and the sample mean. Similar to the mean it is influenced by outlier values. Standard deviations cannot directly be compared since they are dependent on the scale of the values. For example, if two series of distance values were measured in meter and millimeter the latter one would have a higher standard deviation. In order to compare sample variability from different samples, one rather compares the relative standard deviations. This measure is called *coefficient of variation*,

$$cv_n = \frac{s_n}{x}. \tag{13.25}$$

The interpretation of the coefficient of variation is variability relative to location. A more robust measure of variability is the *interquartile range*, IQR, i.e., the difference of the upper and lower quartile of the sample: $\text{IQR}_n = x^{([0.75n])} - x^{([0.25n])}$. Here $[\alpha n]$ denotes the smallest integer that is greater than or equal to αn. Analog to the median another measure is the *median absolute deviation*, MAD,

$$\text{MAD} = \text{median}(|x_1 - x_{med}|, \ldots, |x_n - x_{med}|). \tag{13.26}$$

Both measures of location, $\bar{x}$ and $\bar{x}_m$, are related to their corresponding measure of variability and can be derived as solutions of a minimization procedure. We have

$$\bar{x} \in \arg\min\left\{a; \sum_{i=1}^{n}(x_i - a)^2\right\} \quad \text{and} \quad \bar{x}_{med} \in \arg\min\left\{a; \sum_{i=1}^{n}|x_i - a|^2\right\}$$

The sample characteristics are commonly condensed and visualized by a *box-plot* (Figure 13.2).

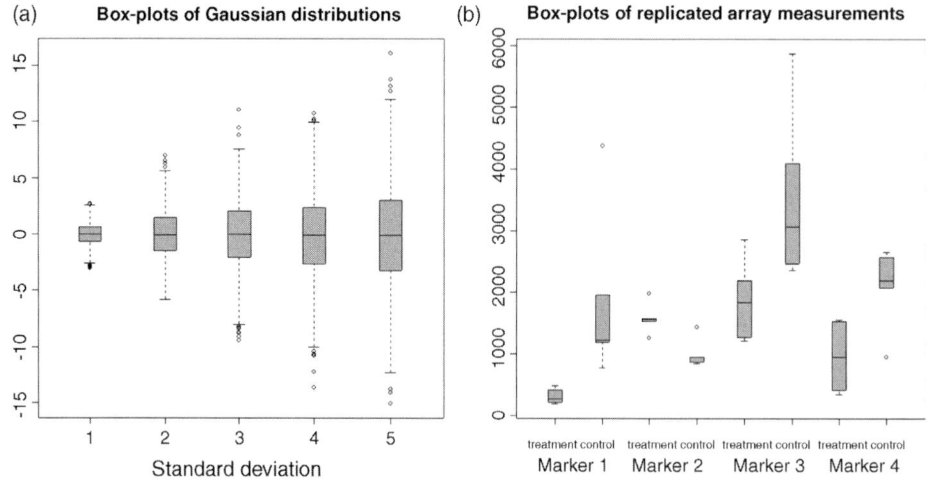

Figure 13.2 Visualization of sample characteristics by box-plots. (a) Five different samples from Gaussian distributions with mean $\mu = 0$ and standard deviations $\sigma = 1, 2, 3, 4, 5$, respectively, were randomly generated. The box displays the interquartile range, the line is the median of the samples. The whiskers denote an area that identifies outliers (circles). Graphics was generated with *R*-statistical software package. (b) Four marker genes determined in a study on Down's syndrome. Samples are based on 6 (treatment) and 5 (control) individuals, respectively. Three markers are down-regulated (markers 1, 3, and 4), one marker gene is upregulated.

13.2.3
Density Estimation

In order to describe the distribution of the sample values across the sample range one commonly defines the *histogram*. Let $I_1, \ldots, I_M$ be disjoint intervals, $I_M = (a_{m-1}, a_m]$, and let $n_m = \{x_i;\ x_i \in I_m\}$ the number of sample values that fall in the respective interval, then the *weighted histogram* statistic

$$f_n(t) = \begin{cases} \dfrac{n_m}{n} \quad \dfrac{1}{a_m - a_{m-1}}, & t \in I_m. \\ 0, & \text{else} \end{cases} \tag{13.27}$$

can be used to estimate the density of the distribution. A fundamental statistic of the sample is the *empirical distribution function*. This is defined as

$$F_n(t) = \frac{1}{n}\sum_{i=1}^{n} 1_{(-\infty,t]}(x_i), \tag{13.28}$$

where $1_{(-\infty,t]}(x_i) = \begin{cases} 1, & \text{if } x_i \leq t \\ 0, & \text{else} \end{cases}$ denotes the indicator function. This function is a real-valued step function with values in the interval [0,1] that has a step at each point x_i. In Section 13.1.4 we showed that the two statistics above converge to the probability density and the distribution function with respect to an underlying probability law.

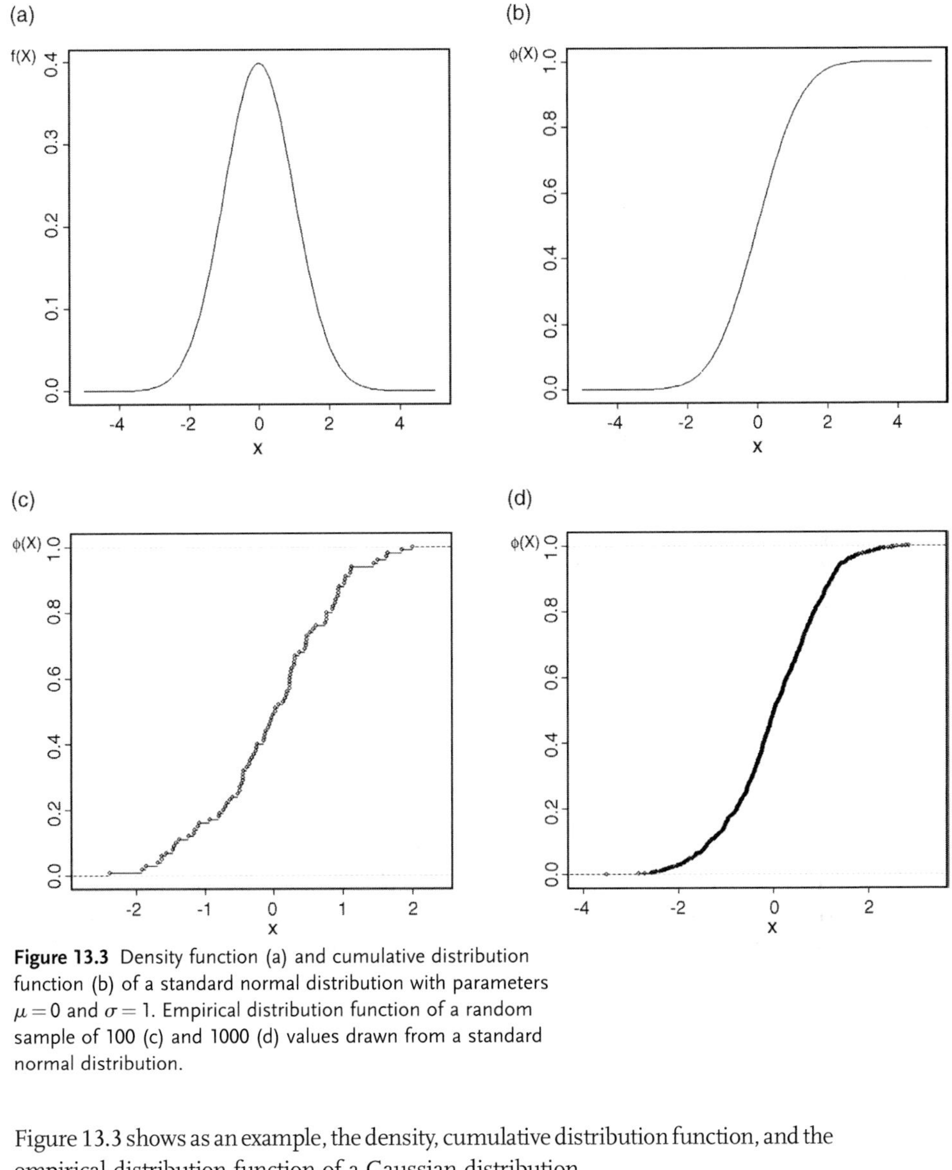

Figure 13.3 Density function (a) and cumulative distribution function (b) of a standard normal distribution with parameters $\mu = 0$ and $\sigma = 1$. Empirical distribution function of a random sample of 100 (c) and 1000 (d) values drawn from a standard normal distribution.

Figure 13.3 shows as an example, the density, cumulative distribution function, and the empirical distribution function of a Gaussian distribution.

13.2.4 Correlation of Samples

So far we have discussed statistics for samples measured on one variable. Let us now consider a sample measured on two variables, i.e., $z_1, \ldots, z_n$, where $z_i = (x_i, y_i)$ is a two-dimensional observation. A fundamental question is whether the two individual samples $x_1, \ldots x_n$ and $y_1, \ldots y_n$ correlate with each other, i.e., have a similar trend.

A measure of correlation is *Pearson's correlation coefficient*. This is defined as

$$\mathrm{PC} = \frac{\sum_{i=1}^{n}(x_i - \bar{x})(y_i - \bar{y})}{\sqrt{\sum_{i=1}^{n}(x_i - \bar{x})^2 \sum_{i=1}^{n}(y_i - \bar{y})^2}}. \tag{13.29}$$

The Pearson correlation measures the linear relationship of both samples. It is close to 1 if both samples have strong linear correlation, it is negative if the samples are anticorrelated and it scatters around 0 if there is no linear trend observable. Outliers can influence the Pearson correlation to a large extent. Therefore, robust statistics for sample correlation have been defined. We call $r_i^x = \#\,\{x_j; x_j \le x_i\}$ the rank of x_i within the sample $x_1, \ldots, x_n$. It denotes the number of sample values smaller or equal to the ith value. Note that the minimum, the maximum, and the median of the sample have ranks, 1, n, and $\frac{n}{2}$, respectively and that the ranks and the ordered sample have the correspondence that $x_i = x^{(r_i^x)}$. A more robust measure of correlation than Pearson's correlation coefficient is *Spearman's rank correlation*

$$\mathrm{SC} = \frac{\sum_{i=1}^{n}(r_i^x - \bar{r}^x)(r_i^y - \bar{r}^y)}{\sqrt{\sum_{i=1}^{n}(r_i^x - \bar{r}^x)^2 \sum_{i=1}^{n}(r_i^y - \bar{r}^y)^2}}. \tag{13.30}$$

Here, $\bar{r}^x$ denotes the mean rank. SC is derived from PC by replacing the actual sample values by their ranks within the respective sample. Another advantage of this measure is the fact that SC can measure other relationships than linear ones. For example, if the second sample is derived from the first by any monotonic function (square root, logarithm) then the correlation is still high (Figure 13.4). Measures of correlation are extensively used in many algorithms of multivariate statistical analysis such as pairwise similarity measures for gene expression profiles (Chapter 9).

13.3 Testing Statistical Hypotheses

Many practical applications imply statements like "it is very likely that two samples are different" or "this fold change of gene expression is significant." Consider the following problems:

1. We observe the expression of a gene in replicated measurements of cells with a chemical treatment and control cells. Can we quantify whether a certain observed fold change in gene expression is caused by the treatment?
2. We observe the expression of a gene in different individuals of disease and a control group. Is the variability in the two groups equal?
3. We measure gene expression of many genes. Does the signal distribution of these genes resemble a specific distribution?

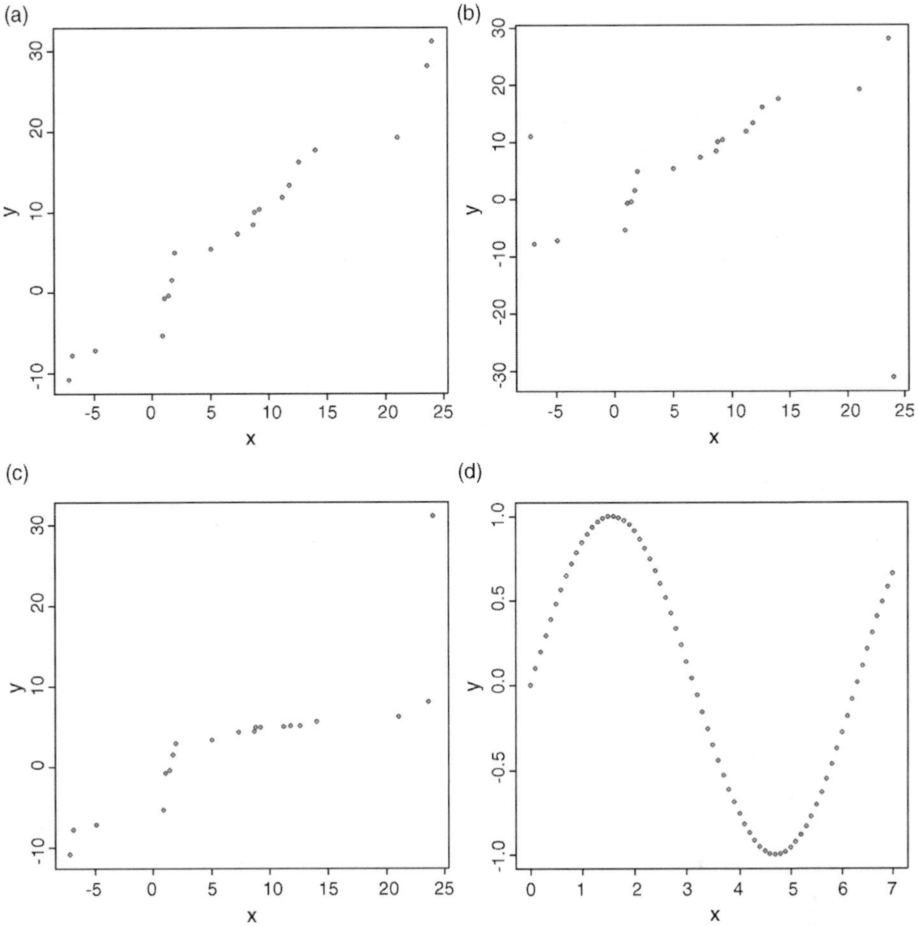

Figure 13.4 Correlation plots and performance of correlation measures. (a) Linear correlation of two random variables (PC = 0.98, SC = 1.00); (b) presence of two outliers (PC = 0.27, SC = 0.60); (c) nonlinear, monotonic correlation (PC = 0.83, SC = 1.00); (d) nonlinear, nonmonotonic correlation (PC = −0.54, SC = −0.54).

Statistical test theory provides a unique framework to tackle these questions and to determine the significance of these differences.

13.3.1
Statistical Framework

Replicated measurements of the same object in a treatment and a control condition typically yield two series of values, $x_1, \ldots, x_n$ and $y_1, \ldots, y_m$. The biological problem of judging differences from replicated measurements can be formulated as statistical hypotheses, the null hypothesis, H_0, and the alternative, H_1.

An important class of tests is the two-sample location test. Here, the null hypothesis states that the quantities represented by two samples have identical mean values, whereas the alternative states that there is a difference.

$$H_0 : \mu_x = \mu_y \text{ versus } H_1 : \mu_x \neq \mu_y,$$

where μ_x, μ_y are the mean values of the quantities represented by the respective samples.

A very simple method would be to calculate the averages of the two series and compare the difference. However, this would not allow judging whether a difference different from zero stems from an actual difference between the quantities or just from random scatter of the samples. If we make some additional assumptions we can describe the problem using an appropriate probability distribution. We regard the two series as realizations of random variables $x_1, \ldots, x_n$ and $y_1, \ldots, y_m$. Statistical tests typically have two constraints: (i) It is assumed that repetitions are independent and (ii) that the random variables are identically distributed within each sample. Test decisions are based upon a reasonable test statistic, a real-valued function T, on both samples. For specific functions and using the distributional assumptions it has been shown that they follow a quantifiable probability law given the null hypothesis H_0. Suppose that we observe a value of the test statistic $T(x_1, \ldots, x_n, y_1, \ldots, y_m) = \hat{t}$. If T can be described with a probability law we can judge the significance of the observation by prob(T more extreme than $\hat{t}$). This probability is called a *P-value*. Thus, if one gives a *P*-value of 0.05 to a certain observation this means that under the distributional assumptions the probability of observing an outcome more extreme than the observed one is 0.05 given the null hypothesis. Observations with a small *P*-value typically give incidence that the null hypothesis should be rejected. This makes it possible to quantify statistically if the result is significant by using a probability distribution. In practice, confidence levels of 0.01, 0.05, and 0.1 are used as upper bounds for significant results. In such a test set up, two types of error occur: error of the first kind and of the second kind:

	H_0 is true	**H_1 is true**
Test does not reject H_0	No error (TN)	Error of the second kind (FN)
Test rejects H_0	Error of the first kind (FP)	No error (TP)

The *error of the first kind* is the *false positive rate* of the test. Usually, this error can be controlled by the analysis by assuming a significance level α and judging only those results as significant where the probability is lower than α. The *error of the second kind* is the false negative rate of the test. The *power* of a test (given a significance level α) is defined as the probability of rejecting H_0 across the parameter space that is under consideration. It should be low in the subset of the parameter space that belongs to H_0 and high in the subset H_1. The quantities $\frac{TP}{TP+FN}$ and $\frac{TN}{FP+TN}$ are called *sensitivity* and *specificity*, respectively. An optimal test procedure would give a result of 1 to both quantities.

13.3.2
Two Sample Location Tests

Assume that the elements of both samples are independently Gaussian distributed, $N(\mu_x, \sigma^2)$ and $N(\mu_y, \sigma^2)$, respectively, with equal variances. Thus we interpret the sample values x_i as outcomes of independent random variables that are Gaussian distributed with the respective parameters (y_i likewise). We want to test the hypothesis whether the sample means are equal, i.e.,

$$H_0 : \mu_x = \mu_y \text{ versus } H_1 : \mu_x \neq \mu_y,$$

Under the above assumptions the test statistic

$$T(x_1, \ldots, x_n, y_1, \ldots, y_m) = -\frac{\bar{x} - \bar{y}}{\sqrt{\frac{(n-1)s_x^2 + (m-1)s_y^2}{n+m-2}}\sqrt{\frac{1}{n} + \frac{1}{m}}}, \tag{13.31}$$

(compare Sections 13.2.1 and 13.2.2) is distributed according to a *t*-distribution with $m + n - 2$ degrees of freedom. The test based on this assumption is called *Student's t-test.*

For a calculated value of the *T*-statistic, $\hat{t}$, we can now judge the probability of having an even more extreme value by calculating the probability $P(|T| > |\hat{t}|) = 2P(T > |\hat{t}|) = \int_{\hat{t}}^{\infty} f_{T,p}(z)dz$, where

$$f_{T,p}(z) = \frac{\Gamma\left(\frac{p+1}{2}\right)}{\Gamma\left(\frac{p}{2}\right)\Gamma\left(\frac{1}{2}\right)\sqrt{p}}\left(1 + \frac{z^2}{p}\right)^{-(p+1)/2}, \tag{13.32}$$

is the probability distribution of the respective *t*-distribution with p degrees of freedom. Here, $\Gamma(z) = \int_0^{\infty} t^{z-1}e^{-t}dt$ is the *gamma function.*

For most practical applications the assumptions of Student's *t*-test are too strong since the data are often not Gaussian distributed with equal variances. Furthermore, since the statistic is based on the mean values, the test is not robust against outliers. Thus, if the underlying distribution is not known and in order to define a more robust alternative, we introduce the *Wilcoxon test.* Here, instead of evaluating the signal values, only the ranks of the signals are taken under consideration. Consider the combined series $x_1, \ldots, x_n, y_1, \ldots, y_m$. Under the null hypothesis this series represents $m + n$ independent identically distributed random variables. The test statistic of the Wilcoxon test is

$$T = \sum_{i=1}^{n} R_i^{x,y}, \tag{13.33}$$

where $R_i^{x,y}$ is the rank of x_i in the combined series. The minimum and maximum values of T are $\frac{n(n+1)}{2}$ and $\frac{(m+n)(m+n+1)}{2} - \frac{n(n+1)}{2}$, respectively. The expected value under the null hypothesis is $E_{H_0}(T) = \frac{mn}{2}$ and the variance is $\mathrm{Var}_{H_0}(T) = \frac{mn(m+n+1)}{12}$. Thus, under the null hypothesis, values for T will scatter around the expectation and unusually low or high values will indicate that the null hypothesis should be rejected. For small sample sizes P-values of the Wilcoxon test can be calculated exactly, for larger sample sizes we have the following approximation:

$$P\left(\frac{T-\frac{mn}{2}}{\sqrt{\frac{mn(m+n+1)}{12}}} \leq z\right) \rightarrow \Phi(z) \quad \text{for} \quad n, m \rightarrow \infty. \tag{13.34}$$

The P-values of the Wilcoxon test statistic can be approximated by the standard normal distribution. This approximation has been shown to be accurate for $n + m > 25$.

In practice, some of the series values might be equal, for example because of the resolution of the measurements. Then, the Wilcoxon test statistic can be calculated using *ties*. Ties can be calculated by the average rank of all values that are equal. Ties have an effect on the variance of the statistic, which is often underestimated and should be corrected in the normal approximation. The correction is calculated by replacing the original variance by

$$\mathrm{Var}_{H_0,corr}(T) = \mathrm{Var}_{H_0}(T) - \frac{mn}{12(m+n)(m+n+1)} \sum_{i=1}^{r} (b_i^3 - b_i). \tag{13.35}$$

Here, r is the number of different values in the combined series of values and b_i is the frequency.

Example 13.12

Expression of a specific gene was measured in cortex brain tissue from control mice and Ts65Dn mice – a mouse model for Down syndrome [1]. Repeated array hybridization experiments yield the following series of measurements for control mice:

$$2434, 2289, 5599, 2518, 1123, 1768, 2304, 2509, 14820, 2489, 1349, 1494$$

and for trisomic mice

$$3107, 3365, 4704, 3667, 2414, 4268, 3600, 3084, 3997, 3673, 2281, 3166.$$

Due to two outlier values in the control series (*5599* and *14820*) the trisomic versus control ratio is close to 1, 1.02, and the P-value of Student's t-test is not significant, $p = 9.63 \times 10^{-1}$. For the Wilcoxon statistic, we get $T = \sum_{i=1}^{n} R_i^{x,y} = 14 + 16 + 22 + 18 + 8 + 21 + 17 + 13 + 20 + 19 + 5 + 15 = 188$, $E_{H_0}(T) = 72$, $\mathrm{Var}_{H_0}(T) = 300$ and for the Z-score we have $z = \frac{116}{\sqrt{300}} \sim 6.70$, which indicates that the result is significant. The exact P-value of the Wilcoxon test is $p = 2.84 \times 10^{-2}$.

13.4 Linear Models

The general linear model has the form $\boldsymbol{y} = \boldsymbol{X\beta} + \boldsymbol{\varepsilon}$, with the assumptions $E(\boldsymbol{\varepsilon}) = \boldsymbol{0}$ and $\mathrm{Cov}(\varepsilon) = \sigma^2 \boldsymbol{I}$. Here y is an n-dimensional vector of observations, $\boldsymbol{\beta}$ is a p-dimensional vector of unknown parameters, $\boldsymbol{X}$ is an $n \times p$ dimensional matrix of known constants (the design matrix), and $\boldsymbol{\varepsilon}$ is a vector of random errors. Since the errors are random, y is a random vector as well. Thus, the observations are separated in a deterministic part and a random part. The ratio behind linear models is that the deterministic part of the experimental observations (dependent variable) is a linear function of the design matrix and the unknown parameter vector. Note that linearity is required in the parameters but not in the design matrix. For example, problems such as $x_{ij} = x_i^j$ for $i = 1,\ldots,n$ and $j = 0,\ldots,p-1$ are also linear models. Here, for each coordinate i we have the equation $y_i = \boldsymbol{\beta}_0 + \sum_{j=1}^{p-1} \boldsymbol{\beta}_j x_j^i + \boldsymbol{\varepsilon}_i$ and the model is called *polynomial regression model.*

The goal of linear models is testing of complex statistical hypotheses and parameter estimation. In the following sections we introduce two classes of linear models, analysis of variance and regression.

13.4.1 ANOVA

In Section 13.3.2 we introduced a particular test problem – the two-sample location test. Purpose of this test is to judge whether two samples are drawn from the same population or not by the comparison of the centers of these samples. The null hypothesis was H_0: $\mu_1 = \mu_2$ and the alternative hypothesis was H_1: $\mu_1 \neq \mu_2$, where μ_i is the mean of the ith sample. A generalization of the null hypothesis is described in this section. Assume n different samples where each sample measures the same factor of interest. Within each sample, i, the factor is measured n_i times. This results in a table of the following form:

x_{11}	x_{21}	$\ldots$	x_{n1}
$\ldots$	$\ldots$	$\ldots$	$\ldots$
$x_{1_{n1}}$	$x_{1_{n2}}$	$\ldots$	$x_{1_{nN}}$

Here, the columns correspond to different individual samples and the rows correspond to the individual repetitions within each sample (the number of rows within each sample can vary!). The interesting question now is, whether there is any difference in the sample means, or, alternatively, whether the samples represent the same population. We thus test the null hypothesis H_0: $\mu_1 = \mu_2 \ldots = \mu_n$ against the alternative H_1: $\mu_i \neq \mu_j$ for at least one pair, $i \neq j$. This question is targeted by the so-called *one-way ANOVA*. As in the case of Student's t-test, additional assumptions on the data samples are necessary:

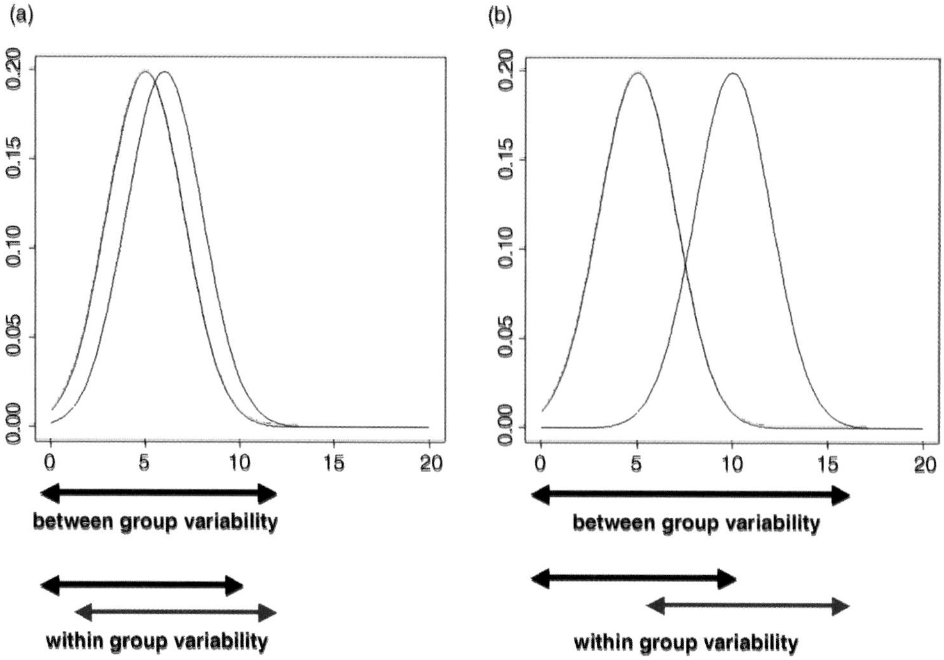

Figure 13.5 ANOVA test for differential expression. (a) Two normal distributions with means $\mu_1 = 5$, $\mu_2 = 6$ and equal variances. The variability between the groups is comparable with the variability within the groups. (b) Two normal distributions with means $\mu_1 = 5$, $\mu_2 = 10$ and equal variances. The variability between the groups is higher than the variability within the groups.

1. The n samples are drawn independently from each other representing populations with mean values $\mu_1, \mu_2, \ldots, \mu_n$.
2. All population variances have the same variance σ^2 (*homoscedasticity*).
3. All populations are Gaussian distributed, $N(\mu_i, \sigma^2)$.

Although the one-way ANOVA is based on the analysis of variance, it is essentially a test for location. This is exemplified in Figure 13.5. The idea of ANOVA is the comparison of between- and within-group variability. If the variance between the groups is not different from the variance within the groups we cannot reject the null hypotheses (Figure 13.5(a), if the variances differ we would reject the null hypothesis and conclude that the means are different (Figure 13.5(b)).

The calculation of the one-way ANOVA is based on the partition of the sample variance $\sum_{i=1}^{n}\sum_{j=1}^{n_i}(x_{ij}-\bar{x})^2$ into two parts that account for the between- and within-group variability, i.e.,

$$SS_{\text{total}} = \sum_{i=1}^{n}\sum_{j=1}^{n_i}(x_{ij}-\bar{x}..)^2 = \sum_{i=1}^{n}\sum_{j=1}^{n_i}(\bar{x}_{i.}-\bar{x}..)^2 + \sum_{i=1}^{n}\sum_{j=1}^{n_i}(x_{ij}-\bar{x}_{i.})^2$$

$$= SS_{\text{between}} + SS_{\text{within}} \tag{13.36}$$

We choose the test statistic $T = \frac{SS_{\text{between}}}{SS_{\text{within}}} \frac{M-n}{n-1}$, where $M = \sum_{i=1}^{n} n_i$. It can be shown that under the null hypothesis M is distributed according to an *F distribution* with degrees of freedom $\nu_1 = n-1$ and $\nu_2 = M-n$, respectively. The multiplicative constant accounts for the degrees of freedom of the two terms. Thus, we can quantify experimental outcomes according to this distribution. If μ_i are not equal, SS_{between} will be high compared to SS_{within} and conversely, if all μ_i are equal, then the two factors will be similar and T will be small.

13.4.2
Multiple Linear Regression

Let $\boldsymbol{y}$ be an n-dimensional observation vector (dependent variables) and let $\boldsymbol{x}_1, \ldots, \boldsymbol{x}_p$ be the independent n-dimensional variables. We assume that the number of observations is greater than the number of variables, i.e., $n > p$. The standard model here is

$$\boldsymbol{y} = \boldsymbol{X\beta} + \boldsymbol{\varepsilon}, \tag{13.37}$$

where, $\boldsymbol{E}(\boldsymbol{\varepsilon}) = 0$ and $\sum_{\boldsymbol{\varepsilon}} = \sigma^2 \boldsymbol{I}_n$. In our model we are interested in an optimal estimator for the unknown parameter vector $\boldsymbol{\beta}$. The *least-squares method* defines this optimization as a vector $\hat{\boldsymbol{\beta}}$ that minimizes the Euclidean norm of the residuals, i.e.,

$$\hat{\boldsymbol{\beta}} \in \operatorname{argmin}\{\boldsymbol{\beta}; ||\boldsymbol{y} - \boldsymbol{X\beta}||^2\}.$$

Using partial derivatives we can transform this problem into a linear equation system by

$$\boldsymbol{X}^{\mathrm{T}}\boldsymbol{X}\hat{\boldsymbol{\beta}} = \boldsymbol{X}^{\mathrm{T}}\boldsymbol{y}, \tag{13.38}$$

and, if the inverse exists, get the solution

$$\hat{\boldsymbol{\beta}} = (\boldsymbol{X}^{\mathrm{T}}\boldsymbol{X})^{-1}\boldsymbol{X}^{\mathrm{T}}\boldsymbol{y}. \tag{13.39}$$

The solution is called the *least-squares estimator* for $\boldsymbol{\beta}$. The least-squares estimator is unbiased, i.e., $\boldsymbol{E}(\hat{\boldsymbol{\beta}}) = \boldsymbol{\beta}$ and the covariance matrix $\sum_{\hat{\boldsymbol{\beta}}}$ of $\hat{\boldsymbol{\beta}}$ is equal to $\sum_{\hat{\boldsymbol{\beta}}} = \sigma^2(\boldsymbol{X}^{\mathrm{T}}\boldsymbol{X})^{-1}$. Through the estimator for $\boldsymbol{\beta}$ we have an immediate estimator for the error vector $\boldsymbol{\varepsilon}$ using the residuals

$$\hat{\boldsymbol{\varepsilon}} = \boldsymbol{y} - \boldsymbol{X}\hat{\boldsymbol{\beta}} = \boldsymbol{y} - \boldsymbol{X}(\boldsymbol{X}^{\mathrm{T}}\boldsymbol{X})^{-1}\boldsymbol{X}^{\mathrm{T}}\boldsymbol{y} = \boldsymbol{y} - \boldsymbol{P}\boldsymbol{y}. \tag{13.40}$$

Geometrically, $\boldsymbol{P}$ is the projection of $\boldsymbol{y}$ in the p-dimensional subspace of $\Re^n$ that is spanned by the columns vectors of X. An unbiased estimator for the unknown standard deviation of the residuals is given by

$$s^2 = \frac{||\boldsymbol{y} - \boldsymbol{X}\hat{\boldsymbol{\beta}}||^2}{n-p}, \tag{13.41}$$

thus $E(s^2) = \sigma^2$.

Example 13.13: Simple linear regression

An important application is the simple linear regression of two samples $x_1, \ldots, x_n$ and $y_1, \ldots, y_n$. Here Eq. (13.37) reduces to $\begin{pmatrix} y_1 \\ \vdots \\ y_n \end{pmatrix} = \begin{pmatrix} 1 & x_1 \\ \vdots & \vdots \\ 1 & x_n \end{pmatrix} \begin{pmatrix} \beta_1 \\ \beta_2 \end{pmatrix} + \begin{pmatrix} \varepsilon_1 \\ \vdots \\ \varepsilon_n \end{pmatrix}$ and the parameters of interest are β_1, β_2 the intercept and the slope of the regression line. Minimizing the Euclidean norm of the residuals computes the line that minimizes the vertical distances of all points to the regression line. Solving according to Eq. (13.39) gives

$$X^T X = \begin{pmatrix} n & \sum_{i=1}^n x_i \\ \sum_{i=1}^n x_i & \sum_{i=1}^n x_i^2 \end{pmatrix} \text{ and } X^T y = \begin{pmatrix} \sum_{i=1}^n y_i \\ \sum_{i=1}^n x_i y_i \end{pmatrix} \text{ and thus we have}$$

$$\hat{\beta} = \frac{1}{n\sum_{i=1}^n x_i^2 - \left(\sum_{i=1}^n x_i\right)^2} \begin{pmatrix} \sum_{i=1}^n x_i^2 & -\sum_{i=1}^n x_i \\ -\sum_{i=1}^n x_i & n \end{pmatrix} \begin{pmatrix} \sum_{i=1}^n y_i \\ \sum_{i=1}^n x_i y_i \end{pmatrix}$$

$$= \frac{1}{n\sum_{i=1}^n x_i^2 - \left(\sum_{i=1}^n x_i\right)^2} \begin{pmatrix} n\sum_{i=1}^n x_i^2 \sum_{i=1}^n y_i & -\sum_{i=1}^n x_i \sum_{i=1}^n x_i y \\ n\sum_{i=1}^n x_i y_i & -\sum_{i=1}^n x_i \sum_{i=1}^n y_i \end{pmatrix}.$$

Thus, the slope of the regression line is the correlation of the samples divided by the variance of the dependent variables. The slope of the regression line is called *empirical regression coefficient*.

13.5 Principal Component Analysis

Principal component analysis (PCA) is a statistical method to reduce dimensionality and to visualize high-dimensional data in two- or three dimensions. Consider an $n \times p$ expression matrix X, where rows correspond to genes and columns correspond to experiments. Thus, each gene is viewed as a data vector in the p-dimensional space. In general not all dimensions will contribute equally to the variation across the genes so that we can hope to reduce the overall dimension to the most relevant ones. The idea of PCA is to transform the coordinate system to a system whose axes display the maximal directions of variation of the data sample [2].

Figure 13.6(a) shows an example for $p = 2$. Here, essentially one dimension contains the variation of the sample and thus the dimensionality can be reduced to 1 after transforming the coordinate system appropriately.

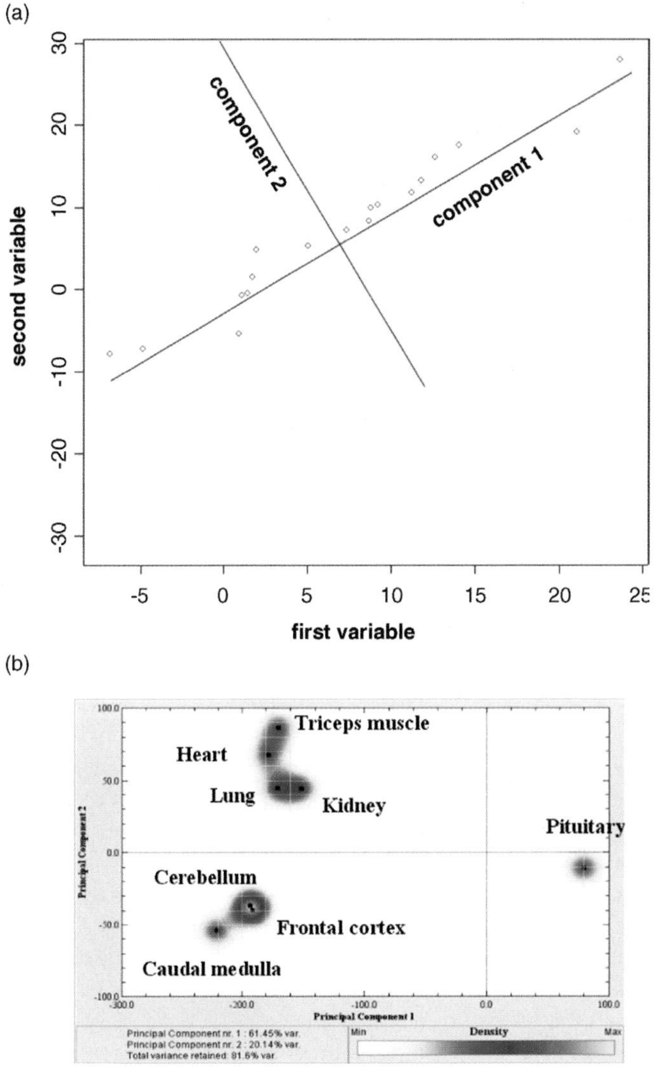

Figure 13.6 PCA performance. (a) A two-dimensional example of dimension reduction. The scatter plot shows highly correlated data samples that show significant variation with respect to the coordinate axes. Applying PCA will replace the original axes by principal components centered at the mean data vector whose directions determine the data variation. In the new coordinate system component 1 explains most of the data variation. (b) Practical example of PCA-based visualization of gene expression in eight bovine tissues. Gene expression was measured with DNA arrays and a subset of probes was preselected that separates these tissues appropriately. PCA allows the display using only two main directions and explaining 82% of the variance. Analysis was generated with *J-Express Pro* (Molmine, Bergen Norway).

Consider now more generally n p-dimensional data vectors $\boldsymbol{x}_1, \ldots, \boldsymbol{x}_n$ with component-wise mean vector $\bar{\boldsymbol{x}}$. PCA is computed with a decomposition of the $p \times p$-dimensional *empirical covariance matrix* of the sample (compare formula (13.6))

$$S = \frac{1}{n-1}\sum_{i=1}^{n}(\boldsymbol{x}_i-\bar{\boldsymbol{x}})(\boldsymbol{x}_i-\bar{\boldsymbol{x}})^{\mathrm{T}}. \tag{13.42}$$

Since the matrix $\boldsymbol{S}$ is symmetric and positive semidefinite there exist p nonnegative *eigenvalues* $\lambda_1 \geq \cdots \geq \lambda_p \geq 0$ (which we may assume to numerate in decreasing order, cf. Section 3.1.2). Let $\boldsymbol{r}_1, \ldots, \boldsymbol{r}_p$ be the corresponding *eigenvectors* such that

$$\boldsymbol{r}_j^{\mathrm{T}}\boldsymbol{r}_k = \begin{cases} 1, & \text{if } j = k \\ 0, & \text{if } j \neq k \end{cases} \qquad \boldsymbol{S}\boldsymbol{r}_j = \lambda_j \boldsymbol{r}_j. \tag{13.43}$$

If we denote with $\boldsymbol{R}$ the $p \times p$-dimensional matrix whose columns are composed of the p eigenvectors of $\boldsymbol{S}$ and if $\Lambda = \begin{pmatrix} \lambda_1 & 0 & 0 \\ 0 & \ddots & 0 \\ 0 & 0 & \lambda_p \end{pmatrix}$ denotes the $p \times p$-dimensional diagonal matrix whose diagonal elements are the p eigenvalues we get the decomposition

$$\boldsymbol{S} = \boldsymbol{R}\Lambda \boldsymbol{R}^{\mathrm{T}}. \tag{13.44}$$

Geometrically, the eigenvectors of $\boldsymbol{S}$ are the main axes of dispersion of the data set $\{\boldsymbol{x}_1, \ldots, \boldsymbol{x}_n\}$. The dispersion is maximal high in the first principal component, second highest with the second principal component, etc. The dispersion in each principal component, i, equals $\sqrt{\lambda_i}$. Suppose now that an eigenvalue λ_k is close to zero. This means that there is not much variance along that principal component at all and that the kth-coordinate of the vectors $\boldsymbol{x}_i$ are close to zero in the transformed coordinate system. Thus, this dimension does not contribute much to the overall dispersion of the data and can be neglected without essential loss of information. Similarly, this holds for $j = k+1, \ldots, p$ since we assumed the eigenvalues to be sorted in decreasing order. Thus, we have replaced the original p dimensions into $k-1 < p$ dimensions that explain the relevant variance of the data sample.

An important question is how many principal components are needed to explain a sufficient amount of the data variance. Denote each vector by its coordinates $\boldsymbol{x}_i = (x_{i1}, \ldots, x_{ip})^{\mathrm{T}}$ and let $\bar{x}_j$ be the jth coordinate of the mean vector $\bar{\boldsymbol{x}}$. A suitable measure for the total variance of the sample is the sum of the variances of the p coordinates given by

$$\sum_{j=1}^{p}\frac{1}{n-1}\sum_{i=1}^{n}(x_{ij}-\bar{x}_j)^2 = \mathrm{Trace}(\boldsymbol{S})\sum_{j=1}^{p}\lambda_j. \tag{13.45}$$

Thus, for each $k < p$ the relative amount of variance explained by the first k principal components is given by

$$\frac{\sum_{j=1}^{k}\lambda_k}{\sum_{j=1}^{p}\lambda_p}. \tag{13.46}$$

In gene expression analysis, for instance, PCA is widely used to reduce the gene expression matrix or its transpose matrix, the condition expression matrix, to two or three dimensions. Formula (13.46) is widely used in practice to characterize the computed dimension reduction. If the amount of variance explained is high then such a reduction makes sense otherwise the data set is too complex to be visualized with PCA.

Example 13.14: PCA examples

Figure 13.6(b) shows a display after PCA for eight different bovine tissues that were screened with a cDNA array. 600 cDNAs were filtered from the total set of 20,000 cDNAs in order to represent the tissues in a suitable way. Criteria were fold changes between tissues and reliable expression differences. PCA shows that the brain regions (cortex, cerebellum) form a tissue cluster separated from the others. The selected first two principal components explain approximately 82% of the data variance indicating that the visualization by PCR is an appropriate presentation of the whole dataset.

References

1 Kahlem, P. *et al.* (2004) Transcript level alterations reflect gene dosage effects across multiple tissues in a mouse model of down syndrome. *Genome Res*, **14**, 1258–1267.

2 Jolliffe, I.T. (1986) *Principal Component Analysis*, Springer, New York.

14
Stochastic Processes

Summary

A random process describes a system that can move randomly between different states in a state space, where time and state space can be discrete or continuous. Random processes serve, for instance, to describe thermal motion of particles or molecule numbers in chemical reaction systems. In Markov processes, the system's state in a given moment completely determines the probabilities for its future random behavior. The probability distribution of states in such processes can change in time: its time evolution can be computed, depending on the type of process, by the Master equation and the Fokker–Planck equation. The Langevin equation represents a random process in continuous time and state space. Formally, it appears like an ordinary differential equation with an additional noise term.

14.1
Basic Notions for Random Processes

A *random process* [1, 2] – also called stochastic process – describes a system that can move randomly between different states x in a state space $\mathcal{X}$. The states may describe the coordinates of a diffusing particle in space, but also the configurations of a complex system, like the molecule numbers in a biochemical network. The system states x and the time variable t can be discrete (e.g., described by positive integer numbers), continuous (e.g., real numbers), or both. The movements from one state to the other follow a stochastic law: in each time point t, the state is described by a random variable $X(t)$, and the random variables for different time points follow a joint probability distribution. So mathematically, the random process X is a collection of $\mathcal{X}$-valued random variables $X(t)$ indexed by a time variable $t \in T$.

Alternatively, a random process can also be seen as a collection of possible histories of the system called *realizations* of the process together with their probabilities.

Systems Biology: A Textbook. Edda Klipp, Wolfram Liebermeister, Christoph Wierling, Axel Kowald, Hans Lehrach, and Ralf Herwig

ISBN: 978-3-527-31874-2

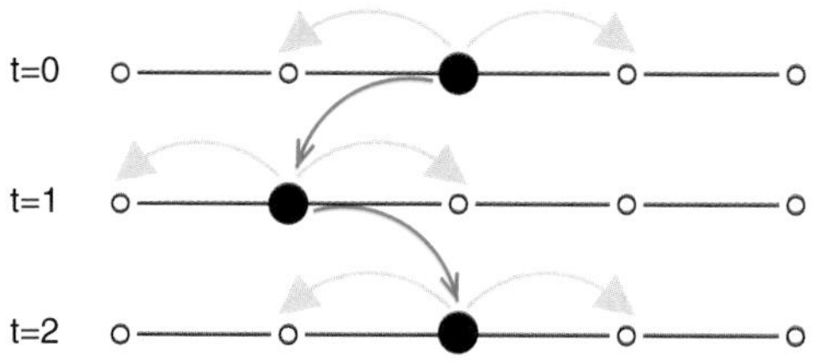

Figure 14.1 Random walk in discrete time and space. In each time step t, the walker can stay at its place or make a step left or right (possible jumps shown in gray, actual jumps in red).

If time is discrete $t = 1,2, \ldots$, each realization consists of a series of states $\{x(t)\}$ with a certain probability to occur in the process. For processes in continuous time $t \in \mathbb{R}$, the realizations are functions $x(t)$, each characterized by a probability density. *Stochastic simulation* can be used to determine the statistical properties of a random process and to visualize its dynamics. It produces different realizations of the process according to their probabilities (for discrete processes) or probability densities (for continuous processes) and can be seen as a form of Monte Carlo sampling.

Example 14.1: Discrete random walk

Figure 14.1 shows a simple random process, the discrete random walk. A random walker moves on a one-dimensional grid; in each time step, he can stay at his position or make a random step to the left or to the right, according to the following scheme:

Step	Transition	Probability
Right	$x \to x+1$	q_+
Left	$x \to x-1$	q_-
Stay	$x \to x$	$1-q_+-q_-$

(14.1)

Choices at different time points are statistically independent. In addition, we specify an initial distribution $p(x,0)$ for the position of the walker. If the walker starts at position $x=0$, this distribution would read $p(0,0) = 1$, $p(x,0) = 0$ for all $x \neq 0$. The initial distribution, together with the probabilities for individual jumps, define a joint distribution for all possible paths. To picture this random process, we may imagine a large number of random walkers (a so-called *ensemble*), each one taking different random decisions and thus realizing a different path.

The discrete random walk can be used to model *Brownian motion*, the thermal movement of a microscopic particle. An alternative random model would be the *Wiener process*, a random process with continuous space and time.

Example 14.2: The Wiener process

The Wiener process $W(t)$ describes a continuous variable $w \in \mathbb{R}$ in continuous time $t \in \mathbb{R}_+$. It is defined by the following properties:
(i) $W(t)$ starts in the state $W(0) = 0$.
(ii) almost all realizations of $W(t)$ are continuous functions of time t.
(iii) for time points $0 \leq t_1 \leq t_2$, the increments $W(t_2) - W(t_1)$ follow a Gaussian distribution with mean 0 and variance $t_2 - t_1$.
(iv) increments are independent of increments in the past, so for $t_1 \leq t_2 \leq t_3 \leq t_4$, the increments $W(t_2) - W(t_1)$ and $W(t_4) - W(t_3)$ are independent random variables.

The Wiener process can be seen as a limiting case of the discrete random walk: we can associate the space and time points in the discrete random walk with a grid in continuous space and time (interval sizes Δt and Δx). If we make the intervals smaller and smaller while keeping $\Delta t/\Delta x^2$ constant, the discrete random walk will approximate the Wiener process.

Figure 14.2 shows realizations of the discrete random walk, a random walk in discrete space and continuous time, and the Wiener process.

14.1.1 Reduced and Conditional Distributions

A random process determines a joint probability for the system states at all time points. If we consider a subset of n time points only, the states $X(t_1),\ldots, X(t_n)$ at these time points form an n-dimensional random vector with joint probability $p(x_\omega,t_n;\ldots x_\alpha,t_1)$. In particular, the system state at a time point t is described by the probability distribution $p(x,t)$. Figure 14.3 illustrates this for the Wiener process: all realizations start at a value $x(0) = 0$; at later time points, the distribution $p(x, t)$ becomes broader (Figure 14.3(a)). We can see this from the standard deviations (Figure 14.3(b)) and from the histograms at different time points (Figure 14.3(c)). The Wiener process consists of random movements relative to the current position. Once a realization has reached a position x above average, it tends to stay above average at later times. Therefore, the positions at different time points are positively correlated (Figure 14.3(d)). From the joint distribution at two time points t_1 and t_2, we can determine the *transition probability*

$$p(x_\alpha, t_2|x_\beta, t_1) = \frac{p(x_\alpha, t_2; x_\beta, t_1)}{p(x_\beta, t_1)}. \tag{14.2}$$

It describes the probability of ending up in state x_α at t_2 provided that the system was in state x_β at t_1. A process is called *stationary* if the ensemble as a whole is not affected by shifts of the time variable, $t \to t + \Delta t$; however, individual realizations of the process can still depend on time. In a stationary process, the transition probabilities $p(x_\alpha,t_2|x_\beta,t_1)$ only depend on time differences $t_2 - t_1$, and the distribution $p(x,t)$ is independent of time.

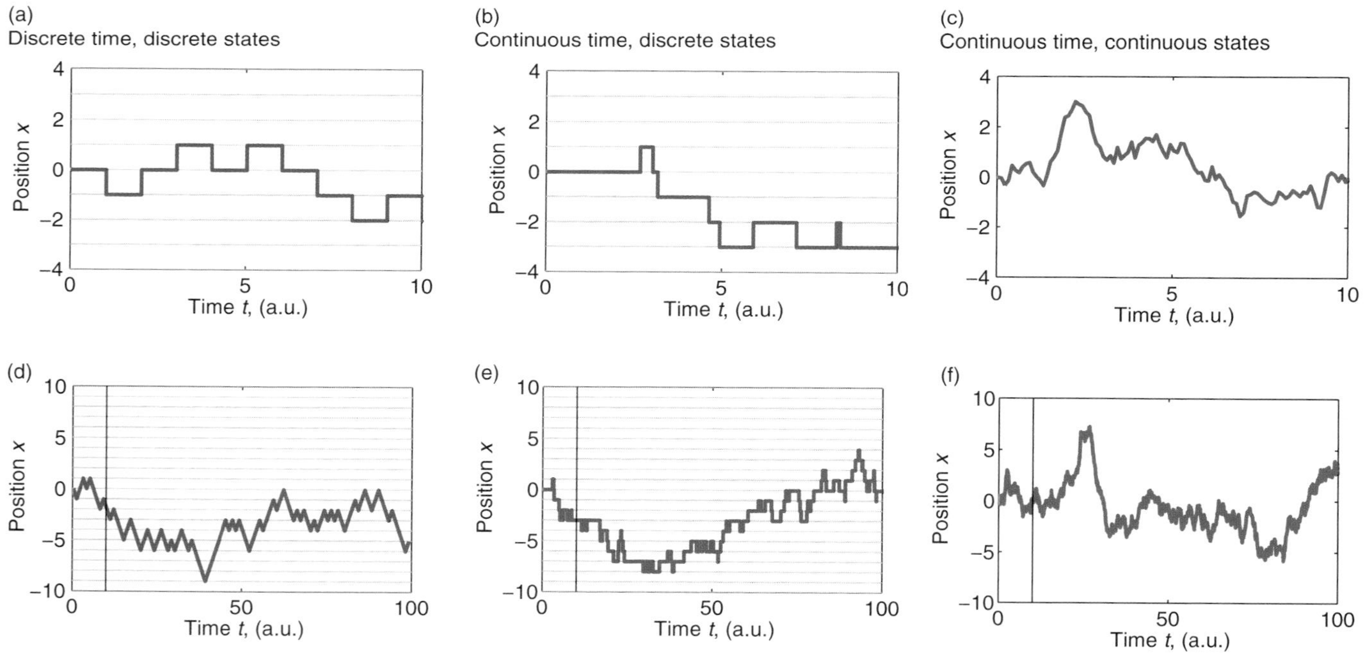

Figure 14.2 Realizations of three random processes. (a) Random walk with discrete space and time intervals $\Delta x = 1$ and $\Delta t = 1$ (see Figure 14.1). At each tick of the clock, the walker makes a random step right or left (here: up or down) with probabilities $q_{\pm} = 1/2$. (b) In a random walk in continuous time (no clock ticks), steps can happen at any moment with equal rate (i.e., probability per time) $w_{\pm} = 1/2$. (c) The Wiener process (see Example 14.2 and Section 14.4) describes random motion in continuous space and time. The bottom panels (d), (e), and (f) show the same realizations, plotted on a longer timescale. Vertical lines indicate the detail shown in the top row pictures.

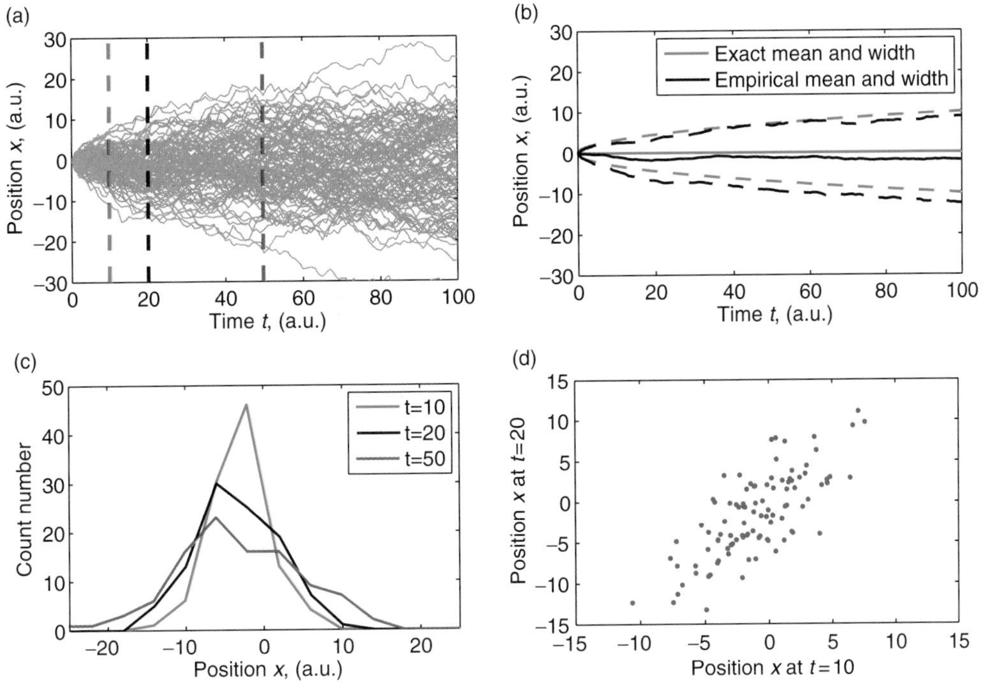

Figure 14.3 Statistical properties of the Wiener process. (a) 100 realizations of the Wiener process W (see Figure 14.2, right and Example 14.2). (b) Time-dependent mean value and standard deviations can be estimated from the realizations (solid lines). The exact ensemble averages $\langle W(t) \rangle = 0$ and standard deviation $\sqrt{\langle W(t)^2 \rangle} = \sqrt{t}$ for the process are shown by dashed lines. (c) Empirical distribution of states $W(t)$ at two different time points, $t = 10$, $t = 20$, and $t = 50$ (compare dashed lines in (a)). (d) A scatter plot for states at $t = 10$ and $t = 20$ shows the temporal correlations.

14.2 Markov Processes

Is the future behavior of a system determined by its current state, or does it additionally depend on the system's past? In models with delay equations, e.g., $dx(t)/dt = f(x(t-\tau))$, the time derivative of a variable at time t is computed from the system state at past time points $t-\tau$. In differential equation models, on the other hand, the future behavior of a system depends only the current state, without any additional dependence on states in the past. This is an important and strong model assumption; it implies that the model state is a complete description of the system (i.e., sufficiently complete to predict the future from it).

The same feature – the so-called *Markov property* – also plays an important role in random processes: here we assume that the *transition probabilities* between the current state and future states depend only on the current state, without any further dependence on states in the past. Mathematically, *Markov processes* are defined by the following condition:

$$p(x_\alpha, t_{n+1}|x_\beta, t_1; \ldots, x_\omega, t_n) = p(x_\alpha, t_{n+1}|x_\omega, t_n) \tag{14.3}$$

for all time points $t_1 < t_2 < \ldots < t_n < t_{n+1}$. In other words: given the state at time t_n, the state at later times $t_{n+1} > t_n$ is conditionally independent of all earlier states. A Markov process can be fully specified by its initial probability distribution $p(x,t_0)$ and the transition probabilities $p(x_\alpha,t_2|x_\beta,t_1)$ for all times $t_2 > t_1 \geq t_0$. Depending on the nature of the time and space variables (discrete or continuous), we distinguish between Markov chains, Markov jump processes, and continuous Markov processes.

14.2.1 Markov Chains

The discrete random walk (14.1) is an example of a *Markov chain*, a Markov process with discrete time points $t = 1,2, \ldots,$ and discrete or continuous states x. A Markov chain is determined by the initial probabilities $p(x_\alpha,0)$ and by the transition probabilities $q_{\alpha\beta}(t) = p(x_\alpha,t+1|x_\beta,t)$. Different states are labeled by Greek subscripts, and we will assume here that the values $q_{\alpha\beta}$ are constant in time.

Realizations $\{x(t)\}$ of a Markov chain can be obtained by stochastic simulation: we first draw an initial state $x(0)$ from the distribution $p(x_\alpha,0)$. Then, we move from state to state, choosing each new state $x(t+1)$ randomly with the probabilities $p(x_\alpha,t+1|x(t),t)$ based on the previous state $x(t)$. We can use a similar iterative procedure to compute the time-dependent distribution $p(x_\alpha,t)$: starting from the initial distribution $p(x_\alpha,0)$, we compute each distribution $p(x_\alpha,t+1)$ iteratively by the formula

$$p(x_\alpha, t+1) = \sum_\beta q_{\alpha\beta} p(x_\beta, t) = q_{\alpha\alpha}\, p(x_\alpha, t) + \sum_{\beta \neq \alpha} q_{\alpha\beta}\, p(x_\beta, t) \tag{14.4}$$

Equation (14.4) shows that the transition probabilities $q_{\alpha\beta}$ have to be normalized to $\sum_\alpha q_{\alpha\beta} = 1$, otherwise the updated probabilities would not sum up to 1. It can also be written in vectorial form: with the vector $\boldsymbol{p}(t)$ containing all probabilities $p(x_\alpha,t)$ at time t, Eq. (14.4) becomes

$$\boldsymbol{p}(t+1) = \boldsymbol{Q}\,\boldsymbol{p}(t). \tag{14.5}$$

The distribution $\boldsymbol{p}(t)$ can be computed by applying this formula t times to the initial distribution $p(x,0)$, so for a constant transition matrix $\boldsymbol{Q}$, we obtain $\boldsymbol{p}(t) = \boldsymbol{Q}^t\boldsymbol{p}(0)$. Furthermore, we can define the *invariant distribution* $\boldsymbol{p}_\infty$, an eigenvector of $\boldsymbol{Q}$ with the eigenvalue 1, satisfying $\boldsymbol{p}_\infty = \boldsymbol{Q}\,\boldsymbol{p}_\infty$. If the system starts with the invariant distribution $\boldsymbol{p}(0) = \boldsymbol{p}_\infty$, this distribution will remain constant in time. In the stationary case, the individual realizations of the process still show random jumps, but the probability flows between different states are exactly balanced.

Example 14.3: Probability distribution in the discrete random walk

In the discrete random walk, the distribution $p(x,t)$ can be computed by enumerating all possible paths leading from position 0 (at time 0) to position x (at time t). In the case with symmetric and obligatory jumps, $q_{\pm} = 1/2$, each possible path has simply the probability $(1/2)^t$. At time point t, the walker has made t jumps, among them Y jumps to the right. The random number Y follows a binomial distribution $p(y,t) = \binom{t}{y}(1/2)^t$ and determines the current position by $X = 2Y - t$. The transition probabilities can be computed similarly: the probability to move from x_β (at time t_1) to x_α (at time t_2) only depends on the differences $t_2 - t_1$ and $x_\alpha - x_\beta$ because the probabilities for single jumps are time-invariant and do not depend on the absolute position. We can therefore compute the transition probabilities from the distribution $p(x_\alpha,t)$ by $p(x_\alpha, t_2|x_\beta, t_1) = p(x_\alpha - x_\beta, t_2 - t_1)$.

14.3 Jump Processes in Continuous Time: The Master Equation

In some stochastic models, e.g., population models for plants or animals, discrete time steps (of years) may be a natural assumption. For chemical reaction systems, however, it is more plausible to consider continuous time. In a *Markov jump process*, state transitions occur in continuous time $t \in \mathbb{R}_+$, while the states x themselves are still discrete. An example is shown in Figures 14.2(b) and (e).

Instead of discrete time steps as in a Markov chain, we now consider small time intervals $[t, t + \Delta t]$. We assume that for very small intervals $\Delta t \to 0$, the probability for a transition within the interval is proportional Δt. With the proportionality constant $w_{\alpha\beta}(t)$ for a transition $x_\beta \to x_\alpha$, called the *transition rate*, we can approximate the transition probability by $w_{\alpha\beta}(t)\Delta t$.

The transitions will lead to temporal changes of the state probabilities $p(x,t)$, and these will follow a system of differential equations called the *Master equation*. To derive it, we first consider the joint probability $p(x_\alpha,t_2;x_\beta,t_1) = p(x_\alpha,t_2|x_\beta,t_1)p(x_\beta,t_1)$ at two time points $t_1 < t_2$.

$$\begin{aligned} p(x_\alpha, t_2) &= p(x_\alpha, t_2; x_\alpha, t_1) + \sum_{\beta \neq \alpha} p(x_\alpha, t_2; x_\beta, t_1) \\ &= \left(1 - \sum_{\beta \neq \alpha} p(x_\beta, t_2|x_\alpha, t_1)\right) p(x_\alpha, t_1) \\ &\quad + \sum_{\beta \neq \alpha} p(x_\alpha, t_2|x_\beta, t_1) p(x_\beta, t_1). \end{aligned} \tag{14.6}$$

We now set $t_1 = t$ and $t_2 = t + \Delta t$. For small time differences $\Delta t = t_2 - t_1$, we can approximate $p(x_\alpha,t + \Delta t|x_\beta,t) \approx w_{\alpha\beta}(t)\Delta t$ and obtain

$$p(x_\alpha, t + \Delta t) \approx p(x_\alpha, t) + \left[\sum_{\beta \neq \alpha} w_{\alpha\beta}(t) p(x_\beta, t) - w_{\beta\alpha}(t) p(x_\alpha, t)\right] \Delta t. \tag{14.7}$$

In the limit $\Delta t \rightarrow 0$, we obtain the differential equation

$$\frac{dp(x_\alpha, t)}{dt} = \sum_{\beta \neq \alpha} \left[w_{\alpha\beta}(t) p(x_\beta, t) - w_{\beta\alpha}(t) p(x_\alpha, t) \right], \tag{14.8}$$

for the probability of state x_α. The first, positive term counts all transitions from other states to x_α, while the second, negative term counts all transitions from x_α to other states; we can interpret the terms as probability flows between different states. The equations (14.8) for all states x_α form a system of linear first-order differential equations, called the *Master equation.*

In practice, the number of states – which determines the size of the equation system – can be very large. In a biochemical system of m molecule species, each described by a particle number between 0 and n, a state would be determined by a specific choice of all these particle numbers. Altogether, we obtain m^{n+1} possible states, and each of them contributes one differential equation. In many real-world problems, it is impossible to solve the Master equation analytically [3]; however, the behavior of the random process can be computed by stochastic simulation or, in some cases, from the generating function (see the web supplement).

14.4 Continuous Random Processes

Continuous Markov processes like theWiener process can be used to model complex systems; e.g., the state of a metabolic system described by a number of real-valued substance concentrations.

14.4.1 Langevin Equations

Some continuous Markov processes can be written symbolically as *Langevin equations.* In its appearance, a Langevin equation

$$\frac{dX(t)}{dt} = f(X(t)) + \xi(t) \tag{14.9}$$

resembles an ordinary differential equation, but it contains a stochastic term $\xi(t)$ on the right-hand side. Accordingly, it does not specify a function, but a random process. A common choice of $\xi(t)$ is *Gaussian white noise,* a hypothetical random process with mean zero and covariance function

$$\mathrm{cov}(\xi(t_1), \xi(t_2)) = \langle \xi(t_1)\xi(t_2) \rangle = \delta(t_1 - t_2). \tag{14.10}$$

The simple Langevin equation

$$\frac{dX(t)}{dt} = \xi(t) \tag{14.11}$$

is solved by the Wiener process $W(t)$, so the white noise term, integrated over time, corresponds to Gaussian-distributed random increments. We can use this fact to simulate Langevin equations by the *stochastic Euler method*: the continuous process (14.9) is approximated by a time-discrete process

$$X(t_{i+1}) \approx X(t_i) + f(X(t_i))\Delta t + \Delta W, \tag{14.12}$$

in which each step corresponds to an original time interval Δt. The random term ΔW is a Gaussian random number with mean 0 and variance Δt; it can be interpreted as the time increment of a Wiener process, which justifies this method. The Euler method (14.12) is not exact because it approximates the term $f(X(t))$ by a constant value within each time interval; however, its accuracy can be tuned by the interval length Δt.

14.4.2
The Fokker–Planck Equation

Given a random process $X(t)$, we may ask how the probability density $p(x,t)$ of the states x will change in time. For discrete state spaces and continuous time, this question is answered by the Master equation (14.8); for a Langevin equation with continuous states $x \in \mathbb{R}^n$, we can use the *Fokker–Planck equation*

$$\frac{\partial p(x,t)}{\partial t} = \left[-\sum_{i=1}^{n} \frac{\partial}{\partial x_i} g_i(x,t) + \sum_{i=1}^{n}\sum_{j=1}^{n} \frac{\partial^2}{\partial x_i \partial x_i} D_{ij}(x,t) \right] p(x,t), \tag{14.13}$$

a partial differential equation specified by a drift vector $\mathbf{g}(x)$ and a diffusion tensor $\boldsymbol{D}(x)$. Both quantities are directly related to terms in the Langevin equation: for instance, let us consider a Langevin equation for a vectorial process $X(t)$

$$\frac{\mathrm{d}X(t)}{\mathrm{d}t} = \boldsymbol{f}(X(t),t) + \boldsymbol{B}(X(t),t)\,\xi(t), \tag{14.14}$$

with a vector $\boldsymbol{f}(\boldsymbol{x},t)$, a matrix $\boldsymbol{B}(\boldsymbol{x},t)$, and uncorrelated white noise inputs $\xi_i(t)$ satisfying $\langle \xi_i(t_1)\xi_k^{\mathrm{T}}(t_2)\rangle = \delta_{ik}\delta(t_2 - t_1)$. The resulting probability density $p(\boldsymbol{x},t)$ follows from a Fokker–Planck equation (14.13) with the drift and diffusion terms

$$\begin{aligned} \mathbf{g}(x,t) &= \boldsymbol{f}(x,t) \\ \boldsymbol{D}(x,t) &= \frac{1}{2}\boldsymbol{B}(x,t)\boldsymbol{B}^T(\mathrm{x},t). \end{aligned} \tag{14.15}$$

If we imagine the probability distribution $p(\boldsymbol{x},t)$ as a cloud in state space, the cloud will move in time according the deterministic part of the Langevin equation, while its width will increase according to the noise term. For simple Brownian motion in one dimension, the Fokker–Planck equation becomes

$$\frac{\partial}{\partial t} p(x,t) = D \frac{\partial^2}{\partial x^2} p(x,t), \tag{14.16}$$

with diffusion constant D and a vanishing drift term. Equation (14.16) describes the probability distribution for the position of a single particle; it is closely related to the diffusion equation for substance concentrations (see Section 3.4.3).

References

1 Honerkamp, J. (1994) *Stochastic Dynamical Systems*, John Wiley and Sons, Inc., New York.

2 Trigger, G.L. (ed.) (2005) *Mathematical Tools for Physicists*, Wiley-VCH, Weinheim.

3 Jahnke, T. and Huisinga, W. (2007), Solving the chemical master equation for monomolecular reactions systems analytically. *Journal of Mathematical Biology*, **54**, 1–26.

15
Control of Linear Systems

Summary

Control theory describes the response of dynamical systems to external perturbations and provides ways to stabilize or to control their behavior. Linear differential equation systems define a mapping between temporal input signals and temporal output signals. Output signals can be described in terms of responses to simple (pulse-like or oscillatory) input signals. These two descriptions are summarized by the impulse response and the frequency response function, respectively. Temporal random signals can be characterized by mean values and spectral densities. For linear systems, the spectral density of the output signals follows from the spectral density of the input signals and the frequency response of the system. Two important properties of linear control systems, controllability and observability, can be judged by the Gramian matrices.

15.1
Linear Dynamical Systems

Control theory studies how a given dynamical system can be controlled by external intervention. An important application is the design of feedback systems that stabilize a given system against perturbations caused by external influences or by unreliable parts. A variety of methods have been developed for linear systems of the form

$$\begin{aligned} \frac{d\boldsymbol{x}(t)}{dt} &= \boldsymbol{A}\boldsymbol{x}(t) + \boldsymbol{B}\boldsymbol{u}(t) \\ \boldsymbol{y}(t) &= \boldsymbol{C}\boldsymbol{x}(t) + \boldsymbol{D}\boldsymbol{u}(t) \end{aligned} \tag{15.1}$$

for time points $t \geq 0$. The equations describe a number of internal state variables x_i, input variables u_j, and output variables y_l, and are specified by constant matrices $\boldsymbol{A}$, $\boldsymbol{B}$, $\boldsymbol{C}$, and $\boldsymbol{D}$.

Systems Biology: A Textbook. Edda Klipp, Wolfram Liebermeister, Christoph Wierling, Axel Kowald, Hans Lehrach, and Ralf Herwig

ISBN: 978-3-527-31874-2

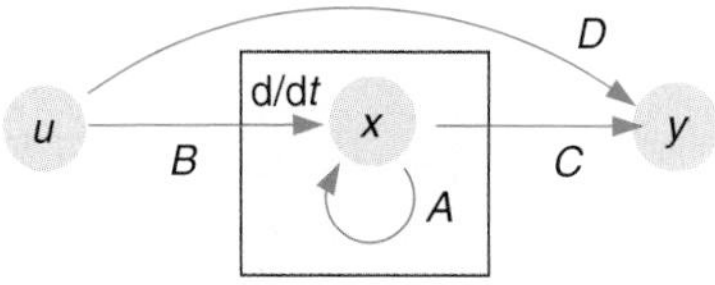

Figure 15.1 Linear dynamical system. According to Eq. (15.1), the time derivative of the internal state vector $\boldsymbol{x}$ depends on both $\boldsymbol{x}$ itself and on the input vector $\boldsymbol{u}$. This input can represent external regulation or random perturbations. The output vector $\boldsymbol{y}$, which can be observed from the outside, is computed from $\boldsymbol{x}$ and $\boldsymbol{u}$. The system is specified by the matrices $\boldsymbol{A},\boldsymbol{B},\boldsymbol{C}$, and $\boldsymbol{D}$.

In the model, the state variables x_i respond to their own current values and to the input values u_j, while the output variables y_l are linear combinations of the state variables x_i and the inputs u_j (see Figure 15.1). In the model – just like in real systems – the state variables are not necessarily accessible from the outside, but they can be influenced via the input vector $\boldsymbol{u}$ and observed via the output vector $\boldsymbol{y}$. A particular solution of the system depends on the initial condition $\boldsymbol{x}(0) = \boldsymbol{x}_0$ and on the external input $\boldsymbol{u}(\cdot)$. Here the symbol $f(\cdot)$ denotes the function as a whole, in contrast to a particular value $f(t)$ of the function at time t.

Linear systems like Eq. (15.1) can be obtained by linearizing a kinetic model around a steady state. In this case, the matrices $\boldsymbol{A}$, $\boldsymbol{B}$, $\boldsymbol{C}$, and $\boldsymbol{D}$ result from linear approximations of the local dynamics (see Sections 4.3 and 7.1.6).

If the input variables vanish (constant $\boldsymbol{u}(\cdot) = 0$), the system (15.1) has a fixed point at $\mathrm{x} = 0$. By adding a constant term in the differential equation, the fixed point could easily be shifted to other values, representing, for instance, the steady state of a metabolic model. In the following, we always assume that the system (15.1) is asymptotically stable, i.e., all eigenvalues of A have strictly negative real parts.

15.2
System Response

In the linear system (15.1), a given temporal input $\boldsymbol{u}(\cdot)$ together with the initial condition $\boldsymbol{x}(0) = \boldsymbol{x}_0$ uniquely defines the temporal output $\boldsymbol{y}(\cdot)$. As the equations (15.1) are linear, the dynamics arising from an initial value $\boldsymbol{x}(0)$ and an input $\boldsymbol{u}(\cdot)$ is the sum of two terms: (i) the behavior that would arise with a vanishing input (i.e., the given value of $\boldsymbol{x}(0)$ and $\boldsymbol{u}(\cdot) = 0$) and (ii) the behavior arising from $\boldsymbol{x}(0) = 0$ and the given time course $\boldsymbol{u}(\cdot)$. In particular, if we set $\boldsymbol{x}(0) = 0$, the system (15.1) directly maps input time courses $\boldsymbol{u}(\cdot)$ to output time courses $\boldsymbol{y}(\cdot)$. This *input–output relation* depends only on the matrices $\boldsymbol{A}$, $\boldsymbol{B}$, $\boldsymbol{C}$, and $\boldsymbol{D}$. For simplicity, we shall assume in the following that $\boldsymbol{x}(0) = 0$ and $\boldsymbol{D} = 0$ if not stated differently.

For the linear system (15.1) with $\boldsymbol{x}(0) = 0$, the responses to different inputs are additive, so we can linearly combine them. If the system maps an input $\boldsymbol{u}^{(1)}(\cdot)$ to an output $\boldsymbol{y}^{(1)}(\cdot)$ and an input $\boldsymbol{u}^{(2)}(\cdot)$ to an output $\boldsymbol{y}^{(2)}(\cdot)$, it will also map the linear combination $\alpha\boldsymbol{u}^{(1)}(\cdot) + \beta\boldsymbol{u}^{(2)}(\cdot)$ to the respective linear combination $\alpha\boldsymbol{y}^{(1)}(\cdot) + \beta\boldsymbol{y}^{(2)}(\cdot)$.

Responses to complicated inputs can be co-bined from responses to simpler inputs. Therefore, it is instructive to study the responses to two simple types of input, namely pulses and oscillatory signals.

1. The response to short input pulses is described by the *impulse response function.* Assume that one of the input variables, u_j, shows an infinitesimally short pulse with a time integral of 1, while all other input variables are zero. Such a pulse can be represented by a Gaussian function of width ε and height $1/\varepsilon$ located at $t=0$. For small $\varepsilon \to 0$, this function will approximate a Dirac delta distribution $\delta(t)$. In this limit, the system's response (with initial condition $x(0)=0$ and with $\mathbf{D}=0$) is given by the *impulse response function* (also called "kernel" or "Green's function")

$$\mathbf{K}(t) = \mathbf{C}\, e^{\mathbf{A}t}\mathbf{B}, \quad t \geq 0\,, \tag{15.2}$$

where the matrix exponential is defined by the Taylor series

$$e^{\mathbf{A}t} = \mathbf{I} + \mathbf{A}t + \frac{1}{2}(\mathbf{A}t)^2 + \cdots. \tag{15.3}$$

Using the impulse response (15.2), the system response to bounded, integrable inputs $\mathbf{u}(\cdot)$ of arbitrary shape can be written as a convolution integral

$$y(t) = \int_{-\infty}^{t} \mathbf{K}(t-t')\, \mathbf{u}(t')dt'. \tag{15.4}$$

2. On the other hand, we can consider an oscillatory input

$$\mathbf{u}(t) = \tilde{\mathbf{u}}\, e^{i\omega t} \tag{15.5}$$

with circular frequency $\omega = 2\pi/T$ (where T is the oscillation period); here we assume that the time $t \in \mathbb{R}$ can also be negative. The input (15.5) will induce forced oscillations

$$\mathbf{x}(t) = \tilde{\mathbf{x}}\, e^{i\omega t}, \quad y(t) = \tilde{y}\, e^{i\omega t} \tag{15.6}$$

of the same frequency, where the complex amplitudes in the vectors $\tilde{\mathbf{u}}, \tilde{\mathbf{x}}$, and $\tilde{y}$ describe the amplitudes and phases of the oscillating variables. We can prove this in two ways: using (15.4), we obtain

$$y(t) = \int_{-\infty}^{t} \mathbf{K}(t-t')\mathbf{u}\, e^{i\omega t'}\mathrm{d}t', \tag{15.7}$$

and by a substitution $\tau = t-t'$

$$y(t) = \int_{0}^{\infty} \mathbf{K}(\tau)\mathbf{u}\, e^{i\omega(t-\tau)}\mathrm{d}\tau. \tag{15.8}$$

Then we have

$$y(t) = \left(\int_{0}^{\infty} \mathbf{K}(\tau)e^{-i\omega\tau}\mathrm{d}\tau\right)\mathbf{u}e^{i\omega t}. \tag{15.9}$$

On the other hand, by inserting Eq. (15.6) as an ansatz into the system equation (15.1) with the simplifying assumption $\mathbf{D}=0$, we obtain

$$\tilde{y} = C(i\omega I - A)^{-1} B \tilde{u}. \tag{15.10}$$

A comparison between Eqs. (15.10) and (15.9) shows that the matrix

$$H(i\omega) = C(i\omega I - A)^{-1} B, \tag{15.11}$$

called the *frequency response function*, is nothing but the Fourier transform of the impulse response.

The system responses to pulses and wave-like inputs are therefore related to each other by the Fourier transformation. The convolution integral (15.4) describes the input–output relation for temporal signals, but the same signals can also be described in frequency space by their Fourier transforms. This allows us to avoid the complicated evaluation of the convolution integral. As a convolution in the time domain corresponds to multiplication in the frequency domain, we can compute the Fourier components of $y(\cdot)$ by multiplying the Fourier components of $u(\cdot)$ with the frequency response function

$$\tilde{y}(\omega) = H(i\omega)\tilde{u}(\omega), \tag{15.12}$$

which is nothing else than Eq. (15.10), or the Fourier transform of Eq. (15.4). Equation (15.12) also has a practical interpretation: a time-invariant linear system (15.1) can be seen as a filter that specifically dampens or amplifies the Fourier components of a signal.

15.2.1
Random Fluctuations and Spectral Density

To study how the system (15.1) would respond to random noise inputs, we assume that the input signal u does not represent a mathematical function, but a stationary Gauss–Markov random process (see Section 14.4). An important special case is the white noise process, which appears in the chemical Langevin equation (see Section 7.1.4). As initial conditions, we specify $x(t_0) = 0$ at time point t_0 and consider the limit $t_0 \to -\infty$. Due to the random input u, the output y will also follow a random process. Both processes can be described by mean values and cross-correlations, or alternatively, by their frequency-dependent spectral densities.

By averaging over all realizations of a random process, we obtain its ensemble average $\langle x(t) \rangle$ If the process is stationary – as we assume – this average is constant in time. Individual realizations may deviate from the mean behavior: the deviations $\Delta x(t) = x(t) - \langle x(t) \rangle$ consist of (short-term) fluctuations within a realization and (long-term) differences between the realizations. In general, the deviations $\Delta x(t)$ at different time points will show statistical correlations, and in a stationary process, these correlations only depend on the time difference τ between the moments for which the deviations are compared. We can quantify the strength of fluctuations by the matrix-valued covariance function

$$C_x(\tau) = \langle \Delta x(\tau) \Delta x^{T}(0) \rangle. \tag{15.13}$$

Again, we can describe the process in the frequency domain by using the Fourier transformation: the Fourier transform of the covariance function,

$$\Phi_x(\omega) = \int_{-\infty}^{\infty} C_x(\tau)e^{-i\omega t}d\tau, \tag{15.14}$$

called the *spectral density matrix*, describes a random process in terms of fluctuations at different frequencies. The covariance function can be obtained from the spectral density by an inverse Fourier transformation

$$C_x(\tau) = \frac{1}{2\pi}\int_{-\infty}^{\infty} e^{i\omega t}\Phi_x(\omega)d\omega. \tag{15.15}$$

According to Eq. (15.15), the stationary covariance

$$C_x(0) = \frac{1}{2\pi}\int_{-\infty}^{\infty} \Phi_x(\omega)d\omega. \tag{15.16}$$

summarizes noise contributions from all frequencies.

For a linear process of the form (15.1) with random input $\boldsymbol{u}(\cdot)$ and output $\boldsymbol{y}(\cdot)$, the spectrum of input and output variables – as well as the correlations between them – is represented by the spectral density matrices $\Phi_u(\omega)$ and $\Phi_y(\omega)$ (for an example, see Section 7.2.3). As in the case of deterministic inputs, the system acts as a filter: the output spectral density can be computed from the input spectral density and the frequency response function by the formula

$$\Phi_y(\omega) = \boldsymbol{H}(i\omega)\Phi_u(\omega)\boldsymbol{H}(i\omega)^{\dagger}, \tag{15.17}$$

where the symbol † denotes the matrix adjoint (= conjugate transpose). If a system is driven by white noise (with a spectral density $\Phi_u(\omega) = 1$), the output spectral density $\Phi_y(\omega) = \boldsymbol{H}(i\omega)\boldsymbol{H}(i\omega)^{\dagger}$ is just determined by the frequency response $\boldsymbol{H}(i\omega)$ of the system.

15.3 The Gramian Matrices

To design control mechanisms for a given system, two central questions have to be addressed: to what extent can the system state be manipulated via its inputs? And will observations of the outputs allow us to reconstruct the system's internal state? Ideally, a system is both controllable and observable, as defined next. A system is *controllable* if it can be steered from any initial state $x^{(0)}$ to any final state x within an appropriate time interval and by an appropriately chosen input signal $\boldsymbol{u}(\cdot)$. A system is *observable* if its internal state $x(t_0)$ at time point t_0 can be inferred from its input values $\boldsymbol{u}(\cdot)$ and output values $\boldsymbol{y}(\cdot)$, observed in a time interval $[t_0,t_1]$ following this time point.

For the system (15.1), controllability and observability are determined by two matrices, the *controllability Gramian* $\mathbf{W}_c$ and the *observability Gramian* $\mathbf{W}_o$:

$$\mathbf{W}_c(t_1) = \int_0^{t_1} e^{At} \boldsymbol{B}\boldsymbol{B}^T e^{A^T t} dt, \quad \mathbf{W}_o(t_1) = \int_0^{t_1} e^{A^T t} \mathbf{C}^T \mathbf{C} e^{At} dt. \tag{15.18}$$

The Gramian matrices describe which internal variables (or linear combinations of them) can be controlled and observed – and to what extent. A system with matrices $\boldsymbol{A}$ and $\boldsymbol{B}$ is controllable if $\mathbf{W}_c(t)$ is regular (i.e., invertible) for some (and hence any) time $t > 0$. Likewise, a system with $\boldsymbol{A}$ and $\mathbf{C}$ is observable exactly if $\mathbf{W}_o(t)$ is regular for some (and hence any) time $t > 0$.

The Gramian matrices are related to the so-called input and output energies: a given input signal is characterized by an *input energy*

$$E_u = \int_0^{t_1} \boldsymbol{u}^T(t)\boldsymbol{u}(t)dt. \tag{15.19}$$

In problems of optimal control, we may interpret the input energy as the effort that has to be invested to influence the system. Suppose that the system should be steered from state $x(t_0{=}0) = 0$ to the state $\boldsymbol{x}_1$ at time point t_1 with a minimal amount of input energy. If the matrix $\mathbf{W}_c$ is invertible, the optimal input is given by

$$\boldsymbol{u}(t) = \boldsymbol{B}^T e^{A^T(t_1-t)} \mathbf{W}_c^{-1}(t_1)\boldsymbol{x}_1, \tag{15.20}$$

and the corresponding energy value reads $\boldsymbol{x}_1^T \mathbf{W}_c^{-1}(t_1)\boldsymbol{x}_1$. In analogy, the *output energy*

$$E_y = \int_0^{t_1} \boldsymbol{y}^T(t)\boldsymbol{y}(t)dt. \tag{15.21}$$

scores the outputs of a system that starts in $\boldsymbol{x}_1$ at $t_0 = 0$ and then evolves at an input $\boldsymbol{u}(t) = 0$. The output energy can also be written as $\boldsymbol{x}^T \mathbf{W}_o(t_1)\boldsymbol{x}$. For asymptotically stable systems, the infinite-time Gramian matrices $\mathbf{W}_c$ and $\mathbf{W}_o$ are defined by

$$\mathbf{W}_c = \int_0^{\infty} e^{At} \boldsymbol{B}\boldsymbol{B}^T e^{A^T t} dt, \quad \mathbf{W}_o = \int_0^{\infty} e^{A^T t} \mathbf{C}^T \mathbf{C} e^{At} dt. \tag{15.22}$$

They can be computed by solving the two Lyapunov equations

$$\begin{aligned} \boldsymbol{A}\mathbf{W}_c + \mathbf{W}_c\boldsymbol{A}^T + \boldsymbol{B}\boldsymbol{B}^T &= 0, \\ \boldsymbol{A}^T\mathbf{W}_o + \mathbf{W}_o\boldsymbol{A} + \mathbf{C}^T\mathbf{C} &= 0. \end{aligned} \tag{15.23}$$

The infinite-time controllability Gramian $\mathbf{W}_c$ has another important interpretation: it represents the covariance matrix of the internal state x that results from uncorrelated white-noise input signals $u_j(t) = \xi_j(t)$. The Gramian matrices can also be used for model reduction by balanced truncation (see the web supplement).

16
Databases

Summary

With the rapid increase of biological data, it has become even more important to organize and structure the data in a way so that information can easily be retrieved. As a result, the number of databases has also increased rapidly over the past few years. Most of these databases have a web interface and can be accessed from everywhere in the world, which is an enormously important service for the scientific community. In the following, various databases are presented that might be relevant for systems biology.

Moreover, the journal *Nucleic Acids Research* offers a database issue each year in January dedicated to factual biological databases and in addition to this a web server issue each year in July presenting web-based services.

16.1
Databases of the National Center for Biotechnology

The National Center for Biotechnology (NCBI) (http://www.ncbi.nlm.nih.gov/) provides several databases widely used in biological research. Most important are the molecular databases, offering information about nucleotide sequences, proteins, genes, molecular structures, and gene expression. Besides this, several databases comprising scientific literature are available. The NCBI also provides a taxonomy database that contains names and lineages of more than 130,000 organisms. For more than 1000 organisms, whole genomes (either already completely sequenced or for which sequencing is just in progress) and corresponding gene maps are available, as along with the tools for their inspection. A full overview of the databases provided by the NCBI can be found under http://www.ncbi.nlm.nih.gov/Sitemap/index.html. All these databases are searchable via the Entrez search engine accessible through the NCBI homepage.

Among the nucleotide sequence databases, the Genetic Sequence database (GenBank), the Reference Sequences database (RefSeq), and UniGene can be found.

Systems Biology: A Textbook. Edda Klipp, Wolfram Liebermeister, Christoph Wierling, Axel Kowald, Hans Lehrach, and Ralf Herwig

ISBN: 978-3-527-31874-2

GenBank (Release 164.0, from April 2008) comprises 85.7 billion nucleotide bases from more than 82 million reported sequences. The RefSeq database [1, 2] is a curated, nonredundant set of sequences including genomic DNA, mRNA, and protein products for major research organisms. In UniGene, expressed sequence tags (ESTs) and full-length mRNA sequences are organized into clusters, each representing a unique known or putative gene of a specific organism. (For molecular biological analyses, e.g., sequencing or expression profiling, the mRNA of expressed genes is usually translated into a complementary DNA [cDNA, copy DNA], since this is more stable and feasible for standard biotechnological methods.) An EST is a short – approximately 200–600-bp long – sequence from either side of a cDNA clone that is useful for identifying the full-length gene, e.g., for locating the gene in the genome.

In addition to nucleotide sequences, protein sequences can be searched for at the NCBI site via Entrez-Proteins. Searches are performed across several databases, including RefSeq, Swiss-Prot, and Protein Data Bank (PDB).

The Entrez database (http://www.ncbi.nlm.nih.gov/Entrez) offers diverse information about specific genetic loci (the location of a specific gene). Thus, Entrez provides a central hub for accessing gene-specific information of a number of species, like human, mouse, rat, zebrafish, nematode, fruit fly, cow, and sea urchin.

Among the literature databases are PubMed and OMIM (Online Mendelian Inheritance in Man). PubMed is a database of citations and abstracts for biomedical literature. Citations are from MEDLINE (http://medline.cos.com) and additional life science journals. OMIM is a catalog of human genes and genetic disorders with textual information and copious links to the scientific literature.

Thus, the databases at the NCBI are one of the major resources for sequence data, annotations, and literature references. They can be used to determine what is known about a specific gene or its protein, or to get information about the sequences, its variants, or polymorphisms. In addition to this, the NCBI also offers a database on gene expression data (Gene Expression Omnibus, GEO).

Besides all these databases, the NCBI also provides tools mostly operating on sequence data. These include programs comparing one or more sequences with the provided sequence databases.

16.2
Databases of the European Bioinformatics Institute

The European Bioinformatics Institute (EMBL-EBI) also offers several biologically relevant databases (http://www.ebi.ac.uk/Databases). This includes databases on nucleotide sequences, genes, and genomes (EMBL Nucleotide Database, Ensembl automatic genome annotation database), a database on alternative splicing sites (ASTD), a database of protein modifications (RESID), a database on protein families and protein domains (InterPro), a database on macromolecular structures (PDBe), and a database on gene expression data (ArrayExpress). The protein databases Swiss-Prot, TrEMBL, and UniProt will be discussed in separate sections below.

16.2.1
EMBL Nucleotide Sequence Database

The EMBL Nucleotide Sequence Database (http://www.ebi.ac.uk/embl) incorporates, organizes, and distributes nucleotide sequences from public sources and synchronizes its data in a daily manner with the DNA Database of Japan (DDBJ) and GenBank, which are the two other nucleotide sequence databases most important worldwide [3].

16.2.2
Ensembl

The Ensembl project (http://www.ensembl.org/) is developing and maintaining a system for the management and presentation of genomic sequences and its annotation for eukaryotic genomes [4–6]. What does annotation mean in this context? Annotation is the characterization of features of the genome using computational and experimental methods. In the first place, this is the prediction of genes, including structural elements like introns and exons, from the assembled genome sequence and the characterization of genomic features, like repeated sequence motifs, conserved regions, or single nucleotide polymorphisms (SNPs). SNPs (pronounced "snips") are common DNA sequence variations among individuals, where a single nucleotide is altered. Furthermore, annotation includes information about functional domains of the proteins encoded by the genes and the roles that the gene products fulfill in the organism.

The central component of Ensembl is a relational database storing the genome sequence assemblies and annotations produced by Ensembl's automated sequence-annotation pipeline, which utilizes the genome assemblies and data from external resources for this purpose. In April 2008, Ensembl provided genomic annotations for several vertebrates (among are human, chimp, mouse, rat, pufferfish, zebrafish, and chicken), arthropods (among are mosquito, honeybee, and fruitfly), and others. Annotations, such as genes with their intron-/exon-structure, SNPs, etc., can be viewed along the assembled sequence contigs using the Ensembl ContigView, which is accessible via the organism-specific webpages.

16.2.3
InterPro

InterPro (http://www.ebi.ac.uk/interpro/) is a protein signature database comprising information about protein families, domains, and functional groups [7, 8]. It combines many commonly used protein signature databases and is a very powerful tool for the automatic and manual annotation of new or predicted proteins from sequencing projects. In addition, InterPro entries are mapped to the Gene Ontology (GO, see Section 16.6) and are linked to protein entries in UniProt (see Section 16.3).

16.3
Swiss-Prot, TrEMBL, and UniProt

In addition to several nucleotide sequence databases also a variety of protein sequence databases exist, ranging from simple sequence repositories to expertly curated universal databases that cover many species and provide a lot of further information. One of the leading protein databases is Swiss-Prot (http://www.expasy.ch/sprot). As of April 2008 (release 55.0), it contains 356,194 protein sequence entries. Swiss-Prot is maintained by the Swiss Institute of Bioinformatics (SIB) and the European Bioinformatics Institute (EBI) and offers a high level of annotation comprising information about the protein origin (gene name and species), amino acid sequence, protein function and location, protein domains and sites, quaternary structure, references to the literature, protein-associated disease(s), and many further details. In addition, Swiss-Prot provides cross-references to several external data collections such as nucleotide sequence databases (DDBJ/EMBL/GenBank), protein structure databases, databases providing protein domain and family characterizations, disease-related databases, etc. [9].

Since the creation of fully curated Swiss-Prot entries is a highly laborious task, another database called TrEMBL (Translation from EMBL) was introduced, which uses an automated annotation approach. TrEMBL contains computer-annotated entries generated by *in-silico* translation of all coding sequences (CDS) available in the nucleotide databases (DDBJ/EMBL/GenBank). The entries offered at TrEMBL do not overlap with those found in Swiss-Prot.

The world's most comprehensive catalog providing protein-related information is the UniProt database (http://www.uniprot.org). UniProt is composed of information of Swiss-Prot, TrEMBL, and PIR (http://pir.georgetown.edu). One part of UniProt, UniParc, is the most comprehensive publicly accessible nonredundant protein sequence collection available [10].

16.4
Protein Databank

Biological macromolecules, i.e., proteins and nucleic acids, fold into specific three-dimensional structures. Using techniques such as X-ray crystallography or nuclear magnetic resonance (NMR), these structures can be solved and the three-dimensional coordinates of the atoms can be determined. Obviously, such information is extremely valuable for understanding the biological activity of the molecules and their interaction with possible reaction partners. The PDB is the main repository for three-dimensional structures of biological macromolecules [11]. As of April 2008, the databank holds more than 50,000 structures and the number is growing exponentially.

The PDB website (http://www.rcsb.org) offers extensive search and browse capabilities. In the most simple case, one can enter a PDB ID, a four-character alphanumeric identifier, to get straight to a specific structure. 1B06, for instance, brings up the information for the superoxide dismutase of *Sulfolobus acidocaldarius*, a thermophilic archaebacterium. The resulting page gives essential information about the protein-like literature reference, quality parameters for the crystal structure, and GO terms. Via the available pull down menus, further functions can be reached. The most important are probably downloading structure (PDB or mmCIF format, macromolecular Crystallographic Information File) or sequence (FASTA format) files, and accessing different three-dimensional viewers. Some viewer, like KiNG or WebMol, only require a Java-enabled web browser, while others, like Rasmol or Swiss-PDB viewer, need a special browser plug in.

16.5 BioNumbers

For many biological properties, concrete values are hard to find. Most quantitative properties in biology depend on the context or the method of measurement, the organism, and the cell type. Often, however, the order of magnitude is already very useful information for modeling. BioNumbers (bioNumbers.org) is a database of useful biological numbers. It enables you to find easily many common biological numbers that can be important for your research, such as the rate of translation of the ribosome or the number of bacteria in your gut. BioNumbers is a community effort to make quantitative properties of biological systems easily available and with full reference.

16.6 Gene Ontology

The accumulation of scientific knowledge is a decentralized, parallel process. Consequently, the naming and description of new genes and gene products is not necessarily systematic. Often gene products with identical functions are given different names in different organisms or the verbal description of the location and function might be quite different (e.g., protein degradation vs. proteolysis). This, of course, makes it very difficult to perform efficient searching across databases and organisms.

This problem has been recognized, and in 1998 the *Gene Ontology* (GO) project (http://www.geneontology.org) was initiated as a collaborative effort of the Saccharomyces Genome Database (SGD), the Mouse Genome Database (MGD), and FlyBase. The aim of the GO is to provide a consistent, species-independent, functional description of gene products. Since 1998, the GO project has grown considerably and now includes databases for plant, animal, and prokaryotic genomes. Effectively, GO consists of a controlled vocabulary (the GO terms) used to describe the biological function of a gene product in any organism. The GO terms have a defined parent–child relationship and form a directed acyclic graph (DAG). In a DAG, each node can have multiple child nodes, as well as multiple parent nodes. Cyclic references, however, are omitted. The combination of vocabulary and relationship between nodes is referred to as ontology. At the root of the GO are the three top-level categories, *molecular function, biological process,* and *cellular component,* which contain many levels of child nodes (GO terms) that describe a gene product with increasing specificity. The GO consortium, in collaboration with other databases, develops and maintains the three top-level ontologies (the set of GO terms and their relationship) themselves, creates associations between the ontologies and the gene products in the participating databases, and develops tools for the creation, maintenance, and use of the ontologies.

Let us look at a practical example to see how the concept works. The enzyme superoxide dismutase, for instance, is annotated in FlyBase (the *Drosophila melanogaster* database) with the GO term *cytoplasm* in the cellular component ontology, with the GO terms *defense response* and *determination of adult life span* in the biological process ontology and with the terms *antioxidant activity* and *copper, zinc superoxide dismutase activity* in the molecular function ontology. The GO term cytoplasm itself has the single parent *intracellular,* which has the single parent *cell,* which is finally connected to cellular component. The other GO terms for superoxide dismutase are connected in a similar hierarchical way to the three top categories.

To use the GO effectively, many different tools have been developed that are listed on the GO website (http://www.geneontology.org/GO.tools.html). The repertoire encompasses web-based and standalone GO browsers and editors, microarray-related tools, and programs for many specialized tasks. In the remainder of this section, we will only take a quick look at three such tools. Our first candidate is AmiGO (http://amigo.geneontology.org), which is a web-based GO browser maintained by the GO consortium (Figure 16.1(a)). First of all, AmiGO can be used to browse the terms of the ontologies. The numbers in parenthesis behind the GO terms show how many gene products in the currently selected database are annotated to this term. The seven-digit number behind GO is the GO-ID that links each GO term to a unique identifier. One or more species and one or more data sources can be selected to restrict the results of the search. A click on a leaf of the GO hierarchy (like biological_processes unknown) brings up a window that lists the genes in the selected databases that have been annotated to this term. Instead of browsing the GO tree, one can also search for specific GO terms and get to the gene products associated with these terms or search for gene products and find the connected GO terms. Finally, it is also possible to get a *Graphical view,* showing where the selected term is located within the ontology tree.

AmiGO's search options are quite limited, since it is only possible to search for several terms that are connected via the OR function (under advanced query). The

Figure 16.1 (a) AmiGO, a web-based GO browser developed by the GO consortium. It allows us browsing the GO hierarchy and searching for specific GO terms or gene products in different databases. The numbers in brackets behind the GO terms indicate how many gene products have been annotated to this term in the selected database. (b) GoFish, a Java applet, can also connect to several databases and allows the user to search for gene products using complex Boolean expressions for GO terms.

(a)

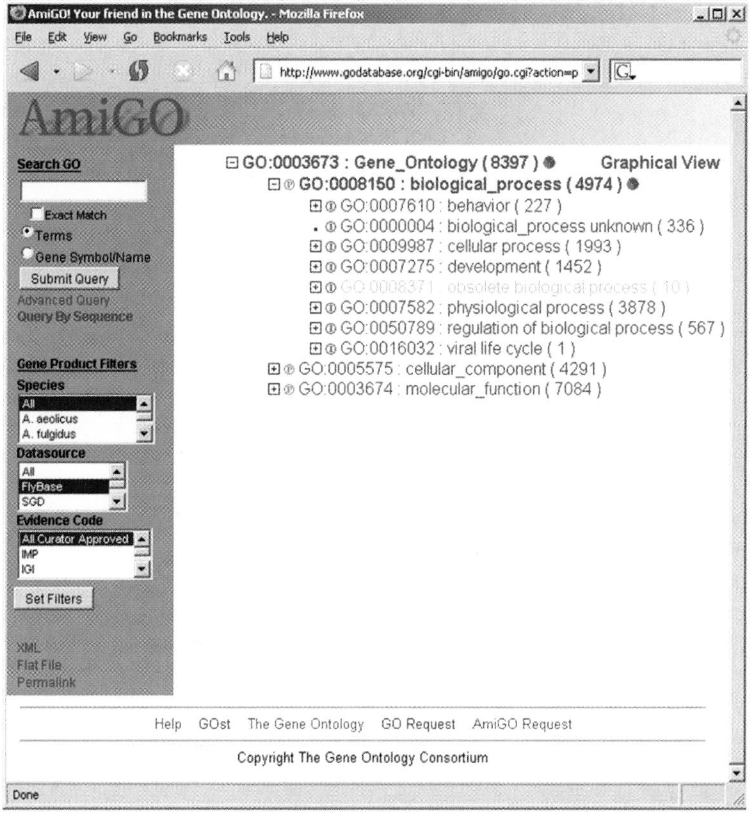
AmiGO! Your friend in the Gene Ontology. - Mozilla Firefox
File Edit View Go Bookmarks Tools Help
http://www.godatabase.org/cgi-bin/amigo/go.cgi?action=p
AmiGO
Search GO
Exact Match
Terms
Gene Symbol/Name
Submit Query
Advanced Query
Query By Sequence
Gene Product Filters
Species
All
A. aeolicus
A. fulgidus
Datasource
All
FlyBase
SGD
Evidence Code
All Curator Approved
IMP
IGI
Set Filters
XML
Flat File
Permalink
GO:0003673 : Gene_Ontology (8397)
Graphical View
GO:0008150 : biological_process (4974)
GO:0007610 : behavior (227)
GO:0000004 : biological_process unknown (336)
GO:0009987 : cellular process (1993)
GO:0007275 : development (1452)
GO:0008371 : obsolete biological process (10)
GO:0007582 : physiological process (3878)
GO:0050789 : regulation of biological process (567)
GO:0016032 : viral life cycle (1)
GO:0005575 : cellular_component (4291)
GO:0003674 : molecular_function (7084)
Help GOst The Gene Ontology GO Request AmiGO Request
Copyright The Gene Ontology Consortium
Done

(b)

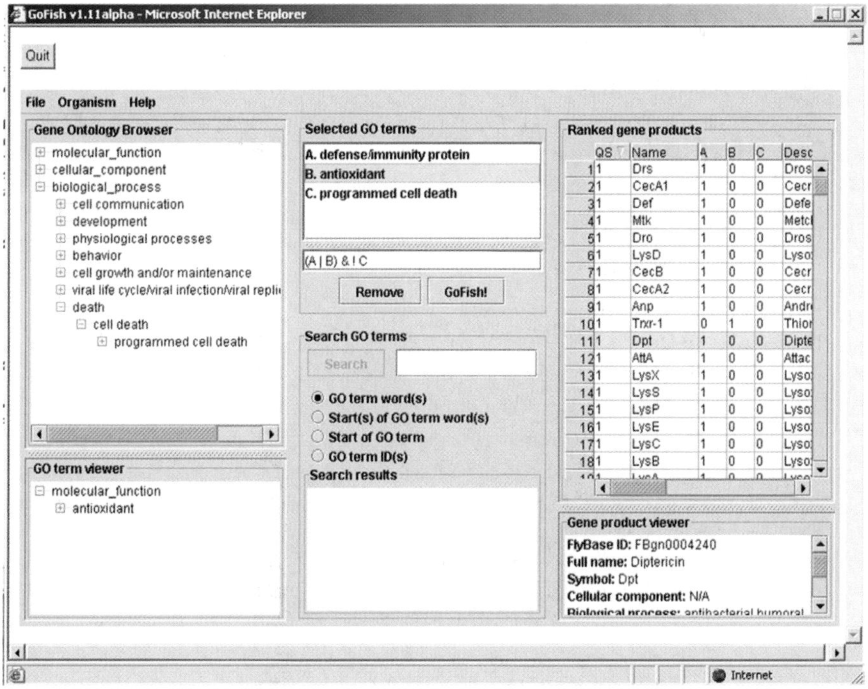
GoFish v1.11alpha - Microsoft Internet Explorer
Quit
File Organism Help
Gene Ontology Browser
molecular_function
cellular_component
biological_process
cell communication
development
physiological processes
behavior
cell growth and/or maintenance
viral life cycle/viral infection/viral repli
death
cell death
programmed cell death
GO term viewer
molecular_function
antioxidant
Selected GO terms
A. defense/immunity protein
B. antioxidant
C. programmed cell death
(A | B) & ! C
Remove
GoFish!
Search GO terms
Search
GO term word(s)
Start(s) of GO term word(s)
Start of GO term
GO term ID(s)
Search results
Ranked gene products
QS Name A B C Desc
1 1 Drs 1 0 0 Dros
2 1 CecA1 1 0 0 Cecr
3 1 Def 1 0 0 Defe
4 1 Mtk 1 0 0 Metc
5 1 Dro 1 0 0 Dros
6 1 LysD 1 0 0 Lyso
7 1 CecB 1 0 0 Cecr
8 1 CecA2 1 0 0 Cecr
9 1 Anp 1 0 0 Andr
10 1 Trxr-1 0 1 0 Thior
11 1 Dpt 1 0 0 Dipte
12 1 AttA 1 0 0 Attac
13 1 LysX 1 0 0 Lyso
14 1 LysS 1 0 0 Lyso
15 1 LysP 1 0 0 Lyso
16 1 LysE 1 0 0 Lyso
17 1 LysC 1 0 0 Lyso
18 1 LysB 1 0 0 Lyso
Gene product viewer
FlyBase ID: FBgn0004240
Full name: Diptericin
Symbol: Dpt
Cellular component: N/A
Internet

Java applet GoFish v1.11 (http://llama.med.harvard.edu/~berriz/GoFishWelcome.html) is a good alternative for such cases (Figure 16.1(b)). Different GO terms can be selected from a GO tree (left side), which can then be combined into complex Boolean expressions (top window in the middle). In the case shown here, we are searching for gene products in the FlyBase that are antioxidants or involved in defense/immunity but are not concerned with programmed cell death. When the user selects a specific database, the applet downloads the GO terms and associations for this database and, therefore, the response time of GoFish is normally faster than for AmiGO.

The recently developed high-throughput techniques like DNA-chips enable researchers to measure the expression profile of thousands of genes in parallel. Often one is interested whether the genes that are over- or underexpressed share biological function. The web-based program GOstat (http://gostat.wehi.edu.au/) makes use of the GO to test if certain GO terms are statistically over- or underrepresented in a group of genes of interest. GOstat can compare the list of genes either against a user-supplied control list or against the complete list of genes in a selected database. It then uses Fisher's Exact Test or the chi-square test to determine whether the observed differences of the frequencies of GO terms is significant or not. The output is a list of p-values that state how specific the associated GO terms are for the list of genes provided. The list can then be obtained as text or html file.

This was only a brief introduction of three of the many available programs that make use of GO annotations. Furthermore, it is always possible to develop own programs, since all GO-related files like lists of GO definitions or database annotations can be downloaded at http://www.geneontology.org.

16.7 Pathway Databases

The development of models of biochemical reaction networks requires information about the stoichiometry and topology of the reaction network. Such information can be found in databases like KEGG and Reactome (cf. Section 2.4.4.1). Often pathway databases cover a specific scope, e.g., metabolic pathways, signal transduction pathways, or gene regulatory networks. An integration of such pathway data into a comprehensive database is done by the ConsensusPathDB.

16.7.1 ConsensusPathDB

ConsensusPathDB [12] (http://cpdb.molgen.mpg.de) is a database integrating human functional interactions. Currently the database integrates the content of 12 different interaction databases with heterogeneous foci comprising a total of 26133 distinct physical entities and 74289 distinct functional interactions covering 1738 pathways. The database comprises protein–protein interactions, biochemical reactions, and gene regulatory interactions. ConsensusPathDB has a sophisticated interface for the visualization of the functional interaction networks. Furthermore, the database provides functionalities for the over-representation analysis. It is also possible to expand existing networks provided in BioPAX, SBML, or PSI-MI format.

Exercises and Problems

1. What are the basic types of information relevant to systems biology that can be obtained from public databases and how can those data be used for modeling?
2. Which database can be used for the development of a model prototype describing the reaction network topology of a metabolic pathway such as glycolysis? Where can you find kinetic parameters for such a model?
3. Visit the web site of ConsensusPathDB (http://cpdb.molgen.mpg.de). How many biochemical reactions and physical reactions have been imported from Reactome and how many of them are also present in KEGG? How many physical entities do these two databases share?
4. Search in ConsensusPathDB for the protein Bcl-XL. In how many source databases is the protein present? How many functional interactions does this protein have? Select several physical interactions and biochemical reactions involving this protein and visualize them as an interaction network.

References

1 Maglott, D.R. *et al.* (2000) NCBI's LocusLink and RefSeq. *Nucleic Acids Res*, **28**, 126–128.

2 Pruitt, K.D. *et al.* (2007) NCBI reference sequences (RefSeq): a curated non-redundant sequence database of genomes, transcripts and proteins. *Nucleic Acids Res*, **35**, D61–D65.

3 Kulikova, T. *et al.* (2004) The EMBL nucleotide sequence database. *Nucleic Acids Res*, **32**, D27–D30.

4 Hubbard, T. *et al.* (2002) The Ensembl genome database project. *Nucleic Acids Res*, **30**, 38–41.

5 Birney, E. *et al.* (2004) An overview of Ensembl. *Genome Res*, **14**, 925–928.

6 Flicek, P. *et al.* (2008) Ensembl 2008. *Nucleic Acids Res*, **36**, D707–D714.

7 Biswas, M. *et al.* (2001) Application of InterPro for the functional classification of the proteins of fish origin in SWISS-PROT and TrEMBL. *J Biosci*, **26**, 277–284.

8 Mulder, N.J. *et al.* (2002) InterPro: an integrated documentation resource for protein families, domains and functional sites. *Brief Bioinform*, **3**, 225–235.

9 Boeckmann, B. *et al.* (2003) The SWISS-PROT protein knowledgebase and its supplement TrEMBL in 2003. *Nucleic Acids Res*, **31**, 365–370.

10 Apweiler, R. *et al.* (2004) UniProt: the Universal Protein knowledgebase. *Nucleic Acids Res*, **32** (Database Issue), D115–D119.

11 Berman, H.M. *et al.* (2000) The protein data bank. *Nucleic Acids Res*, **28**, 235–242.

12 Kamburov A., Wierling C., Lehrach H. and Herwig R. (2009) ConsensusPathDB – a database for integrating human functional interaction networks. *Nucleic Acids Research*, **37** (Database issue), D623–D628.

17
Modeling Tools

Summary

Databases and high-throughput experiments are a rich source of data for modeling in systems biology. Many different tools in the form of programming languages and software packages are required and available to process and visualize these large quantities of data. The tools can roughly be divided in general purpose and specialized programs. General-purpose tools, like Mathematica, Matlab, or R, are enormously powerful packages for the numerical, symbolical, and visual analysis of arbitrary mathematical problems. However, their generality can also be a limitation, since they have a very steep learning curve, requiring considerable effort to get started.

Therefore, many specialized tools have been developed that are very restricted in their application range, but are much easier to use. Typical areas of specialization are the construction of biochemical reaction networks, the analysis of reaction networks (stability, flux analysis, metabolic control theory) including parameter fitting, or the simulation of stochastic reactions.

A problem that arose with the multitude of tools was the lack of model compatibility. A model developed with one program had often to be reimplemented for use with a different tool. This important problem is now tackled with the development of model exchange languages. The Systems Biology Markup Language (SBML) is rapidly developing into a *de facto* standard with more than 100 tools supporting it.

17.1
Introduction

The databases described in the last chapter are huge repositories for the biological data that have been gathered by various techniques. The information in the databases represents raw material for most types of modeling efforts. Modeling tools help to formulate theoretical ideas and hypotheses and to extract information relevant to these hypotheses from the raw material stored in the databases. Section 2.4 provided the first overview of the most popular modeling tools and data formats. However, there are of course many more. In this chapter, we want to briefly describe a few more

Systems Biology: A Textbook. Edda Klipp, Wolfram Liebermeister, Christoph Wierling, Axel Kowald, Hans Lehrach, and Ralf Herwig

ISBN: 978-3-527-31874-2

as showcases for special techniques or approaches. Mathematica® and Matlab®, for example, are general-purpose tools for solving mathematical problems analytically or numerically and visualizing the results using a large number of different graphics types. Although enormously powerful and flexible, general-purpose tools have a steep learning curve and require some effort to get used to. While the majority of existing mathematical models still use deterministic techniques, it has been recognized in recent years that some phenomena can only be understood if stochasticity is taken into account. "Dizzy" is one of the tools that can perform various types of stochastic simulations and is used to highlight this type of modeling. Finally, we describe the Systems Biology Workbench (SBW) as a unique type of tool, which tries to provide an integrating framework for other tools.

The number of available tools is simply too large to provide a description for all of them. However, for more than 80 tools essential details are given in a listing at the end of this chapter.

17.2
Mathematica and Matlab

Mathematica® and Matlab® are two extensive general-purpose tools for the computation and visualization of any type of mathematical model.

Mathematica is produced by Wolfram Research (http://www.wolfram.com) and exists currently as version 6 for the operating systems Microsoft Windows, Macintosh, Linux, and several Unix variants. The Mathematica system consists of two components, the kernel that runs in the background performing the calculations and the graphical user interface (GUI) that communicates with the kernel. The GUI has the form of a so-called notebook that contains all the input, output, and graphics. Apart from its numerical calculation and graphics abilities, Mathematica is renowned for its capability to perform advanced symbolic calculations. Mathematica can either be used by interactively invoking the available functions or by using the built-in programming language to write larger routines and programs, which are also stored as or within notebooks. For many specialized topics, Mathematica packages (a special kind of notebook) are available that provide additional functionality. J/Link, .NET/Link and MathLink, products that ship with Mathematica, enable the two-way communication with Java, .NET, or C/C++ code. This means that Mathematica can access external code written in one of these languages and that the Mathematica kernel can actually be called from other applications. The former is useful if an algorithm has already been implemented in one of these languages or to speed up time-critical calculations that would take too long if implemented in Mathematica itself. In the latter case, other programs can use the Mathematica kernel to perform high-level calculations or render graphics objects. Apart from an excellent help utility, there are also many sites on the Internet that provide additional help and resources. The site http://mathworld.wolfram.com contains a large repository of contributions from Mathematica user all over the world. If a function or algorithm does not exist in Mathematica, it is worthwhile to check this site before implementing it yourself. If questions and problems arise during the use of Mathematica, a valuable source of help is also the newsgroup news://comp.soft-sys.math.mathematica/.

The major rival of Mathematica is Matlab 7.5, produced by MathWorks (http://www.mathworks.com). In many respects, both products are very similar and it is up to the taste of the user which one to prefer. Matlab is available for the same platforms as Mathematica, has very strong numerical capabilities, and can also produce many different forms of graphics. It also has its own programming language, and functions are stored in so-called M-files. Toolboxes (special M-files) add additional functionality to the core Matlab distribution and like Mathematica, Matlab can be called by external programs to perform high-level computations. A repository exists for user-contributed files (http://www.mathworks.com/matlabcentral/fileexchange and http://www.mathtools.net/MATLAB/toolboxes.html) as well as a newsgroup (news://comp.soft-sys.matlab) for getting help. But albeit those similarities, there are also differences. Table 17.1 gives a very short, superficial, and subjective list of important differences.

Let us have a look at Mathematica and Matlab using a practical example. The superoxide radical, $O_2^{\bullet -}$, is a side product of the electron transport chain of mitochondria and contributes to the oxidative stress a cell is exposed to. Different

Table 17.1 Important differences between Mathematica and Matlab.

Topic	Mathematica	Matlab
Debugging	Before version 6 cumbersome and difficult. No dedicated debugging facility. Version 6 provides basic debugging capabilities.	Dedicated debugger allows to single step through M-files using breakpoints.
Add-ons	Many standard packages ship with Mathematica and are included in the price.	Many important toolboxes have to be bought separately. See http://www.mathworks.com/products/product_listing.
Deployment	User needs Mathematica to perform the calculations specified in notebooks.	Separately available compiler allows to produce stand-alone applications.
Symbolic computation	Excellent built-in capabilities.	Possible with commercial toolbox.
Storage	All input, output, and graphics are stored in a single notebook.	Functions are stored in individual M-files. A large project can have hundreds of M-files.
Graphics	Graphics is embedded in notebook and cannot be changed after its creation.	Graphic appears in a separate window and can be manipulated as long as the window exists.
Ordinary differential equation (ODE) model building	Differential equations are specified explicitly.	Dynamical processes can be graphically constructed with Simulink, a companion product of Matlab.

forms of the enzyme superoxide dismutase (SOD) exist that convert this harmful radical into hydrogen peroxide, H_2O_2. This causes itself oxidative stress and further enzymes, like catalase (cat) or glutathione peroxidase, exist to convert it into water. If we want to describe this system, we can write down the following reaction scheme and set of differential equation:

$$\xrightarrow{c_1} O_2^{\bullet -} \xrightarrow[SOD]{c_2} H_2O_2 \xrightarrow[cat]{c_3} H_2O$$

$$\frac{dO_2^{\bullet -}}{dt} = c_1 - c_2 \cdot SOD \cdot O_2^{\bullet -}$$

$$\frac{dH_2O_2}{dt} = c_2 \cdot SOD \cdot O_2^{\bullet -} - c_3 \cdot cat \cdot H_2O_2$$

17.2.1 Mathematica Example

First, we define the differential equations (and assign them to the variables eq1 and eq2) and specify the numerical values for the constants.

```
eq1 = O2' [t] == c1 - c2*SOD*O2[t];
eq2 = H2O2' [t] == c2*SOD*O2[t] - c3*cat*H2O2[t];
par = {c1→6.6 x 10^-7, c2→1.6 x 10^9, c3→3.4 x 10^7,
SOD→10^-5, cat→10^-5}.
```

Now we can solve the equations numerically with the function NDSolve and assign the result to the variable "sol." As boundary conditions, we specify that the initial concentrations of superoxide and hydrogen peroxide are zero and instruct NDSolve to find a solution for the first 0.01 s. NDSolve returns an interpolating function object, which can be used to obtain numerical values of the solution for any time point between 0 and 0.01. We see that at 0.01 s, the concentrations are in the nanomolar range and the level of H_2O_2 is approximately 50-fold higher than the concentration of superoxide. Finally, we use plot to produce a graphic showing the time course of the variable concentrations (Figure 17.1). We specify several options like axes labels and colors to make the plot more informative (some details of the plot command are specific for version 6 of Mathematica).

```
sol = NDSolve[{eq1, eq2, O2[0]==0, H2O2 [0]==0}/.par,
{O2, H2O2}, {t,0,0.01}]
{O2 [0.01], H2O2 [0.01]}/.sol ⇒ {{4.125 x 10^-11,
1.84552 x 10^-9}}
Plot[Evaluate[{O2[t],H2O2[t]/50}/.sol],{t,0,0.01},
PlotRange->All, FrameLabel -> {"time","concentra-
tion"}, Frame -> True, LabelStyle -> Directive
[FontSize->14], Epilog -> {Text[Style["O2",Large],
{0.001,3.8 x 10^-11}], Text[Style["H2O2",Large],
{0.006,2.5 x 10^-11}]}]
```

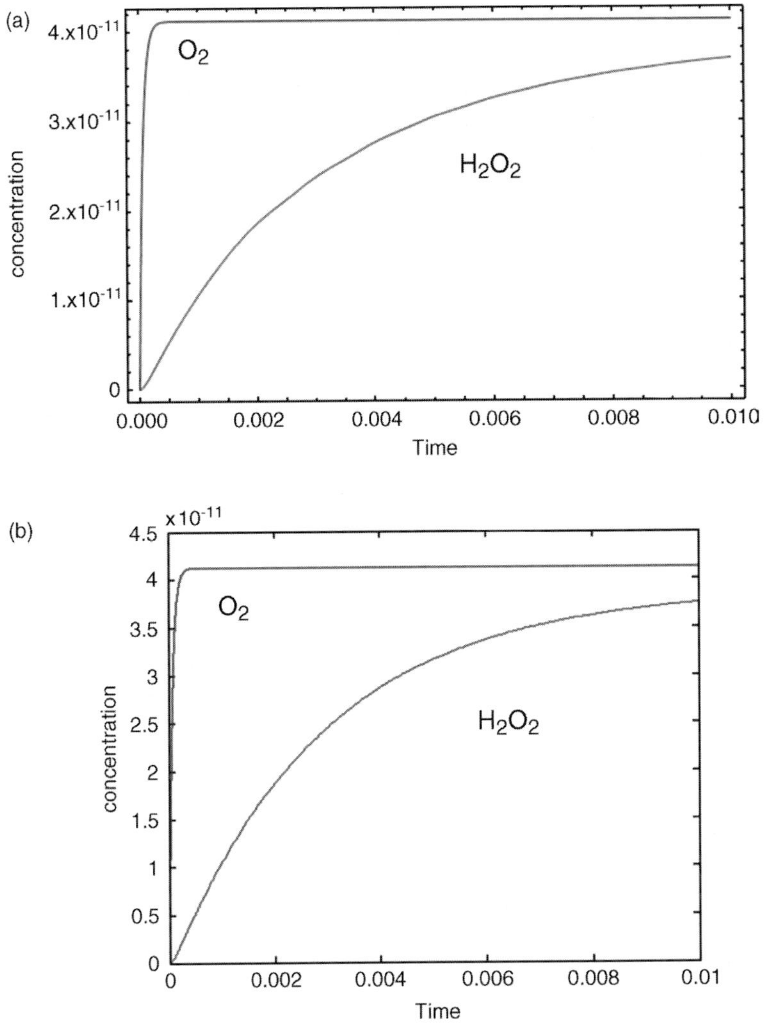

Figure 17.1 Graphical output generated by the software packages (a) Mathematica and (b) Matlab. The diagrams show the solution of a system of two differential equations describing the reactions of SOD and catalase with superoxide and hydrogen peroxide.

17.2.2
Matlab Example

In Matlab, the routine that solves the ODE system requires as one of its arguments a function that evaluates the right-hand side of the ODE system for a given time and variable values. Because the example system is so small, we can define this function as an *inline function* and avoid writing a separate M-file. Next the options for the ODE solver are defined. The absolute values of the solution are very small and, therefore, the absolute tolerance has to be very small.

```
dydt=inline('[c1-c2*SOD*y(1);c2*SOD*y(1)-c3*cat*y
(2)]', 't', 'y', 'tmp', 'SOD', 'cat', 'c1', 'c2', 'c3');
options = odeset('OutputFcn', [ ], 'AbsTol',
1e-30, 'RelTol', 1e-6);]]
```

Now ode45 is called, which solves the ODE system for the specified time span. In addition to d*y*d*t* that evaluates the derivatives, we also supply the starting concentrations of the variables and the numerical values for the constants that are used in d*y*d*t*. ode45 is only one of a whole set (ode45, ode23, ode113, ode15s, ode23s, ode23t, and ode23tb) of possible solvers with different properties (differing in accuracy or suitability for stiff problems). The function returns a vector, *t*, holding time points for which a solution is returned and a matrix, *y*, that contains the variable values at these time points. To find out which concentration exists at a given time, the function interp1 can be used that also interpolates between existing time points if necessary. Finally, the resulting time course is plotted and the axes are labeled appropriately.

```
[t, y] = ode45(dydt, [0,0.01], [0;0], options,
1e-5, 1e-5, 6.6e-7, 1.6e9, 3.4e7);
interp1(t,y,0.01) ⇒ 4.125 x 10^-11, 1.84552 x 10^-9
plot(t, y(:,1), t, y(:,2)/50)
xlabel('time' )
ylabel('concentration')
text(0.001,3.8 x 10^-11,'O2')
text(0.006,2.5 x 10^-11,'H2O2')]]
```

17.3 Dizzy

Simulations using differential equations assume that the number of molecules in the described system is so large that it can be treated as a continuous variable. A second assumption of ODE modeling is that the system is completely deterministic. Random fluctuations do not occur. The smaller the number of molecules, the more unrealistic those assumptions become. Most molecules in a cell exist in large numbers, but some are very rare. Transcription factors, for example, exist in notoriously low numbers in cells. There are for instance only approximately 10 molecules of the Lac repressor in an *Escherichia coli* cell [1]. Proteins involved in signal transduction pathways are also very rare, as are defective mitochondria that might be relevant for the aging process. Under those circumstances, it becomes important that four or five molecules might be in a cell, but not 4.325 (as assumed by ODEs). Of special importance can be the difference between 0 and 1 items, if this item is a self-reproducing object like a defective mitochondrion. If modeled with ODEs, it is practically impossible to obtain zero defective mitochondria, since a small amount (well below one) will always remain. Because of their self-reproducing property, a population of defective mitochondria could always regrow from this artifact. If modeled stochastically, all defective organelles disappear (zero concentration) once the last one is destroyed and, thus, they cannot regrow. If the simulated system has more than one possible steady state, there can also be qualitative differences between a deterministic simulation with differential equations and a stochastic simulation that takes random effects into account. In an ODE model, the system will settle into one of the possible steady states and remain there forever. If modeled stochastically, however, the system can jump from one steady state to the other if they are close enough together.

The stochastic simulation tool Dizzy has been developed by Stephen Ramsey from the Institute for Systems Biology in Seattle and is freely available from http://magnet.systemsbiology.net/software/Dizzy. This software is written in Java and is, therefore, available for all platforms with a Java virtual machine. The use of Dizzy is straightforward as shown in Figure 17.2. Models can be imported either in SBML format or in

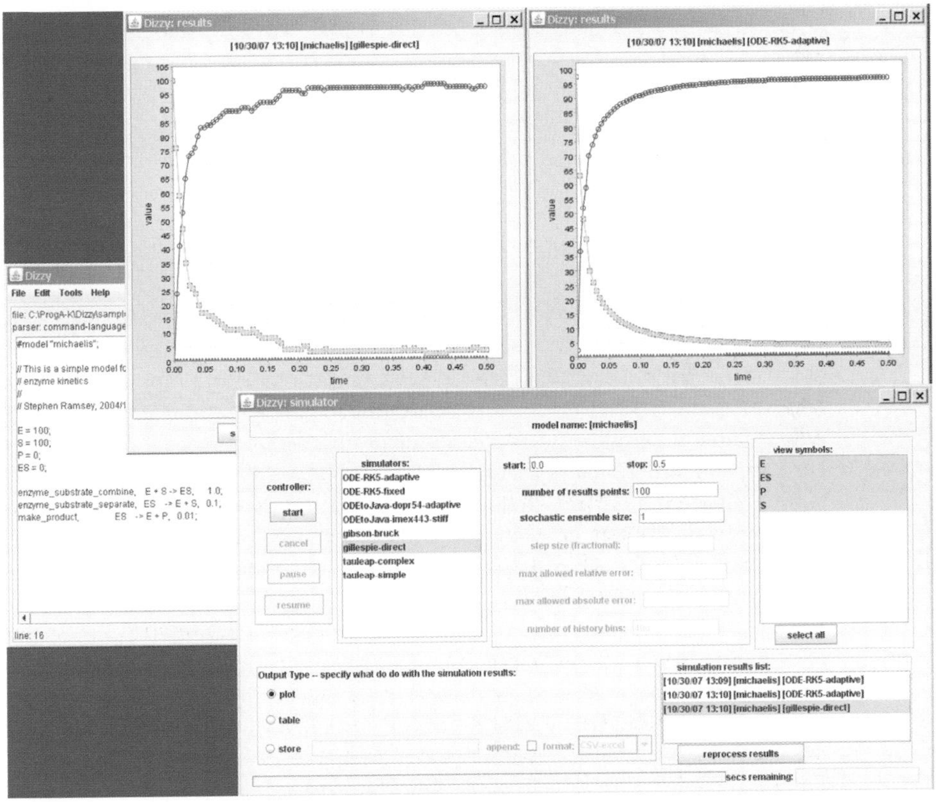

Figure 17.2 Dizzy is a simulation tool for stochastic models. The software can import and export models written in SBML or a special model definition language (left). Several deterministic and stochastic simulators are available (bottom), and the results can be displayed graphically (top), as table or saved into a file.

a proprietary scripting language. Once loaded, the model can be simulated by a variety of stochastic and deterministic algorithms, which is actually a very valuable feature. Stochastic simulation runs normally take a much longer time and many runs are required to obtain statistically meaningful results. A deterministic simulation, based on interpreting the underlying elementary reactions as differential equations, is therefore a quick way to get a first feeling for the model behavior. Dizzy can be controlled using a GUI, but it can also be started from the command line, since GUI and the number crunching machinery are separated. For a complex model describing the accumulation of defective mitochondria [2], we performed 1000 time-consuming repetitions of the model simulation on our Linux cluster, using the command-line version of Dizzy. Although SBML is emerging as *de facto* standard for models in systems biology, the model definition language of Dizzy has powerful features for handling arrays of variables and defining large number of similar reactions that make it interesting for specialized problems. Using these special language constructs, we were able to define 4950 reactions with only five lines of code for the above mentioned mitochondrial model.

Finally, it should be mentioned that also Copasi (www.copasi.org) can perform stochastic and deterministic simulations and might, therefore, be a possible alternative to Dizzy. For purely stochastic simulations, the package STOCKS2 (www.sysbio.pl/stocks) is another, although less powerful, simulator.

17.4 Systems Biology Workbench

So far we have already discussed quite a number of different modeling tools, and many more are listed in the following sections. One reason for this multitude of simulation tools is that no single tool can provide all the possible simulation methods and ideas that are available. This is especially true since new experimental techniques and theoretical insights constantly stimulate the development of new ways to simulate and analyze biological systems. Consequently, different researchers have written different tools in different languages running on different platforms. A serious problem of this development is that most tools save models in their own format, which is not compatible with the other tools. Accordingly, models cannot easily be exchanged between tools, but have to be reimplemented by hand. Another problem is the overhead involved with programming parts of the tool that are not part of the actual core function. That means although a program might be specialized in analyzing the topology of a reaction network, it also has to provide means for the input and output of the reaction details.

Two closely related projects aim at tackling these problems. One is the development of a common format for describing models. This resulted in the development of the Systems Biology Markup Language (SBML), which is described in Section 2.4. The other project is the Systems Biology Workbench (SBW) [3], which is a software system that enables different tools to communicate with each other (http://www.sys-bio.org). Thus, SBW-enabled tools can use services provided by other modules and in

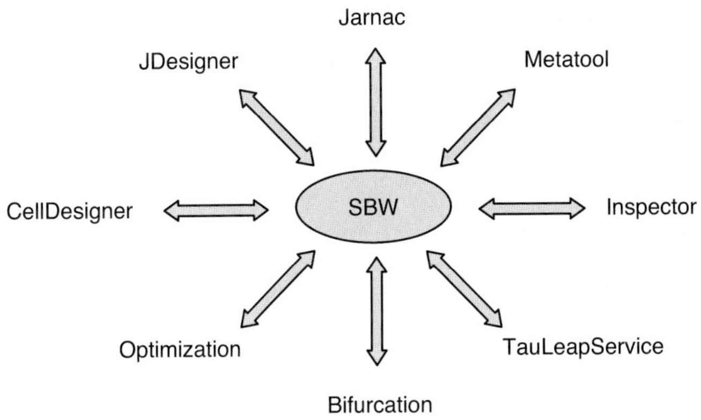

Figure 17.3 The SBW and SBW-enabled programs. The SBW broker module (in the center) forms the heart of the SBW and provides message passing and remote procedure invocation for SBW-enabled programs. The programs can concentrate on a specialized task like graphical model building (JDesigner, CellDesigner) or simulation and analysis (Jarnac, TauLeapService, Metatool, Optimization, Bifurcation) and otherwise use the capabilities of already existing modules.

turn advertise their own specialized services. Figure 17.3 gives an overview of SBW and some of the currently available SBW-enabled programs. At the center of the system is the SBW broker that receives messages from one module and relays them to other modules. Let us have a quick look at this mechanism using JDesigner and Jarnac, two modules that come with the SBW standard installation. JDesigner is a program for the graphical creation of reaction networks (similar to CellDesigner), and Jarnac is a tool for the numerical simulation of such networks (time course and steady state). Jarnac runs in the background and advertises its services to the SBW broker. JDesigner contacts the broker to find out which services are available and displays the found services in a special pull down menu called SBW. A reaction model that has been created in JDesigner can now be send to the simulation service of Jarnac. A dialog box opens to enter the necessary details for the simulation and then the broker calls the simulation service of Jarnac. After a time-course simulation finishes, the result is transmitted back to JDesigner (via the broker) and can be displayed. Further technical details of the SBW system are given in Sauro *et al.* [4].

The list of SBW-enabled programs shown in Figure 17.3 contains programs specialized in the graphical creation of reaction networks (JDesigner and CellDesigner), simulation tools (Jarnac and TauLeapService), analysis and optimization tools (Metatool, Bifurcation and Optimization), and utilities like the Inspector module, which provides information about other modules.

SBW and SBML are very interesting developments that might hopefully help to facilitate the exchange of biological models and thus stimulate the discussion and cooperation among modelers. The more tool developers adopt the SBML format and render their applications SBW aware, the more powerful this approach will be.

17.5 Tools Compendium

To provide the reader with a rough overview of the many other tools that exist and could not be discussed here, we have included here a listing that is mainly based on a survey of modeling tools used by the systems biology community [5]. However, it has been edited slightly and a brief description of the main purpose of the tools has been added. Most of the listed tools support SBML.

13C Flux www.simtec.mb.uni-siegen.de/software/13cflux
13C-FLUX is a universal software system for the modeling, simulation, and evaluation of carbon-labeling experiments (CLE).

BASIS www.basis.ncl.ac.uk
"*B*iology of *a*geing e-science integration and *si*mulation *s*ystem"; carry out simulations remotely, store models and results, easy to get data for export, and easy to make changes to models.

Berkeley Madonna www.berkeleymadonna.com
A Windows application written in C for the fast and convenient simulation of ODEs, difference equations, and discrete simulations using conveyors, ovens, and queues.

BIOCHAM contraintes.inria.fr/BIOCHAM
BIOCHAM is a programming environment for modeling biochemical systems, making simulations, and querying the model in temporal logic. It has a simulator for Boolean and numerical models that can be accessed via a GUI. Versions exist for Windows, Linux, and Max OS X.

BioCharon rtg.cis.upenn.edu/mobies/charon
Charon is a language for modular specification of interacting hybrid systems based on the notions of agent and mode. Written in Java.

BioCyc www.biocyc.org
BioCyc is a collection of 371 Pathway/Genome Databases. Each Pathway/Genome Database in the BioCyc collection describes the genome and metabolic pathways of a single organism, which can be queried for various types of information.

BioModels www.biomodels.net
The BioModels.net project is an international effort to (1) define agreed-upon standards for model curation, (2) define agreed-upon vocabularies for annotating models with connections to biological data resources, and (3) provide a free, centralized, publicly accessible database of annotated, computational models in SBML and other structured formats.

ByoDyn diana.imim.es/ByoDyn

ByoDyn has been designed to provide an easily extendable computational framework to estimate and analyze parameters in highly uncharacterized models. It includes a set of tools to (1) integrate ODEs, including systems with events, rules (differential algebraic equations), and delays built from a given biological model; (2) globally optimize the parameters that fit the provided experimental information and evaluate the sensitivity of the model with respect to the different parameters; and (3) include the sensitivity of the parameters in an optimal experimental design pipeline.

BioNetGen cellsignaling.lanl.gov/bionetgen

BioNetGen is a tool for automatically generating mathematical models of biological systems from user-specified rules for biomolecular interactions. Rules are specified in the BioNetGen language, which enables precise, visual, and extensible representation of biomolecular interactions. The language was designed with protein–protein interactions in mind. A user can explicitly indicate the parts of proteins involved in an interaction, the conditions upon which an interaction depends, the connectivity of proteins in a complex, and other aspects of protein–-protein interactions.

Bio Sketch Pad biocomp.cis.upenn.edu/biosketch.php3

Bio Sketch Pad is an interactive tool for modeling and designing biomolecular and cellular networks with a simple, easy-to-use, graphical front end, leveraging powerful tools from control theory, hybrid systems, and software engineering.

BioSens www.chemengr.ucsb.edu/~ceweb/faculty/doyle/biosens/BioSens.htm

BioSens provides a simulation and sensitivity analysis toolkit for Bio-SPICE through the BioMat Bridge. Sensitivity analysis investigates the changes in the system outputs or behavior with respect to the parameter variations, which are quantified by the sensitivity coefficients. Mathematically, the sensitivity coefficients are the first-order derivatives of the outputs with respect to the system parameters.

BioSPICE Dashboard biospice.sourceforge.net

Bio-SPICE, an open-source framework and software toolset for Systems Biology, is intended to assist biological researchers in the modeling and simulation of spatiotemporal processes in living cells. The core of the Bio-SPICE application is called the Dashboard. The Bio-SPICE Dashboard has an Update Center and allows for different tool functionality to be downloaded, data to be specified, and both to be integrated into tool chains and work flows for modeling, analysis, and simulation. The Dashboard is a Java-based toolkit, but the integrated tools can be written in any language.

BioTapestry www.biotapestry.org

BioTapestry is an interactive tool for building, visualizing, and simulating genetic regulatory networks. BioTapestry is designed around the concept of a developmental network model and is intended to deal with large-scale models with consistency and clarity. It is capable of representing systems that exhibit increasing complexity over time, such as the genetic regulatory network controlling endomesoderm development in sea urchin embryos.

BioUML www.biouml.org

BioUML is a Java framework for systems biology. It spans the comprehensive range of capabilities including access to databases with experimental data, tools for formalized description of biological systems structure and functioning, as well as tools for their visualization and simulations.

BSTLab bioinformatics.musc.edu/bstlab

BSTLab is a Matlab toolbox for biochemical systems theory (BST). The toolbox implements functions common to BST-based studies and is designed to integrate easily into the widely used Matlab environment, automate many common tasks, and allow expansion and customization by the user. The toolbox also includes functions needed to reformulate and transport models that are written in SBML.

CADLIVE www.cadlive.jp

CADLIVE is a comprehensive computational tool that analyzes and rationally designs large-scale biochemical networks at the molecular interaction level. It consists of a GUI network constructor, database, a pathway search module for knockout mutants, a network layout module, and the dynamic simulator that automatically converts biochemical network maps into mathematical models.

CellDesigner celldesigner.org

CellDesigner is a structured diagram editor for drawing gene-regulatory and biochemical networks. Networks are drawn based on the process diagram, with graphical notation system proposed by Kitano, and are stored using the SBML, a standard for representing models of biochemical and gene-regulatory networks (GRN). Networks are able to link with simulation and other analysis packages through SBW.

Cellerator www.cellerator.org

Cellerator™ is a Mathematica® package designed to facilitate biological modeling via automated equation generation. Cellerator was designed with the intent of simulating essential biological processes such as signal transduction networks (STN); cells that are represented by interacting STN; and multicellular tissues that are represented by interacting networks of cells that may themselves contain internal STNs.

CellML2SBML sbml.org/software/cellml2sbml

CellML and SBML are XML-based languages for storage and exchange of biological models. CellML 1.1 and SBML L2V1 use a similar subset of the MathML specification to describe the mathematical aspects of the models. CellML2SBML can convert a valid CellML 1.1 model into a valid SBML L2V1 model.

CellNetAnalyser www.mpi-magdeburg.mpg.de/projects/cna/cna.html

CellNetAnalyzer is a package for MATLAB and provides a comprehensive and user-friendly environment for structural and functional analysis of biochemical and cellular networks. CellNetAnalyzer facilitates the analysis of metabolic as well as signaling and regulatory networks solely on their network topology, i.e., independently of kinetic mechanisms and parameters. The core concept of visualization and interactivity is realized by interactive network maps where the abstract network model is linked with network graphics. CellNetAnalyzer provides a powerful collection of tools and algorithms for structural network analysis, which can be started in a menu-controlled manner within the interactive network maps. CellNetAnalyzer is the successor and further development of FluxAnalyzer 5.3.

Cellware www.bii.a-star.edu.sg/research/sbg/cellware

A simulation tool designed to conduct modeling and simulation of gene-regulatory and metabolic pathways, which also offers an integrated environment for diverse mathematical representations, parameter estimation, and optimization. Developed by the Bioinformatics Institute, Singapore.

CL-SBML common-lisp.net/project/cl-sbml

A "Common Lisp" binding for SBML.

CLEML sg.ustc.edu.cn/MFA/cleml

CLEML is the abbreviation of carbon-labeling experiment markup language, a SBML dialect format for representation and exchange of ^{13}C metabolic flux analysis models. CLEML extends SBML through the annotation tag, so it is not only completely compatible with SBML Level 1 and SBML Level 2, but also fully supports carbon-labeling experiment based metabolic flux analysis (^{13}C MFA). CLEML allows for describing a CLE by defining the structure and stationary states of a metabolic system, e.g., metabolites, reactions, carbon atom transition, flux constraints, and measurement data.

COPASI www.copasi.org

Complex pathway simulator (COPASI) is an application for the simulation and analysis of biochemical networks. It features stochastic and deterministic time-course simulation, steady-state analysis, metabolic control analysis, parameter scans, optimization of arbitrary target functions, parameter estimation using experimental data, and import and export of SBML. Versions exist for Windows, Linux, MacOS X, and Solaris.

CPN Tools wiki.daimi.au.dk/cpntools/cpntools.wiki

CPN Tools is a tool for editing, simulating, and analyzing Colored Petri Nets. The GUI is based on advanced interaction techniques, such as toolglasses, marking menus, and bimanual interaction. Feedback facilities provide contextual error messages and indicate dependency relationships between net elements. The tool features incremental syntax checking and code generation, which take place while a net is being constructed. A fast simulator efficiently handles both untimed and timed nets. Full and partial state spaces can be generated and analyzed, and a standard state space report contains information such as boundedness properties and liveness properties. The functionality of the simulation engine and state-space facilities are similar to the corresponding components in Design/CPN, which is a widespread tool for Colored Petri Nets.

Cytoscape www.cytoscape.org

Cytoscape is a bioinformatics software platform for visualizing molecular interaction networks and integrating these interactions with gene expression profiles and other state data. Additional features are available as plug-ins. Plug-ins are available for network and molecular profiling analyses, new layouts, additional file format support, and connection with databases. Plug-ins may be developed using the Cytoscape open Java software architecture by anyone, and plug-in community development is encouraged.

Dizzy magnet.systemsbiology.net/software/Dizzy

Dizzy is a chemical kinetics stochastic simulation software package written in Java. It provides a model definition environment and an implementation of the Gillespie, Gibson-Bruck, and Tau-Leap stochastic algorithms, as well as several deterministic solvers. Dizzy is capable of importing and exporting the SBML model definition language, as well as displaying models graphically using the Cytoscape software system. Dizzy can be used via a GUI or through the command line.

E-CELL www.e-cell.org

E-Cell is an object-oriented software suite for modeling, simulation, and analysis of large-scale complex systems, particularly focused on biological details of cellular behavior.

FluxAnalyzer

www.mpi-magdeburg.mpg.de/projects/fluxanalyzer

Predecessor of CellNetAnalyzer.

Genetic Network Analyser (GNA) www.helix.inrialpes.fr/article122.html

GNA is a computer tool for the modeling and simulation of genetic regulatory networks. GNA consists of a simulator of qualitative models of genetic regulatory networks in the form of piecewise-linear differential equations. Instead of exact numerical values for the parameters, which are often not available for networks of biological interest, the user of GNA specifies inequality constraints. This information is sufficient to generate a state transition graph that describes the qualitative dynamics of the network. The simulator has been implemented in Java 1.5 and has been applied to the analysis of various regulatory systems, such as the networks controlling the initiation of sporulation in *Bacillus. subtilis* and the carbon starvation response in *E. coli*.

Gepasi www.gepasi.org
Predecessor of Copasi.

JACOBIAN numericatech.com/jacobian.htm
A dynamic modeling and optimization software for models written as ordinary or partial differential equations, or as differential algebraic equations. It performs optimization and parameter estimation and can handle hybrid models of discrete and continuous description.

Jarnac www.sys-bio.org
Jarnac is the numerical solver that is part of the SBW.

JavaEvA www.ra.informatik.uni-tuebingen.de/software/JavaEvA
JavaEvA is a framework for Evolutionary and general optimization algorithms implemented in Java. JavaEvA includes evolutionary algorithms (EA) like genetic algorithms (GA), evolutionary strategies (ES), population-based incremental learning (PBIL), and many more. Besides, model-based optimization techniques like methods from the research field of design of experiment, efficient global optimization (EGO), and model-assisted evolution strategies (MAES) are implemented in JavaEvA. The software is divided into two parts: a swing-based GUI (EvAClient) and the optimization kernel (EvAServer), which contains the different optimization algorithms.

JCell www.ra.informatik.uni-tuebingen.de/software/JCell
JCell is a framework for simulating GRN. It is implemented in Java and can be used for two different applications: reverse-engineering and inferring regulatory mechanisms based on the evaluation of given biological and medical data coming from DNA microarray experiments, and simulating cell growth and mitosis by finding GRNs suitable for a given problem (e.g., limited growth).

JDesigner sbw.kgi.edu/software/jdesigner.htm
JDesigner is a Windows application, which allows one to draw a biochemical network and export the network in the form of SBML. JDesigner has an SBW interface that allows it to be called from other SBW compliant modules, for example, Python. In addition, JDesigner has the ability to use Jarnac as a simulation server (via SBW) thus allowing models to be run from within JDesigner. In this mode, JDesigner is both a network design tool and simulator.

JSim www.physiome.org/jsim
JSim is a Java-based simulation system for building quantitative numerical models and analyzing them with respect to experimental reference data. Jsim's primary focus is in physiology and biomedicine; however, its computational engine is

quite general and applicable to a wide range of scientific domains. JSim models may intermix ODEs, PDEs, implicit equations, integrals, summations, discrete events, and procedural code as appropriate. Jsim's model compiler can automatically insert conversion factors for compatible physical units as well as detect and reject unit unbalanced equations. JSim also imports the SBML and CellML model archival formats.

Karyote systemsbiology.indiana.edu/karyote
Karyote is a genomic, proteomic, metabolic cell simulator and based on the numerical solution of a set of reaction-transport equations underlying the kinetics of genomic, proteomic, and metabolic processes. It is integrated with a variety of experimental data types through a novel information theory approach; the result is an automated procedure for tailoring Karyote to a given cell type and that all predictions are accompanied by an assessment of uncertainty.

KEGG2SBML www.sbml.org/kegg2sbml.html
KEGG2SBML is a Perl script, which converts KEGG (Kyoto Encyclopedia of Genes and Genomes) Pathway database files to SBML files.

libSBML www.sbml.org/software/libsbml
LibSBML is a library designed to help you read, write, manipulate, translate, and validate SBML files and data streams. It is not an application itself (though it does come with many example programs), but rather a library you can embed in your own applications. LibSBML is written in ISO C and C++ but as a library it may be used from many different programming languages such as C/C++, Java, Python, Perl, Lisp, or Matlab.

MathSBML sbml.org/software/mathsbml
MathSBML is an open-source package for working with SBML models in Mathematica. It provides facilities for reading SBML models, converting them to systems of ODEs for simulation and plotting in Mathematica, and translating the models to other formats. It supports both Level 1 and Level 2 SBML.

MesoRD mesord.sourceforge.net
MesoRD (mesoscopic reaction diffusion simulator) is a tool for the stochastic simulation of three-dimensional reaction and diffusion systems. In particular, it is an implementation of the Next Subvolume Method, which is an exact method to simulate the Markov process corresponding to the reaction–diffusion master equation. Since version 0.2.0, MesoRD also supports mean-field simulations.

MetaFluxNet mbel.kaist.ac.kr/mfn
MetaFluxNet is a program package for managing information of the metabolic reaction network and for quantitatively analyzing metabolic fluxes in an interactive and customized way, which allows users to interpret and examine metabolic behavior in response to genetic and/or environmental modifications. As a

result, quantitative in silico simulations of metabolic pathways can be carried out to understand the metabolic status and to design the metabolic engineering strategies.

MMT2 www.uni-siegen.de/fb11/simtec/software/mmt2

MMT2 is a software tool for developing a metabolic model from the data extracted from a rapid sampled pulse experiment. MMT2 supports the modeler with the capabilities of setting pools to measured data, fitting parameters, parameter sensitivities, and elementary modes. With an interface to Matlab, its usage and the evaluation of results become fast and easy. MMT2 uses code generation to speed up the process of simulating the metabolic network and, therefore, also significantly speed up the process of parameter fitting.

Narrator narrator-tool.org

Narrator is a graphical modeling tool for the description of the dynamical structure of models. Narrator implements the graph-based formal structure of a co-dependence model. The motivation of co-dependence modeling is to unify a diagrammatical notation tailored to the needs in bioinformatics with an underlying ODE interpretation.

NetBuilder strc.herts.ac.uk/bio/maria/NetBuilder

NetBuilder is an interactive graphical tool for representing and simulating genetic regulatory networks in multicellular organisms. Although the diagrams created in NetBuilder represent biological processes, the underlying concepts have their roots in electronic engineering. In NetBuilder – as in many electronic circuit design packages – pathways are represented as series of linked modules. Each module has specific input–output characteristics. As long as these characteristics conform to experimental observations, the exact transformations occurring 'inside' the modules can be safely neglected. The result is a significant reduction in the number of parameters.

Oscill8 oscill8.sourceforge.net

Oscill8 is a suite of tools for analyzing large systems of ODEs, particularly with respect to understanding how the high-dimensional parameter space controls the dynamics of the system. It features time-course integration, one- and two-parameter bifurcation diagrams, and bifurcation searches. It is written in C++ and runs on Windows, Linux, and MacOS X.

PANTHER Pathways www.pantherdb.org/pathway

PANTHER Pathway consists of over 139, primarily signaling, pathways, each with subfamilies and protein sequences mapped to individual pathway components. A component is usually a single protein in a given organism, but multiple proteins can sometimes play the same role. Pathways are drawn using CellDesigner software, capturing molecular level events in both signaling and metabolic pathways, and can be exported in SBML format. Pathway diagrams are interactive and include tools for visualizing gene expression data in the context of the diagrams.

PathArt jubilantbiosys.com/ppa.htm
PathArtTM Core is a comprehensive collection of curated data from literature as well as public domain databases for more than 2100 signaling and metabolic pathways. PathArtTM includes a database component and dynamic pathway articulator component, which builds directed acyclic graphs from molecular interaction networks.

Pathway Analyser sourceforge.net/projects/pathwayanalyser
PathwayAnalyser (PA) is a software for systems biologists who want to perform flux-based analyses (FBA) and simulations on SBML models. PA affords FBA as well as interfacing with Taylor software for high-precision simulations of ODEs.

PathwayLab innetics.com
PathwayLab is an in silico pathway analysis tool, enabling pharmaceutical R&D to reach their target decisions faster and with higher accuracy. It can create and store reaction objects with user-specified kinetics, perform time-course integration, and metabolic control analysis. Models can be exported to Mathematica, Matlab, and SBML. A 30-day demo version is available.

PET mpf.biol.vt.edu/software/homegrown/pet
PET is a GUI for discovering rate constants of molecular network models, which fit experimental data. It is designed for use by theoretical biologists to build regulatory network models and compare the models to experimental results.

ProcessDB www.integrativebioinformatics.com/processdb.html
ProcessDB is a web-based application that helps molecular cell biologists to manage and test their increasingly complex mechanistic hypotheses. ProcessDB does this with a bio-savvy GUI that helps users formulate, visualize, compare, modify, manage, and test their own mechanistic theories of cellular function. All models in ProcessDB can be automatically combined with user-specified experimental protocols and exported to the Berkeley Madonna solver for testing against experimental data.

PROTON tunicata.techfak.uni-bielefeld.de/proton/web/main.jsp
The interactive modeling environment, PROTON, has been developed to reconstruct biochemical systems from molecular databases in an automated and user-centric way. Providing an intuitive user interface, the fusion of information from distributed databases and the reconstruction of systems is interactively controlled by the user. The approach is based on different layers, which allow the integrative modeling of biochemical systems at multiple levels.

PyBioS pybios.molgen.mpg.de
PyBioS is a web-based application for modeling and simulation of cellular reaction networks (see Section 2.4.2.3). It provides functionalities for the construction, simulation, visualization, analysis and storage of large computer models. For model construction, PyBioS has an interface to external pathway databases such as Reactome, KEGG and ConsensusPathDB. For the interpretation of simulation results PyBioS can plot time course data of a simulation within the automatically generated reaction network of the respective model.

PySCeS pysces.sourceforge.net

This package is written in Python and provides a variety of tools for the analysis of cellular systems. The input is via a text-based model description language. Solvers for time-course integration and steady-state calculations exist. Various modules perform Metabolic Control Analysis (i.e., elasticities, flux, and concentration control coefficients) and bifurcation analysis. PySCeS can import and export SBML and is developed as open-source software.

SAAM II depts.washington.edu/saam2

SAAM II is a powerful compartmental and numerical modeling program developed to assist researchers and practitioners in the pharmaceutical, biomedical, and other scientific fields develop and use models to analyze their data. It helps them create models more easily, design and simulate experiments more quickly, and analyze data more accurately. SAAM II achieves this by creating systems of ODEs from the compartmental model structure, permitting the simulation of complex experimental protocols on the model, and solving the model and fitting it to data using state-of-the-art mathematical and statistical techniques.

SABIO-RK sabio.villa-bosch.de/SABIORK

The SABIO-RK (*s*ystem for the *a*nalysis of *bio*chemical pathways – *r*eaction *k*inetics) is a web-based application based on the SABIO relational database that contains information about biochemical reactions, their kinetic equations and parameters, as well as the experimental conditions under which these parameters were measured. It aims to support modelers in the setting-up of models of biochemical networks, but it is also useful for experimentalists or researchers with interest in biochemical reactions and their kinetics. Information about reactions and their kinetics can be exported in SBML format.

SBML ODE Solver www.tbi.univie.ac.at/~raim/odeSolver

The SBML ODE Solver Library (SOSlib) is both a programming library and a command-line application for symbolic and numerical analysis of a system of ODEs derived from a chemical reaction network encoded in the SBML. It is written in ANSI/ISO C and distributed under the terms of the GNU Lesser General Public License. The package employs libSBML's AST (Abstract Syntax Tree) for formula representation to construct ODE systems, their Jacobian matrix, and other derivatives. SUNDIALS' version of CVODE is incorporated for numerical integration and sensitivity analysis of stiff and nonstiff ODE systems.

SBMLeditor www.ebi.ac.uk/compneur-srv/SBMLeditor.html

The need to build a tool to facilitate the quick creation and edition of SBML files has been growing with the number of users and the increased complexity of the Level2 (and the future Level3). SBMLeditor tries to answer this need by providing a very simple, low-level editor of SBML files. Users can create and remove all the necessary bits and pieces of SBML in a controlled way that maintains the validity of the final SBML file.

SemanticSBML sysbio.molgen.mpg.de/semanticsbml

Combining different models written in SBML by hand can be rather tricky. SemanticSBML tools have been developed to solve this problem. The latest version semanticSBML-0.9.3 comes with a GUI and a scriptable command-line version.

SBML-PET sysbio.molgen.mpg.de/SBML-PET

SBML-PET is an SBML-based *p*arameter *e*stimation *t*ool. This tool has been designed to perform parameter estimation for biological models including signaling pathways, GRNs, and metabolic pathways. SBML-PET supports import and export of models in the SBML format. Currently, it can run on Linux and Cygwin on Windows. Current release version 1.2 of SBML-PET is free for academic use.

SBMLR epbi-radivot.cwru.edu

SBML binding for "R".

SBMLSim www.dim.uchile.cl/~dremenik/SBMLSim

SBMLSim provides a Matlab GUI that allows the user to import a SBML model, simulate it, and visualize the simulations. The GUI allows to control the numerical parameters of the simulations and to easily modify the parameters and initial conditions of the system. It also provides access to the ODE file generated from the SBML model in order that the user be able to directly modify it. The visualization of the simulations consists in the ability to plot any variable or algebraic expression involving the variables and parameters. SBMLSim provides a template that allows the user to define a file for computing the equilibrium of the system.

SBML Toolbox sbml.org/software/sbmltoolbox

The SBMLToolbox is built on top of libSBML and provides a set of functions that allow an SBML model to be imported into Matlab and stored as a structure within the Matlab environment. At present, the toolbox includes functions to translate an SBML document into a Matlab_SBML structure, save and load these structures to/from a Matlab data file, validate each structure (e.g., reaction structure), view the structures using a set of GUIs and to convert elements of the Matlab_SBML structure into symbolic form, and thus allow access to Matlab's symbolic toolbox. There are functions to facilitate simulation using Matlab's ODE solvers, and a function that will output an SBML document from the Matlab_SBML structure definition of a model. Release 2.0.2 includes the function ReadAndValidateSBML, which uses the Xerces XML Parser and the libSBML consistency checks to check the validity of the SBML model being imported prior to translating it into the Matlab_SBML model structure.

SB Toolbox www.sbtoolbox.org

The systems biology toolbox for Matlab offers systems biologists a wide range of functions such as import of SBML models, deterministic and stochastic simulation, steady-state and stability analysis, parameter estimation and sensitivity analysis, bifurcation analysis, optimization, determination of stoichiometric matrix, and simple model reduction.

SBW www.sys-bio.org

The Systems Biology Workbench (SBW) is a software framework that allows heterogeneous application components – written in diverse programming languages and running on different platforms – to communicate and use each other's capabilities via a fast binary encoded-message system. Our goal was to create a simple, high-performance, open-source software infrastructure, which is easy to implement and understand. SBW enables applications (potentially running on separate, distributed computers) to communicate via a simple network protocol. The interfaces to the system are encapsulated in client-side libraries that we provide for different programming languages.

SCIpath www.ucl.ac.uk/oncology/MicroCore/microcore.htm

SCIpath (formerly known as MicroCore) is a pluggable suite of programs specifically designed for the analysis of microarray data. SCIpath and its exponents are programmed in Java2 version 1.4.1 and above. The aim of SCIpath is to map gene expression data measured by DNA microarray and proteomic techniques to cellular pathways and biological processes in a statistically meaningful way.

Sigmoid sigmoid.sourceforge.net

The Sigmoid project is intended to produce a database of cellular signaling pathways and models thereof, to marshal the major forms of data and knowledge required as input to cellular modeling software and also to organize the outputs. To this end, an object schema has been designed that incorporates reactions, reactants, and models. Reactions are further divided into elementary and composite biological processes, and reactants are divided into elementary and composite biological objects such as proteins and protein complexes.

SigPath www.sigpath.org

SigPath is an information system designed to support quantitative studies on the signaling pathways and networks of the cell. The current version of SigPath is a prototype that shows how to address the management of the primary types of biochemical information needed to study cellular signaling.

SigTran depts.washington.edu/ventures/UW_Technology/Emerging_Technologies/CSI.php

Sigtran is software specifically designed to enable biological researchers to carry out large-scale simulations and to analyse complex reactions and interactions, such as signal transduction pathways. Sig Tran operates on documents created with SBML.

SimBiology www.mathworks.com/products/simbiology

SimBiology® extends Matlab® with tools for modeling, simulating, and analyzing biochemical pathways. You can create your own block diagram model using predefined blocks. You can manually enter compartments, species, parameters, reactions, events, rules, kinetic laws, and units, or read in SBML models.

SimBiology software lets you simulate a model using stochastic or deterministic solvers and analyze your pathway with tools such as parameter estimation and sensitivity analysis. A GUI provides access to command-line functionality and lets you create and manage compartments, reactions, events, species, parameters, rules, and units. SimBiology is produced by MathWorks, the manufacturers of Matlab.

Simpathica bioinformatics.nyu.edu/Projects/Simpathica

Simpathica is a set of tools capable of simulating and analyzing biological pathways. It consists of a front end and a back end. The front end is a pathway editor that generates a set of ODEs, which are in turn simulated using Octave (a free Matlab clone). The back end, also known as XSSYS, is a temporal logic analysis tool, which can answer queries about the time course behavior of a set of pathways. A recent addendum to the XSSYS back end is a natural language interrogation interface that can be used in lieu of the pure temporal logic query system.

SloppyCell sloppycell.sourceforge.net

SloppyCell is a software environment for simulation and analysis of biomolecular networks. It has support for much of the SBML level 2 version 3, and can perform deterministic and stochastic dynamical simulations, sensitivity analysis, parameter fitting to experimental data, and stochastic Bayesian analysis of parameter space to estimate error bars associated with optimal fits.

SmartCell smartcell.embl.de

SmartCell has been developed to be a general framework for modeling and simulating diffusion–reaction networks in a whole-cell context. It supports localization and diffusion by using a mesoscopic stochastic reaction model. The SmartCell package can handle any cell geometry, considers different cell compartments, allows localization of species, and supports DNA transcription and translation, membrane diffusion, and multistep reactions, as well as cell growth. Entities are represented by their copy number and location. In order to introduce spatial information, the geometry is divided into smaller volume elements, called voxel, where stochastic events take place. The use of a mesh allows us to consider diffusion as translocation across adjacent volume sites. The user-defined model is translated into an internal core model, where rates are converted into reaction probabilities per unit time. At this stage, reversible processes, diffusion, and complex formation are converted into an equivalent set of unidirectional elementary processes. Finally, each process is translated into as many individual events, as volume elements in the region where the process is defined. The core model is subsequently used by the simulation engine itself.

Snoopy www.dssz.informatik.tu-cottbus.de/index.html?/software/snoopy.html

Snoopy is a software tool to design and animate hierarchical graphs, among others Petri nets.

STELLA www.iseesystems.com/softwares/Education/StellaSoftware.aspx

STELLA is a flexible computer-modeling package with an easy, intuitive interface that allows users to construct dynamic models that realistically simulate biological systems.

StochSim www.pdn.cam.ac.uk/groups/comp-cell/StochSim.html

StochSim provides a general-purpose biochemical simulator in which individual molecules or molecular complexes are represented as individual software objects. Reactions between molecules occur stochastically, according to probabilities derived from known rate constants. An important feature of the program is its ability to represent multiple posttranslational modifications and conformational states of protein molecules. StochSim consists of a platform-independent core simulation engine encapsulating the algorithm described above and a separate GUI.

StochKit www.engineering.ucsb.edu/~cse/StochKit

StochKit is an efficient, extensible stochastic simulation framework developed in the C++ language that aims to make stochastic simulation accessible to practicing biologists and chemists, while remaining open to extension via new stochastic and multiscale algorithms. The beta version contains the popular Gillespie SSA algorithm, explicit tau-leaping, implicit tau-leaping, and trapezoidal tau-leaping methods.

STOCKS www.sysbio.pl/stocks

STOCKS uses Gillespie's direct method to simulate time evolution of the system composed of large number of first- and second-order chemical reactions. The program can perform simulations in the time scale of several cellular generations using linearly growing volume of reaction environment and simple model of cell division. Substances that are in equilibrium resulting from the competition of large number of processes can be modeled as random pools with Gaussian distribution.

Trelis sourceforge.net/projects/trellis

Trelis is a graphical Monte Carlo simulation tool for modeling the time evolution of chemical reaction systems involving small numbers of reactant molecules, as occur in subcellular biological processes like genetic regulatory networks.

VANTED vanted.ipk-gatersleben.de

VANTED stands for *v*isualization and *a*nalysis of *net*works containing *e*xperimental *d*ata. This system makes it possible to load and edit graphs, which may represent biological pathways or functional hierarchies. It is possible to map experimental datasets onto the graph elements and visualize time series data or data of different genotypes or environmental conditions in the context of the underlying biological processes. Built-in statistic functions allow a fast evaluation of the data (e.g., *t*-test or correlation analysis).

Virtual Cell www.vcell.org

The Virtual Cell consists of a biological and mathematical framework. Scientists can create biological models from which the software will generate the mathematical code needed to run simulations. Mathematicians may opt to use the math framework, based on the Virtual Cell Math Language, for creating their own mathematical descriptions. The simulations are run over the Internet on 84 servers with 256 GHz total CPU power.

Xholon primordion.com/Xholon

Xholon is a flexible open-source tool for multiparadigm (UML 2, ABM, SBML, NN, GP, PSys, CA, ...) modeling, simulation, design, execution, and transformation. Generic Java and XML building blocks are extended into multiple domains, and woven into loosely organized systems. Xholon is especially appropriate for event-driven systems, or any system in which objects move around, are regularly created, destroyed and modified, need to change their class at runtime, or even need to dynamically create new classes and new instances of those classes. While some Xholon applications, such as the example elevator controller, have very deterministic behavior and can be statically validated, the tool is especially designed to allow very open-ended systems that organize themselves at runtime and cannot be completely pinned down to a specific UML metamodel or XML schema. The goal of the Xholon project is to enable building of systems that approach the complexity of biological systems, using many of the same principles that have made biological systems so adaptable, successful, and long-lived.

XPPAUT www.math.pitt.edu/~bard/xpp/xpp.html

XPPAUT is a tool for solving differential equations, difference equations, delay equations, functional equations, boundary value problems, and stochastic equations. XPPAUT contains the code for the popular bifurcation program, AUTO. Thus, you can switch back and forth between XPPAUT and AUTO, using the values of one program in the other and vice versa.

yEd www.yworks.com/en/products_yed_about.htm

yEd is a very powerful graph editor that is written entirely in the Java programming language. It can be used to quickly and effectively generate drawings and to apply automatic layouts to a range of different diagrams and networks. yEd can be used to automatically lay out complex graph structures. Several highly sophisticated layout algorithms have been implemented and shipped with yEd. They can be used either to automatically arrange the items or to support the user when undertaking a manual layout.

Exercises and Problems

1. When and why should a system be modeled stochastically instead of deterministically?
2. Which development of the last years is important for the exchange of models between different simulation tools?

3. What is the purpose of libSBML?
4. Is it possible to develop models in (a) Mathematica or (b) Matlab that support SBML?
5. Use CellDesigner to model the irreversible reaction S → P using a Michaelis–Menten kinetics. Draw the diagram, specify the kinetics (for $K_m = 2$ mmol/l, $V_{max} = 5$ mmol/(l*s), $S_{t=0} = 100$ molecules, and $P_{t=0} = 0$ molecules) and run a time-course simulation.
6. Export the model as SBML and import it into Copasi. Run a time-course simulation to see if it is identical to the one from CellDesigner.
7. Use the following three time/substrate concentration data points for model fitting: $P_1 = 5$ s/60 mMol, $P_2 = 10$ s/50 mmol, $P_3 = 15$ s/20 mmol. What are the values of K_m and V_{max} after fitting?
8. Import the CellDesigner SBML model into Dizzy and run a stochastic simulation. Do you see any differences to the deterministic solution?

References

1 Levin, B. (1999) *Genes VII*, Oxford University Press, Oxford.

2 Kowald, A. *et al.* (2005) On the relevance of mitochondrial fusions for the accumulation of mitochondrial deletion mutants: A modelling study. *Aging Cell*, **4**, 273–283.

3 Hucka, M. *et al.* (2002) The ERATO Systems Biology Workbench: enabling interaction and exchange between software tools for computational biology. *Pacific Symposium on Biocomputing*, 450–461.

4 Sauro, H.M. *et al.* (2003) Next generation simulation tools: the Systems Biology Workbench and BioSPICE integration. *OMICS*, **7**, 355–372.

5 Klipp, E. *et al.* (2007) Systems biology standards – the community speaks. *Nature Biotechnology*, **25**, 390–391.

Index

Systems Biology: A Textbook. Edda Klipp, Wolfram Liebermeister, Christoph Wierling, Axel Kowald, Hans Lehrach, and Ralf Herwig

ISBN: 978-3-527-31874-2

d

h